Sourcebook of Treatment Programs for Sexual Offenders

APPLIED CLINICAL PSYCHOLOGY

Series Editors:

Alan S. Bellack
University of Maryland at Baltimore, Baltimore, Maryland

Michel Hersen
Pacific University, Forest Grove, Oregon

Current volumes in this Series

A BEHAVIOR ANALYTIC VIEW OF CHILD DEVELOPMENT
Henry D. Schlinger, Jr.

CONJOINT BEHAVIORAL CONSULTATION
A Procedural Manual
Susan M. Sheridan, Thomas R. Kratochwill, and John R. Bergan

CONTEMPORARY ISSUES IN BEHAVIOR THERAPY
Improving the Human Condition
Edited by Joseph R. Cautela and Waris Ishaq

FUNDAMENTALS OF BEHAVIOR ANALYTIC RESEARCH
Alan Poling, Laura L. Methot, and Mark G. LeSage

GUIDEBOOK FOR CLINICAL PSYCHOLOGY INTERNS
Edited by Gary K. Zammit and James W. Hull

INTRODUCTION TO SCIENTIFIC PSYCHOLOGY
Henry D. Schlinger, Jr. and Alan Poling

KEY CONCEPTS IN PSYCHOTHERAPY INTEGRATION
Jerold R. Gold

PSYCHOLOGICAL ASSESSMENT IN MEDICAL SETTINGS
Ronald H. Rozensky, Jerry J. Sweet, and Steven M. Tovian

THE SCIENTIFIC PRACTICE OF PROFESSIONAL PSYCHOLOGY
Steven J. Trierweiler and George Stricker

SOURCEBOOK OF ADULT ASSESSMENT STRATEGIES
Nicola S. Schutte and John M. Malouff

SOURCEBOOK OF TREATMENT PROGRAMS FOR SEXUAL OFFENDERS
Edited by William Lamont Marshall, Yolanda M. Fernanadez,
Stephen M. Hudson, and Tony Ward

A Continuation Order Plan is available for this series. A continuation order will bring delivery of each new volume immediately upon publication. Volumes are billed only upon actual shipment. For further information please contact the publisher.

Sourcebook of Treatment Programs for Sexual Offenders

Edited by

William Lamont Marshall
Yolanda M. Fernandez

Queen's University
Kingston, Ontario, Canada

and

Stephen M. Hudson
Tony Ward

University of Canterbury
Christ Church, New Zealand

Plenum Press • New York and London

Library of Congress Cataloging-in-Publication Data

Sourcebook of treatment programs for sexual offenders / edited by
  William Lamont Marshall ... [et al.].
      p.   cm. -- (Applied clinical psychology)
  Includes bibliographical references and index.
  ISBN 0-306-45730-X
  1. Sex offenders--Mental health services. 2. Sex offenders-
-Rehabilitation.   I. Marshall, William L.   II. Series.
RC560.S47S68 1998
362.2'7--dc21   98-21057
                                                              CIP

ISBN 0-306-45730-X

©1998 Plenum Press, New York
A Division of Plenum Publishing Corporation
233 Spring Street, New York, N.Y. 10013

http://www.plenum.com

10 9 8 7 6 5 4 3 2 1

Printed in the United States of America

"... the doctrine that you can't change human nature has a larger purpose: defense of the existing social arrangements."

—Barrows Dunham
Man against Myth, 1947

Contributors

Gene G. Abel • Behavioral Medicine Institute of Atlanta, Atlanta, Georgia 30327

Jocelyn Aubut • University of Montréal and Philippe Pinel Institute of Montréal, Montréal, Quebec, Canada H1C 1H1

Kathryn A. Baker • Shenandoah Valley Sex Offender Treatment Program, Harrisonburg, Virginia 22801

Howard E. Barbaree • Forensic Division, Clarke Institute of Psychiatry, Toronto, Ontario, Canada M5T 1R8

Richard Beckett • Department of Forensic Psychology, Fair Mile Hospital, Wallingford, Oxfordshire, England OX10 9HH

Surya R. Bhate • Kolvin Unit, Newcastle General Hospital, Newcastle-upon-Tyne, England NE4 6BE

John M.W. Bradford • Forensic Service and Sexual Behaviours Clinic, Royal Ottawa Hospital, Ottawa, Ontario, Canada K1Z 7K4

Gergory M.S. Canfield • Justice Resource Institute, Bridgewater, Massachusetts 02324

Emily Coleman • Clinical and Support Options, Greenfield, Massachusetts 01302

Franca Cortoni • Sexual Offenders' Program, Kingston Penitentiary, Kingston, Ontario, Canada K7L 4V7

Enny Cramer • Joseph J. Peters Institute, Philadelphia, Pennsylvania 19102

Denise M. Cull • Victim and Offender Assessment and Treatment Services Ltd., Claremont, Western Australia 6010

Mario J.P. Dennis • Shenandoah Valley Sex Offender Treatment Program, Harrisonburg, Virginia 22801

Anthony Eccles • Forensic Behaviour Services, Kingston, Ontario, Canada K7L 1A8

Hilary Eldridge • The Lucy Faithfull Foundation, Birmingham, England B48 7EA

Lawrence Ellerby • Forensic Behavioral Management Clinic, Native Clan Organization, Winnipeg, Manitoba, Canada R3C 0A1

Dewey J. Ertz • The Manlove Psychiatric Group, Rapid City, South Dakota 57701

Yolanda M. Fernandez • Department of Psychology, Queen's University, Kingston, Ontario, Canada K7L 3N6

Dawn Fisher • Psychology Department, Llanarth Court Psychiatric Hospital, Llanarth, Nr. Raglan, Gwent, Wales NP5 2YD

Arthur Gordon • Sex Offender Treatment Program, Twin Rivers Corrections Center, Monroe, Washington 98272

Finlay Graham • Kolvin Unit, Newcastle General Hospital, Newcastle-upon-Tyne, England NE4 6BE

David M. Greenberg • Forensic Service and Sexual Behaviours Clinic, Royal Ottawa Hospital, Ottawa, Ontario, Canada K1Z 7K4

Don Grubin • Department of Forensic Psychiatry, St. Nicholas' Hospital, Gosforth, Newcastle-upon-Tyne, England NE3 3XT

James Haaven • Oregon State Hospital, Salem, Oregon 97310

David Hillman (Tuhoe) • Te Piriti Special Treatment Unit, Psychological Services, Department of Corrections, Albany, New Zealand

Gerald Hover • Sex Offender Treatment Program, Twin Rivers Corrections Center, Monroe, Washington 98272

Stephen M. Hudson • Department of Psychology, University of Canterbury, Christchurch, New Zealand

Alan Jenkins • NADA Counselling, Consulting, and Training, Stirling, South Australia 5152

Toni Cavanagh Johnson • 1101 Fremont Avenue, Suite 101, South Pasadena, California 91030

Robin L. Jones • Project RAP, Center for Community Alternatives, New York, New York 10011

Elymar Kacin • Project RAP, Center for Community Alternatives, New York, New York 10011

Andrew F. Kelly • Clergy Consultation and Treatment Services, Outpatient Mental Health Services, St. Vincent's Westchester, Harrison, New York 10528

Bernadette Lamoureux • Philippe Pinel Institute of Montréal, Montréal, Quebec, Canada H1C 1H1

Jillian Larsen • Te Piriti Special Treatment Unit, Psychological Services, Department of Corrections, Albany, New Zealand

Joseph Maher • Joseph J. Peters Institute, Philadelphia, Pennsylvania 19102

Barry M. Maletzky • The Sexual Abuse Clinic, Portland, Oregon 97202

Ruth E. Mann • Program Development Section, HM Prison Service, Abell House, London, England SW1P 4LH

William L. Marshall • Department of Psychology, Queen's University, Kingston, Ontario, Canada K7L 3N6

Jane Kinder Matthews • Transition Place, Minneapolis, Minnesota 55414

André McKibben • Philippe Pinel Institute of Montréal, Montréal, Quebec, Canada H1C 1H1

Pablo E. Moro • Arlington County Juvenile Sexual Offenders Program, Child and Family Services Division, Arlington, Virginia 22205

Jules Mulder • Dr. Henri van der Hoeven Kliniek, Forensic Psychiatric Institute, 3500 AD Utrecht, The Netherlands

Candice A. Osborn • Behavioral Medicine Institute of Atlanta, Atlanta, Georgia 30327

Edward J. Peacock • Warkworth Sexual Behaviour Clinic, Warkworth Institution, Campbellford, Ontario, Canada K0L IL0

Derek Perkins • Psychology Department, Broadmoor Hospital, Crowthorne, Berkshire, England RG45 7EG

Darlene Pessein • Joseph J. Peters Institute, Philadelphia, Pennsylvania 19102

Robert Prentky • Joseph J. Peters Institute, Philadelphia, Pennsylvania 19102

Jean Proulx • University of Montréal and Philippe Pinel Institute of Montréal, Montréal, Quebec, Canada H1C 1H1

Graeme Richardson • Kolvin Unit, Newcastle General Hospital, Newcastle-upon-Tyne, England NE4 6BE

Paul Robertson (Kai Tahu) • Auckland Regional Office, Psychological Services, Department of Corrections, Auckland, New Zealand

William N. Salloway • Project RAP, Center for Community Alternatives, New York, New York 10011

Barbara K. Schwartz • Justice Resource Institute, Bridgewater, Massachusetts 02324

Michael Seto • Forensic Division, Clarke Institute of Psychiatry, Toronto, Ontario, Canada M5T 1R8

Lloyd G. Sinclair • Wisconsin Sex Offender Treatment Network, Inc., Madison, Wisconsin 53719

Alec Spencer • HM Prison, Peterhead, Aberdeenshire, Scotland AB42 6YY; *present address:* HM Prison, Edinburgh, Scotland EH11 3LN

Cynthia Steinhauser • The Sexual Abuse Clinic, Portland, Oregon 97202

John Stonechild • Forensic Behavioral Management Clinic, Native Clan Organization, Winnipeg, Manitoba, Canada R3C 0A1

David Thornton • Program Development Section, HM Prison Service, Abell House, London, England SW1P 4LH

Daan van Beek • Dr. Henri van der Hoeven Kliniek, Forensic Psychiatric Institute, 3500 AD Utrecht, The Netherlands

David S. Wales • Kia Marama Special Treatment Unit, Rolleston Prison, Rolleston, New Zealand

William Walker • Forensic Behaviour Services, Kingston, Ontario, Canada K7L 1A8

Tony Ward • Department of Psychology, University of Canterbury, Christchurch, New Zealand

Brent W. Warberg • Behavioral Medicine Institute of Atlanta, Atlanta, Georgia 30327

David M. Wehner • Sex Offender Treatment Unit, Ministry of Justice, Northbridge, Western Australia 6003

Marsha Weissman • Project RAP, Center for Community Alternatives, New York, New York 10011

Mark X. Winkler • Project RAP, Center for Community Alternatives, New York, New York 10011

James R. Worling • SAFE-T Program, Thistletown Regional Centre for Children and Adolescents, Toronto, Ontario, Canada M9V 4L8

Ray Wyre • The Lucy Faithfull Foundation, Birmingham, England B48 7EA

Preface

A tradition has been defined, somewhat facetiously, as something we did last year, enjoyed, and therefore have decided to do again. This volume fits that tradition in that, just as the *Handbook of Sexual Assault* (Marshall, Laws, & Barbaree, 1990) was conceived over a meal at the annual meeting of the International Academy of Sex Research held in Amsterdam in 1986, this present volume arose from discussions during the 1994 Association for the Treatment of Sexual Abusers conference held in San Francisco. One of the benefits of attending such meetings is the chance to crystallize thoughts. It seemed clear to us in San Francisco that what was missing from the literature on sexual offenders was guidance on how to implement treatment in the quite different, and often difficult, settings in which it is offered and how to provide treatment to the increasingly diverse subgroups of sexual offenders that are seen in all settings. We decided to do our best to fill that gap.

Looking back over the history of our collective attempts to treat men who behave in sexually aggressive ways, we can only be impressed by the creative energy that has been expended. The early behavioral approaches, born from a sense of optimism created by behavior therapy's success in assisting chronically psychiatrically disabled people lead happier more fulfilled lives, have been augmented by the broader social learning approaches. These in turn have been extended by the development of the now most commonly used theory of treatment: relapse prevention. While this approach to structuring interventions is not without its problems, it has become the touchstone against which any competing intervention is evaluated. Most critically it has articulated optimism, at least for therapists, and has very usefully served to place our focus on the dynamic process of offending.

One of the major issues for the area has centered around whether treatment is the most rational response to sexual abuse. Some members of the professional community (e.g., Quinsey, Rice, Harris, & Lalumière, 1993) have espoused sceptical views of the value of treatment. They have quite rightly pointed out that the extant treatment outcome literature has methodological weaknesses that preclude definitive conclusions. We (Marshall, 1993; Marshall & Pithers, 1994; Marshall, Ward, Jones, Johnston, & Barbaree, 1991), on the other hand, have taken a more optimistic view and have read into this same literature encouraging signs of the potential of treatment. In addition, we are further encouraged by the growing body of research indicating that similar cognitive–behavioral programs produce positive benefits among nonsexual offenders (Andrews et al., 1990). In any event, whatever position is assumed with regard to treatment efficacy, it is clear that many clinicians worldwide are engaging in interventions with sexual offenders aimed at reducing their propensity to reoffend.

Given the rather low base rates of reoffending among sexual offenders and the associated difficulty in demonstrating treatment effects, it may be some time before any program has generated enough treatment graduates at risk for a sufficient period of time to demonstrate any effects (Barbaree, 1997). In the meantime, the pressing questions for practitioners have more to do with how we go about treating sexual offenders and what sort of adjustments we have to make in our programs to address the unique features of both our clients and the settings in which we work. What are the particular problems that therapists face in treating sexual offenders in prisons, in psychiatric facilities, and in community settings? In what ways do we need to modify our programs and educate ourselves in order to effectively treat differing populations of sexual offenders? Are juveniles, women, professionals, aboriginals, and disabled offenders all responsive to the same treatment approach, or must we make changes to our programs to accommodate their special needs?

Our goal in this volume is to offer some answers to these questions by selecting authors who have experience and expertise in working with these diverse populations in different settings and in different countries. In this way, we hope that readers will not have to individually reinvent the wheel, but rather will be given guidance not only about the specific features that need to be addressed in treatment but also about the likely problems they may face and how they might deal with these difficulties. Since resources are typically in short supply, there is seldom the luxury of having several months available to develop the structure and content of a program prior to seeing the first client. We therefore hope that the present volume will provide guidance that will allow practitioners to more rapidly develop a sound approach to their particular population or circumstance.

The broad settings we have chosen are meant to be illustrative of the creativity that currently abounds. We have included programs operating in prison settings, psychiatric hospitals, and in the community, as well as programs dealing with special populations, including juveniles, women, clergy, professionals, variously disabled offenders, and aboriginal offenders. We also have secured representative authors from different countries who describe their programs in order to illustrate the unique circumstances and opportunities provided by each country. Despite this diversity, what is perhaps most surprising is the relative uniformity of the basic aspects of each program described in this volume. The unique features of each program are built into a core, which is essentially the cognitive–behavioral program that has been evolving in North America over the past 20–30 years, with relapse prevention as the latter-day integrative perspective.

With so many programs operating worldwide and with most of them based on the same approach, we should be in a far better position, some 10 years hence, to make a clearer estimate of the value of treating sexual offenders. However, simply counting the number of treated offenders who recidivate will never tell us the real value of treatment. It is the reduction in the number of innocent victims who are so disastrously damaged by sexual abuse that is the real key to evaluating treatment programs for sexual offenders, as well as the financial savings to society. It is already clear that for treatment to be valuable in these terms, it does not have to be dramatically successful. Preventing only 1 or 2% of sexual abusers from reoffending has a real impact on the integrity of the lives of possible victims and saves society (i.e., the taxpayers) a significant amount of money (Marshall, 1992; Prentky & Burgess, 1991). Most treatment providers apparently have a more optimistic view than this minimum would suggest of the effectiveness of their treatment.

We hope that the present volume will encourage clinicians to see that neither the physical circumstances in which treatment is delivered nor the specifics of any given offender group are insurmountable obstacles to implementing effective programs for sexual offenders. We also hope that this volume will encourage greater international cooperation and communication between treatment providers. We think that each of our authors has done an excellent job in describing their program, its difficulties, and their solutions, and hopefully their experience will assist others in developing their own programs.

W. L. Marshall
Yolanda M. Fernandez
Stephen M. Hudson
Tony Ward

REFERENCES

Andrews, D. A., Zinger, I., Hoge, R. D., Bonta, J., Gendreau, P., & Cullen, F.T. (1990). Does correctional treatment work? A clinically relevant and psychologically informed meta-analysis. *Criminology, 28,* 369–417.

Barbaree, H. E. (1997). Evaluating treatment efficacy with sex offenders: The insensitivity of recidivism studies to treatment effects. *Sexual Abuse: A Journal of Research and Treatment, 9,* 111–128.

Marshall, W. L. (1992). The social value of treatment for sexual offenders. *Canadian Journal of Human Sexuality, 1,* 109–114.

Marshall, W. L. (1993). The treatment of sex offenders: What does the outcome data tell us? A reply to Quinsey et al. *Journal of Interpersonal Violence, 8,* 524–530.

Marshall, W.L., Laws, D. R., & Barbaree, H. E. (Eds.). (1990). *Handbook of sexual assault: Issues, theories, and treatment of the offender.* New York: Plenum Press.

Marshall, W.L., & Pithers, W. D. (1994). A reconsideration of treatment outcome with sex offenders. *Criminal Justice and Behavior, 21,* 10–27.

Marshall, W. L., Ward, T., Jones, R., Johnston, P., & Barbaree, H. E. (1991, March). An optimistic evaluation of treatment outcome with sex offenders. *Violence Update,* pp. 1–8.

Prentky, R.A., & Burgess, A. W. (1991). Rehabilitation of child molesters: A cost-benefit analysis. *American Journal of Orthopsychiatry, 60,* 108–117.

Quinsey, V. L., Rice, M. E., Harris, G.T., & Lalumière, M. L. (1993). Assessing treatment efficacy in outcome studies of sex offenders. *Journal of Interpersonal Violence, 8,* 512–523.

Acknowledgments

Primarily, we would like to thank our authors for their contributions. All are active clinicians or program directors who have so many other tasks that it is remarkable they were able to give up the time to describe their programs. We heartily thank them.

Thanks also are due to Kathleen Lucadamo, our editorial help at Plenum Publishing, for her guidance and patience, and Val Angus, who provided valuable typing assistance with the edited manuscripts.

More generally, we acknowledge the support and encouragement of our family, friends, and colleagues, who made the task easier.

Contents

SECTION C: PSYCHIATRIC SETTINGS

PART II: DIVERSE POPULATIONS

I

Adult Male Offenders

A. Prison Settings

The Twin Rivers Sex Offender Treatment Program

Arthur Gordon and Gerald Hover

Many American state governments and departments of corrections are challenging the usefulness of prison-based sexual offender treatment programs. Legislatures, the media, and the public feel that providing such treatment is being "soft on crime." Claims are often made that treatment does not work, and that most if not all sexual offenders will reoffend after their release from prison. These claims, although having little basis in fact, have encouraged some jurisdictions to eliminate prison-based sexual offender treatment programs (e.g., Virginia, California) or to not offer such services (e.g., Arizona, Idaho). These same beliefs have also encouraged legislatures to pass increasingly harsh punitive measures for sexual offenders, including, in Washington State, life sentences after two felony sexual offenses. However, it remains the case that the vast majority of incarcerated sexual offenders will eventually return to the community and that treatment is an effective component of a comprehensive strategy that can help reduce and manage risk.

Prison-based sexual offender programs typically face many challenges beyond those of designing and delivering high-quality treatment. Programs often work with the highest-risk offenders, who are often resistant to change. We are beginning to understand that dealing with the brutal acts committed by sexual offenders can have profound negative effects on therapists. This stress can be exacerbated by the prison environment, which may not be well equipped for or supportive of treatment activities. In fact, other prison staff may be hostile toward treatment staff and their efforts and may attempt to sabotage their efforts. Hiring new staff typically must follow personnel policies that do not always allow managers to choose among candidates—those who have the training, skills, and temperament needed for this specialized and demanding task. As if this were not enough, the current political and social climate demands that programs demonstrate that they are accountable, cost efficient, and effective. Increasingly, long-term survival demands that programs help educate the public and policymakers about sexual offenders and the value of treatment in helping to protect the community. The fact that there are over 120 prison-based sexual offender programs currently operating in American prisons is a testament to the perseverance of many dedicated professionals. The sexual offender treatment program at the

Arthur Gordon and Gerald Hover • Sex Offender Treatment Program, Twin Rivers Corrections Center, Monroe, Washington 98272.

Sourcebook of Treatment Programs for Sexual Offenders, edited by Marshall et al. Plenum Press, New York, 1998.

Twin Rivers Corrections Center in Washington State has faced many issues and crises, including a 1994 decision by the state legislature to eliminate the program. This chapter describes some of these problems and the strategies we have adopted to provide a first-rate clinical service, while trying to ensure our long-term survival.

The Twin Rivers program was born in the midst of political and social turmoil. The Washington State legislature created the program in 1986 (Engrossed Substitute House Bill 1598) and it began operation in 1988. Prior to this time, the courts could send convicted sexual offenders to one of two state psychiatric hospitals for treatment; Western State Hospital in Fort Steilacoom, Washington, offered one of the first comprehensive programs for sexual offenders in the world. Treatment staff largely determined when an offender could be returned to the community. In the mid-1980s, two released offenders committed particularly brutal offenses. Spurred by public outrage, the legislature decided that treatment should be provided by and the offender controlled by the Department of Corrections. The Twin Rivers program is the only prison-based treatment program for adult male sexual offenders in Washington State.

The Twin Rivers program is one of the finest programs the first author has encountered in his 20 years experience in this field. Much of the credit is due to Dr. Barbara Schwartz and the staff who initially designed the program and steered it through its early development. This chapter describes some of the clinical and operational challenges the program has faced since 1993. We begin with a description of the program itself and discuss some of the key issues that all prison-based programs must face. We then address some of our relatively unique problems and our attempts at solutions.

THE TWIN RIVERS PROGRAM: INTRODUCTION

The Twin Rivers Corrections Center is an 816-bed medium-security prison. Two hundred beds and 27 staff are dedicated to the sexual offender treatment program. The program is structured around teams, each with a team leader and four to six therapists. Staff, who are recruited according to personnel policies of the Department of Corrections, represent a wide range of academic and clinical training ranging from high school graduates and 2-year community college degrees, through masters of social work and PhDs in psychology. The program treats all volunteer offenders including those who are developmentally disabled or who suffer from a variety of physical handicaps. Most recently, services for unilingual Spanish-speaking offenders have been offered.

The program seeks to achieve three main goals: (1) to provide state-of-the-art treatment to help incarcerated sexual offenders avoid future offending; (2) to help manage the offender's risk by communicating relevant and timely information to key partners in corrections and the community; and (3) to evaluate all aspects of treatment to ensure that the program is meeting its goals. We have found that stressing the importance of helping the community manage the offender has helped the public and legislators better understand the role of treatment. Acknowledging that we cannot cure offenders but rather can help better manage risk will hopefully reduce the perception that every reoffense reflects the overall failure of treatment.

The program uses cognitive behavioral treatment techniques within a relapse prevention framework. Rather than serving as the last component of treatment, relapse prevention serves as the core of all clinical decisions and activities. Thus, offenders are expected to define their crime cycle at the outset of treatment and it is information from the cycle that helps define what skills the offender must learn to prevent future offending.

More recently, we have adopted the principles of effective correctional treatment described by Andrews and his colleagues (Andrews & Bonta, 1990; Andrews et al., 1990) to help guide program development. Based on a series of meta-analyses on the effects of treatment on recidivism in general criminal populations, Andrews has determined a set of factors associated with optimizing treatment impact. The risk, need, and responsivity principles are most relevant to the Twin Rivers program.

The risk principle states that correctional treatment will be most effective with higher-risk offenders. That is, although higher-risk offenders are by definition more likely to reoffend, treating these offenders is most likely to significantly reduce recidivism. The need principle states that treatment will reduce recidivism if it targets factors that are directly related to criminal behavior. Although some treatment targets (e.g., insight about childhood traumas) may be clinically defensible, treatment will be most effective if it focuses on elements of behavior that research has shown are related to future offending (e.g., attitudes supporting the criminal behavior). The responsivity principle states that treatment must be delivered in a manner that is consistent with the learning and personality style of the offender. Although these principles have not been as well researched with sexual offenders, they have proven a valuable framework to help us resolve a number of issues.

TREATMENT STRUCTURE AND CONTENT

Offenders typically follow a series of prescribed steps during the treatment process. However, we maintain sufficient flexibility at each stage to allow for unique needs and circumstances. Above all, and consistent with the responsivity principle, we adapt conditions and procedures to ensure that all offenders who wish treatment can receive it.

Screening and Eligibility

All offenders enter the Department of Corrections through the Washington Corrections Center where they are assessed and assigned to other facilities. During this reception process, one staff screens all convicted sexual offenders to determine if they wish to receive treatment. The eligibility criteria are deliberately broad: The offender must acknowledge that he has committed a sexual offense, must not be acutely mentally ill, and must volunteer. We do not insist that the offender acknowledge every offense on record or that he take full responsibility for his actions. Rather, we see one purpose of treatment as dealing with issues of motivation, minimization, and denial. We do not exclude offenders on the basis of intelligence, physical handicaps, or literacy skills. Rather, we have adapted treatment to meet the special needs presented by these offenders. Similarly, although we would prefer that the offender enter treatment at least 18–24 months before his release, we will accept an offender with as little as 6 months on his sentence in the hope that some treatment (that may lead to community-based therapy) is better than none. Historically, approximately 50% of eligible offenders volunteer for treatment.

Although state law specifies that treatment be made available to inmates currently serving time for a sexual offense, we also consider offenders who are not currently convicted of a sexual crime but have a relevant history, or whose offense had a sexual component although the official offense may be nonsexual (e.g., murder), or who report to prison staff sexually aggressive behaviors that have not resulted in convictions. Such cases can be admitted through an override by the Twin Rivers' superintendent. The current waiting list of 950 offenders represents an increase of over 100% in the last 3 years. This growth has demanded that we provide quality treatment as efficiently as possible so all willing offenders can receive treatment before their release.

Local state legislators and the public have recently questioned whether high-risk recidivistic offenders should be eligible for treatment, arguing that only first-time and low-risk offenders deserve the opportunity. In submissions to the legislature, we have described the risk principle and have successfully argued that higher-risk offenders are most likely to benefit from treatment. Indeed, we see our community-protection role as being best served by working with high-risk offenders, even if that means we will face more public scrutiny as some of our offenders commit new crimes.

The risk principle can be interpreted as saying that since treatment is not likely to reduce recidivism in low-risk offenders, resources should not be provided to them. However, a number of local victim service providers have argued that many victims, particularly of intrafamilial abuse, might be reluctant to report the offender or help with his prosecution if they believe the offender will not receive treatment. We therefore accept all offenders who volunteer regardless of their risk. However, to better manage our scarce resources, we are developing a triage model that provides more intensive and lengthier treatment to higher risk offenders, and shorter-term treatment to lower risk men.

Admissions and Orientation

Periodically, groups of offenders (serving the least time to release) are transferred to Twin Rivers Corrections Center to begin an orientation period. During this time, offenders sign consent forms and complete extensive interviews and formal testing. These initial assessments serve to help define relevant areas for clinical intervention, provide for calculation of actuarial risk, and establish a baseline to evaluate treatment impact.

The test battery is quite comprehensive in focusing on sexual-offender-specific information (e.g., the Multiphasic Sex Inventory), as well as on a variety of behavioral dimensions (attitudes, aggression, social competence). Although we support the value of plethysmography, resource limitations (i.e., one technician) means that we must reserve such testing primarily for pedophiles whose arousal patterns seem more directly related to their offending. Once they have completed orientation, offenders are absorbed into the formal program as space becomes available.

It is important that offenders adjust to the treatment program as quickly and productively as possible. To this end, we are evaluating a number of strategies to improve adjustment. While they are in orientation, offenders may attend a weekly, unstructured group session that serves to acclimatize them to the demands of treatment; 20–40 offenders attend these sessions weekly. We have begun a short series of information sessions on topics such as relapse prevention, crime cycles, and so forth. Finally, we are developing a system to match offenders and therapists rather than creating matches randomly. It has been our experience that each therapist develops more effective therapeutic relationships with different types of offenders (e.g., more aggressive, more criminalized, more mental health concerns, etc.). In line with the responsivity principle, we expect that matching offenders with therapists will result in more productive treatment and better outcomes.

Program Content

Most treatment occurs in a group format. Each therapist carries 12–14 cases split into two smaller primary groups that meet 5 to 8 hours per week throughout treatment. The primary group seeks to: (1) resolve issues of minimization and accepting responsibility; (2) define the offender's crime cycle; (3) define and monitor individualized treatment goals; (4) teach relapse prevention information and skills; and (5) help the offender integrate content from other groups and classes. The primary group also provides basic skills training (e.g., communication skills, victim empathy, anger management, stress management, healthy sexuality) as these are relevant to the group members.

The program provides a range of time-limited psychoeducational groups to teach specific skills that offenders may require. What groups are offered changes over time to reflect the current needs of group participants. Some groups are compulsory (e.g., understanding sexual assault, critical thinking), while the offender is assigned to others (e.g., anger management, living skills) if he requires more training than the primary group can provide. All offenders also attend a community transition group toward the end of treatment. This group is led by community therapists and guests (e.g., the police detective who oversees all sexual offenders released to Seattle, former clients who are adjusting to the community). The transition group addresses issues of community adjustment, treatment maintenance, and legal requirements the offender must follow.

Each offender also receives individual therapy to deal with issues that are more efficiently resolved in this format (e.g., phobias, sexual arousal conditioning). The frequency of such sessions varies over time and with individual needs. We have resisted taking the common philosophical stance that all treatment must occur in groups (lest, in part, the offender "grooms" the therapist). Rather, we adopt strategies that will achieve relevant treatment goals as rapidly and effectively as possible.

Treatment Completion

Determining when an offender should leave the Twin Rivers program remains a problem. At one time, offenders had to "pass" a number of courses and groups. We have rejected this approach as being overly academic in its focus and not necessarily indicating relevant progress for each offender. Rather, we have defined a series of more universal goals that we expect each offender to achieve. That is, by the end of treatment, we hope that the offender:

1. Can recognize and understand the factors that contribute to his crime cycle
2. Is able to detect potential changes in himself and the environment that indicate he is at increased risk
3. Has learned skills that allow him to avoid, cope with, and escape from high-risk situations
4. Has developed the motivation and ability to apply his monitoring and intervention skills in a timely and effective manner

Consistent with the responsivity principle and clinical experience, we recognize that our offenders vary considerably in terms of motivation, learning style, and ability. Thus, we do not expect that all offenders will equally achieve each of these goals in an optimal manner. We therefore continue treating an offender until, in our judgment, he has achieved as much as he is willing or able to do. The final treatment summary can then describe each offender's achievement or lack thereof.

The very notion of treatment completion has proven problematic. There is often an unwarranted perception among corrections personnel, parole officials, and the public that an offender who has "completed treatment" is no longer at risk to reoffend. Moreover, decision makers often demand a simple label (e.g., treatment completer, graduate) to guide their tasks. At the suggestion of our advisory committee, we completed a survey of all prison-based treatment programs in the United States. Despite the low response rate, we were able to conclude that: (1) most programs face similar problems in labeling an offender's status; and (2) no solutions are available. We have tried, with varying degrees of success, to educate decision makers to read the details of the treatment summary rather than relying on a categorical label. In addition, we are developing more formal ratings of the offenders progress on a series of specific dimensions.

Community Follow-up

We recognize the importance of long-term maintenance treatment when the offender returns to the community. If organized properly, such treatment can also improve the community corrections officer's ability to effectively monitor and control the offender. The Department of Corrections has assigned five community corrections positions to provide treatment at no cost to the offender. These treatment staff work closely with the Twin Rivers program but report to the Division of Community Corrections. Working across jurisdictions often requires close monitoring and networking to ensure shared expectations and plans.

Program Evaluation

A recent report by Song and Lieb (1995) provided outcome data on the first 4 years of the Twin Rivers program. The authors clearly stated that their data were preliminary and did not reflect a valid evaluation of the program. Nonetheless, the fact that sexual offense recidivism was only marginally less for treated versus comparison offenders (11 vs. 12%) led a number of legislators to conclude publicly that "treatment does not work." Although we were able to head off that challenge, it is clear that evaluating our efforts remains a top priority if we are to survive; indeed, the legislature has demanded that we do so as quickly as possible. Unfortunately, no additional resources have been provided for this task.

We introduced a comprehensive evaluation strategy in 1994. This strategy includes evaluating the clinical impact of each group (primary and psychoeducational) and of the program overall. Results to date are encouraging, suggesting that offenders are achieving the short-term clinical changes that we expect. Ultimately, we must evaluate the impact of treatment on recidivism. This task is made more difficult as we must collect relevant data from a variety of data bases (e.g., state patrol, FBI, county) to determine an accurate estimate of arrests and convictions. To date, we have reported data only from the Department of Corrections database, which defines recidivism as offenders who have returned to a Department of Corrections facility. As of July, 1996, 11.4% of the 132 released offenders who completed treatment between 1988 and 1992 had returned for a new sexual offense; these data are consistent with those reported by Song and Lieb (1995). However, of the 235 released offenders who completed treatment between 1993 and 1995, only 4.3% had returned to prison for a sexual offense. We are optimistic that the full evaluation, including a comparison group matched on risk, will help demonstrate the value of the program.

CHALLENGES AND SOLUTIONS

Over time, the Twin Rivers program has undergone considerable change, as do many programs in our evolving field. Much of the change has been generated by the program itself in order to take advantage of current research and internal reviews. External feedback (from legislatures, the courts) or critical comments from colleagues have also helped identify concerns. As many of the problems we have faced are common to those faced by other programs, a review of our solutions and their impact may be useful.

Like many similar programs, the Twin Rivers program generates monthly statistics on variables such as the number of program participants, treatment completers, terminations and reasons, days to completion and termination, and so forth. In many programs, such data are collected and forgotten. However, when examined over time, these data can help define problems as well as provide a baseline to evaluate the impact of solutions. Table 1.1 summarizes data illustrating the discussion that follows.

Treatment Terminations

One disturbing trend in the data through 1993 was that the vast majority of offenders were not completing treatment. This is a serious concern for several reasons. First, there is growing evidence that offenders who fail to complete treatment are two to six times more likely to reoffend. Second, it can be argued that the program is simply eliminating possible failures, thus reducing the validity of positive outcome evaluations. Third, we can fairly question the value of any treatment that apparently meets the needs of only a minority of the intended audience. Fourth, a high treatment termination rate may reflect a program that is not presenting itself in a way that is understandable or accessible to its clients (i.e., not following the responsivity principle).

A review of the Twin Rivers program suggested several problems. First, there was little recognition that early treatment termination was a problem. Staff saw their role as giving offenders access to treatment as it had been designed. If the requirements made little sense to the offender, or if he objected to specific program elements, he was allowed to fail. Such failure is typically attributed to the offender's manipulation and lack of motivation; the possibility that we (as staff) have failed to be good teachers may not be considered. We therefore began to promote a philosophy that made the offender's success our primary goal. Staff were encouraged to collaborate with the offender to determine goals and solutions. If an offender objected to a specific task (e.g., satiation therapy), we tried to find alternate strategies (e.g., arousal control training, covert sensitization) that might achieve the same result.

TABLE 1.1
Operating Data for the Twin Rivers Program

	1993	1994	1995	1996
Completed TRCC treatment	44	52	110	170
Terminated from treatment	130	74	29	21
Percent completed treatment	25%	41%	79%	89%
Days to complete treatment	NA	979	712	542

A second problem appeared to be the highly confrontational nature of treatment. While there is little question that staff (and other offenders) must confront the offender's distorted beliefs and perceptions, it appeared that such confrontations had reached the level of "shark attacks." We observed group meetings where an offender was made to stand in the center of a large circle, while seated staff and offenders attacked every statement. We realized that, as staff, we would not readily change our behavior if supervisors used that approach with us. Rather, we would either quit our jobs (as many of our offenders chose to do) or we would learn to say the expected things (as long as we were being observed) to escape or avoid such attacks. While this latter strategy might keep our paychecks (or our program status), it would not likely promote genuine behavior change.

This second problem was relatively easy to change. Most staff used excessive confrontation because they thought their supervisors expected them to do so. As our stated expectations changed, so did staff behavior. And as staff began modeling more appropriate challenging, other offenders began adopting similar approaches. Interestingly, while most offenders reported feeling much more willing to be open in group, some offenders, generally the more prison-wise, felt that this softer approach was not as productive and certainly not as exciting.

A third problem with early terminations seemed to be related to staff's use of power and control. It is commonly said that sexual offenders abuse their power and control over others in the commission of their offenses and that helping the offender learn to use power responsibly is a major goal of treatment. It is therefore somewhat ironic that there are few clinical settings that provide therapists with as much power and the opportunity to abuse such power as does a prison environment. Staff can give orders, write infractions (charges), terminate offenders from treatment, influence transfer to another prison, and above all can help determine when and if an offender will be released from prison. If power is an important treatment issue, it is extremely important that staff model how they use their power responsibly. Some of the strategies noted above (e.g., negotiating treatment tasks, helping offenders succeed) have helped in this regard. Offenders now sign off on their final treatment report and are invited to submit written rejoinders that become a permanent part of their case file. We are also initiating a more extensive termination process, including widespread case conferences for problematic offenders in an attempt to find clinical solutions before termination is used as a last resort.

As Table 1.1 shows, fewer than 15% of offenders currently fail to complete treatment. Of these, approximately half are self-terminated (usually shortly after they arrive) and 20% leave for nonprogram reasons (e.g., death, terminations for security reasons). Not surprisingly, the learning environment has improved with the reduction in early terminations.

Treatment Completions

A second feature of interest in Table 1.1 is the number of offenders completing treatment and the time it takes to do so. In 1993, only 44 men finished treatment. Although time-to-completion data were not being collected, it appeared that most of these men had been in treatment for more than 3 years. Given the cost of providing treatment and faced with a waiting list of over 900 offenders, such low productivity was clearly unacceptable. Several features of our operation seemed to be contributing to these problems.

The main problem appeared to be that there was no expectation that treatment would be completed in a timely manner. The program had adopted the common but unsubstantiated belief that treatment lasting less than 2–3 years could not be effective with sexual offenders. There was a tendency to retain offenders until every possible clinical issue had been addressed. Many offenders, particularly more manipulative men, could easily prolong their stay by generating new clinical issues as needed.

We first addressed this issue by redefining the purpose and nature of treatment. We concluded that our goal was to help offenders learn skills and attitudes that would help them control their behavior and avoid offending. This premise has at least two implications. First, all skill acquisition follows a learning curve in which skills improve most rapidly early in training. Once the learning curve asymptotes, behavior can improve but each increment takes longer to achieve. Therefore, prolonging treatment beyond the offender's asymptote is a very inefficient use of resources. Our task became to help each offender reach his asymptote, recognizing that each offender's maximal level and rate of learning would be different.

A second implication of our definition of treatment is that only those treatment components that could reasonably be expected to help the offender avoid offending should be included in the program. At one time, the program provided over 25 psychoeducational groups and classes, and most offenders completed all of them. Although all offerings may have been clinically sound for some populations and problems, the real question was how many of these were *necessary* to help the offender avoid relapsing. Streamlining program content is always a difficult task, as most of us are reluctant to drop program elements that are comfortable.

To rationalize program content and organization, we completed a zero-base program review. A zero-base review requires redesigning the program from the ground up, justifying each component on the basis of research evidence and accepted principles and goals; including a component because "we've always done it that way" is not acceptable. Although we retained many aspects of the existing program, the zero-base exercise resulted in the more streamlined program described above.

As Table 1.1 shows, the treatment completion rate has increased steadily since 1993, while the time required has been reduced by 43%. As far as we can tell from the recidivism data reviewed earlier, these changes have not been associated with increased reoffending.

Treatment Consistency

Large programs involving numerous treatment staff have many advantages. Staff bring a variety of experiences and skills that add to the diversity of available resources. However, this diversity can also lead to reduced treatment consistency across all therapists. This was illustrated for the Twin Rivers program during a court hearing in which many staff were asked to describe the treatment an offender had completed. It became apparent that each staff was describing a very different program. Although this testimony likely did not affect the outcome of the hearing, it did raise concerns about what treatment was actually being provided.

A lack of treatment consistency and standardization can arise for many reasons. Staff may see themselves as independent clinicians with a professional duty to impose their understanding of sexual deviance on the treatment process with their clients. While private practice allows the therapist to operate in this manner, interstaff differences in treatment philosophy, goals, and procedures can be disruptive in a large, multistaff program. However, it would be equally unrealistic and inappropriate to have all staff act as clones. Indeed, trying to adhere to the responsivity principle requires that staff be creative and innovative in tailoring treatment to each offender's needs and learning styles.

Program structure can also contribute to treatment consistency. Some programs, like Twin Rivers, tend to modularize treatment so that each offender must complete all or some of the available groups and classes. In such a system, each staff may work with each offender only during one or more such modules and no staff may be responsible for overseeing each offender's overall treatment. This system is akin to an academic setting in which students choose and complete courses, but no single faculty member need be aware of the student's overall progress or individual needs. At Twin Rivers, we realized that this system has several drawbacks. Some offenders were taking groups and classes that were not relevant to their clinical and criminogenic needs. Other offenders had completed over a year of treatment without having defined their crime cycle. Above all, staff found it difficult to write comprehensive and informative final treatment reports and typically resorted to listing comments submitted by the leaders of the various groups the offender had taken. In short, each staff saw the program from the perspective of their role as group trainer rather than therapist.

The most important step to resolve these problems was the bolstering of the primary groups and defining the primary therapist as the case manager. Moreover, most of the core programming (e.g., defining crime cycles, teaching relapse prevention) is now delivered through the primary group. Each primary therapist can better define their offender's needs and can both focus more group time to these areas and direct the offender to relevant psychoeducational modules. As the case manager, the primary therapist is in an ideal position to prepare a comprehensive and useful final treatment report.

A second element of treatment consistency that we continue to debate is the extent to which activities within the primary groups should be driven by a treatment manual as are the psychoeducational groups. While a fixed curriculum can provide greater interstaff consistency, it can also limit the therapist's ability to adapt to the range of offenders and their needs. We have adopted a compromise approach in which the primary groups are driven by a set of common goals (e.g., offense disclosure, accepting responsibility, defining the crime cycle, etc.) rather than procedures. Our treatment manual is largely made up of strategies and curricula staff have used to achieve each goal, problems they have encountered, and solutions they have tried. In this way, staff can adopt and adapt cognitive behavioral approaches that best meet the current needs of their caseload. At the same time, adopting common goals allows for evaluating offender progress across therapists and groups.

Final Treatment Summaries

Determining what information should be included in a final treatment report and who should have access to this information can be a problem for many prison-based programs. Some programs report to health care, and all documents are considered highly confidential. In such cases, many individuals who must help manage the offender (e.g., community corrections) may have trouble getting access to relevant treatment information. Moreover, the content of the treatment reports may avoid useful detail for fear of breaching confidentiality. At the same time, criminal justice systems are often criticized, especially during investigations of a reoffense, for not sharing relevant information that may have helped prevent a new crime.

This problem was effectively resolved in Washington State with the passage of the Sentencing Reform Act in 1991. This legislation effectively mandated that the Twin Rivers program share all relevant information with stakeholders that have a need to know. In

Washington State, this includes an end-of-sentence review board who determine if the offender will be referred for potential civil commitment as a sexual predator and local and county police who determine the degree to which the community will be informed of the offender's presence. Thus, our final treatment summaries are, for all practical purposes, not at all confidential. This lack of confidentiality is clearly detailed in the treatment consent form and does not appear to be an impediment to treatment for many offenders (i.e., our waiting list has over 900 names); it is less clear how many of the 50% of eligible offenders who refuse treatment do so because of confidentiality concerns.

The widespread distribution of treatment reports also raised concerns about their content. At one time, our final treatment summaries focused largely on a social history, comments about the offender's participation in various groups, and a brief clinical statement of the offender's risk to reoffend. While this format may keep more sensitive clinical information confidential, feedback from the users of the reports suggested that they were not useful and were rarely read. To ensure that our reports usefully contribute to decision making and offender management, we have chosen to focus our final treatment summaries on issues such as static and dynamic risk, the offender's crime cycle, high-risk situations, and behavioral signs that the offender's risk may be increasing. Most importantly, we offer recommendations regarding the offender's management (e.g., conditions of release, need for further services), including strategies we have found to work and not work in gaining the offender's compliance. In short, we consider the final treatment summary to be a blueprint to help the reader monitor and evaluate the offender's behavior and intervene in a timely manner.

Feedback from users (e.g., community corrections officers) suggests that this information is much more useful than social histories and treatment performance when it comes to actively managing the offender. Indeed, we have documented numerous cases where community corrections officers and treatment providers used information from a final treatment summary to prevent what appeared to be imminent relapse. Moreover, we have instituted a series of postmortems on offenders who do reoffend or are revoked to determine if and how we could have prevented relapse. We are also investigating how accurately our description of the offender's crime cycle describes actual lapses and relapses.

PROGRAM SUPPORT

Prison-based treatment programs rarely control their own destiny. Such programs exist within a complex prison system whose priorities and philosophies may shift over time. Prison systems themselves operate within the public arena and are susceptible to changing demands from legislators. However, while complete control may not be possible, treatment programs can and must proactively prepare to deal with potential challenges.

One common source of stress for a prison-based program can come from the host prison itself. Many programs report to managers who are several steps removed from the superintendent, making it difficult to compete for scarce resources or the resolution of ongoing problems. It is often the case that prison staff, like the public generally, think negatively of sexual offenders and view treatment as being "soft on crime," a waste of resources, and clearly not related to the true purpose of prisons—that is, secure confinement. In some settings, staff may try to sabotage treatment actively or passively. At the same time, nontreatment (e.g., custody) staff are trained to observe behavior and can monitor the offender's behavior and attitudes when the social demands of the therapist's presence are not operating.

The Twin Rivers program is very fortunate in many respects. The program director reports directly to the superintendent, Janet Barbour, who is extremely supportive of the program, as are the other senior managers. On numerous occasions, the superintendent has personally intervened within the institution, at Department of Corrections headquarters, and with the legislature to help resolve problems. The importance and value of open communication between the program and senior managers cannot be overestimated.

The line staff at Twin Rivers are generally a very professional and competent group of individuals. The program has made a concerted effort to form working alliances with the prison staff by providing information about our activities (e.g., through periodic newsletter articles, informational and social open houses), taking active part in events that are of importance to the staff at large (staff-of-the-year ceremonies), contributing our expertise to nonprogram projects (e.g., screening emergency response team members, hostage negotiation training), and generally contributing to the prison as a whole. We have encouraged treatment staff to approach correctional officers on their posts to get information about our offenders. Program staff who have initiated this contact have generally been received very positively and have had access to a wealth of information. Our ongoing challenge is to encourage treatment staff to make time for these consultations. The results of our various efforts have stopped short of the program being universally respected and valued. However, we have reached a working accommodation with most prison staff who, if they are not our strongest allies, have done little to interfere with the program's operation.

In 1995, the Twin Rivers program faced a major crisis when the legislature eliminated program funding from the state budget. As noted earlier, this decision was based in part on an outcome evaluation (Song & Lieb, 1995) that did not show a statistical advantage for treatment. Although the authors of the report clearly stated that the results were preliminary and should not be taken as a true reflection of the worth of the program, some legislators immediately concluded that treatment had failed.

Because the budget deliberations were nearing completion, the Twin Rivers program had little time to react. Within days, key legislators received letters and personal visits from well over 100 local professionals and the public, as well as input from national and international sexual offender treatment experts. While all of this input clearly had an impact, the most influential support came from the victim treatment community, the police, and prosecutors. Each of these groups identified themselves as natural allies of the Twin Rivers program and persuasively argued that treating sexual offenders was an important part of a comprehensive societal reaction to the problem of sexual abuse. Within 2 weeks, the Twin Rivers program had been returned to the budget.

As a result of these events, the Twin Rivers program has taken a number of steps to better prepare for similar future challenges. During our response to the legislature, it became apparent that many legislators were largely uninformed about the program and were making decisions based on what they had heard from others. We have since hosted a series of open houses for legislators and their staff, including opportunities to meet with offenders. We began issuing an annual report that includes statistical information about program accomplishments and directions. We have met with the editorial boards of the larger local newspapers to discuss the program and more general issues involving sexual offenders. More generally, we have remained open to enquiries and requests from the media and now average over 50 such contacts per year. Although our message does not always appear as we had intended, we cannot fairly expect the public to support our program if they know nothing about it.

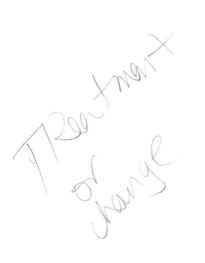

to emphasize the role of the Twin Rivers program
) share the goal of protecting society from sexual
etwork with these others groups, the Twin Rivers
iittee to ensure that the perspective of various
or managers from the Department of Corrections,
esentation from victim advocates, sexual offender
ors and defense attorneys, academia, and the state
to challenge the program and provide suggestions
l concerns. As a result of their input, the program
th our offenders' victims and their therapists, is
mily reunification is better controlled, and has
on measures. Although the committee meets only
ource of ongoing advice and support on a range of
the occasion arise, we expect that committee
owledgeably about the program and its integrity.

CONCLUSIONS

Operating effective sexual offender treatment programs in prisons remains a challenging and rewarding task. The need to resolve problems arising from changing prison and government policies, legal challenges, staff morale and performance issues, and public confidence and support seems constant. In addition, research is increasingly showing that therapists who treat sexual offenders suffer considerably more stress than is found with other clinical populations. At times, it seems that dealing with often resistant offenders may be the easiest part of the job. It is therefore essential that programs take proactive steps to create a positive work and treatment environment for staff and inmates, while attending to issues of accountability and community support. Given the relatively short history of systematic approaches to treating this difficult problem, we can reasonably expect to become increasingly effective over time. A strong belief that our efforts are contributing to public safety and the satisfaction of being able to demonstrate positive change in offenders and the program make many of the daily frustrations more tolerable.

REFERENCES

Andrews, D.A., Zinger, I., Hoge, R., Bonta, J., Gendreau, P., & Cullen, F. (1990). Does correctional treatment work? A clinically relevant and psychologically informed meta-analysis. *Criminology, 28,* 369–404.

Andrews, D.A., & Bonta, J. (1990). Classification for effective rehabilitation: Rediscovering psychology. *Criminal Justice & Behavior, 17,* 19–52.

Song, L., & Lieb, R. (1995). *Washington State sex offenders: Overview of recidivism studies.* Olympia: Washington State Institute for Public Policy.

2

A. Prison Settings

Kia Marama

A Treatment Program for Child Molesters in New Zealand

Stephen M. Hudson, David S. Wales, and Tony Ward

The Kia Marama special treatment unit was established in late 1989, in response to a confluence of a number of factors. By 1986, the high rates of reoffending among child molesters released from New Zealand prisons (approximately 25%) had been identified by local research. Second, the Psychological Service of the New Zealand Department of Justice (now Department of Corrections) had developed an explicit mission statement involving a commitment to reducing future offending. There was also a developing sense of optimism with respect to the ability of cognitive–behavioral-oriented interventions to reduce the reoffending rate of sexual offenders. The early proposal for the unit was modeled on the Atascadero Sex Offender Treatment and Evaluation Program; however, Marshall devised the original program and trained the first group of staff.

The Kia Marama unit consists of rectangular row of 60 self-contained rooms that face an open, grassed compound, all of which is surrounded by a 5-m perimeter fence. A ratio of approximately 1 : 10 is kept between custodial staff (prison officers) and inmates. Together with their custodial duties, prison officers seek to maintain an environment that is maximally conducive to therapeutic gains. Officers are assigned to each therapy group and are encouraged to provide support and monitoring of the therapeutic progress of group members.

Only men convicted of child sexual offenses are contained within this unit. The benefits of separate institutions for sexual offenders are seen as being reduced harassment from other offenders and the possibility of creating a more therapeutic environment. The residents have freedom of movement within the compound to encourage both social and therapeutic interchanges. We also hope that contact between those about to start the program and those further along will also foster a broad therapeutically oriented milieu.

Stephen M. Hudson and Tony Ward • Department of Psychology, University of Canterbury, Christchurch, New Zealand. **David S. Wales** • Kia Marama Special Treatment Unit, Rolleston Prison, Rolleston, New Zealand.

Sourcebook of Treatment Programs for Sexual Offenders, edited by Marshall et al. Plenum Press, New York, 1998.

THE PROGRAM

Referral

Referrals to the program are made by the psychological service staff from eligible volunteers within 11 prisons situated in the South Island and lower half of the North Island. The remaining seven prisons refer to a second program, Te Piriti, opened in Auckland in 1994. One half of the total of 3.6 million people in New Zealand live in the region we serve. Admission to the program is clearly voluntary; a significant amount of information is provided to any potential client prior to the transfer to the unit. The inmate first provides informed consent to the assessment process, and only subsequent to this does he provide further informed consent to treatment. The transfer to Kia Marama is typically made as close to the commencement data of the relevant program as possible and is typically toward the end of the offender's sentence. We have debated the utility of entry early in the sentence, where motivation is arguably maximal, against the deterioration that we believe is likely to occur if significant periods of time intervene between the completion of the program and release to the community. Given that the central aim of the program is to reduce the risk of reoffense in the community, we have opted for a more seamless transition to aftercare. An educationally oriented group, which meets once per week, is provided for those men transferred prior to the start of their particular program.

Entry requirements include a medium- or minimum-security classification and the inmate must have been convicted of, or admit to, sexual offense(s) against a person under 16 years of age (i.e., the legal definition of childhood in new Zealand). This does not exclude men who have also offended against adult women; indeed, we have admitted such men to the program. However, the presence of these men has required specific safety plans to be developed for the protection of female staff. Due to the cognitive content of the program, volunteers are required not to be intellectually disabled, which is defined for practical purposes as an IQ less than 70. They are also required to be free of active mental illness, although depression is relatively common during the program. Finally, they do not need to have admitted the offenses for which they were convicted at least initially; the paradox of volunteering for a treatment program while in denial is usually a reflection of both ambivalence and a positive expectation of treatment completion with respect to parole hearings. However, persistent total denial that survives the "Understanding Your Offending" and "Victim Impact and Empathy" modules (see below) result in the man being discharged from the program. These entry criteria are liberal compared to many of the documented programs overseas.

Assessment

The program starts with a 2-week period devoted to assessment. This process culminates in a clinical formulation that serves to guide the customization of the program content to the individual. It includes a series of clinical interviews, beginning with the man's view of his offending and the factors and processes that led up to these instances and going on to cover issues of social competency. More specifically, these interviews cover details regarding the offender's general life management skills; his ability to use leisure effectively; his interpersonal goals and ability to form satisfying intimate relationships; his beliefs and attitudes about self; his ability to regulate his affect, particularly negative emotions; his capacity for empathy and perception of victim harm; his sense of responsibility for the offenses and the extent to which he is still minimizing some aspects of his offending; his views regarding sex, particularly his own entitlement, the appropriateness of sexual contact between adults and children, and what needs he considers are satisfied by his deviant and nondeviant sexual activity; and, finally, his use of both pornography and intoxicants. Due to the tight scheduling of the assessment phase, we encourage the men to write social, sexual, and emotional histories prior to commencing assessment. These can be used by therapists to structure assessment interviews around significant themes.

All clients undergo phallometric testing to identify the presence or absence of deviant attraction to either children and/or aggressive themes. We are aware of the controversy surrounding phallometric assessment and are seeking to develop alternative measures of sexual interest. However, until these are fully available, we believe there to be sufficient utility in this process, at least for child molesters, to justify its continuance. We see this as an essential component of the assessment process and it is explicitly covered in the consent form. Refusal to participate would mean being declined entry into the program. Most men accept the therapist's explanation that it is needed in order to adequately set treatment goals and to help reduce their risk of reoffending. The link between deviant sexual arousal and offending is also drawn explicitly in the "Understanding Your Offending" module (see below).

The resident also completes a series of 16 self-report scales that cover the following domains: sexual attitudes, beliefs, and behaviors, including views of sexual activity between an adult and a child, attitudes and fantasies about various sexual activities, hostile attitudes, and acceptance of violence toward women; emotional functioning, particularly anger, anxiety, and depression; interpersonal competence, particularly issues of self-esteem, intimacy, and loneliness; and personality. Both the scales and the phallometric assessment are repeated at the completion of treatment. We also have the therapists complete a psychopathy assessment at the end of treatment, as this forms part of our risk assessment.

Treatment

Overall Structure

The program is almost entirely group based, with individual therapy kept to a minimum, sufficient only to enable a resident to participate in group. Group treatment is more effective both in terms of use of time (more men can be dealt with at once) and, we believe, in terms of efficacy in that processes such as credible challenges by other offenders and vicarious learning are not available in individual treatment. Groups are selected on the basis of release dates and currently consist of eight men with one therapist. We have previously had up to ten men in a group. There are five therapists on staff: three psychologists, one nurse therapist, and one social worker therapist. They all administer a standard program. The full program, described below in terms of the series of modules it comprises, runs for 31 weeks with groups meeting for three 2.5-hour sessions per week (see Table 2.1 for an overview). Nontherapy time is spent engaged in homework assignments, therapy-related activities, prison work (e.g., kitchen or garden), or at leisure.

Recent changes in legislation has enabled some incarcerated inmates to be released at one third of their full sentence, which in New Zealand is typically a fixed period rather than a range; the exceptions to this are a life sentence and preventative detention. It was also identified that a proportion of referrals to the program did not require the full program,

TABLE 2.1
Components of Program Used at Kia Marama

Module	Duration	Content
Assessment	2 weeks	Clinical interviews Written social, sexual and emotional histories Psychometric Plethysmographic
Norm building	6 sessions	Establishment of group rules Disclosure of personal details Introduction to principles of relapse prevention
Understanding your offending	17 sessions	Disclosure of offense preconditions Completion of offense chain Identification of factors contributing to offending Disclosure of own experiences of abuse Challenging dysfunctional cognitions
Arousal reconditioning	6 sessions	Covert sensitization Masturbatory reconditioning: Directed masturbation and satiation
Victim impact and empathy	12 sessions	Impact of offending on victims Readings from victim accounts Videos portraying victim experiences Discussion with guest speaker (abuse survivor) "Autobiography" from own victim's point of view Role play between self and victim
Mood management	12 sessions	Cognitive behavioral model of mood Identification of mood emotions associated with offending Physiological, cognitive and behavioral skills to manage these
Relationship skills	12 sessions	Intimacy Establishing and maintaining intimate relationships Sexuality
Relapse prevention	12 sessions	Identification of relapse chain Identification of skills to manage relapse issues Identification of support people Presentation of personal statement
Reassessment	2 weeks	Re-administration of psychometrics and plethysmographic assessment

specifically those modules designed to increase social competency skills. Hence, a shortened version of the program was developed that consisted of what we see to be the core modules of "Understanding Your Offending," "Victim Impact and Empathy," and "Relapse Prevention." Only a small number of referrals for this modified program were received and we have now reverted to assigning all referrals to the full program.

Finally, the Department of Corrections is committed to policies that reflect our obligations, under the Treaty of Waitangi, to Maori people. The Te Piriti program (see Chapter 26, this volume) has adopted a different structure in order to more appropriately reflect local population demographics. It incorporates a greater emphasis on cultural factors in treatment delivery, including the involvement of *whanau* (family) and the employment of a full-time cultural consultant. The Kia Marama program has access to a part-time cultural consultant who has assisted therapists with individual clients and has developed culturally appropriate welcoming and departure ceremonies.

Module 1: Norm Building

The primary aim for this module is to establish the rules of conduct that are essential if the group is to function effectively and to provide an overview of the treatment philosophy, that is the "the big picture." Although each group generates its own set of rules that are in a sense unique to the group, most groups typically include rules covering confidentiality (prohibiting the discussion of issues raised in group concerning other group members with people outside the group) and communication procedures (using "I" statements, one person speaking at a time, speaking to each other not about each other, and demonstrating active listening skills). Additional rules emphasize the importance of accepting responsibility for one's own issues (by facing up to challenges and by asking questions when something is not understood) and challenging other members constructively and assertively rather than aggressively or by colluding. The unit operates a strict nonviolence policy both within and out of groups. Any resident threatening or using violence is immediately dismissed from the program. This policy is made explicit on arrival.

We get each of the men to disclose personal details, such as his family structure and a developmental and recent social history, with the general aim of establishing appropriate patterns of the group working. Group members are encouraged to discuss how they reached the decision to attend the program, what their reasons are for being in the program, what obstacles they can identify that might inhibit their progress, and what behaviors (e.g., anger, aggression, or withdrawal) might prevent others from aiding them to change. As well as initiating the process of shaping disclosure, risk taking, and honesty, these questions are aimed at eliciting self-motivated statements.

Finally, our belief is that the use of the relapse prevention framework, despite the need for significant theoretical refinement (Ward & Hudson, 1996), has considerable advantages for these clients. It articulates a very positive view of their offending in so far as rather than events that just happen, as they often perceive their offending to be, relapse prevention describes a series of identifiable steps or a chain that constitute the problem behavior process (see, for example, Ward, Louden, Hudson, & Marshall, 1995). This view explicitly allows for the possibility of control at multiple points (i.e., escape or avoidance), and thus termination of the behavior chain. In essence it provides a compensatory view of a habit process, where the man is not held responsible for the vulnerability factors that we believe underlie his offending, but he is liable for managing them. Our belief is that if the man has a grasp of this overall framework, however rudimentary, all that is required of him in treatment makes sense, and this, in turn, assists motivation as well as comprehension.

Module 2: Understanding Your Offending

The primary aim of this module is for the man to come to fully understand his offense chain. This inevitably contains the notions of a cyclical or repetitive, but stepwise, progression through fundamentally predictable stages. It is critical that the therapist be very well informed about each man's history and offense details prior to the session in which he presents his "story." This means the therapist needs to have read prison files, especially any presentence material such as probation report, summary of facts, judicial sentencing notes, victim impact statements (although the recent Privacy Act makes these more difficult to obtain), in addition to material gained by way of interviews, questionnaires, phallometry, or discussions with significant others.

We base this process on the understanding we have developed regarding the typical offending pathways (Ward et al., 1995). Using a collaborative approach, with help from group members, the client is expected to develop an understanding of how background factors, such as low mood, lifestyle imbalances, sexual difficulties, and intimacy difficulties set the scene for offending. We make a very clear distinction between historical facts and the resulting or current thoughts, feelings, and behaviors that the man has developed in response to those factors. Thus, chain links are expressible in statements such as "I allowed myself to …" "I convinced myself that.…"

This distinction is particularly useful, but not exclusively so, where the man has a history of being sexual victimized. Research suggests that such histories are common among sexual offenders. We believe a therapeutic conundrum exists to the degree that men frequently use this abuse history as an explanation for their own abusive behavior. Our response to this involves three related steps. First, the compensatory model mentioned above is presented; that is, they remain responsible for managing their current behavior. Second, a modification is introduced into their view of the causal link; early abuse can cause offense supportive attitudes and beliefs that persist into the "here and now," so that while they cannot change the fact that the abuse occurred, they can change the current sequelae. Finally, we believe that abusive men with histories of being abused are as entitled to help with their own victimization as those who have not abused others; to deny them access to assistance seems unduly punitive. However, we spend limited time on this aspect treatment in order for the focus to be on the issues not the excuses. Further work postrelease is frequently recommended.

The next two sections of the chain—distal planning and entering the high-risk situation (in which both proximal planning and the offense behaviors occur)—are distinguished by the presence of a potential victim or being in a situation where the presence of a potential victim is highly probable (e.g., being in a park shortly after children get out of school). The final part of the chain involves a description of the types of reactions the man has to having offended and how these reactions inevitably add to his difficulties and therefore increase the likelihood of the chain continuing. Each man completes this task during one group session. After receiving feedback from the therapist and other group members he then has a further opportunity to refine his understanding during a further session. Each man then identifies and highlights the essential components in his offense process, typically three links in each of the distal planning and high-risk phases. He then specifies the specific treatment goals related to each link. Conventional cognitive restructuring, particularly the challenging of distortions, remains a major part of the intervention through this entire process.

This module is seen as being fundamental to the program, as the remainder of therapy is based on an adequate understanding of the offense process. Therefore, during the final session of this module, we have the man's comprehension of his offense chain "tested" by the program director. This adds an extrinsic element to motivation, as well as providing a validity check for the adequacy of progress.

Module 3: Arousal Reconditioning

Sexual arousal to children is seen by most authors as at least partly causing the man to behave in sexually inappropriate ways with children and is typically described as an important part of the problem behavior process. Even where there is no phallometric evidence of sexual arousal to children, our belief is that any extensive pairing of orgasm and children means that it is likely that under circumstances of risk (e.g., a negative mood state and the presence of a potential victim) the man will experience deviant sexual arousal. In our experience many of the men participating in treatment find this module very difficult, and consequently therapists need to be very clear about the rationale for these procedures. The major reason we offer for the need to modify deviant arousal is to point to the central role that sexual arousal has played in at least the proximal phase of past offending and the need to attend to this in order to reduce future risk. Our experience is that with adequate explanation, together with handouts describing the procedures and their scientific basis, the majority of the residents participate fully.

There are three components to this intervention. Covert sensitization comprises the first of these. Each man identifies the process or sequence involved in his most recent or most typical sexual assault and operationalizes this by preparing a personalized fantasy divided into four parts: (1) a neutral scene involving boredom; (2) a scene involving gradual buildup to hands-on contact with a victim, but which ends before sexual contact is actually made; (3) a scene of negative consequences involving detection, arrest, going to jail, and the associated humiliation and loss; and (4) an escape scene involving "coming to his senses" and getting out of the situation, feeling relieved and "very pleased with himself." These scenes are then written on pocket-sized cards. He is required to regularly review these behavior sequences. Scenes 1 and 2 are repeatedly paired with both scenes 3 and 4. The men are encouraged to activate the escape scene at progressively earlier points in the previous scenes. Repeated practice of this type is meant to encourage thinking about negative consequences earlier rather than simply after the offense, as is usually the case. The man's familiarity with and use of these cards are reviewed frequently during the remainder of the program. The men are encouraged to carry these cards with them at all times, including postrelease.

The remaining components in this module are designed to both decrease deviant sexual arousal and to strengthen sexual arousal to appropriate images and thoughts. Directed masturbation, where the man is encouraged to become aroused by whatever means is necessary, but once aroused to masturbate to consensual images involving an adult, is designed to pair arousal with thoughts of appropriate sexual activity in order to strengthen these associations. Once the man has ejaculated and becomes at least relatively refractory to sexual stimulation, he is asked to carry out a modification of the satiation procedures suggested by Marshall (1979). These involve the man repeatedly verbalizing components of his deviant sexual fantasies, for at least 20 minutes, while in this state of minimal sexual arousal. This pairing of deviant sexual material with both low arousal and relative unresponsiveness is likely to reduce its positive valence. In keeping with the relapse prevention philosophy espoused by the program, men are led to expect that they will continue to have occasional thoughts of sex with children. It is how they respond to these lapses that is seen to be critical. What they are instructed to do is reinstate the conditioning procedures or contact their therapist.

Module 4: Victim Impact and Empathy

A lack of empathy for their victims and an inability or refusal to seriously consider the traumatic effects of sexual abuse appear to be common features of sexual offenders. We enhance each man's understanding of the impact of offending on victims by having the group "brainstorm" immediate effects, postabuse effects and long-term consequences. Any gaps in understanding are filled by the therapist.

A general deficiency in the capacity to be empathic is often seen as facilitating offending, where things that are manifestly harmful are done to others. It is most likely that the deficit is quite selective to the man's own victim, and as such most likely reflects dysfunctional cognitions specifically related to his own offending. The victim impact material is intended to reinstate their capacity to empathize with potential victims and reduce future risk of reoffending.

To enhance this process we have the men engage in several other tasks. We have them read aloud accounts of sexual abuse and view videotapes of victims describing their experiences. We also have an abuse survivor come in to the group, as a guest speaker; she facilitates a discussion about the impact of abuse, both in general and specifically to her. They then write an "autobiography" from their own victim's perspective. This covers the distress they suffered and the ongoing consequences to having been abused. Finally, we have the man role-play both roles between himself and his victim. The group assists in these processes, challenging and suggesting additional material, and provides, along with the therapist, final approval.

Marshall, O'Sullivan, and Fernandez (1996) have provided evidence indicating that these procedures produce significant improvements in reported empathic responding specifically focused on the men's own victims. However, this work needs to be replicated across other groups. Additional work is also needed with respect to the issues of maintaining this change and the problem that it is seldom skill deficits that underlie performance deficits; the motivation to use these skills or perspectives in high-risk situations is what finally counts.

Module 5: Mood Management

Negative mood states are a frequent precipitating stimulus for the offense chain, usually depression or feelings of rejection, or more rarely anger. Indeed, Pithers' (1990) version of the relapse prevention model is based entirely on this pathway to offending. Therefore, deficiencies in affect regulation are a critical part in the management of risk. The men are presented with a cognitive–behavioral model of mood as an overarching framework. They are taught to identify and distinguish between a range of affects, including anger, fear, and sadness. They are then asked to identify particular moods that are, for them, especially associated with their offending process. Next we teach them the physiological, cognitive, and behavioral skills to manage these moods. For example, physiological skills include training in relaxation. Men are provided with information on how diet and exercise can influence mood. Cognitive strategies include techniques aimed at challenging or interrupting negative thoughts as well as developing positive coping strategies. Behavioral techniques include teaching and role-playing effective communication styles for expressing emotions, including assertiveness training, anger management, and conflict resolution techniques. Last, problem-solving and time management strategies are briefly introduced.

Module 6: Relationship Skills

This module constitutes the second broad aspect of social competency addressed by the program. It is our belief that a significant factor in the various motivations that cause these men to offend derives from their difficulties establishing emotionally satisfying relationships with other adults. Many offenders cite the need for closeness as a primary reason for sexual offending. Not only do these difficulties in relating to others result in unmet needs, they also relate to difficulties in regulating affect. It is therefore of considerable importance to enhance interpersonal functioning.

In this module we focus particularly on intimate relationships, first establishing their benefits and then examining ways in which they can be enhanced. The four main areas we focus on here involve: conflict and its resolution; the constructive use of shared leisure activities; the need to be communicative, supportive, and rewarding of each other; and finally, intimacy, which is the key issue around which all the others revolve. Sexual offenders are deficient in their capacity for intimacy (Seidman, Marshall, Hudson, & Robertson, 1994) and have problems in the attachment styles they have adopted to establish relationships (Ward, Hudson, & Marshall, 1996). We have also shown that sexual offenders display negative emotional states, such as loneliness and anger, that are related to intimacy deficits (Hudson & Ward, 1997).

We play attention to the relationship style described or exhibited by each man and identify aspects that may serve to block the development of an intimate relationship. We then examine approaches to relationships that might more effectively serve to develop intimacy. This is completed through the use of brainstorming, role-playing, discussion of prepared handouts, and homework assignments. Therapy staff have developed a group exercise that requires men to respond to a series of interpersonal dilemmas in ways that enhance intimacy and satisfactorily resolve conflict.

We also traverse issues relevant to sexuality and sexual dysfunction as part of this module, providing educational material, through handouts and videos, as required to correct misinformation or challenge unhelpful attitudes. We discuss sexuality as an aspect of intimacy and consider attitudes and behaviors that make for a mutually fulfilling encounter. Last, for a limited number of men, we address their confusion regarding adult sexual orientation. While emphasizing the importance of resolving such confusion as a means of reducing risk, we acknowledge that many of the factors contributing to such confusion are of a long-standing nature, and therefore are likely to require therapeutic attention over an extended period. We encourage men who remain unclear about their adult orientation to continue to examine it throughout the program, and make available to them further therapy at the completion of the program.

Module 7: Relapse Prevention

The overarching framework of the program is that of a relapse prevention view of offending, and we introduce these constructs early in treatment. In this sense the final intervention module of the program comes as no surprise to the men and forms a natural extension of the earlier components. The distinction between internal and external management has utility and we make use of it in structuring this module.

The internal management component involves the man presenting his ever-more refined understanding of his offense chain that he developed during the first module and describing the skills he has acquired to manage the relapse issues inherent in his chain. This whole approach embodies the belief that there is no cure and that the goal of treatment has been to enhance self-monitoring and control over behavior. The acquisition of the specific behavioral and cognitive skills and attitudes is presented as an aid to the offender in meeting his needs in more prosocial ways. The emphasis on understanding the links in the offending chain is to focus on the self-management skills needed to "break the chain" as early as possible. Thus, this module further assists each offender in identifying the external and internal factors that put him at risk and connecting these to adequate coping responses.

We have each group member identify the ways in which they might get themselves into a high-risk situation, particularly focusing on negative mood states as well as the "seemingly irrelevant choices" that constitute the covert route to high-risk situations. Issues such as lifestyle imbalances, perfectionistic standards, poorly managed interpersonal conflicts, and persistent deviant arousal are also revisited in this context of developing a self-management style that will minimize the risk of relapsing. Offenders also often report that they have deliberately entered a high-risk situation in order to test themselves; we point out the dangers in this strategy.

We also distinguish a lapse from a relapse. A lapse is, in one or another form, a precursor to a relapse (i.e., an actual reoffense). Thus, a lapse may take the form of deviant fantasizing or allowing oneself to enter a high-risk situation. We make this distinction in order to decrease the chances of responding to a lapse with the abstinence violation effect. The negative emotional and motivational consequences to this type of response to a lapse are best avoided. Moreover, we encourage each offender to view lapses as inevitable and as chances to further refine his understanding of the factors that put him at risk. Experience of a lapse also provides a chance to exercise control and to develop an enhanced sense of efficacy with respect to his ability to successfully monitor and manage his behavior.

The external management aspect involves the man in identifying friends or family members who are prepared to support him in his goal of avoiding reoffending. It also requires him to prepare and present his personal statement. This critical component is the bridge between the whole intervention effort and the community in which the man hopes to live the rest of his life. His personal statement articulates the factors or steps in his offending process that move him closer to offending. It covers his plan for how he can avoid risky situations and how to escape from one if it develops. It also covers what observable signs others might detect that may indicate he is behaving in risky ways. This process serves to facilitate good communication between himself and those responsible for his management on release (community corrections officer), as well as those people who have agreed to assist his self-management process.

RELEASE/AFTERCARE

Release plans are discussed and refined throughout the program. A full-time member of the therapy staff, the reintegration coordinator, is responsible for liaison between the resident, community agencies, and appropriate significant others. We aim, where possible, for men to be released back to the community directly from Kia Marama, rather than from a mainstream prison. Men are released to the communities from which they came rather than locally for two main reasons: adverse local community reaction and the need to maximize support during the inevitably difficult transition out of prison.

All residents appear before either a district prisons board or the nationally coordinated prison parole board if their sentence exceeds 7 years. Final release dates and conditions are determined by these statutory bodies. Conditions of release typically include as a minimum requirement residing where directed and regular attendance at community corrections (probation officers) and at the monthly Kia Marama follow-up support group. There may also be conditions regarding ongoing therapy with a psychologist from correction's psychological service. These conditions are enforced for the duration of the parole period, usually

9–12 months. Within the first month of release the man is encouraged to meet with those they have nominated to support them and the probation officer who is responsible for external supervision. The aim of this session is to have him openly discuss his relapse issues, especially what are for him high-risk situations and early warning signs of relapse.

Our policy on reintegration of the offender into a family with children is based on the following conditions: the man must have made adequate progress in treatment; a reliable and robust bond must exist between the child and nonoffending parent; the nonoffending parent accepts that the abuse occurred and that neither she nor the victim are responsible; the nonoffending partner is aware of the man's relapse issues and understands her role in protecting the children; and finally that outside agencies are available to provide both ongoing monitoring and support. If these conditions are met, then the other agencies are contacted with a view to clarifying roles and responsibilities. The typical process involves supervised visits, unsupervised visits of gradually increased length, home visits, overnight stays, and finally moving home with ongoing monitoring.

TREATMENT EVALUATION

To date (November 1996), 335 men have successfully completed the program and have been released back into the community. The mean period "at risk" is 3 years 2 months (range, 0–5 years 9 months). Twelve of these men have been reconvicted of a sexual crime; a reconviction rate of 3.6%, which is substantially less than the expected base rate of between 15 and 20%. More broadly, 361 men have completed the program; 26 men are yet to be released. Their mean age is 40.8 years (SD = 11.9, range, 18–75 years) and they had a mean number of victims each of 8.6 (SD = 22.9, range, 1–300). The mean duration of their offending (date from first conviction) was 8.1 years (SD = 7.8 years, range, 1–40). The most common relationship to their respective victims was father or surrogate father (46%), with another 1% being some other type of relative. Extrafamilial victims were chosen by 43% of the men completing the program, with 8% reporting a combination of both intrafamilial and extrafamilial offending.

CONCLUSIONS

On reflection, the proposal for the Kia Marama unit came at an opportune time. The unit fits with the Department of Corrections' custodial and habilitation needs and is very much in concert with its primary goal of reducing reoffending. Our commitment to an ongoing evaluation of the performance of the program, as well as the positive results so far, facilitates this positive regard.

The national scale of the original unit did create some difficulties in men gaining appropriate access. However, frequent public relations trips by unit staff to the other prisons, both to give talks about the program to custodial staff and to talk to potential participants, has helped in this regard. The opening of Te Pirti unit in Auckland has reduced this problem, but there remains a significant need to facilitate communication between potential clients, referral sources, and the unit. An inmate newsletter has assisted this process and is distributed to all source prisons. We have asked that it be circulated to the inmates as well as staff.

Unit staff have taken the initiative in providing information about the program and its philosophy to the unit's custodial staff. These people are volunteers, usually with a strong interest in habilitation efforts, and as we noted earlier one of the benefits of having just sex offenders in the unit is the possibility of a therapeutic milieu. A close working relationship with the unit custody manager has been maintained and joint policies developed for dealing with management issues such as serious misbehavior. We have carried out training sessions with correctional officers for probation officers who will be responsible for the graduates of the program when they return to their districts. Each treatment group has had a member of the custodial staff assigned to it. However, in practice it tends to be individual prison officers who make links with individual residents. These links are often quite strong with some men, for example, requesting a custodial officer as their support person at family group conferences.

The opening of the Kia Marama unit provided the New Zealand media with a source of expertise regarding sexual aggression. Unit staff have welcomed this and have been helpful in answering many of the questions raised. Two documentaries, similar in nature to "60 Minutes," have provided positive coverage of the unit and its program. We have said often that there is no cure for these types of difficulties, only continued management, and that the only rational expectation is that not all men will be successful. So far, the media has behaved as if they believe these statements.

Finally, the unit, with full departmental support, has been committed to assisting the training of clinical psychologists and social workers. Few workers stay as treatment providers for extended periods of time; hence, training is considered to be very important in the long term.

Overall, the 6 years since the unit was established have been a satisfying experience. There have been a number of challenges to be dealt with and no doubt there will be more in the future. The program has been very well supported; with an average of between 40 and 50 graduates per year and an ongoing commitment to good quality research, it is rightly seen as "delivering the goods."

REFERENCES

Hudson, S. M., & Ward, T. (1997). Intimacy, loneliness, and attachment style in sex offenders. *Journal of Interpersonal Violence, 12,* 323–339.

Marshall, W.L. (1979). Satiation therapy: A procedure for reducing deviant sexual arousal. *Journal of Applied Behavior Analysis, 12,* 10–22.

Marshall, W. L., O'Sullivan, C., & Fernandez, Y. M. (1996). The enhancement of victim empathy among incarcerated child molesters. *Legal and Criminological Psychology, 1,* 95–102.

Pithers, W. D. (1990). Relapse prevention with sexual aggressors: A method for maintaining therapeutic gain and enhancing external supervision. In W. L. Marshall, D. R. Laws, & H. E. Barbaree (Eds.), *Handbook of sexual assault: Issues, theories, and treatment of the offender* (pp. 343–361), New York: Plenum Press.

Seidman, B., Marshall, W. L., Hudson, S. M., & Robertson, P. J. (1994). An examination of intimacy and loneliness in sex offenders. *Journal of Interpersonal Violence, 9,* 518–534.

Ward, T., & Hudson, S. M. (1996). Relapse prevention: A critical analysis. *Sexual Abuse: A Journal of Research and Treatment, 8,* 177–200.

Ward, T., Hudson, S. M., & Marshall, W. L. (1996). Attachment style in sex offenders: A preliminary study. *Journal of Sex Research, 33,* 17–26.

Ward, T., Louden, K., Hudson, S.M., & Marshall, W. L. (1995). A descriptive model of the offense process. *Journal of Interpersonal Violence, 10,* 453–473.

3

A. Prison Settings

Peterhead Prison Program

Alec Spencer

BACKGROUND

Peterhead Prison was built in 1888 to house Scotland's convicts. The location, which juts out onto the North Sea, was chosen so as to enable use of convict labor in the building of a harbor of refuge for the fishing port of Peterhead. Granite was quarried about a mile away by the convicts and conveyed by a special railway line into the prison, where it was broken up, mixed, and poured with concrete to make the huge blocks for the breakwater wall. When finally completed in 1956, the wall enclosed the bay between the prison and the town. As legislation changed, so did the population of the prison, which during much of the second half of the 20th century held long-term prisoners who seemed unwilling to fit into the main prison system. So it was that in the 1980s, the name of Peterhead became synonymous with "hard men," trouble, riots, hostage taking of staff, and arson. It was Scotland's version of Alcatraz. Toward the end of that decade, its governor[1] sought to change the prison and began a dialogue with prisoners. When I arrived to take over the prison in mid-1992, there were only a comparatively small number of these difficult prisoners left, although the staff who dealt with them were still wearing full body armor and helmets for that purpose. Many of the recalcitrant prisoners had been dispersed to other prisons and in their place had come an increasing number of vulnerable prisoners. In fact, the "hard" prisoners who had once ruled the prison were locked up and the vulnerable individuals who had been locked up for their own safety in other prisons were able to associate openly with others like themselves. In 1992, the maximum-security prison held only about 140 inmates. Peterhead Prison, built with extremely thick concrete and granite-shuttered walls, was reckoned to be the most secure accommodation available, and one hall (accommodation unit) was being kept as emergency accommodation for the rest of the prison system. A second hall, "C" hall, was in the process of being refurbished.

By one of those happy coincidences of fate a number of factors came together during the second half of 1992. Peterhead's vulnerable prisoner population comprised mostly sexual offenders. Clearly it was about time something should be done with them. The social work unit within the prison, under the leadership of Philip English, had recognized this problem and had begun a group for a few sexual offenders. A number of staff had also

---

[1]"Governor" is the equivalent of warden or director of a correctional facility.

Alec Spencer • HM Prison, Peterhead, Aberdeenshire, Scotland AB42 6YY; *present address*: HM Prison, Edinburgh, Scotland EH11 3LN.

Sourcebook of Treatment Programs for Sexual Offenders, edited by Marshall et al. Plenum Press, New York, 1998.

expressed an interest in working with sexual offenders and received some training, supported by one of the junior governors, Bill Millar, who also understood the need. Bill Marshall, who had visited both the English and Scottish prison services, was spending 3 days at Peterhead to assist with staff training. Although I was not due to start at Peterhead for another month, I traveled specially to be with Bill. Those 3 days, when he taught by day and we discussed by night, were to change my own and the prison's life. After a lot of activity over the following 8 months and hard work by the program manager, Bob McConnell, the prison was ready to start. C hall, which had been refurbished, was opened in January 1993, specifically for sexual offenders, and took 60 prisoners.

ABOUT THE "STOP" PROGRAM

We first thought about delivering a Sex Offender Treatment Program or SOTP. This was not a useful acronym and juggling the letters we got STOP. More importantly, we did not want to use the term *treatment* to describe the work undertaken. *Treatment*, as a medical model, implies two things: first, that having diagnosed some malady there is a *cure*, and second, that *something can be done to the patient* to provide the cure. Sexual offending, like other manifestations of behavioral problems, addictions, or obsessions cannot be cured. That is, there is no certainty that having undertaken a course of treatment, the outcome is guaranteed. Whatever is done, it is the individual who must come to internalize inhibitors, understand the harm he causes victims, and learn about his cycle of offending so that he can intervene before a lapse leads to a relapse. The work delivered is thus a program of intervention. We came to realize that we were delivering a program designed to break the pattern of offending behavior exhibited by sexual offenders. STOP, therefore, is not an acronym but represents the aspiration of attempting to prevent reoffending behavior.

Aims of the STOP Program

The aims of the program are threefold: (1) to engender acceptance of personal responsibility; (2) to address the consequences of offending behavior for both self and victim(s), including secondary victims, e.g., family and friends; and (3) to develop personal strategies that will assist the exercising of self control and avoid situations likely to lead to reoffending. In order to achieve these goals, the program has three distinct components.

Assessment

Staff assess each offender through a series of interviews and standard banks of questions to establish the nature of his offending behaviors, the pattern of offending, how he selects and views his victims, his attitude to the offense, and other personal factors. These then provide some basis for risk assessment and decisions about the nature of the intervention to be tried. The analysis of the information gained might usefully be categorized as follows:

- Scale and pattern of offending and associated thinking errors
- Personal history
- Sexual history
- Social functioning and self-image

- Ability to develop victim awareness and empathy
- Perspective taking ability and attributional style
- Sexual attitudes and arousal patterns
- Self-control
- Verbal intelligence and ability to work in group
- Overall measure of risk assessment (from high to low)

These interviews also begin the process of challenging denial.

There is also the opportunity to undertake some parallel and preparatory work, which is available to offenders either before joining the program or while already involved with the groupwork. Examples are the cognitive skills groups and life skills classes.

The STOP Groupwork Program

The STOP program is delivered in two phases with a break halfway. Each phase consists of 40 sessions. Groups are composed of eight to ten offenders who have been convicted of sexual offenses against children and/or adults. Groups meet twice per week and each of the 80 sessions lasts approximately 2½ hours, with additional wind down time over a cup of coffee built into the timetable. Each group is led by prison staff and, in some, jointly with social workers. Priority is given to those men who are considered to be at high risk of reoffending. The program beings by focusing on issues such as cognitive restructuring, consent, responsibility, cycles of offending, and the establishment of basic victim empathy. After a break, the second phase continues the development and exploration of the individual's cycle of offending, while using modular work to examine other areas. This forms the basis for the development of an individual plan for relapse prevention.

The program includes:

- Examining responsibility, thinking errors, and defense mechanisms
- Victim awareness
- Issues concerning consent
- Male and female sexuality, and sexual knowledge
- Pornography
- Gender issues
- Social and interpersonal skills
- Filling leisure time
- Triggers and the feeling–thought–action chain
- Cycle of offending behavior
- Relapse prevention

The Maintenance Program

These groups are low level and mix two or three types of offenders: those higher-risk offenders who have already participated in the STOP core program and are its graduates; those low-level-risk prisoners who require minimal intervention programs; and for some higher-risk offenders who might have initial problems being effectively integrated into programs the maintenance group attempt to provide a bridge to enable their future admission to the core program.

The program itself is broadly eclectic in its composition and puts together the fundamental elements to be found in most such programs across the world. What differentiates Peterhead is this: first, the program is owned and principally delivered by basic prison (correctional) staff, and second, at least 85% of the prison population, which is now about 200, are sexual offenders. This allows for a culture to exist that supports the work and makes it one of the central features of the establishment. Indeed, the vision statement of the prison recognizes the importance of the work and the staff's role in its delivery: "To become recognized as a center of excellence through the valuable work undertaken by our staff with sexual offenders."

It was intended that about one third of the sexual offenders should be in groups, with another third waiting to enter, being encouraged by the graduates of the program (the "culture carriers") who should comprise the remaining third. Thus, over a 3- to 4-year cycle all inmates would have the opportunity of becoming involved with the STOP program.

In the buildup to the opening of C hall, a staff notice was published seeking staff interested in working in the hall, which was to be the location for the start of the program. There were many more applicants than anticipated and staff were selected and given some basic training and insight into the work. The first six core workers (four prison officers and two social workers) had already been identified and, especially in the case of the officers, had been given extensive training (see later). Prisoners were also keen to sign up for the program and were required to agree to three preconditions before they were selected for transfer to the hall: (1) a willingness to address their offending behavior; (2) participation in sentence planning and the personal officer schemes; and (3) to maintain a pornography-free environment.

SETTING UP THE PROGRAM

Unlike the general provision for education or work skills courses, where offenders are generally well disposed to it, acknowledge the tutors are doing some good, and if one session is missed it can be slotted in elsewhere, work with sexual offenders is not so easy. No one likes the inmates or their crimes, the staff who work with them often are treated badly by their colleagues, and consistent attendance at group sessions is vital for the success of the group and the individuals involved. Thus, setting up a program for sexual offenders demands a high level of sustained commitment from management and some organizational and structural changes to support the viability of the program. At Peterhead we realized that a number of changes were necessary to our approach.

Management Support

Management had to ensure the integration of the various players delivering offense-specific programs, principally, prison officers (correctional officers), social workers, and psychologists. Initially, some specialists were somewhat protective of their own area of operation and management had to work to create a cohesive team that shared common values and worked in a coordinated and focused way. It is worth noting that in Scotland, social workers and psychologists are employed by other agencies and their services are hired by the prison. During 1996, the Scottish Prison Service began to recruit some of its own psychologists to act as "theme leaders" in order to provide a range of support to the organization, including support for the delivery of specialized programs.

Correctional Officers Are Central

In my view, an intervention program for sexual offenders is only sustainable in prison on a large scale if delivered by mainstream staff, that is, by prison officers. This view is based on a number of considerations. First, sexual offender work *is* part of the prison's core business and yet work undertaken by specialists (and visiting professionals) tends, initially, to be seen as marginal. Second, initiatives are more likely to succeed if they are delivered by staff who have a vested interest in their success or who have the power to diminish the chances of success. Of course, the staff who deliver these programs require the active support of other prison officers. Those staff who are delivering the programs need to acquire a range of skills, and if we were to have only specialists as the main providers of the program, the acquired skills would not so easily be transferred to other staff and would consequently be lost when the specialist moved away. Finally, if we use only specialists, the volume of delivery would be determined by the number of specialists employed; hence, it would be limited by resources and their availability. In view of these considerations, it seemed best to use specialists to support the work of core prison staff.

Delivered in Groups

The work is undertaken in groups of eight to ten offenders. There are a number of reasons why it is best to deliver such programs within the setting of a therapeutic group:

1. It is less resource intensive to run groups than to engage in one-to-one offense specific work.
2. The "experts" on sexual offending are the offenders themselves. It therefore makes good sense to let them challenge other offenders who are trying to deceive themselves or those around them.
3. The groups are not always comfortable for those offenders being challenged, but one-to-one therapy depends on a degree of rapport being built between the therapist and offender, which can all too easily become too cozy or even collusive at times. Beckett, Beech, Fisher, and Fordham (1994) also make the point that it is less likely that therapists will enter collusive relationships with their clients within a group format. Thus, offenders may use one-to-one situations as an excuse to avoid tackling real issues and there is a danger that the offender may start to manipulate, target, or groom the therapist.
4. Groups should be heterogeneous (a range of offending behaviors) so that the challenges are made from differing viewpoints and sustained.
5. Groups contribute to the resocialization process of its members, helping them to develop interpersonal skills and appropriate cognitive processes.
6. By joining a group, a sexual offender publicly acknowledges his need to change.
7. Group members can provide out-of-group support for other members who are going through a difficult time and can, where necessary, help resolve issues before the next session.
8. Challenges by other offenders within the group also help to share the load of the therapist.

Working in the Right Environment

Groups should feel comfortable enough to get on with the important matters, that is, deal with their offending behavior. The physical conditions should support the work. At Peterhead, we converted an area into a purpose-built set of rooms: a group room with comfortable chairs, flip charts, and notice boards; a smaller room with one-way mirror for filming the group sessions for training and record purposes; and next to it a general purpose area for relaxing with tea or coffee after the groups. These rooms were isolated when groups took place to prevent interruptions. The investment by management in the building and equipment needs was recognized as a tangible commitment and paid handsome dividends. A second similar facility within Peterhead has been created since.

Creating a Supportive Environment

Innovative programs are never easy to introduce into traditional prisons, which have established routines and structures. Even more so with sexual offender programs, which cut across some of the established cultures and inmate hierarchies. Therefore, in order for it to be successful, it has to become central to the work of the prison and form part of the culture and core business. To achieve this, we made certain that the following eight conditions were met:

1. All staff were made aware that the program was central to the work of the prison and that they should support it. The work is demanding and is an emotional drain on staff and they require support and not cynicism from their colleagues.

2. Prison management organized staffing and resources to facilitate the programs. To be able to have regular group meetings, old traditions had to go and the core staff were not permitted to be taken away for emergencies as they arose. Similarly, the inmate's attendance at groups had to have priority over other demands staff might make. The organization of the prison had to serve the needs of the program and not vice versa. In Peterhead, between 1993 and mid-1995, all 480 sessions were held for the first six groups.

3. All staff had to have some understanding of the nature of sexual offending and how the groups tackle this problem. They all undertook awareness training to raise their consciousness and harness their support for the core staff and to ensure that they would not inadvertently collude with sexual offenders and their faulty belief systems.

4. The general regime of the prison had to be consistent with the sexual offender work. Staff were trained and encouraged to act as personal officers to inmates, who themselves were encouraged to join in the sentence planning scheme, which provides a method of developing self-awareness over a range of personal issues. (The Scottish Prison Service introduced the sentence planning initiative in 1990 to foster personal development of inmates and provide opportunities for them to take greater responsibility for their own lives.) Staff were also encouraged to undertake counseling and welfare work with the prisoners.

5. Good staff–inmate relationships were considered to be essential. In particular, the prison staff involved with the core work of delivering the intervention program had to establish trust with the prisoners. The work within the group was to remain confidential and initially progress was slow while the group gained confidence and tested out what happened to new information.

6. The environment had to be made conducive to such work. In general, the regime we established was one in which staff worked with offenders in a "non-put-down" environment that was supportive but not collusive. This milieu was difficult to achieve.

Without an approach that valued our inmates as individuals and that treated them as people of worth, our attempts to undertake therapeutic or cognitive group work with individuals whose self-esteem was low and who felt a threat to their personal safety would not likely lead to much progress. The need to develop an approach that enhanced the self-esteem of the offenders cannot be overstated. Marshall (1995) states, "We have found that increasing the offenders' sense of self-worth is critical to changing all other features of them" (p. 3). In particular, inmates had to be able to feel safe from both physical threats and taunts.

7. Other parts of the prison were to complement the work of the program by providing a range of supporting groups and classes. These helped in a number of ways. They created the right sort of milieu in the prison, which became accepting of counseling and intervention work; they enabled the offender to look at his own attitudes and values; they began to acclimatize him into the group and discursive environment; and they provided additional skills to improve communication, expression, and reasoning. At Peterhead, specialists and prison staff deliver a range of complementary groups that promote the development of the individual and the culture of the establishment. These groups include:

- *Cognitive reasoning.* This involves looking at thinking processes, problem solving, and interpersonal skills, and equips offenders with the skills necessary to avoid making pro-offending choices.
- *Sentence planning and counseling by the personal officer.* This is a national scheme that facilitates the development of self-awareness through a modular package and examines a range of lifestyle issues such as education, work, the criminal process, relationships, and spare time.
- *Aggression in the family/anger management.* This group examines why men use violence and why they accept it as a normal part of their lives; this is particularly useful for those who have committed offenses of violence, baby battering, and wife abuse.
- *Life and social skills.* This is aimed at equipping inmates to cope more effectively with the difficulties of everyday living.
- *Women, men and society.* Here we examine gender issues and the traditional roles of men and women in society, by looking at attitudes, values, and issues of power.
- *Substance abuse.* The aim of the groups that address these issues (alcohol and drug awareness) is not necessarily to produce abstinence, but rather to develop knowledge and control over behavior.
- *Dance and drama.* This provides an opportunity to improve expression, communications skills, and the confidence of participants, which is valuable for sexual offenders contemplating group work in developing expression, self-esteem, and confidence in front of others.
- *Prerelease program.* Here, an examination is undertaken of the issues to be faced, such as employment, social security benefits and entitlements, budgeting, and how the community may respond to their return.

8. Finally, it was noted that inmates in offense-specific programs may require additional support from time to time. This was offered in terms of caring by staff, psychologists, or social workers but did not replace or excuse the challenges to be found in group therapy work. For example, if an offender declared in group that he himself was abused as a child, the matter of dealing with that issue, working through problems, and giving support would be undertaken outside the context of the group. Otherwise, there was a danger of using such claims as an excuse to avoid taking responsibility for personal actions, and the purpose of

the group could become muddied. Also, the offer to provide individual offense-specific work was resisted and the offender continued to be challenged in groups for the reasons outlined earlier. There was a need to create clear boundaries and identify when therapy stopped. It was not the intention to provide round-the-clock, 24 hours-a-day, 7 days-a-week intervention programs and therapy. Other staff who also dealt with the inmate had to ensure that they understood and were clear about the role of the core group worker and distinguished it from the very different but supportive role of other prison officers, psychologist, social workers, or teaching staff. These other staff could deal with a whole host of personal and situational issues, but they had to be careful not to stray into the offense-specific work or attempt to continue the work of the core groups.

Ground Rules Have to Be Established

Group members had to understand what would be done when "new" information was revealed to the group. Discussion of the index offense or revealing nonspecific, general, or vague information would not be transmitted out of the group because it served no purpose. However, specific information that enabled other past offenses to be identified, information about other named offenders (such as active pedophile rings), and details about further victims would be passed on to the appropriate authorities (principally the police and/or social services departments). All participants were made aware of this condition, which was agreed on before each group program commenced.

Pornography

Work with offenders in a community setting would not be expected to occur in an environment that displays pornography. The same should apply in a prison setting; otherwise, one type of message is being given during the offense-specific group work and the opposite message is presented when prisoners return to other areas such as their cells, where they see pornography with its message of objectification, dehumanization, and submission. We decided that our programs for sexual offenders would occur in a pornography-free environment, and so all pornography was banned within that part of the prison for both staff and inmates. At the time of my departure from the prison, a total ban was being considered, with prisoners who were being transferred to Peterhead for the STOP program having to sign a contract specifically agreeing to maintain a pornography-free environment.

Family Contact and Visiting

Sexual offenders, unlike any other type of offender, create turmoil and trauma within the family by their actions. If the offense is nonfamilial, such as the rape of an adult female, there are tremendous tensions created between the offender and his partner which might never be resolved. If the offense occurred within the family (e.g., incest), then not only is it likely that the nonoffending mother blames herself for allowing events to have taken place, but all trust is destroyed. The offender may not be suitable for return to the family home, since contact with the victim is likely to perpetuate the abuse. It is within this context that visiting and other family contacts, such as letters and telephone calls, have to be seen. This is a problem area, and if the victim is permitted to visit the offender, special precautions have to be taken. If such visits are not recognized for what they are and properly managed, it might allow the offender the opportunity to perpetuate the abuse and victimization of the child and the equally harrowing transference of guilt and responsibility to the nonoffending mother. The focus and primary consideration should been given to the victim, who should not be brought to such a meeting until he or she has received positive help and the offender has undertaken therapy and, importantly, until the victim feels ready for such contact. We have established these conditions at Peterhead, and when we allow visits between the offender and the victim, they take place in the presence of a counselor or social worker who monitors what is being said and done. It should also be remembered that it is possible for the offender to continue the process of grooming other children even if the primary victim is kept away. We are very aware of and careful to avoid the potential dangers from even short and supervised visits.

NEED FOR TRAINING AND SUPPORT OF STAFF

Training of staff and providing effective support at all levels has been crucial to the delivery of our offense-specific program and, we believe, is essential if the program is to have any meaningful chance of success. For the core workers the training is a lengthy process, with the initial phase alone taking several months, and includes a variety of training experiences. Staff have to understand that they are entering an area that will present difficulties for them. The work they do inevitably leads them to examine their own attitudes and beliefs in a variety of areas. They may even question their own sexuality and motives. Also, they typically find it difficult to "leave behind" their work when they go home. The images that are conveyed by offenders remain with them, often affecting the way they view their partners and children and sometimes causing them to draw back from quite normal situations, like bathing their children and sitting the kids on their laps, for fear of some resonance with what has been said in the group. It is important that staff understand these pressures and how things may affect them; they need to be able to network with other staff and get appropriate support when necessary.

In addition, we selected the staff on the basis of their apparent personal resilience. They need strong "stomachs" when listening to some of the details of the offending behaviors; some issues can call into question the very basis of their own beliefs and behaviors. Things may be said that start to stir in the staff events shut out of their own minds through time. They have to be prepared for such eventualities. Sexual offenders who deny their actions are practiced at manipulating others. They may try to score points, prove other people are wrong and confused, or simply to turn the spotlight away from themselves and their own unwillingness to accept responsibility. Worse, some offenders will try to humiliate and even ruin staff. Some of our offenders have written anonymous letters to outside agencies and the media, suggesting that the staff themselves have been involved in abuse and offending. These campaigns were undertaken by offenders who did not want to engage in looking at their own offending and were willing to do anything to destroy the therapeutic process and the staff. Luckily, these allegations were easily disproved. But staff have to be aware that this sort of attack can occur and management at all levels (whether on a confidential basis or otherwise) has to give total support.

It is worth noting that in some ways social workers or probation staff, who are usually seen by prisoners as being the more caring type of individuals, are particularly disliked and become targets of sexual offenders' malevolence, especially by offenders convicted of offenses against children. Unfortunately, these staff not only have involvement with offense-specific work inside the prison, but they are also involved in writing reports on prisoners that may affect their future position with their families. These additional duties arise because social workers and probation officers are not directly employed by the prison but are employed by local authority social work departments where they have also statutory duties in relation to child protection legislation and access to children. Some offenders hold social work staff directly responsible for questions of access, and offenders blame them for the difficulties created with their families. Of course, in reality this should be expected, since such offenders who deny responsibility for their own actions can only turn to others and blame them for the consequences.

Both the training and support of staff are vital. In Peterhead, it has be given in a number of ways and to a number of differing groups of staff.

Forms of Training

Generalized Training for All Staff

It seemed necessary to us that all staff be given some "awareness" training in order to understand the process and issues faced by staff and prisoners engaging in offense specific work with sexual offenders. This training examines their attitudes, values, and beliefs, explores the roles of men and women in society, looks at the effects on victims, gives a brief outline of offenders distorted thinking, and considers the effects of pornography. In addition, all staff are made aware of the nature and difficulties of the work undertaken by program staff and they are reminded of the need to support those who are participating in the program. Other issues that are discussed include the need to create a working environment with the offenders that is not a put-down but is also noncollusive; understanding the boundaries between what goes on in group sessions, what can take place in informal discussions, and clarifying the difference in roles between the residential officer and the core worker; and, finally, the need to maintain good liaison between the group workers and personal officers. At Peterhead, at the time of this writing, about 90% of all staff, including industrial, maintenance crew, and administrative staff, have received such training. Input is also provided at the end of the specialized sentence planning course, for all personal officers, relating the program to the sentence planning initiative. The normal 3-day course, addressing attitudes, values, and beliefs, has been delivered by a variety of in-house and guest speakers and is organized by the staff training unit. These generalized courses seek to raise the consciousness of all staff, including managers, who provide the context within which the offense focused groups run, and harness their support for those directly involved in group work. These courses also contribute to the general ethos of the establishment, group and counseling work, and the equal opportunities policy of the prison service. Once trained and experienced, the core staff also contribute to the general training of other staff.

An important message to emphasize is the priority attached by all staff, from senior management down, to the success of the program. This cannot be achieved if prisoners are prevented by other staff from attending the groupwork sessions (e.g., by being kept back in a workshop to finish an important contract). Therefore, despite there being a high level of industrial activity in the workshops, prisoners being required to attend education, needed for interviews, or to participate in physical education, and so on, the core STOP program has taken precedence.

Specialized Training for Core Staff

The core workers received extensive training including social work placements in the community and courses in group dynamics, interviewing and assessment, criminal personality, and profiling. They have attended conferences, meetings, and workshops and received training from a psychologist in group dynamics and group work techniques to deal with offense-specific material. They have received some training from an expert on pedophiles and have had a seminar on pornography from a member of the police obscene publications branch, which was considered to be of particular value.

In addition, all core workers received on-the-job training and live supervision while engaged in the delivery of the program, for 4 days per month during 1993, from our visiting consultant–trainer (Hilary Eldridge). This has been achieved using a competency-based curriculum that focuses on both process and content. Training is aimed at increasing knowledge of sexual offending behavior patterns and also encouraging the development of a personally suitable therapeutic style. Bill Marshall provided additional training during his 1-month consultancy visit to Peterhead. The core staff were also given the opportunity to attend the Gracewell Clinic in England, which was a community-based facility primarily for pedophiles, for 1 week and to participate in the work of the groups. Two of our staff (one core worker and one social worker) spent 3 weeks of specialized training with Bill Marshall in Canada during May 1994. Current training is ongoing and further training will be provided to develop a greater appreciation of the experiences and problems faced by victims.

Developing the skills and enlarging the numbers of core workers continues. The process is undertaken in five ways:

1. *Training program for core staff.* A basic training program was devised by Allan Boath and John Duncan, STOP trainers, and is presented on a modular basis to those staff identified as suitable for participation in sexual offender group work. It particularly gives in-depth focus to interviewing and group-working techniques. The program content includes discussions on gender issues, a look at attitudes and value systems; an exploration of the basic issues of sexual offenders and offending and an examination of assumptions about offending, interviewing techniques; the purpose of group work, theoretical models and practice issues, victim awareness, discussions on empathy, giving and receiving feedback in order to make the process constructive rather than destructive, thus allowing workers to become comfortable with criticism and to learn from observations of others; an outline of the STOP program content, including its underlying philosophy and aims; the availability and use for prisoners of complementary and supporting programs; maintenance programs and cognitive reasoning processes; team-building exercises and networking and support; a research project; and finally, a review.

2. *The process of osmosis.* Trainee core workers become involved by sitting in groups as observers and watching the processes work. They then have an opportunity to discuss these with core staff later. Much of the work by staff happens outside the group, for example, reading records of prisoners, watching videotaped recordings of sessions, discussing what occurred in the group, and planning for future groups. The trainees shadow core staff, sit in on meetings, and become involved in discussions.

3. *On the job training and support.* This has been a critically important aspect of the development of our staff. At times, a consultant trainer is available to watch the STOP groups and provide advice, suggestions, and training to staff. On a more consistent basis, support and guidance are provided from two sources: first, by an experienced supervisory officer, who is well versed in this type of work, has line responsibility for their work, and provides supervision and support on an ongoing basis; and second, by the head of the social work unit who has expertise in this subject and is also involved as one of the core workers. In addition, the other social workers involved with the core group have provided support and training to prison officer staff.

4. *Individual reading and study.* Staff are encouraged to develop their own knowledge base, skills, and competencies. The establishment's staff training library has been gathering materials, and core staff are welcome to use them. Many staff display an impressive knowledge of the subject gained from reading and discussions, and it is known that they spend a considerable amount of their own time broadening their understanding of the subject.

5. *Networking and conferences.* Some employers apparently believe that if their staff are away at conferences, they are not doing the "real job" and are only there to get away from work, relax, socialize with others, and have a good time. Of course, staff who give so much of themselves in the group setting and who are committed to this intensive and specialized work should be able to relax from time to time. More importantly, however, conferences provide the opportunity to discuss and network with other practitioners about the work and also about how they feel. Looking after themselves and not burning out are important issues, and having the opportunity to share problems and issues with others at meetings, workshops, and conferences should not be missed or its value underestimated. Finally, conferences, seminars and the like provide unique opportunities for staff to learn about the work of others, discuss issues for practitioners and gain knowledge in the subject. That is why the National Offender Treatment Association–UK (NOTA) and the Association for the Treatment of Sexual Abusers–North America (ATSA) are so important. At Peterhead, we encourage and try to facilitate staff being members of NOTA and attending seminars and conferences. "Attending conferences by people working in this field is not a luxury but an essential component to their development" (Marshall, 1994, p. 5).

General Training for the Pool of Potential Core Staff

With all such programs, some staff who are not involved become interested in the work and express a willingness to become involved. At Peterhead, a number of staff indicated that they too would like to be given the opportunity of delivering intervention programs. They applied to be considered and were interviewed to assess potential and aptitude. These staff, in addition to receiving the general awareness training given to all staff, have received offense-specific sessions from a number of our visiting guest speakers and specialists. They have also undertaken training in group dynamics and have to comprehend the manipulative tactics of sexual offenders. They are expected to participate in interviewing exercises in discussions about risk assessment. Should these staff show a continuing interest in the work, feel comfortable with it, and display the appropriate aptitudes and motivation, they can then be further selected for core training. During this process, such staff have been able to use their involvement in training as a period during which they can decide to opt out if they wish. This type of work is not suited to all staff, and some find the issues involved too disturbing. Yet others themselves may have been a victim of some type of inappropriate behavior, and the discussions and insights gained may open up for them, perhaps for the first time, very difficult areas. Finally, there may be a few staff who find the challenges to their own value systems and beliefs too close for comfort.

SUPPORT MECHANISMS

Support for those staff delivering the programs is crucial if the program is to be sustained and developed. The nature of the work creates stress and demands a huge amount of emotional stamina. Without a range of support mechanisms in place, delivery of a meaningful program would be impossible. At Peterhead, support has been given in a number of ways:

1. *Debriefing.* The team gets together for debriefing sessions. Core staff have their own office accommodation where they keep records and where they meet together to discuss the progress being made and support issues. The staff are free to discuss any issues, and problems or concerns can be discussed in private. The staff also get together at other times to plan and review the work, and they function very much as a supportive team.

2. *Management support.* This is demonstrated through consistent commitment and public statements as to the necessity of the program. Line management support and supervision is given by the group manager, who also has helped by acting as a facilitator within the accommodation block setting where the offenders live. First-line management and support is provided by the supervisory officer. The primary task of this officer is the support of the groupwork team members.

3. *Systems for delivery of programs and support of core staff.* In addition to the processes identified above, management support has been provided through an investment of management time and commitment and by giving clear and consistent signals. The feeling that "we were in it for real" was also signaled with a financial investment in equipment, rooms, and training. In addition, management have been "up front" in talking to all staff about these issues. A steering group was established, initially chaired by the governor, to implement and guide the program and clear policy lines were given with backing for the core work. Other staff were instructed that they must support and not hinder the work of the core staff and groups. It cannot be overemphasized that in establishing a program in any institution, it is not merely a matter of delegation of tasks. For a new initiative to succeed, especially one where staff require consistent support and can feel vulnerable, a clear, consistent, and continuing message has to be given by top management as to the value and need of the work undertaken. Anything less can jeopardize the whole process. As indicated earlier, it is also important for the various specialists to jell as a team. The report of our visiting trainer–consultant indicates positive results:

> The relationships between social workers and uniformed staff has worked well. They have developed a team identity and there is mutual respect. The uniformed staff recognise and value the expertise of the social workers and the supervision they receive from them. (Eldridge, 1994, p. 4)

4. *Emotional support.* This is also provided by the supervisory officer, who has regular contact and discussions with his team. There are regular meetings between the core workers, the program manger, and the coordinator every 4 to 6 weeks for general discussions and an examination of feelings and needs. Support is also available from members of the social work team as and when required by operating an open-door policy for core workers. More professional support can also be provided by the prison's psychologist, who is a member of the steering group.

5. *On-the-job training and supervision support.* Some description of this process has already been given earlier. Core workers work with "experts" for parts of the program. During the first year, a consultant (Hilary Eldridge) was available for 4 days each month to review how staff worked and she was present during sessions. Since in-house expertise has now reached sufficiently satisfactory levels, the consultant visits on a less frequent basis. There is additional support provided by the head of the social work unit, who attends therapy groups from time to time. Bill Marshall, who has visited Peterhead on a number of

occasions as a visiting consultant, has also provided support and training at those times. Finally, some training for staff trainers has been given to enable support from them to core and other staff.

6. *Demands on work time.* Although staff are expected to carry out a range of duties as part of their employment, it would be unrealistic to expect them to carry out all their normal duties (as a custodial prison officer) as well as the highly intensive and demanding functions of a core worker. In fact, they are excused such duties as night shifts and are not rostered for leave during the period of the 40-session blocks in order to avoid breaking the continuity of group sessions. With cooperation of the trade unions at Peterhead, the staff have been largely disengaged from such routine work so that they can spend the time in groups, discussions, training and review, and on providing reports on the progress made by prisoners in groups. However, they do continue to be based in the residential hall and have certain other less demanding duties placed on their time. There are and always will be inherent conflicts in the relationships prison staff have with offenders, social workers have with their clients, or indeed parents have with their children. The conflict arises between enforcing control and exercising care, support, and advice. Staff must never forget their position and their responsibilities in relation to security and good order, yet matters should be so organized that the burdens of ordinary work do not interfere with the valuable contribution they can make to the work with sexual offenders.

7. *Organizational support.* A steering group meets on a monthly basis to review the work of the groups, looks at problems relating to the delivery of the program, and provides future direction and development. It is composed of the program manger, senior social worker, psychologist, groupwork support supervisor, and a core worker. When required, the steering group can meet with the governor in charge of the establishment and also with the representative of outside social work line management. There also is the facility to discuss issues at the monthly senior prison management meeting to ensure cooperation from all parts of the prison and ensure that the strategic planning of the establishment and STOP program developments are aligned.

Advice/Support to Management

Management support needs to be consistent. But management itself must be well informed if it is to make decisions and policies that facilitate and develop the sexual offender work. Management have received training about the process of creating and maintaining a therapeutic environment. Our visiting consultant (Hilary Eldridge) has provided advice at Peterhead and both she and Bill Marshall have written critical and evaluative reports to advise us on how to take the program forward. Senior staff also try to familiarize themselves with the work of the groups and understand the objectives of the STOP program. Administrative staff must share the values and be able to speak the language of intervention programs. For this propose, attending seminars and conferences is also an aid to their understanding and further evidence of their commitment to staff.

INTEGRATION OF PROGRAM
WITH OTHER PRISONS AND AGENCIES

It is particularly important that if the work with sexual offenders is to be effective, then what is done in one place needs to fit into a cohesive framework. In Scotland, there are now clear guidelines for the role of social workers located in prison and in community offices (Social Work Services Group, 1994). Prisons also operate under parallel instructions. These require a proper flow of information from court to prison, so that the social worker can become involved in assessment and in intervention while the inmate is in prison, and then from prison to the outside, so that information can be passed on prior to release, by notifying the relevant local authorities (relating to both offender and victim) and by establishing provision for throughcare. The need for developing good relationships with child protection agencies is recognized, and social workers are expected to attempt to arrange for adequate supervision and support on release. Since it is not easy to organize complete integration in a prison system where many of the other inmates, and perhaps some staff, are hostile to sexual offenders, specialized units have to be developed for those vulnerable offenders both at induction and later on in their sentence. In Scotland, two further prisons, Barlinnie Prison in Glasgow and Shotts Prison in Lanarkshire are engaging, respectively, short-term and long-term prisoners with this work and they too are developing strong links with outside agencies. In the case of long-term prisoners convicted of sexual offending, there is the additional problem of their integration and onward movement within the prison system.

One of the problems with establishing treatment in institutions is that there is no "right time" to commence an intervention program. Ideally, it should be ongoing throughout the sentence. Judgments have to be made about when it is most appropriate to deliver such a program. It makes sense that such work is most effective and best undertaken in the period prior to release or to potential release on parole, so that the benefits of the core work can be maintained by low-level groups continuing in other establishments. Short-term inmates pose other problems. There is a need to begin work in earnest because they will only spend a short time in prison. The initial work with them must begin to make them realize they have a problem that requires further help on release, and that preparations should be made that link them to that care. Many of these sexual offenders, who serve only short-term sentences, are not subject to compulsory supervision on release, and so the initial work undertaken with them must attempt to "hook" them into voluntary aftercare.

At the time of this writing, a national policy for prisons is under consideration. This policy will have to bring together the requirement for a multiagency approach, the need for good throughcare, information flow, risk assessment, and program timing and delivery to short- and long-term sentenced prisoners and ensure that if such prisoners are moved, they are linked into adequate support or maintenance provision.

ARE WE HAVING ANY EFFECT?

One of my regrets in setting up the program was that we did not build research and evaluation into the process from the start. I suppose that getting the program established was a big enough task and we thought that we could not tackle everything at once. We could also have had greater discourse with the judiciary, attempted to arrange with social work departments in the community how they could support our "graduates," and met with colleagues from other prisons to establish a system of movement between prisons; in fact, a national system! However, if we had tried to do all that, maybe we would never have started. Now, because the work is underway, other prisons and agencies are responding and national policy is being considered. The same is true of research, which is also currently being proposed.

The real evaluative test, however, is the measurement of reoffending. This cannot be undertaken with any degree of credibility until at least a significant number of offenders have satisfactorily completed the program and have been released for a sufficient period of time. Before we have such numbers, there is the likelihood of reaching false conclusions if we attempt to do so too quickly. In the first year, 20 inmates entered the STOP program. Now, after 3 years, with four groups running, 100 inmates have gone through the program and 80 have completed all phases. So far, only 43 have been released back into the community. So, it is too early to complete an evaluation. To date, however, three have been reconvicted, but only one for a sexual offense. Nevertheless, we have not ignored the necessity to prepare for evaluation. In planning for future research, full records have been kept comprising lists, details, and reports of those inmates participating in the STOP program. This will provide the initial database for research. Evaluation is important because it can provide assessments on: how well the program is operating; the consistency of the program over different groups; how others (such as prison staff, parole board members, social service staff, and offenders) feel about the program; how well the program is meeting its objectives (e.g., overcoming denial, accepting responsibility, development of victim empathy, developing sound relapse prevention plans); and, whether or not reductions in reoffending rates have been produced.

We already have a feel for some of the issues. Although comparative studies are not easily undertaken and it is also too soon to evaluate the success of the STOP program, an early assessment was undertaken by Jack and Mair (1993) of the actual shift in offender attitudes, using standardized tests derived from Hogue (1992). The results indicate that a good start had been made. Both our visiting consultants also endorsed this view:

> At present Peterhead provides a quality programme for a realistic number of offenders. It has chosen this approach as opposed to a short programme for a larger number of offenders. In doing so it has established itself as a leader in the field.... The STOP programme has developed remarkably well in a short space of time. It is now an established part of the prison's working life. It is a well planned programme operating in line with current research. (Eldridge, 1994, p. 12)

> My conclusion is that the program has made excellent progress in the short time it has been in operation and it is in far better shape than any other program I have seen at this same stage of implementation. (Marshall, 1995, p. 4)

Finally, the prison was subject to inspection by the chief inspector of prisons for Scotland during 1995. It is worth quoting from his introductory remarks:

> Peterhead has changed from a prison concerned mainly with the containment of convicted sexual offenders and other vulnerable prisoners to one which actively seeks to promote long-term change in individual attitude and response through participation in offending behaviour programmes which are aimed at reducing crime and recidivism. Though much of the prison's exterior and indeed public image has altered little, we were in effect encountering an entirely new regime and ethos. Our opinion after inspection was that some of the current provision in relation to sexual offender programmes was amongst the most innovative which had been taking place in the Scottish Prison Service in recent years ... and that these developments had enhanced the potential for public safety throughout the country. (Her Majesty's Chief Inspector of Prisons for Scotland, 1996, pp. 1, 81).

There is already some anecdotal evidence from staff and other inmates telling us that some of the other prisoners who have been released but did not engage in the program have already reoffended. As noted, so far, there has been only one failure among those who completed the program. (The case notes at the time indicated that this prisoner had not really wanted to engage, had derived little benefit from the program, and was likely to remain a high risk. He was released at the end of his sentence without parole or supervision.) We have also received positive feedback from external social work agencies who have perceived our "graduates" to be better participants in continuing throughcare work.

One piece of research was undertaken during the first half of 1994, by McIvor, Campbell, Rowlings, and Skinner (1997). This examined how the program was implemented, its impact on the inmates at Peterhead, the attitudes of staff and inmates to the program, and the effect such attitudes had on the operation of the program. The researchers, who interviewed 94 individuals, found that officers who were directly involved in the program perceived STOP in a very positive light, as it made their job more interesting, increased their job satisfaction, provided an opportunity to learn and utilize new skills, and increased their understanding of offending behavior. Most of the officers interviewed who were not directly involved in the program also identified personal benefit, including greater insight into sexual offending and increased job satisfaction arising from improved relationships between staff and inmates. The introduction of the program was also felt by many prisoners to have had a positive impact on the prison in general and this was evidenced through a change in staff attitudes enabling them to understand and work more effectively with prisoners. They also found that the majority of prisoners who participated in the STOP program had felt it was an extremely painful experience, but, despite this, most had felt that the program had made a significant impact on their understanding of their offending and had also helped them to identify other problem areas in their behavior.

Also, the report is illuminating in highlighting the anxieties faced by staff and inmates when such programs are being set up, and makes extensive use of direct quotations from individuals to illustrate more vividly the views and attitudes held.

WHY BEGIN THIS PROCESS IN PRISON?

Nothing would suit many sexual offenders better than for everybody to ignore their offenses while they serve their sentences, and it would make life easier for them inside if other inmates did not know about their crimes. However, if we were to ignore their offending we would be tacitly colluding with them and allowing them to reinforce their distorted self-perceptions and fantasies, and would contribute to the continuation of their own distorted value systems. Time spent in prison can provide an ideal opportunity for the offender to be challenged about his behavior and accept responsibility for what he has done. Once the offender is released and the controls over him recede, he may become reluctant to accept that he has done anything at all or he may consider that since he has served his sentence he does not need to do any more to address his offending behavior. He would therefore remain a significant risk to the public.

So, the primary motivation of the staff at Peterhead is to try to make society a safer place by reducing the propensity for reoffending among sexual offenders. That is why they have willingly given their support to the program. There can be no clearer example of this commitment than that shown by the local branch of the Prison Officers Union at Peterhead, who worked with management to free up extra staff from within existing resources in order to deliver the program. That support has allowed the staff and program to flourish; the excellence of the work, commitment, and dedication of the core group-work staff was recognized in 1996, when the Princess Royal presented the STOP Team with the United Kingdom Prison Services' Butler Trust Top Group Award. Marshall, Laws, and Barbaree (1990) urge us to never forget the bottom line—our reason why we undertake such work:

> Sexual assaults have devastating effects on innocent victims, so that any reduction in the rate of offending should be viewed as beneficial. In fact, an often neglected aspect of offering treatment to offenders is the real reduction in suffering that occurs when even a few of these men are prevented from reoffending. The rate of reoffense among sexual offenders is known to be very high; it is known that in some subgroups the majority of offenders eventually reoffend. Whenever treatment, no matter how unsophisticated, reduces reoffending by any degree, it saves innocent victims much suffering. (p. 6)

That is why prison staff are so keen to undertake such work. I believe that for those of us working in prisons, we can make a positive contribution in reducing the numbers of people at risk and in attempting to minimize harm by providing programs for sexual offenders. It is not a lot, but at least it is a start.

REFERENCES

Beckett, R., Beech, A., Fisher, D., & Fordham, A.S. (1994). *Community-based treatment for sex offenders: An evaluation of seven treatment programmes.* A report for the Home Office (England and Wales) by the STEP Team, London.

Eldridge, H. (1994, January). *Report on Consultancy/Supervised Practice January–December 1993.* Report to the Governor, HM Prison, Peterhead.

Her Majesty's Chief Inspector of Prisons for Scotland. (1996). *Report on HM Prison Peterhead, 1995.* Edinburgh: Scottish Office Home Department.

Hogue, T.E. (1992). *Sex Offence Information Questionnaire (SOIQ), and Individual Clinical Rating Form.* Unpublished manuscript, Psychology Unit, HM Prison Dartmoor.

Jack, A.M., & Mair, K.J. (1993). *Evaluation of the STOP Programme.* Unpublished manuscript, Psychology Unit, HM Prison, Peterhead.

Marshall, W.L. (1994, February). *Appraisal of the sex offenders' treatment program at Peterhead Prison.* Report to Scottish Prison Service, Edinburgh.

Marshall, W.L. (1995, April). *Report on current status and future development of sex offender program at Peterhead and suggestions for a Scottish national policy.* Report to Scottish Prison Service, Edinburgh.

Marshall, W.L., Laws, D.R., & Barbaree, H.E. (1990). Issues in sexual assault. In W.L. Marshall, D.R. Laws, & H.E. Barbaree (Eds.), *Handbook of sexual assault: Issues, theories, and treatment of the offender* (p. 6). New York: Plenum Press.

McIvor, G., Campbell, V., Rowlings, C., & Skinner, K. (1997). *The STOP programme: The development and implementation of prison-based group work with sex offenders.* Report to the Scottish Office Home and Health Department, Edinburgh: Scottish Prison Service Occasional Papers 2/1997.

Social Work Services Group. (1994, October). *Child protection: The imprisonment and preparation for release of prisoners convicted of offences against children.* Circular Instruction SW/11/1994, Social Work Services Group, Scottish Office, Edinburgh.

4

A. Prison Settings

The Evolution of a Multisite Sexual Offender Treatment Program

Ruth E. Mann and David Thornton

In June 1991, the Home Secretary announced that Her Majesty's Prison Service of England and Wales would introduce a national strategy for the treatment of imprisoned sexual offenders. Sexual offenders would be concentrated in a smaller number of prisons that would offer a unified group treatment program that would be designed in line with research about effective treatment for this type of offender, and the program would be centrally designed, monitored, evaluated, and refined (Grubin & Thornton, 1994; Thornton & Hogue, 1993). Since 1991, the Sex Offender Treatment Program (SOTP) has been established in 25 penal establishments, ranging from the highest security to the lowest, and is situated in every part of the country, from Northumbria to Devon.

SOTP consists of a family of group work modules designed in line with current knowledge about criminogenic factors relevant to sexual offending. The program takes a cognitive–behavioral approach and uses a variety of treatment methods, including role-play, modeling, disputing of irrational thoughts, and so forth. The central element of SOTP is the core program, which, in its current form, takes about 180 hours to deliver. The core program tackles issues common to all sexual offenders, whatever the nature of their offending or the gender or age of their victims; that is, reducing denial and minimization of their behavior, promoting recognition of harm caused to victims, and developing relapse prevention skills.

The core program is supplemented by three additional programs. The first of these, the thinking skills program, is an integrated cognitive–behavioral skills training package, which takes about 50 hours to complete and is designed to improve decision making, perspective taking, and some interpersonal skills. It is seen as contributing to the effectiveness of participants' relapse prevention strategies and as relevant for most sexual offenders. The second is the extended program. This originally consisted of an array of shorter modules, to be undertaken on an as-needed basis. Presently, the extended program is being

Ruth E. Mann and David Thornton • Program Development Section, HM Prison Service, Abell House, London, England SW1P 4LH.

Sourcebook of Treatment Programs for Sexual Offenders, edited by Marshall et al. Plenum Press, New York, 1998.

revised so that in future it will comprise a single 40- to 50-session group work module, supplemented by some individual therapy. It will address the management of negative emotions, relationships (and especially conflicts in relationships), and offense-related fantasy. These elements, which we have previously dealt with separately, are now seen as intrinsically interwoven in the psychology of most offenders [e.g., with conflicts leading to moods that trigger particular fantasies (Proulx, McKibben, & Lusignan, 1996)] and so better dealt with through a more integrated approach.

The third supplementary module is the booster (relapse prevention) program. The booster program is intended for prisoners serving long sentences who have undertaken the core program earlier in their sentence and are now soon to be released. It focuses primarily on the development and strengthening of relapse prevention strategies to create a realistic release plan. The booster program also repairs any attenuation in treatment gains that may have taken place since the completion of the core program. The duration of the booster program is between 50 and 70 hours, depending to some extent on how much "repair work" is needed.

The core program is preceded by an extensive assessment process comprising clinical interviews, psychometric testing, and (in eight establishments) penile plethysmography. The purpose of the assessment process is to identify each offender's individual treatment needs and to establish a set of baseline measures from which progress in treatment can be measured. The assessment procedure is repeated on completion of the core program, and relevant components of it are also retaken after completion of each subsequent program.

About 1400 males are received into prison every year in England and Wales with sentences of at least 2 years imposed for a sexual offense. Not all of these men will agree to participate in treatment; currently about half of those who are offered treatment accept the offer. Thus, the potential demand for the core program is somewhere between 700 and 1400 places per annum. The intention is to build up treatment capacity until a place can be provided for all those who are willing to take part. Table 4.1 shows the number of prisoners completing the core program per annum.

There are five aspects of SOTP that we believe make it unusual in comparison with other programs: (1) its multisite implementation; (2) its commitment to systematic evolution guided by its own short-term evaluations and other research information; (3) the use of lay therapists in the delivery of treatment; (4) the emphasis on therapist style as well as program content; and (5) a system of annual external accreditation of quality of content and delivery.

This chapter will discuss each of these areas in turn and will also consider some of the challenges that have been encountered during the design, implementation, and monitoring of the program.

TABLE 4.1
Program Completions

Year	Prisons offering SOTP	Prisoners completing core program	Prisoners completing booster program
1991–1992	0	0	0
1992–1993	17	284	0
1993–1994	20	439	0
1994–1995	22	554	0
1995–1996	25	406	33
1996–1997	25	565	108

UNIQUE ASPECTS OF SOTP

Multisite Implementation

Operating in 25 separate sites, SOTP is believed to be the largest sexual offender treatment program in the world. The maintenance of consistent treatment delivery across these sites is one of the greatest challenges presented by the program. Central coordination of SOTP is handled from Program Development Section, situated in prison service headquarters, where three psychologists share the task of monitoring and developing treatment across the country. SOTP in each site is managed by a tripartite team of whom one (the treatment manager) is responsible for the maintenance of treatment integrity; that is, for ensuring the program is delivered as intended. Treatment managers receive specialized training in addition to the standard core program training and meet together quarterly to discuss issues of treatment monitoring and supervision. The staff selected for this role are normally forensic psychologists. The other members of the tripartite team are the program manager (normally a prison governor) who is responsible for the practical aspects of program delivery, and a senior probation officer who is responsible for the throughcare of program participants.

Central monitoring is provided by the program development section in various forms such as the viewing of videotapes of group sessions from each site, through audits carried out at each site annually, and the analysis of treatment "products" (such as offense accounts, cognitive–behavioral chains, and relapse prevention plans).

Commitment to Program Evolution

SOTP is committed to evolution guided by in-house, short-term clinical impact evaluations as well as by research from elsewhere and advice from an independent panel of expert advisers. By 1994, it had become clear that the first version of the core program was effective in undermining the distorted thinking typically demonstrated by sexual offenders to excuse and justify their offending (Program Development Section, 1996), but that the victim empathy and relapse prevention components were too limited. Accordingly, these parts of the program were completely rewritten using techniques adapted mainly from the California and Vermont programs (e.g., Marques, Day, Nelson, & Miner, 1989; Nelson & Jackson, 1989; Pithers, 1994).

At the time of writing, it appears that the relapse prevention element of the core program still requires further development. Although there is some evidence that relapse prevention skills do improve substantially as a result of attending the core program (Mann, 1996), relapse prevention plans tend to rely too heavily on behavioral rather than cognitive strategies and to be deficient in the variety and number of strategies drawn up for each risk factor. In addition, feedback from therapists and group members suggests that the relapse prevention sessions are perceived as too theoretical and cognitive (relying too heavily on written preparation and group discussion as treatment methods). Accordingly, work is underway to further revise this portion of the core program, incorporating creative behavioral methods designed to encourage group members to develop comprehensive and realistic coping plans.

Use of Lay Personnel

From the outset, SOTP was designed so that it could be delivered by lay therapists or paraprofessionals who would be trained in the theory and skills necessary for the able

tutoring of the program. This decision was made partly for economic reasons but principally because previous experiences of group work in prisons involving multidisciplinary
teams had demonstrated that professional background was less important than personal
qualities in shaping a person's ability to deliver group work. As Grubin and Thornton
(1994) note, prison officers in particular have the advantage of being able to observe and
interact with offenders outside the treatment setting, and their involvement in the program
reduces suspicion and noncooperation with treatment by other discipline staff within a
prison. Perhaps even more important, because prison officers are the people with whom
prisoners interact most in their daily lives, their potential to act as positive nonoffending
role models is particularly useful. In practice, it is clearly the case that nonspecialists make
excellent treatment providers and that taking on this work has greatly enhanced the prison
officers' role for those involved. For example, in a survey of SOTP tutors (Turner, 1992),
96% reported that involvement in the program had greatly improved their job satisfaction.
More than any other factor, the enthusiasm and commitment of the lay therapists delivering
SOTP has probably ensured its effective implementation.

Having said this, it is obviously not the case that all nonspecialists make effective
therapists (just as it is the case that not all specialists do). Consequently, it has been
important to develop a comprehensive procedure for selecting staff who are to train as
therapists. Research by Sacre (1995) identified the personal competencies of an effective
sexual offender therapist, and this research has enabled the design of a comprehensive
selection procedure for tutors. Those staff who pass the selection procedure attend a
centrally run training course during which their skills and understanding of sexual offender
treatment are closely assessed by the trainers (who are particularly experienced therapists)
in line with Sacre's identified competencies. Only those trainees who demonstrate a
suitable level of skill by the end of training are recommended to undertake the work.

Care is also taken to pair newly trained staff with those who have treatment experience. The treatment team working with a given group of offenders will almost always
include at least one psychologist or probation officer; that is, professionals with a background in therapeutic work with offenders. The treatment manager closely monitors newly
trained staff and seeks to provide additional support and training until they are satisfied that
an adequate level of treatment skill is being displayed.

Our ability to use lay personnel is also facilitated by very detailed treatment manuals.
Thus, our staff are expected to deliver a predefined program rather than to develop the
content of their own treatment sessions. This reduces the level of professional judgment and
the depth of academic knowledge required.

Emphasis on Therapist Style

Descriptions of other sexual offender programs have rarely made mention of the issue
of therapist style. SOTP has always emphasized the importance of style, and the approach
taught is the Socratic method, drawn from the work of Miller (Miller, 1983; Miller &
Rollnick, 1991) and Overholser (1993a,b, 1994, 1995). This approach involves the use of
probing questions, asked in a tone of genuine enquiry, which are designed to encourage the
offender to think for himself. This is the style implicitly recommended by Murphy (1990),
in his analysis of methods for undermining cognitive distortions.

The *method* is the framing of the questions asked; the *style* is the tone of genuine
enquiry. The Socratic method is used because: (1) it communicates respect (important in
working with a client group who are fearful of the consequences of full and honest

disclosure of their behavior and motivations); (2) it diffuses resistance and denial (again, because of the nature of the behavior under discussion and the usual sanctions that result from admitting to sexual offending, a common problem with this client group); and (3) it encourages offenders to think for themselves and teaches them to challenge their own thinking, thereby teaching implicitly the skill of disputing.

The importance of this sort of therapist style has recently been validated by research. Beech and Scott Fordham (1997), in a study of community sexual offender programs in Britain, found that the most successful programs were those where the therapists were perceived as warm and supportive and in control without being overly directive. Research from our program (Thorne, 1996) has replicated this finding by showing that improvements on a measure of victim harm recognition were associated with lower levels of leader control.

Accreditation

In 1996, the prison service decided to make completion of offending behavior treatment programs a national key performance indicator in the evaluation of prisons. The international expert advisory panel to SOTP was redesignated the SOTP accreditation panel and set standards for both content and delivery of SOTP. All sites delivering the program undergo an annual audit of delivery standards, clustered into six key areas: (1) institutional support, (2) selection and training of staff, (3) selection and initial assessment of participants, (4) products, (5) quality of delivery, and (6) communication with aftercare agencies. Each site is assigned an implementation quality rating (IQR) based on the audit report and examination by the panel of treatment products. In 1996–1997, 22 out of 25 SOTP sites received an IQR of 100%.

UNPREDICTED PRACTICE ISSUES

Over the 5 years since SOTP was introduced, a variety of challenges have presented themselves that were not or could not have been predicted during the preparation phase of the program. Some of these are described here, along with an explanation of the ways in which we have responded.

Effects on Therapists

Turner (1992), studying 82 SOTP tutors working in 16 different sites, identified a range of ways in which those staff delivering SOTP felt their experience had affected their emotional and personal lives. One third of the tutors felt that their intimate relationships had been affected and described various ways in which this had happened. For instance, some found it difficult to communicate about their work and they felt they should protect partners from the unpleasant details, while others felt continually preoccupied over group issues in a way that disturbed their family life. A minority of tutors (4% of postal respondents but 30% of interviewees) described loss of interest in sex and even sexual impotence as a result of working with these offenders.

Thirty-nine percent of tutors who had children felt that their parenting had been negatively affected. Many felt that they had become overprotective of their children and wanted to limit their activities outside the home. Also, they felt self-conscious about their own behavior with their children and started to wonder if it had a hidden meaning. Some tutors felt unable to play with their children in a physical way or to bathe them in case this was interpreted as sexual. Some found themselves thinking about child sexual abuse so much that they started to worry in case this meant they were "turning into an abuser."

Other personal problems were also described. Some tutors had themselves been victims of sexual abuse. Unresolved aspects of that experience came to the fore as a result of SOTP. Other tutors described wanting to avoid or reject certain sexual offenders. Some tutors, finding group work difficult and progress slow, began to lose self-confidence, feeling that they were not able to be effective. Many reported feeling angry at group members and not knowing how to deal with that anger. Some found they were distancing themselves from their group members, a symptom of the battle between being supportive and being collusive. Wanting to avoid collusion at all costs, tutors went to the opposite extreme and took pains to keep a psychological, even physical, distance between themselves and their group members. Adverse effects did not seem to be related to the tutor's professional background. Those with years of professional training in psychology or social work seemed just as vulnerable as those without.

In order to deal with these issues, we adopted a two-pronged approach, seeking first to forewarn tutors of the possible effects they may experience, and then taking steps to strengthen the quality of support provided to tutors. First, we introduced a system where, at the point of their application to become tutors (i.e., before they entered the selection procedure), prospective tutors would receive a summary of the research described above and would be asked, as part of their selection, how they felt about what they had read. This procedure was intended to assess whether or not would-be tutors were able to accept the likelihood of their being affected by the work, assuming that those who could not accept that possibility would find problems harder to deal with if they did occur. This was supplemented by including a session in the tutor training course that described the research results again, with the aim of preparing them for the work and increasing their motivation to make use of support facilities.

We also established an independent personal support service to provide all tutors with access to a professional counselor. Each tutor is required to attend three such sessions during the course of a core program. The purpose is to enable them to monitor and explore their personal reactions to the group work as a preventive measure against more serious long-term problems. The service is compulsory as the culture of the prison service may otherwise make it difficult for staff to admit a need, or even a wish, for counseling.

Informed Program Management

Turner (1992) also reported that tutors required more support from their managers than they were currently receiving. This was also observed by program development section staff during audit visits. It seemed that some managers lacked an understanding of the program and consequently were not allowing tutors any wind-down time after groups ended, but were requiring them to move immediately to other duties such as serving lunch or patrolling the prison.

Further research by Attrill (1995) asked tutors how they would define supportive behaviors by their managers and nontutoring colleagues (i.e., other prison officers and specialist staff not involved in delivering sexual offender treatment). Prison officers responded that they wanted more sympathetic "detailing" (the process by which they are assigned to particular tasks throughout a shift) that allowed them time to prepare for and debrief from group sessions. They wanted managers to understand the stresses they were under and to communicate more of an interest in sexual offender treatment by simple behaviors such as asking questions about how their group was going.

Program development section staff then began to offer an awareness course for managers of SOTP staff (including, but not only, the program management team in each prison). This 2-day course aims to enlighten managers about the nature of the work by demonstrating a variety of key treatment sessions (namely, a session aimed at moving a group member toward taking greater responsibility for his behavior and a session using role-play methods to develop victim empathy) as well as explaining the key treatment concepts and the rationale behind the program. This course has been particularly well received by managers who feel it brings the core program "out from behind the closed doors of the group work room" and enables them to feel more confident about discussing SOTP with their staff. Anecdotal evidence from tutors suggests that managers' behavior after attending the managers' course becomes significantly more supportive.

Throughcare

The prison service does not have any authority to determine what happens to an offender after release. Responsibility for supervising offenders in the community rests with the probation service, which, while being part of the Home Office, is managed independently from the prison service. To make matters even more complicated, the probation service is not a national organization but is split into 54 geographical areas, each of which is again independently managed.

A recent survey of community treatment by the probation service (Proctor, 1996) reported that specialist sexual offender programs were available in most probation areas. The majority of programs are similar in content to the core program in that they are general programs aimed at developing responsibility for offending. There are comparatively few programs that have a specific relapse prevention monitoring–maintenance focus, which would be the ideal approach for post-SOTP offenders after release. Some offenders resent the idea that they have to essentially repeat their treatment program rather than receiving structured group support on maintenance issues.

Given that the prison service can only have a limited influence on probation service practice, our efforts have concentrated on establishing effective methods of communication with supervising probation officers. A standard letter is sent to each supervising probation officer when a prisoner enters treatment along with a leaflet that describes the aims and structure of the program. When the program has been completed, a substantial treatment summary document is produced by the treatment team. The supervising probation officer is invited to attend a case conference where progress in treatment is discussed and further treatment goals are agreed on.

Sexual Murderers

Within the English criminal justice system, any person found guilty of murder receives a mandatory life sentence. Responsibility for releasing a mandatory life sentence prisoner rests ultimately with the Home Secretary, whose decision is based on recommendations made by prison service staff and the parole board. All life prisoners serve a minimum sentence based on a recommendation made by the trial judge, and once that time (known as the "tariff") has expired, their release is dependent on an assessment determining that they pose an acceptable level of risk (i.e., that they are unlikely to reoffend). Therefore, life sentence prisoners are under particular pressure to undertake work focusing on their offending behavior. There are about 2500 life sentence prisoners currently in prison in England and Wales.

Many of these prisoners have committed a murder where there appears to have been some sexual contact with the victim. In some cases (but these are a minority) there is a conviction for a sexual offense along with the murder conviction. Mostly this is not the case, but the details of the offense, usually the forensic evidence, imply that a sexual offense was committed as well as the murder.

These prisoners present a difficult challenge in terms of assessment and treatment. Commonly, they deny the sexual aspect of the offense, and where the risk assessments are carried out by staff who have no training in understanding sexual offending, this denial is often accepted as a fair version of events. It is only in recent years, since the introduction of SOTP, that many life sentence prisoners are starting to be identified as possible sexual offenders.

A case example may be the best way to illustrate the complex assessment issues in such cases:

> Charlie is convicted of the murder of a 12-year-old boy. The boy was found drowned in a river, with a bruise to his penis and some tearing around the anus. Charlie's version of events says that he and the boy were kicking a football around when during a particularly rough tackle, the boy fell to the ground unconscious. Charlie's explanation of the bruise to the penis is that it must have happened during this tackle when he accidentally kicked the boy in the groin. Fearing that he had "accidentally" killed the boy, he dumped the body in a river. He suggests that tearing to the anus must have been caused by rocks in the river.

In cases where the victim is dead, there is no alternative version of events such as that which usually would be provided by a victim's statement to the police. Thus, cases such as Charlie's demand particular therapeutic skill in undermining the denial and uncovering the true version of events, which otherwise can only be surmised from the forensic evidence.

Training in risk assessment has been provided to the section of the prison service that administers life sentence prisoner casework and to the parole board (the body that recommends release or continued imprisonment to the Home Secretary). However, there has been the continuing issue that many of the staff in penal establishments who are providing risk assessment reports on lifers such as Charlie do not have specialist knowledge in understanding sexual offending. In response, a pool of assessors is being created, all of whom will have received training in the special issues involved in determining the presence of a sexual element in a homicide. Sets of guidelines have been evolved to help this group operate consistently.

In addition, a number of treatment centers have begun to specialize in working with this group. The most evolved example of this is a residential unit that is totally dedicated to the assessment and treatment of life sentence prisoners with a sexual element in their offenses. Particular care was taken in setting up this unit. Managed by a psychologist with particular experience in working with this group, most staff on the unit have undergone specialist training in risk assessment of sexual murderers and all have completed the standard SOTP training. The unit offers the core and thinking skills programs. Although this unit has only been open for a short period, it has already demonstrated an ability to make breakthroughs with offenders who have resisted treatment elsewhere.

Dealing with Difficult Sexual Offenders

A survey of SOTP tutors (Mann, 1995) identified three groups of sexual offenders with whom delivery of SOTP was particularly difficult: offenders who were disruptive group members, offenders with low intelligence, and those who completely denied their offending.

Disruptive group members are not peculiar to sexual offender treatment but are found in all types of therapeutic group work. In response to the identification of this problem, the SOTP tutor training course was modified to include additional training in understanding group process and dealing with difficult group members.

Separate treatment strategies have been formulated for the other two problematic groups. The core program excludes sexual offenders with IQs less than 80, who may have particular cognitive deficits (such as difficulties in sequencing and articulating emotions) that would impair their response to a verbal treatment style. A National Health Service clinic, specializing in the treatment of offenders with learning disabilities, has completed an adaption of the core program for us, and this has now been introduced in three prisons.

Recent research into treatment of sexual offenders who deny their offending suggests that such offenders can be successfully treated (Maletzky, 1996) or can, through specially designed programs, become willing to admit to their offending (O'Donohue & LeTourneau, 1993; Schlank & Shaw, 1996). Research conducted on our own prisoners (Lord, Schofield & Willmot, 1996) examined ex-deniers and found that five elements were necessary to facilitate admission of offending: (1) a trustful climate; (2) ex-denier role models; (3) removal of fear of negative consequences; (4) recognition of positive outcomes of admission; and (5) encouragement to admit. As a result, a seven-session course for deniers has been developed and is currently being piloted.

EVALUATION

Evaluative research from other programs has played a key role in the evolution of SOTP, and doubtless will continue to do so, but evaluation of this kind of initiative is not a simple business. The scale of SOTP makes some kinds of evaluation easier while others become more difficult.

Short-term evaluation of the clinical impact of the program (i.e., do the procedures achieve their goals) is relatively easy and the large numbers involved mean that a clear-cut result can be produced quite rapidly. Long-term evaluation (i.e., recidivism of released offenders) is both easier and more difficult than it would be for a smaller program. The large scale of the program means that an adequate sample of "treated cases" can easily be generated for a reconviction study. The problem is that the wide availability of the program means that there are too few comparable untreated sexual offenders against whom to compare the results for treated offenders. Untreated offenders are currently either those assigned a low priority because they were thought to present a lower risk, those whose sentence was too short to complete a program before release (and who therefore will have been sentenced for what the court viewed as less serious offenses), or those who were unwilling to take part in treatment.

It had been hoped that we could use the cohort of untreated sexual offenders who had been discharged before SOTP was introduced as a comparison group. Unfortunately, the reconviction rate for untreated sexual offenders is known to have decreased substantially during the 1980s. This occurred at the same time as changes in the ratio between crimes known to the police and numbers convicted or cautioned also changed. Both of these changes coincided with various changes in the criminal justice system, and so probably reflect a reduced effectiveness in catching and convicting sexual offenders.

These difficulties have led us to adopt a variety of less direct approaches. We plan to combine four strategies: (1) using nonequivalent comparison groups and relying on statistical techniques to equate them for risk of sexual and violent reconviction; (2) comparing outcomes of treated subjects before and after major changes were introduced in the program (so far there has been one major change involving a doubling of the length of the program); (3) comparing reconviction rates for treated offenders who have achieved specified treatment goals to the reconviction rates of those who failed to achieve these goals; and (4) comparing reconviction rates for those who participated in poorly run groups to the reconviction rates of those who participated in better run groups (as judged on the basis of ratings of session videotapes and other indices). None of these methods will give as decisive a result as could be obtained with a proper controlled trial using random allocation. However, although less conclusive in terms of whether the program has any long-term effect, they will actually provide the kind of information that can be used to guide the future development of treatment. For example, the results of such studies could indicate that the attainment of some treatment goals is really important while the attainment of others is less critical.

CONCLUSION

We believe that the major lessons we have learned from the experience of introducing national sexual offender treatment programs are:

1. It is possible to introduce a sexual offender treatment program on a large scale and to maintain consistency and quality of delivery over a large number of sites.
2. Lay personnel can be used effectively to carry out therapeutic work with sexual offenders provided they are carefully selected, trained, and supervised.
3. For such a program to survive, both management and treatment issues need to be attended to with equal care.
4. Sexual offender treatment affects those who carry it out. The size of our program and the number of staff involved have made it clear that adverse effects are widespread and not linked to professional background or previous pathology.
5. Sexual offender treatment must be an evolutionary process. That is, as treatment providers we should continually monitor and research our practice, in order that we can identify and learn from our inadequacies or mistakes. Sustaining our commitment to evolution is, we believe, our greatest asset.

REFERENCES

Attrill, G. (1995). *The dimensions of staff support of the sex offender treatment program: Why, what, who and how?* Unpublished M.Sc. thesis, University of London.

Beech, A., & Scott Fordham, A. (1997). Therapeutic climate of sex offender treatment programs. *Sexual Abuse: A Journal of Research and Treatment, 9,* 219–223.

Grubin, D., & Thornton, D. (1994). A national program for the assessment and treatment of sex offenders in the English prison system. *Criminal Justice and Behaviour, 21,* 55–71.

Lord, A., Schofield, C., & Willmot, P. (1996, September). *"How I gave up denial and learned to love treatment": Working with sex offenders who deny their offending*. Paper presented at NOTA Annual Conference, Chester, England.

Maletzky, B.M. (1996). Editorial. *Sexual Abuse: A Journal of Research and Treatment, 8*, 1–5.

Mann, R.E. (1995, May). *What's difficult about working with sex offenders?* Paper presented to the Annual Conference of the British Society of Criminology, Loughborough, England.

Mann, R.E. (1996, November). *Measuring the effectiveness of relapse prevention intervention*. Paper presented at the 15th Annual Research and Treatment Conference of the Association for the Treatment of Sexual Abusers, Chicago.

Marques, J.K., Day, D.M., Nelson, C., & Miner, M. (1989). The Sex Offender Treatment and Evaluation Project: California's relapse prevention program. In D.R. Laws (Ed.), *Relapse prevention with sex offenders* (pp. 247–267). New York: Guilford Press.

Miller, W.R. (1983). Motivation for treatment: A review with special emphasis on alcoholism. *Psychological Bulletin, 98*, 84–107.

Miller, W.R., & Rollnick, S. (1991). *Motivational interviewing: Preparing people to change addictive behavior*. New York: Guilford Press.

Murphy, W.D. (1990). Assessment and modification of cognitive distortions in sex offenders. In W.L. Marshall, D.R. Laws, & H.E. Barbaree (Eds.), *Handbook of sexual assault: Issues, theories and treatment of the offender* (pp. 331–342). New York: Plenum Press.

Nelson, C., & Jackson, P. (1989). High-risk recognition: The cognitive–behavioral chain. In D.R. Laws (Ed.), *Relapse prevention with sex offenders* (pp. 167–177). New York: Guilford Press.

O'Donohue, W., & LeTourneau, E. (1993). A brief group treatment for the modification of denial in child sexual abusers: Outcome and follow-up. *Child Abuse and Neglect, 17*, 299–304.

Overholser, J. (1993a). Elements of the Socratic method I: Systematic questioning. *Psychotherapy, 30*, 67–74.

Overholser, J. (1993b). Elements of the Socratic method II: Inductive reasoning. *Psychotherapy, 30*, 75–85.

Overholser, J. (1994). Elements of the Socratic method III: Universal definitions. *Psychotherapy, 31*, 286–293.

Overholser, J. (1995). Elements of the Socratic method IV: Disavowal of knowledge. *Psychotherapy, 32*, 283–292.

Pithers, W.D. (1994). Process evaluation of a group therapy component designed to enhance sex offenders' empathy for sexual abuse survivors. *Behaviour Research and Therapy, 32*, 565–570.

Proctor, E. (1996). *Community based interventions with sex offenders organised by the probation service: A survey of current practice*. Unpublished report, Association of Chief Officers of Probation, London.

Program Development Section. (1996). *The core programme: Evidence of effectiveness*. Internal H.M. Prison Service document.

Proulx, J., McKibben, A., & Lusignan, R. (1996). Relationships between affective components and sexual behaviours in sexual aggressors. *Sexual Abuse: A Journal of Research and Treatment, 8*, 279–289.

Sacre, G. (1995). *Analysis of the role of the tutor on the national SOTP: A competency based approach*. Unpublished M.Sc. thesis, University of London.

Schlank, A.M., & Shaw, T. (1996). Treating sexual offenders who deny their guilt: A pilot study. *Sexual Abuse: A Journal of Research and Treatment, 8*, 17–23.

Thornton, D., & Hogue, T. (1993). The large-scale provision of programs for imprisoned sex offenders: Issues, dilemmas and progress. *Criminal Behaviour and Mental Health, 3*, 371–380.

Thorne, I. (1996). *Sex Offender Treatment Program: An evaluative study of the victim empathy blocks*. Unpublished M.Sc. thesis, University of London.

Turner, C. (1992). *The experience of staff conducting the core programme*. Unpublished M.Sc. thesis, University of London.

5

A. Prison Settings

Ontario Penitentiaries' Program

Howard E. Barbaree, Edward J. Peacock, Franca Cortoni, William L. Marshall, and Michael Seto

The present chapter will describe the treatment programs for incarcerated sexual offenders sponsored by the correctional services of Canada (CSC) in the Ontario regional penitentiaries. The chapter will describe sexual offender treatment in Ontario penitentiaries in general terms and then it will focus on two programs in particular: the Warkworth Sexual Behaviour Clinic and the Bath Institution Sex Offenders' Program.

A BRIEF HISTORY

From 1973 until 1983, all sexual offenders in Ontario under the jurisdiction of the CSC who received treatment did so at the Regional Treatment Centre Ontario (RTC), a maximum-security inpatient facility, located within the walls of the Kingston Penitentiary. To receive treatment, offenders were transferred from their home institution to the RTC for the period of their treatment. The program was a combination of nonbehavioral psychotherapy and behavioral or cognitive–behavioral treatments. A group therapy program was led by a consulting psychiatrist and involved confrontation, role-play, and general discussion. Cognitive–behavioral components of therapy, conducted in both group and individual therapy formats, included sex education, treatment of deviant sexual arousal, and social skills training. The inpatient unit was staffed by psychiatric nurses, and these staff were involved in all aspects of treatment. In 1983, a satellite program was established at the protective custody unit at Kingston Penitentiary. Together, from 1973 until 1989, these two programs completed treatment with approximately 300 participants, but this did not fully meet the needs of the numbers of offenders seeking treatment.

After a series of serious reoffenses by sexual offenders on parole and with increasing demand for availability of programs for sexual offenders, including a pending lawsuit brought by several inmates at Warkworth Institution, the CSC began a period of program expansion, implementation, and development, both in the correctional facilities and in the

Howard E. Barbaree and Michael Seto • Forensic Division, Clarke Institute of Psychiatry, Toronto, Ontario, Canada M5T 1R8. **Edward J. Peacock** • Warkworth Sexual Behaviour Clinic, Warkworth Institution, Campbellford, Ontario, Canada K0L IL0. **Franca Cortoni** • Sexual Offenders' Program, Kingston Penitentiary, Kingston, Ontario, Canada K7L 4V7. **William L. Marshall** • Department of Psychology, Queen's University, Kingston, Ontario, Canada K7L 3N6.

Sourcebook of Treatment Programs for Sexual Offenders, edited by Marshall et al. Plenum Press, New York, 1998.

larger communities in the province. In 1989, the Warkworth Sexual Behaviour Clinic was established, and this program has treated an average of approximately 80 sexual offenders each year since. During the years 1990–1992, community-based sexual offender treatment programs were established in Toronto, Hamilton, Ottawa, and Kingston. By now, there are numerous other programs and clinical services available in the smaller communities in Ontario. In 1991, a sexual offender program was established at the minimum-security Bath Institution. While Bath Institution has recently been upgraded to medium security, other treatment programs for sexual offenders have been established in two minimum-security institutions in the Kingston area during the past 2 years. At present, all sexual offenders in the Ontario region are offered treatment while they are incarcerated.

INSTITUTIONAL AND LEGAL CONTEXT

In 1996, there were approximately 1200 sexual offenders under the jurisdiction of the CSC in the province of Ontario. These men had been sentenced to 2 years or more in a federal penitentiary for serious sexual crimes, including rape and penetrative sexual assaults against children, and murder and attempted murder where there were sexual components to the offense. Of the 1200 sexual offenders, almost 1000 were incarcerated in one of the correctional facilities and the remainder were under parole supervision in the community.

The federal penitentiaries in Ontario are divided into three levels of security. Table 5.1 presents a list of the federal correctional facilities in Ontario by level of security and the numbers of sexual offenders incarcerated in each. In maximum security, offenders are housed in single locked cells or on a small range of cells housing compatible inmates. In medium security, the institution has a secure perimeter, with controlled movement within the facility. In a minimum security facility, movement beyond a fenceless boundary is prohibited. Within facilities, changes in the level of security can be affected at the discretion of the warden; for example, when it is felt that a man is a danger to himself or others, he may be held in a segregation cell for a period of time, or offenders may be given escorted or unescorted passes to the community for brief periods for the purpose of family visitation, bereavement, and to attend hospital or medical appointments. In the community, there are three levels of security. At the first level, the community correctional centers are single locked residential facilities from which offenders on parole are released to the community for work, family visits, treatment, and other daily activities. At the second level, the community-based residential facility, the offender may be required to report his movements to the staff at the facility on a regular basis. Finally, in the third and least restrictive level of security, men are released to the community, often with requirements to abstain from substance use and to attend treatment and the obligation to report to their parole offender and the police on a regular basis.

In Canada, determinate sentences are divided into thirds. At the end of the first third of a sentence, the inmate is eligible for parole. However, in actual practice, because of recent public outrage over sexual reoffenses committed by parolees, fewer sexual offenders receive parole at this early stage. At the end of the second third of a determinate sentence, inmates are normally released into the community at what is referred to as their statutory release date. These men then serve the latter third of their sentence in the community on parole. In 1992, the Corrections and Conditional Release Act was amended to allow the "detention of some offenders at their Statutory Release Date, holding these offenders in custody until the end of their sentences." Initially, detention applied to offenders whose

TABLE 5.1
Institutional Group Therapy Programs

Institution and programs	Focus on stage	Sessions per week	Length per session (hours)	Duration (months)	Total group contact (hours)	Individual therapy sessions[a]	Deviant arousal	Anticipated enrolment 1996–1997	Sexual offenders currently in institution
Maximum									
RTC (Ontario)		5	2	5	215	2/wk	Y	60	38
Kingston Penitentiary		7	2.5	5–7	300	N	Y	24	204
Millhaven Assessment									117
Medium									
Warkworth								112	324
Long-termers	1	1	3	8	100	N	N	12	
Full prerelease	1,2	5	3	6	325	N	Y	88	
Advanced	2	4	3	5	200	N	Y	12	
Bath								79	126
Moderate/high risk	1,2	3	3	4	144	N	N	10	
Low risk (closed)	1,2	2	3	3	72	N	N	21	
Low risk (open)	1,2	2	3	Open	Minimum 72	N	N	48	
Joyceville									106
Collins Bay									6
Minimum									
Pittsburgh	2	2	1.5	Open		N	Y	40	20
Frontenac	2	1	2	Open		N	N	75	24
Beaver Creek									17
Community									230
Total Spring 1996									1212

[a]N, no; Y, yes.

index offense caused death or serious harm to another person, and where there were reasonable grounds to believe that the offender was likely to do so again before the expiration of his sentence. Then, in 1995, the Act providing for detection was amended further to apply to any offender who had assaulted a child and was thought likely to do so again before the expiration of his sentence.

For men on indeterminate sentences, the only chance for release to the community is through parole, and parole can only be sought after a parole eligibility date determined by the court at sentencing. Men on indeterminate sentences are either serving "life" terms after convictions for murder, or they have been designated as a "dangerous offender." In Canada, at sentencing, the prosecuting attorney has the option, when the offender has committed very serious crimes or has been persistently offending over many years, to make application to the court to designate the convicted offender as a dangerous offender. After a judicial hearing, and if the application is successful, the offender is given a life sentence. A dangerous offender can apply for parole after a short period of incarceration, but practically speaking, he does not get a realistic chance at parole until after approximately 17 years of incarceration.

Within this context, all sexual offenders are motivated to do what they can to increase their chances for parole and to avoid detention. They will work hard to achieve a release to the community. Even within the prisons, men can work toward an improved quality of life through transfer to lower levels of security. At any time, inmates are eligible for transfer to a lower level of security, and these transfers are greatly desired because at lower levels of security there are fewer restrictions, greater freedoms, and more valued privileges. This movement to lower levels of security is referred to as "cascading." These features, of course, provide incentives for sexual offenders to participate in treatment, since potential release or cascading are contingent on these offenders having been judged to have been effectively treated. Not surprisingly, the majority of sexual offenders do participate in treatment.

Within the prisons, the institutional case management officer (CMOI) is responsible for assisting the inmate in planning all rehabilitative programs, and the CMOI is responsible for all recommendations regarding release and transfer. All decisions concerning release to the community are made by the national parole board. Decisions regarding transfers are usually made by the wardens of the sending and receiving institutions. All recommendations and decisions regarding transfer and release take into consideration the assessments and recommendations of the treatment professionals regarding risk to reoffend, treatment needs, and the offender's likelihood of success in the community or in a lower security prison.

Upon admission to the penitentiary system, all inmates are sent to the Millhaven Assessment Unit for initial assessment. The purpose of the assessment is to determine the appropriate institutional placement for the offender, the offender's security requirements (e.g., protective custody), and risk for reoffense and to determine in general terms his treatment requirements. At this stage, the emphasis is on assessment of static risk factors. From the Millhaven Assessment Unit, inmates are sent to one of the regional correctional facilities. The majority (approximately 60%) are sent to a medium-security prison, and most of these are sent to Warkworth Institution. Approximately 25% are sent to maximum security, primarily for their own protection, and the remainder are sent to minimum security. Upon completion of treatment, they may cascade down to lower levels of security or they may stay at the same level until they are released to the community.

Offenders are offered treatment according to a system of prioritization based on their statutory release date; those with the earlier statutory release dates have higher priority. Most often this means that men are offered treatment approximately 12–18 months prior to their projected date of release. It is currently the goal of the CSC to provide treatment to all offenders by their parole eligibility date, but this has not yet been achieved due to the high numbers of offenders and the relative lack of treatment resources. Sexual-offender-specific treatment programs are available in correctional facilities at all levels of security and in most of the larger communities in Ontario (Chapter 8 describes one of these community programs). Two programs are chosen for particular attention in this chapter: the Warkworth Sexual Behaviour Clinic and the Bath Institution Sex Offenders' Program. These programs share a basic philosophy and follow a similar format, using a cognitive–behavioral approach with a heavy reliance on the principles of relapse prevention.

THE WARKWORTH SEXUAL BEHAVIOUR CLINIC

The Warkworth Sexual Behaviour Clinic (WSBC) was inaugurated in June 1989, as a sexual offender treatment program at Warkworth Institution, a medium-security federal penitentiary located northeast of Toronto. Warkworth Institution is one of Canada's largest penitentiaries, housing over 650 inmates serving sentences of 2 or more years. Approximately half of these offenders were convicted of a sexual offense or a violent offense in which sexual motivation or behavior was considered to be important.

At its inception, the WSBC was funded as a research and service contract between the CSC and Queen's University, to be directed by H.E. Barbaree and W.L. Marshall. The clinic was directed jointly for the first year, and the operation of the clinic was modeled after similar programs set up elsewhere by Barbaree and Marshall. From the beginning of the second year until the present, Barbaree has been the program director. In 1995, the CSC took over administrative responsibility for the clinic, with all full-time staff now employed as regular employees of the CSC, although clinical responsibility has remained with the program director.

Staffing

During its first year of operation, the WSBC treated 60 men. The staff complement included a senior group therapist, a research assessment coordinator, a laboratory technician, a psychometrist, and a clerk–secretary. During the second year of its operation, the WSBC increased its yearly targeted quota of treatment completions to 90. Accordingly, the full-time staffing complement was increased to include three senior therapists, a program coordinator, two laboratory technicians, two case historians, one clerk–secretary. Additionally, three part-time psychometrists assisted with the pretreatment assessment.

Assessment

The WSBC conducts its own assessment of men prior to their entry into treatment. The goals of the assessment are to provide a pretreatment assessment of risk, to determine each offender's treatment needs, and to provide a baseline against which progress in treatment can be evaluated. In the assessment, risk is evaluated by taking into account factors that have been shown in the research literature to predict sexual recidivism (Barbaree & Marshall, 1988; Serin & Barbaree, 1993).

A novel feature of the WSBC program is the use of a "multifactorial assessment of sex offender risk for reoffense" (MASORR). At the time the WSBC was implemented, a comprehensive review of the literature on the prediction of reoffense among sexual offenders was conducted and formed the basis of MASORR. This review indicated that four factors were predictive of sexual reoffense: (1) a history of sexual offending; (2) deviant sexual arousal; (3) a history of antisocial behavior and other indicators of an antisocial personality (as measured by the Psychopathy Checklist-Revised); and (4) social competence (estimated from apparent intelligence level and socioeconomic status).

The MASORR is therefore based on static predictors of reoffense. It was initially implemented as a pretreatment assessment of risk. Later, however, it was modified for use as a posttreatment assessment of risk to incorporate two dynamic factors reflecting the man's performance while in treatment. These dynamic factors were "motivation for treatment" and "degree of behavior change achieved." An overall clinical impression based on the man's involvement with the WSBC was also incorporated into the posttreatment risk evaluation. These various factors were combined to form overall ratings of risk for reoffense, first at pretreatment (static factors only) and again at posttreatment (initial risk score modified by consideration of the dynamic factors).

The assessment process is composed of two phases. The first phase consists of a comprehensive file review that examines all available information on the offender. The information is entered into a computerized database designed to ensure that all aspects of an offender's functioning are covered. This includes, but is not limited to, childhood history, education, work history, family relationships, marital relationships, offense history, and institutional adjustment. This database provides both coding of the information for future research and written descriptions of all inputted information. This information is then subsequently used to complete the assessment report. In addition, the file review provides all relevant information for the therapist once the man enters treatment.

The second part of the assessment process consists of a 2-hour semistructured interview. This interview provides the information required to obtain an index of the man's criminal personality through the use of the Psychopathy Checklist-Revised (PCL-R) (Hare, 1991). The interview, which is an extended version of the interview recommended for use with the PCL-R, also provides the opportunity for the man to present his current thinking and functioning and his version of his sexual offense(s). This process permits an evaluation of the offender's level of denial and minimization of his offense(s), the presence of cognitive distortions, his readiness for treatment, and the presence of other problems that may be related to his sexually offending behavior. These other problems include the presence of general criminal behavior, social functioning, marital problems, substance abuse problems, and psychological or psychiatric problems. The information obtained through both phases of the assessment is then fully detailed in the pretreatment assessment report, including an identification of the source of the information. The report also details the level of risk obtained on each factor discussed above. These individual risk factors are then combined to produce the overall pretreatment risk assessment.

An offender entering the assessment process at the clinic is fully apprised of all aspects of his assessment. Before the assessment can proceed, he is required to provide his consent to the assessment for both the file review and the interview. Once the treatment report is completed, the man is provided with the opportunity to review his report and to identify any factual inaccuracy. He is also provided with the opportunity to discuss his report and its finding with one of the psychometrists specifically named as the assessment coordinator. Should he have concerns about his report that were not addressed satisfactorily by the assessment coordinator, the offender then has the option to meet with the program director.

The direct involvement of the offender in all phases of his assessment, including the opportunity to rectify factual errors and discuss his concerns, has established an atmosphere of trust between the offender and the clinical staff. Before this process was in place, the clinic received many complaints about the reports that needed to be addressed by the director. Men also viewed the staff at the clinic with suspicion, and as a result were more resistant to the therapeutic process once in treatment. A notable reduction in complaints about pretreatment reports has been observed since the new process was instituted. Very few offenders have requested further actions once they have met with the assessment coordinator. As well, offenders will often take this opportunity to discuss their feelings toward treatment and their offenses, thereby establishing communication and an atmosphere of trust between the offender and the clinic staff. In turn, this facilitates the therapeutic process of change required for the offender to achieve maximum therapeutic benefits from his contacts with the clinic. Providing treatment for incarcerated offenders can be a challenge, since many offenders feel coerced into treatment and view their consent to the assessment and treatment as immaterial. By involving offenders and providing them with the opportunity for input into their assessment, many of the negative sentiments experienced by the offenders are alleviated. It also provides these men with exposure to appropriate social interactions with the many female staff of the clinic, as well as problem-solving interactions, which they are encouraged to model. This favorably predisposes them toward treatment, therefore increasing the likelihood of success in treatment.

We will present a brief analysis of assessment data compiled from the first 250 cases processed through the clinic. Of these 250 cases, 123 were rapists, 15 were sex killers (men convicted of sex-related homicides), 56 were incest offenders, and 56 were extrafamilial child molesters. At the time of the data analysis, conducted during the summer and fall of 1995, 132 of these 250 offenders had been conditionally released to the community: 23 on day parole, 15 on full parole, and 94 by their statutory release date.

We used a series of crude factor analyses to reduce the large number of quantitative variables in the database (300+) to a more reasonable and manageable number. These analyses reduced the number of historical variables pertaining to the domains of education, occupation, relationships, family history, juvenile antisocial behavior, and adult antisocial behavior into a set of ten historical factors: Child Behavior Problems, Erratic Employment, Previous Treatment, Quality of Early Life, Separation from Family of Origin, Sexual Promiscuity, Alcohol Problems, Severity of Index Offense, Antisocial History, and Criminal History. Behavior during treatment was rated on a number of dimensions and similarly submitted to factor analysis, resulting in three treatment process factors: Treatment Behavior, Treatment Change, and Clinical Impression. The psychological tests included in the pretreatment assessment were also subjected to factor analysis, producing three test factors: Overt Hostility, Covert Hostility, and Social Functioning. An analysis of overall pretreatment risk ratings showed that offender types differed in their initial risk scores; incest offenders were assessed as significantly lower in initial risk than the other types of offenders. After combining the data from the different types of offenders, a further factor analysis revealed two factors as significant predictors of risk: Antisocial History and Criminal History. Together, these two factors explained 23.5% of the variance in pretreatment risk level. Higher-risk subjects had more extensive antisocial and criminal histories.

Treatment

Sexual offenders in the Canadian penitentiaries are not required to submit to treatment; however, some offenders describe a situation in which they feel they are forced or coerced into treatment. From the perspective of the correctional service, sexual offenders are presented with an informed choice regarding treatment. They can choose the natural course through the criminal justice system. In the natural course, there is very little chance for early release. Moreover, as described above, in cases of high-risk offenders, the natural course may include being detained in custody at their statutory release date, to complete their full sentence in prison. As an alternative to the natural course, sexual offenders can choose treatment as an integral part of their correctional plan for rehabilitation. By making this choice and by demonstrating progress in a therapeutic program of rehabilitation, an offender is more likely to receive a favorable evaluation by the treatment professionals, more likely to receive a more favorable recommendation by the CMOI, and will therefore be more likely to achieve a desirable outcome in his parole and transfer applications. As a result of participating effectively in treatment, the offender is more likely to be successful in applying for parole and may be more likely to avoid detention. In short, this informed choice is likely to lead to an earlier release to the community compared to the alternative choice.

Table 5.2 presents the objectives in treatment in our staged model of therapy. In stage 1, participants are required to come to an acceptance of responsibility for their offensive behavior and the harmful effects such behavior has had on their victims. This stage in therapy is designed to engage participants in a long-term treatment process, to encourage compliance with their correctional plan, and to ensure their recognition of the importance of treatment and behavior change in their correction plan. In stage 2, motivated offenders learn about the precursors to their sexual crimes, the chains of behavior leading to their offenses, and the circumstances that place them at high risk for reoffense. Using a framework of relapse prevention, offenders are taught ways to avoid high-risk situations and behaviors and methods they can use to prevent a relapse. Offenders are assessed and treated in the phallometric laboratory, with the aim being their acquisition of control over deviant sexual

---

TABLE 5.2
**Treatment Objectives in a Staged Model
of Therapy for Sexual Offenders**

Stage 1: Developing compliance and motivation for behavior change
- Objective A   Acceptance of responsibility for sexual crimes; treatment targets include denial, minimization, and cognitive distortions
- Objective B   Becoming aware of victim harm and developing empathy

Stage 2: Achieving behavior change
- Objective C   Chains of behavior; developing an awareness of the antecedents and precursors to their sexual crimes
- Objective D   Developing a relapse prevention plan
- Objective E   Eliminating deviant sexual arousal
- Objective F   Finding community supports and resources

Stage 3: Implementation of the relapse prevention plan
- Objective G   Going straight; preventing reoffense while developing a prosocial life in the community

arousal. Also, at this stage, offenders are required to plan their release, with specific planning related to accommodation and residency, employment, social support, and continuing treatment in the community. Therapy in stages 1 and 2 are the focus of institutional treatment programs. In stage 3, participants have successfully completed the first two stages of treatment and have been released to the community on parole. Participants put their relapse prevention plans into operation in a community setting, with the assistance and supervision of their community clinician and their parole officer.

Table 5.1 presents a list of the current sexual-offender-specific institutional treatment programs available in the various institutions in Ontario, at all levels of security. As is evident, different programs focus on different stages of therapy and they vary in intensity with differing numbers of sessions per week, different lengths of treatment sessions, different durations of the program, and different numbers of total treatment contact hours. The program at the RTC (Ontario) offers a significant individual therapy component, while all other programs accomplish as much as possible within a group therapy context. Some programs include the assessment and treatment of deviant sexual arousal and some do not. Table 5.1 includes the current (1996) numbers of sexual offenders in each institution and the expected enrollment in the various programs in this current fiscal year.

The table shows that the WSBC offers three versions of its program, depending on the stage of treatment the program focuses on. For the full prerelease program, offenders complete both within-prison stages, and the group therapy sessions are conducted daily for 3 hours per day, 5 days per week, over a period of 5 months. In the long-termers' program, the focus is on stage 1, with the group therapy sessions being held weekly over a period of 8 months. In the advanced program, the sessions focus on stage 2, and are held 4 days per week, over a 4-month period. The long-termers' program is specifically designed for men who are still some time away from release, so that the intention is to prepare them for later entry into the other two programs. The advanced program is designed for men who have successfully completed the full prerelease program, but who have some time remaining before release and who wish to further develop the skills they have already learned in relapse prevention.

In stage 1, denial minimization is targeted in the following way. The offender is asked to make a disclosure to his therapy group. In his disclosure, the offender describes the offense and his offense history from his perspective. The therapist then provides the offender and his therapy group with a narrative account of the "official" description of the offense and the offender's offense history. The official account is derived from court records, police reports, and victim testimony or statements. Sometimes the offender's disclosure is a good approximation of the official account. Usually, however, there are major discrepancies, with the offender's account being self-serving. Following the presentation of the official version, the therapy group asks the offender to address each discrepancy in turn. Discrepancies might include whether or not he had used a weapon, whether or not the victim had given consent, and so forth. The therapy group then challenges the offender to modify his version of the offense.

We decided early on that we would require offenders to "pass" stage 1 of the program before graduating to stage 2. By "pass" we meant that the offender's version involving denial would be required to demonstrate significant progress toward matching the official version of his offense and offense history, such that we felt he was accepting responsibility for his sexual assaults. When we began the program, our data indicated that over 50% of the offenders who were referred to the program denied that they were a sexual offender, or that they had committed a sexual offense, or that they had problems that required treatment as a sexual offender. Of course, while in denial, offenders would not likely benefit much from treatment. As a consequence, many treatment programs for sexual offenders have made denial an exclusion criterion. Therefore, after stage 1 of therapy, where we felt the offender still was not taking responsibility for his offense(s), we required him to drop out of the treatment program. We felt that with so many offenders in denial, it was our responsibility to try to deal with this as a therapeutic issue. Now, we devote the early part of the program to the treatment of denial and minimization, and we have found that treatment of denial and extreme minimization can be very successful. Over the more than 40 groups of 11 men we have begun in therapy, it is usual to fail 1–2 per group. On average, we fail 10% of the participants in the pretreatment phase of the program. Therefore, pretreatment levels of denial (50%) are reduced by this intervention to 10% at posttreatment.

When men are removed from the program at this stage, they go on 6-weeks of zero pay. This is because the WSBC, at the request of the inmate council, was made an institutional work site. As such, it is subject to the rules and regulations pertaining to inmate employment. One of these is that, if an inmate is fired or quits, he goes on 6-weeks of zero pay. This rule is set out in the treatment consent form that must be signed by each program participant prior to entry into the program.

Case Conferences: Developing a Tripartite Therapeutic Alliance

Early in the history of the program, for the first year or 18 months, we conducted risk assessments both at pretreatment and posttreatment and submitted the reports to the case managers. At the end of the treatment program, inmates were invited to come to the clinic to pick up copies of their posttreatment report. At this time, the offenders read our assessment of their treatment progress and our concluding posttreatment risk assessment for the first time. This method of communication, both to the inmate and the case manager, was found to be inadequate and potentially dangerous in a number of ways. First, for the inmate, expectations concerning the degree to which their involvement in treatment would reduce their risk were often quite unrealistic. These expectations were engendered, in part, by the encouraging feedback they would get from therapists indicating they had done well in the program and that they were to be congratulated on the progress they had made. This feedback led to the impression that this progress would reduce their risk to some very low level. Then, reading their reports for the first time, they were surprised that their risk levels were not reduced to the extent they felt was appropriate. For men who have potential for violence, being angry and upset was a risky situation in the institution. Also, this method of communication had the effect of interfering with the therapeutic alliance we had established with the inmate.

Second, for the case managers, in situations where our assessment of posttreatment risk was quite out of line with what the case manager had in mind, the case manager then had to deal with an unexpected factor in the case. For example, in a case where an inmate would receive a risk assessment of "low" or "low-moderate," and this was out of line with the expectations of the case manager, the inmate would feel strongly that the case manager should nevertheless go forward with a recommendation for parole or transfer to lower security or some kind of gradual release process. Based on other factors, the case manager may not be willing to go forward with that recommendation, but yet has to deal with an inmate with rising expectations.

To solve this problem, we instituted a system of case conferences that were held on two occasions for each inmate in each program: at midterm and at posttreatment. At the midterm conference, held about 2 months into the program, we reviewed the pretreatment risk assessment and the case manager's expectation with respect to options after treatment concerning release or transfer. We reviewed the progress the individual had made in therapy, the problems that had arisen, and we talked about the strengths and weaknesses of the individual inmate. In each conference, these discussions were held first with the inmate absent, then with the inmate present. We try to communicate to the inmate and the case manager our expectations of the outcome of therapy, what the likely risk assessment will be after therapy, and what our recommendations are likely to be for release and transfer. This has the effect of making inmates' expectations more realistic early on in the program. It also has the effect of making our expectations clear to the inmate at midterm concerning what we expect him to accomplish before the treatment program is over. We try to use the midterm case conference as a motivational interview, by establishing some objectives for the inmate and by negotiating an arrangement whereby a certain level of risk assessment and certain recommendations will be made if they meet certain treatment objectives by the end of treatment. For the case manager, these conferences have the effect of informing them early on of our work with the inmate, what our risk assessment has been, and what the likely outcome of treatment might be. The case managers feel they have an opportunity to communicate their concerns and their expectations to us and that they have an influence over the ultimate outcome of therapy.

The case conferences at posttreatment are essentially an endorsement of what has been discussed at the midterm conference. The therapist confirms that the inmate has or has not made the progress expected at the midterm conference and the risk assessment at posttreatment is established and recommendations for transfer and release are communicated to the case manager. Then later the written report reflects essentially a formalization of the decisions and feedback given at the posttreatment case conference.

Treatment of the sexual offender has often been thought of simply as a two-part relationship between the therapist and the inmate. By conducting these case conferences, we have moved toward a three-part therapeutic alliance in which the therapist and the inmate respond to the needs, expectations, and concerns of the case management officer. This often has the result of improving the working relationships between the offender and his case manager.

Outcome

Posttreatment Risk and Release Decisions

One hundred and ninety-three (77.2%) of the 250 subjects in the initial follow-up study completed the treatment program. Treatment completion was unrelated to offender type or whether the offender had committed a sexual offense prior to his current conviction. None of the historical factors emerged as a significant predictor of treatment completion. Men who reported more positive attitudes about treatment and expected to get more out of treatment were more likely to complete the treatment program.

A multiple regression analysis was conducted to identify predictors of posttreatment risk score. The initial risk score was entered first in order to determine if the historical and treatment factors contributed something more to the prediction of posttreatment risk. The regression equation was highly significant, explaining 68.1% of the variance in posttreatment risk score. Significant predictors were initial risk score, Treatment Behavior, Treatment Change, and Clinical Impression. Higher posttreatment risk was associated with higher initial level of risk, poor behavior in treatment, less positive gains over the course of treatment, and poorer overall clinical impression.

As part of the process of reporting to the institutional case manager and the national parole board, WSBC makes specific recommendations for each offender's posttreatment disposition. These recommendations, referred to as the level of management index, are based on the individual's posttreatment risk score and on the various case management options available for that individual (e.g., whether a graduated release to a community residential center would be supported by case management). We found no differences between offender types in the level of management that has been recommended. Three significant predictors emerged from the regression equation, explaining 51.4% of the variance in the recommended level of management: Posttreatment risk, Previous Treatment, and Clinical Impression. In other words, a more restrictive recommendation for management was associated with higher estimated posttreatment risk, previously being involved in treatment, and poorer overall clinical impression.

Data for 215 of the 250 offenders were obtained during a review of national parole board files. Of these 215 offenders, 198 (92.1%) were eligible for conditional release: 1 man died while incarcerated, 12 men were serving a life sentence and were not yet eligible for parole, and 4 men had been designated as dangerous offenders. Of the 198 eligible offenders, 132 (66.7%) were conditionally released; 3 men had passed their parole dates but had not reached their statutory release date, and the remaining 63 men were detained following their statutory release date. A stepwise discrimination function analysis was conducted to identify predictors of detention (i.e., not being released on day parole, full parole, or statutory release). There were 148 valid cases, with 48 (32.4%) of these individuals being detained. Posttreatment level of risk and the recommended level of management were entered in the first block. The treatment process factors were then entered in a stepwise fashion in a second block. There were two significant predictors of being detained: posttreatment level of risk and recommended level of management. In other words, offenders who were assessed as being at higher risk for reoffending at posttreatment and who were given recommendations for more restrictive levels of management were more likely to be detained.

Failure on Conditional Release

Of the 132 subjects who were conditionally released, a total of 42 (31.8%) men failed their conditional release for one of the following reasons: a relapse in which no official action was taken; suspension for the breach of a condition related to their relapse plan; or revocation of their conditional release. Rapists were more likely than child molesters to fail their conditional release (40.7 vs. 25.0%), although this trend was not quite statistically significant. These failure rates are very similar to those found for a sample of 145 sexual offenders recently released on parole with an average follow-up of 1 year, who were identified through the national sex offender census: 42.3% of rapists and 22.5% of child molesters.

The average time at risk for failure during conditional release was approximately 43 months, ranging from 1 week to 5.2 years. Survival analysis showed that 29.1% of the rapists and 14.4% of the child molesters had failed their conditional release conditions after 1 year of follow-up. After 2 years, 47.7% of the rapists and 28.2% of the child molesters had failed, and after 3 years, these proportions were 62.9% and 43.0%, respectively. These results indicate that early on the rapists failed at approximately twice the rate of child molesters, but this difference in failure rate decreased in the third year of follow-up, with the child molesters' risk of failure increasing at a greater rate than the rapists. These results should be considered tentative because only a small number of offenders in the present sample were at risk of failing their conditional release for 3 years and because more than half of the cases were censored at the time of this analysis (i.e., they had not passed their warrant expiry date and were therefore still at risk). We conducted a stepwise discriminant analysis to identify predictors of conditional release failure. The resulting predictors were Antisocial History and Treatment Behavior. In other words, highly antisocial subjects who behaved poorly in treatment were more likely to fail their conditional release.

Recidivism

At the time of the current data analysis, a total of 218 individuals have been released from prison. As noted, 132 of these offenders were conditionally released and the remainder left prison following the expiration of their warrants. One man died after being released and 15 other men were deported from Canada, so the follow-up group was composed of 202 individuals. At the present time, we have identified 13 individuals who committed a new sexual offense and an additional 4 subjects who committed a new violent offense but who did not commit a new sexual offense. A total of 36 individuals committed a new offense of any kind. Therefore, a total of 17 WSBC treatment participants have committed a new serious offense after being released from prison (i.e., violent or sexual reoffense), giving the WSBC a serious recidivism rate of 8.4% and a sexual recidivism rate of 6.4% after an average follow-up period of approximately 2.5 years. These rates compare favorably with the reoffense rates reported by other large treatment programs. However, they were too low to conduct discriminant function or logistic regression analyses. The base rates will presumably be higher and amenable to such analyses as the length of the follow-up period increases.

Problems in the Operation of the WSBC

When we first arrived at Warkworth Institution to discuss the development of a clinic, the warden and senior staff of the institution expressed grave misgivings about what was being proposed. Most felt that serious security issues would arise with the operation of such a clinic in a general population prison. These fears focused on the possibility that nonsexual offender inmates would be able to identify sexual offenders more readily, and that serious persecution or assaults would ensue. Somewhat surprisingly, the outcomes predicted did not materialize. Instead, the implementation of the clinic at Warkworth was made difficult by numerous but more mundane factors, the most important of which were uncertain funding, inadequate resources, and serious difficulties in finding and keeping qualified staff.

Funding

Funding for the clinic was inadequate at the outset, and although some of these inadequacies were addressed when we increased the clinic's capacity at the end of the first year of operation, certain inadequacies continue. First and foremost among these is that each therapy group is run by one senior therapist, and while the new national standards call for coleadership of therapy groups, such has not been possible in the context of the WSBC budget. Additionally, the funding has been uncertain. Contracts have gone from year to year, with many contracts expiring with no new contract to take its place. This uncertainty of funding, together with the toll taken by having sole leadership in group therapy sessions, has led to a significant turnover in staff. Somewhat surprisingly, even with the CSC taking direct administrative control of the clinic, funding remains uncertain and pressure to reduce and limit budgets continues unabated.

Staffing

Recruiting qualified staff has been difficult. As anyone knows who has tried to implement such a program, there is not a pool of experienced sexual offender therapists to draw upon. Our solution has been to recruit the best-qualified generic mental health professionals available, then to train them in the context of the program activities, and to provide close and frequent supervision. For many of our recruits, this method has worked very well. For others, it has become apparent that they have not been suited to the work, and they have left sometimes after only a few months of employment at the clinic.

One problem with staffing that is worthy of special note is the problem of female staff crossing set boundaries with male inmates. We have had a small number of female staff interact with inmate participants in the program in a way that was considered a breach of security, necessitating the termination of their employment. None of these involved explicit "affairs" nor any sexual impropriety, at least as far as we were aware. In one case, a female therapist discussed her difficulties with the administration of the clinic with inmates in her group. In another case, a female therapist had telephone calls from an inmate to her home intercepted by institutional security, yet she did not inform the clinic director of the calls being made. These problems have occurred despite explicit training in security matters at the beginning of employment. Thankfully, these problems have not recurred in the past 4 years, perhaps because of the immediate outcomes in the earlier cases.

Over approximately the last 2 years, the WSBC has undergone a substantial period of administrative transition. It has moved from being funded exclusively as an external contract to it current status of being directly operated by the CSC with a supplemental contract to the program director. When the WSBC was funded entirely through an external contract, it was difficult to recruit and retain full-time staff. This was attributed to the lack of job security as a result of the contract status of the program, the distance of the institution from cities of any size, and the stressful nature of work with sexual offenders, especially in a medium-security federal prison. Now that all full-time staff are government employees, job security has been improved greatly. Although this appears to have reduced staff turnover considerably, the remaining two factors continue to have negative effects on staff recruitment and retention. Further, the public service status of the prisons now means that staff are eligible for transfers to a wide variety of government positions. The allure of such positions has already attracted some clinic staff. Thus, the problem of staff recruitment and turnover has not been eliminated.

As contract employees, our staff often felt isolated from the mainstream of communication and social interactions in the institution, even though there were several other groups of contract staff within the institution. They perceived an immediate and dramatic improvement in acceptance from other employees in the institution once clinic staff became government employees. It became clear that a part of the sense of isolation previously experienced by the WSBC staff was a reflection of the chasm that tends to separate security and treatment–program staff, a difficulty that is found in many institutions and one that is difficult to eliminate entirely. Nevertheless, we learned that in some respects the problem of isolation was not as deep-rooted as originally perceived; it was reduced considerably as a result of improved opportunities to meet and share views with other staff in the institution, primarily in informal settings. In hindsight, we see that there was more that both the clinic and the institution could have done to promote better integration of contract clinic staff within the institution.

Space

Finding adequate space within the institution has been a problem. For the first year, our space was temporary and located in various buildings throughout the institution. Later, we moved into converted space that has been cramped and inadequate. At present, this converted space is being renovated and expanded and will likely provide us, after 8 years of operation, with adequate space. In the meantime, we will spend the fall, winter, and spring months in several construction trailers that have been brought in for the purpose.

Litigation

One new set of problems and our response to them have become a fixture in our day-to-day work at the clinic; namely, the threat of complaints by the inmate participants and the threat of civil litigation by victims of men who have been treated in the clinic. The program director has been named, along with other officials of the CSC, in two lawsuits. In both cases, a former participant in the clinic has escaped custody and in the course of doing so, assaulted new victims. In both cases, the victims and their families have sued, claiming damages and claiming that the clinic was at least in part responsible for their victimization. One case ended after 4 months of trial and the other after several months of negotiation, with the case against the program director being dismissed in both instances. Additionally, the program director has had two complaints laid by inmate participants to his professional college. Both complaints were of the same nature, namely, that the risk assessments done were not representative of their true level of risk and that the men were being coerced into treatment or coerced into participation in research. In one of these cases the complaint was discussed; the other is still pending. Our work at the clinic, the documentation we require of the staff, and the care with which we handle each case, has been influenced by our experience in these lawsuits and complaints.

Standardization

Now that the WSBC is fully integrated into the CSC, it is faced with some new issues. As the number of treatment programs in Canada for federally sentenced sexual offenders has expanded greatly in recent years, there has been increasing pressure for standardization of sexual offender programs across the country. Standardization has the potential for many positive outcomes, including improved mobility of offenders from one treatment program to another, increased understanding of the programs at different institutions, as well as the sharing of information and resources. Nevertheless, such standardization can also have negative consequences. For example, standardization can have negative effects if funding of programs is standardized on the basis of the average cost of programs across the country, without regard to the measured effectiveness of the program or the specific treatment needs of local offenders. Although these have not yet materialized as substantial problems, the possibility of some has been real enough to raise some concerns.

Summary

Arguably, the most important factor contributing to the initial success of the WSBC was its ability to provide quality treatment to a large number of sexual offenders. In large part, this responsiveness resulted from the autonomy afforded by an independent contract and strict adherence to a conceptual model that was heavily based on contemporary research findings. The long-term challenge facing the WSBC will be to maintain program quality and integrity in the face of increasing fiscal restraints and increasing pressure to do more for less money.

BATH INSTITUTION SEX OFFENDERS' PROGRAM

The Bath Institution Sex Offender Program was developed and directed by W.L. Marshall. When the program was initiated (July 1991), Bath Institution was a minimum-security federal penitentiary, but it has since (1995) been upgraded to medium security. However, although the peripheral security features were upgraded, the internal layout is still the open concept of a minimum-security institution. The institution may therefore be best viewed as somewhat of a step down from regular medium security but offering more constraints to the offender than a minimum-security institution. Sexual offenders, whose risk and treatment needs are deemed to be moderate or lower, are sent to Bath Institution either from the Millhaven Assessment Unit or from other institutions such as Warkworth if their risk has been appropriately lowered by treatment. Given this wide range of sexual offender types, the Bath Institution Sex Offender Program offers two levels of treatment. Both levels of treatment aim to reduce the likelihood of reoffending and to prepare the offenders for eventual release through the development of relapse prevention plans. Treatment follows established procedures that have been described elsewhere (Marshall & Eccles, 1995).

Treatment for those offenders deemed by the Millhaven Assessment Unit to be at low or low–moderate risk is far less intensive or extensive than the Warkworth program. The low-risk groups are run on an open format, meaning that each offender proceeds at his own pace, and when he is finished a new offender takes his place. The result of this format is that each group participant is at a different stage in the treatment process, allowing those who have made more progress to valuably assist the new participants. This format also allows us to accommodate to the occasional urgent case. Typically, these low-risk groups have 10–12 participants whose minimum participation is 3 months of two 3-hour sessions per week. The targets in these groups include denial–minimization cognitive distortions, pro-offending attitudes and beliefs, self-esteem, victim harm–empathy, relationship issues, and the preparation of relapse prevention plans (i.e., identifying offense cycles and risk factors, designing plans to avoid or deal with risks and enumerating warning signs). Offenders whose risk levels are moderate or above receive essentially the same treatment program but at a somewhat more extensive and intensive level. This is a closed group format (i.e., all participants start and finish at the same time) running for 4 months with three 3-hour sessions per week. There are typically 8–10 participants per group.

At Bath Institution we do very little in the way of assessment, as this is done very thoroughly at the Millhaven Unit. Evaluation of treatment gains is made by the therapist based on a rating format similar to that used at the Warkworth program. Posttreatment reports include an estimate of risk based on the offender's history plus his determined treatment gains. These reports also stipulate the postrelease conditions that need to be in place to maintain the offender's lowest risk status. Our final reports and the offenders' relapse prevention plans are passed to the case management officer, the national parole board, and both the postrelease supervisory parole officer and the community treatment personnel. It is important to note, however, that postrelease supervision varies quite considerably in quality and many offenders receive no community treatment due to lack of services.

Problems in the Operation of the Bath Program

We have faced very few problems in operating effective treatment programs at Bath Institution. The major initial difficulty was convincing the staff that treating sexual offenders in their institutions would not cause problems. When we started in 1991, there were just over 100 offenders in Bath Institution of whom less than 10% were sexual offenders. Staff (both case management and security staff) thought that offering treatment would identify sexual offenders to the other inmates and chaos and beatings would result. We worked hard to allay these fears, and after 6 months operation none of them were realized; the staff accordingly became fully cooperative. None of this would have happened, however, were it not for the excellent support and enthusiasm of the warden (Sam Brazeau), his deputy (Dave McDonald), and the programs' director (Keir MacMillan). Indeed, all the staff at Bath (including the subsequent wardens) have been and remain fully supportive.

The changes from minimum to medium security, with its attendant physical structural changes, were anticipated with some trepidation, but once again the firm support of all staff made the transition reasonably smooth and did not disrupt our treatment programs. Repeatedly offering brief workshops to staff to outline what we were doing and why (i.e., aiming to reduce the number of future victims), maintaining regular informal contacts with case management staff, and displaying appropriate concern for both security and for the responsibilities and needs of security staff have helped us deliver our programs under as close to optimal conditions as can be achieved within a prison setting.

With the changes in security level, there has also been a marked increase in the institutional population. Bath Institution now has over 300 inmates of whom nearly 50% are sexual offenders. Again, this has not caused any of the anticipated problems. Our funding has increased substantially from an initial support for one therapist (who was and continues to be the director, W.L. Marshall) and one low-risk group, to three therapists running a total of four groups (one moderate–high-risk group, two low-risk groups, and one group that switches between low risk and moderate–high-risk members).

Our initial tentative outcome evaluation on the first 107 men treated and released revealed a 2.7% recidivism rate, but it has been so far impossible to estimate the untreated base rate for our extraordinarily mixed population. For example, in the first four groups we treated, there were three dangerous offenders (i.e., those given a life sentence because of their persistent and dangerous offensive behavior), three sex murderers, eight rapists (four of whom beat their victims so severely they had to be hospitalized for several months), five nonfamilial child molesters with eight or more victims, and, at the other extreme, four incest offenders who were recently convicted of offenses occurring 20 or more years previously (Canada has no statute of limitations).

Perhaps the only significant problem we have encountered has to do with the issue of denial. Of course, we believe that had we not taken the time to assure staff of our good intentions and of our responsibility to their concerns, and had we not been fortunate enough to have such supportive administrators, we would have had considerably more problems. Initially we accepted all deniers into our program with the proviso that admitters (or at least partial admitters) must outnumber deniers in any one group. This worked quite well and our data reveal that we were very effective in overcoming denial and reducing minimization. With the increased demands on our services, we have cut back on the proportion of deniers we accept at initial interview. If they show any sign of some degree of acceptance (e.g., "I must have done it but I can't remember," or "I did have sex but it was consensual"), we will take them into the program, but if they either categorically deny the offense or are appealing the conviction (not the sentence, since we will take men appealing the length of sentence), we turn them away. However, we apprise them of the consequences of denial (i.e., they will be transferred to a less pleasant institution and will probably be denied parole) and, not surprisingly, some weeks later many change their position and accept responsibility for their crimes.

ADDITIONAL PROGRAMS

One important final note is relevant to treatment in both the Bath and Warkworth institutions; that is, each institution has a veritable plethora of other programs to which sexual offenders have access. For example, Bath Institution provides high-quality educational upgrading and occupational retraining, as well as 16 other rehabilitation programs, in addition to sexual-offender-specific treatment. Case management officers implement with the sexual offender a rehabilitation program that includes one of the sexual-offender-specific programs described above plus a selection from the following nonexhaustive list of the 16 available programs: substance abuse, anger management, cognitive skills, parenting skills, and so forth. In addition, almost all inmates complete some educational upgrading. Evaluation of the utility of our sexual offender specific programs is therefore contaminated by the fact that all sexual offenders are involved in one or more (and usually several) of these additional programs. At first glance, our sexual-offender-specific programs may seem somewhat limited until one understands that our offenders are involved in these various other programs.

CONCLUSIONS

The last 8 years have seen a dramatic change and improvement in the treatment available to sexual offenders in the CSC facilities in the Ontario region. Whereas previously inmates had to transfer to the RTC (Ontario) to obtain any treatment, most inmates can now access service in their home institution. This has been accomplished by the implementation of treatment programs in facilities at all levels of security and in most large communities in the Province. These programs are just now beginning to present evaluative research that points to the effectiveness of treatment in decreasing failures on conditional release and recidivism. However, problems remain in terms of the uncertainty of funding, the availability of trained and motivated staff, and an environment of increasing litigiousness among inmate participants and victims of sexual assault.

ACKNOWLEDGMENTS. During the preparation of the chapter, H. Barbaree was supported by a research and service contract from the correctional services of Canada, and M. Seto and H. Barbaree were supported by a research contract from the correctional services of Canada and the Solicitor General for Canada. We are grateful for the financial and other support given. The views and opinions expressed in this chapter are the sole responsibility of the authors and the chapter does not in any way reflect official policy of the correctional services of Canada or the Solicitor General for Canada.

REFERENCES

Barbaree, H. E., & Marshall, W. L. (1988). Deviant sexual arousal, offense history, and demographic variables as predictors of reoffense among child molesters. *Behavioral Sciences & the Law, 6,* 267–280.

Hare, R. D. (1991). *Manual for the Revised Psychopathy Checklist.* Toronto: Multi-Health Systems.

Marshall, W. L., & Eccles, A. (1995). Cognitive–behavioral treatment of sex offenders. In V. B. Van Hasselt & M. Hersen (Eds.), *Sourcebook of psychological treatment manuals for adult disorders* (pp. 295–332). New York: Plenum Press.

Serin, R. C., & Barbaree, H. E. (1993). Decision issues in risk assessment. *Forum of Corrections Research, 5,* 22–25.

6

B. Community Settings

The Lucy Faithfull Foundation Residential Program for Sexual Offenders

Hilary Eldridge and Ray Wyre

The Lucy Faithfull Foundation, named after Baroness Lucy Faithfull, is a child protection agency committed to reducing the risk of children being sexually abused. It runs a residential program for adult male sexual offenders as part of an integrated approach to working with child sexual abuse. The program exists, supported by government funding, as the result of a combination of political support and research showing positive treatment outcome.

HISTORY

Roots and Reasons

The concept of an intensive community-based residential program was first conceived by the second author (Ray Wyre) and initially became reality in 1988, with private backing. It was at that time called the Gracewell Clinic.

Before starting Gracewell, we (both authors) had been running less intensive treatment groups for sexual offenders in prisons and the community. We recognized that for many offenders a full-time residential program was more likely to be effective. In Britain, it was necessary to develop such a project within the criminal justice system rather than in the mental health field. This was because most sexual offenders were not diagnosed as mentally ill and were therefore sent through a criminal justice system that saw punishment and containment alone as the way of dealing with crime. Many sexual offenders were therefore sentenced and subsequently released, still with the same desires, attitudes, and behaviors that had led to the offenses in the first place. A sophisticated prison program for sexual offenders was developed in later years; but although this improved the situation, many offenders in prison still remain untreated.

However, the main impetus for setting up the residential clinic in 1988 came about not because of criminal sentencing issues but as part of the preparation for the 1989 Children

Hilary Eldridge and Ray Wyre • The Lucy Faithfull Foundation, Birmingham, England B48 7EA.

Sourcebook of Treatment Programs for Sexual Offenders, edited by Marshall et al. Plenum Press, New York, 1998.

Act, new legislation over which Lucy Faithfull exerted influence. This Act encouraged the child care system to remove the alleged offender from the home rather than taking the children into care.

Removal of an abuser from the home is insufficient, since untreated abusers may continue to manipulate families. Even when ties are broken, they may join a new family and abuse again. The criminal law is often unable to prosecute due to lack of forensic evidence, and alleged child abuse cases are often addressed solely in civil proceedings. In Britain, these operate on the balance of probability, and hence the same level of evidence is not needed as for criminal cases. In offering a residential facility for abusers and alleged abusers, we provided space for family members within which codes of silence could be broken, grooming could stop, and change could take place. This was particularly important for men and their families for whom the mental health and criminal justice systems could not offer a way forward.

Program Effectiveness

The Gracewell program ran until 1994, and it was positively evaluated by a team of independent researchers, known as the STEP team, who produced a report for the government (Beckett, Beech, Fisher, & Fordham, 1994). Pre- and posttreatment measures, which are described in their report, were used to test a sample of 20 Gracewell residents. Seventy-five percent of these men were categorized by the STEP team as higher deviancy on offense- and personality-related scales. Level of deviancy was identified by the extent to which these men deviated from the STEP team's sample of nonoffenders on a number of their measures. The measures included levels of social inadequacy, lack of empathy for victims of sexual abuse, distorted thinking, sexual obsessions, and emotional identification with children. The men categorized as high deviancy showed clear differences from the nonoffending sample on all the reported measures, while those categorized as low deviancy did not differ so greatly from the nonoffenders on most of the measures.

The high-deviancy group when compared to the low-deviancy group also had tended to commit offenses outside or both inside and outside the family, against boys or both boys and girls, and were nearly twice as likely to have committed a previous sexual offense. These men had a higher risk of reconviction based on Thornton's algorithm, and had a much higher rate of being abused as children (Thornton & Travers, 1991; Fisher & Thornton, 1993).

All 20 of the men in this sample made much greater progress at Gracewell than those similarly categorized in nonresidential community-based programs. Sixty percent of the men in the Gracewell sample who were categorized as higher deviancy reached a normal profile when tested posttreatment, showing a significant treatment effect. Follow-up data indicate that none of the offenders assessed by the STEP team as having been significantly treated had been reconvicted within 2 years. This includes those who were assessed as highly deviant before treatment (Hedderman & Sugg, 1996). An analysis of whether this can be maintained requires a longitudinal study, including reassessment at 5- and 10-year intervals.

Community Problems and Political Solutions

Sadly, the results of the initial research were revealed after Gracewell's enforced closure. Even though careful selection of residents and good monitoring resulted in no resident reoffending while at Gracewell, its location within the community was unpopular and local protest eventually led to closure. The events surrounding this are described elsewhere (Wyre & Tate, 1995).

However, we had developed a clear vision of our future within the context of a new charity, the Lucy Faithfull Foundation. Lucy Faithfull had committed her life to working with children and she believed the best way of protecting children was to treat abusers. The Lucy Faithfull Foundation took over the work of Gracewell, and plans were underway to open another residential clinic. The Gracewell program had already been validated by research and was to be directed by staff who had designed and run it. Hence, what was needed was a location and financial support.

The search for a new clinic proved extremely difficult. Organized and effective protests were encountered whenever we attempted to open. People in city areas recommended a country location and country people recommended the city. It became clear that no one wanted a clinic near them. Most sexual abusers are either not prosecuted or are sentenced and later released, and hence are living freely in the community. While accepting this fact and the need for treatment, people often said, "We would rather not know they are there." Attempts to be open in discussing our work and engaging in consciousness-raising events about offending as a cross-cultural, cross-class issue, were met with comments such as "You've destroyed our innocence." We became increasingly concerned about a society that wishes to live under an illusion of safety.

However, as our founder, Lucy Faithfull, an active politician and lifelong children's advocate, commented: "Democracy sometimes works!" Eighteen months after Gracewell's closure, the Lucy Faithfull Foundation's new residential clinic was eventually established in a hospital setting, following approaches to two government ministries. Appeals were made to leading politicians and top-level government officials who gave financial and moral support to the foundation after a long and determined campaign by Baroness Faithfull.

Our message that work with abusers is about child protection, together with research showing a positive treatment effect, was getting through. As British programs developed generally, the dream of a progressive system was also becoming a reality. Our clinic is complementary to other community-based facilities, especially those run by the probation service. It is also complementary to the prison program, providing an opportunity to extend work started within that program and for offenders to progress from secure, to residential-supervised, and on to nonresidential-supervised intervention.

ETHOS FOR CHANGE: A THERAPEUTIC ENVIRONMENT

The context within which a program exists is at least as important as its content. We continued our work for the Lucy Faithfull Foundation's new clinic on the same principles we had applied at Gracewell. We make these explicit to the offenders who join the program.

We need to create a noncollusive but safe place for change. Offenders need to feel it's safe to relax defenses and allow themselves to be vulnerable. Therefore, the context in which the work is carried out and the relationships therein needs to be challenging but also supportive. A safe place is one built on honesty, not on false promises. Being honest with offenders from the beginning about the parameters for our work is crucial. We work on the basis that honesty begets honesty. Offenders are formally introduced to our principles shortly after arrival. The main principles we follow are described below.

Operating Principles

We are first and foremost agents of child protection. We have a clear policy of close communication and information sharing with other relevant agencies, especially with workers supporting child victims and nonabusing parents. Both at Gracewell and the Lucy Faithfull Foundation we have been proactive in sharing information. The Lucy Faithfull Foundation works with whole families. Out of knowledge of offenders and issues for those on the receiving end of the offender's cycle, we developed an integrated approach that acknowledges individual needs and uses information from work with the offender to free children and other family members from the sense of guilt and responsibility the offender has placed on them. We know that offenders constantly manipulate, not just to gain compliance, but to entrap children and drive a wedge between the children and those who could protect, thereby preventing disclosure. Information about how an offender has managed this can be used to heal rifts he has created within families.

We carry out assessments on offenders so that other agencies including courts can make decisions about their future. We make it clear to the offenders that we are part of that decision-making process, and will pass information on to other agencies.

We do not trust residents to stop offending. Most do not trust themselves, and provided that this issue is addressed sensitively, it can aid the change process. An abuser has probably said many times that he is going to stop abusing, only to abuse again. We want to create a relationship with offenders that avoids "conning games." Offenders need to know that we do not automatically believe what they say. Experience of running weekly groups has taught us that a man may abuse on the way home from a group, and yet each week in group seem very committed. It is important that the men are aware that we know this happens. Each man needs to recognize that creating conning relationships automatically affects the possibility that he can ever change. If he believes that we are accepting without question information he gives, he will know that he has conned us and will in many ways lose hope, as he will have no confidence in our ability to work with him and help create the change within him that is necessary to prevent reoffending. One reason for helping offenders to provide honest information is that it gives them hope for change: using a biblical metaphor, "The truth will set you free." Many offenders do not want to face up to the truth about themselves and their behavior. One of the fears that men have is "if you really knew me, you would hate me." It is important that we give messages that we will be there for them whatever they say, however unpalatable. Working with the information is at times painful but essential if we are to facilitate change.

Challenge is necessary, especially in the early stages of the work when the offender's thinking errors are so powerful. However, familiar therapeutic ideals about respect for the person are adhered to. This, combined with concern to help the abuser build a satisfying offense-free lifestyle for himself, is crucial. The group environment should be one in which the men feel safe to experiment with new ideas, thoughts, and behavior and to take painful steps forward, in the knowledge that they will be appropriately supported. The emphasis is on self-challenge and encouraging residents to work things out for themselves rather than being "told." This produces real change as opposed to parroting the "right" words. We try to ensure that all techniques are used to clear purpose in a positive, facilitating way, which, although challenging of men's beliefs and attitudes, does not belittle, humiliate, or "put down." Interviewing techniques are described in more depth elsewhere (Wyre, 1996).

The work needs to address gender issues and female and male staff have to present a common stance and theme to offenders. Men and women together must present a common front to challenge many of the stereotypical views that are presented by offenders. Sexism, racism, homophobia, and other forms of oppressive attitudes and behaviors are challenged.

We ask each offender to look at that which is abusive in himself. In order to do that, he needs to hold on to and harness that which is good about himself: he may have been a father, a colleague, an employer, he has loved, he has cared, but he has also abused. If he fails to hold onto that which is good, he will see himself as the "animal," the "evil monster." This will not make him safer and may suggest an inability to change, thereby providing another excuse to offend.

We need to know about men's offending both specifically and generally. Some may have abused many children. Vague, general information is not evidence and is of little value in criminal proceedings, but it may assist in the external monitoring component of relapse prevention. As men progress through the change process, they sometimes give the names of previously undisclosed victims in order that those children can receive appropriate help and care. We encourage this and explain that we will notify the relevant authorities. Our experience is that such disclosure does not automatically mean prosecution will follow, but we give no false promises as to how the authorities will deal with it.

The offender is not on a course where at the end he receives a certificate that says he has "made it." The work must be more than just about delaying another offense, and hence each man needs to recognize that his learning and control must go on for the rest of his life. Cure implies sickness. Most sexual offenders are not diagnosed as mentally ill, and therefore the work will usually be done within a criminal framework. The words "intervention" and "control" are more appropriate than "treatment." We believe offenders can change their behavior; they can exercise control and they can be different.

Decisions are not always consistent either within the criminal or children's courts. Decisions regarding family reconstruction or contact are often made on the basis of differential policies between areas and may have little to do with the feelings of family members or a man's progress in therapy. The decisions of the criminal courts seem at times to be affected by other cases that currently have a high media profile. While such anomalies exist, and they always will, discussion about injustice is important. It is a fact of life, but does not provide an excuse to offend.

Offenders need to know that some of our decision making concerns the politics of the work. Most such community-based projects are not wanted by the community. Clinic staff's decisions about the men's access to the community, what they can and cannot do, are made within this context as well as within the context of each man's own actual risk. Explanations and feedback about these issues are essential if an honest relationship between staff and residents is to be maintained. Adherence to the spirit as well as the letter of the strict conditions we impose on offenders is more likely when the decision making is understood.

THE PROGRAM: FROM GRACEWELL
TO THE LUCY FAITHFULL FOUNDATION

Assessment

The original Gracewell program began with a 4-week full-time residential assessment. Using group and individual therapy, standardized questionnaires, and written and video-taped exercises, we identified the nature of the pattern or cycle of offending at a thinking, feeling, and behavioral level. We assessed the offender's ability to challenge his own thinking and learn from the comments of others and his developing motivation to change. Information about his progress was shared with the referrer and, where appropriate, with his family and those working with them.

Twenty-four-hour staff cover enabled ongoing assessment to take place both formally within the daily therapy groups and informally during the evenings and weekends. The staff worked closely together to share information about the congruency of a man's behavior across structured therapy and more informal settings.

Intervention Program

After assessment, men moved into the full-time intervention program for between 6 and 12 months. This included structured modular groupwork, individual therapy, and a more informal evening and weekend residential program.

A multicausal analysis of offending was matched by the use of a range of therapeutic approaches, primarily cognitive and behavioral, but including the use of drama and art to access feelings in a more interactive way. We aimed to address the beliefs, feelings, attitudes, and behavior patterns that legitimized and supported offending. The open-ended nature of the groups ensured that men could act as "culture carriers"; those who had been in the therapy groups for some time could help and challenge those who were at an earlier stage of change.

Therapy took place in a context that addressed attitudes to women and children, power versus intimacy and responsibility in relationships, and perception of self. The prevention of reoffending was our primary aim, and we developed an increasing emphasis on relapse prevention.

The structured daytime group therapy program was modified over time to finally include four core elements that related to the cycle and are crucial in reducing the risk of reoffending. These were victim awareness–empathy development, the role of fantasy in offending patterns, sexuality and relationships, and assertiveness–anger management. Each core element contained four modules. These were led by the same basic aims: namely to restructure the thinking errors of perpetrators, to promote change at an emotional as well as intellectual level, to challenge abusive behavior patterns, and to foster links between new learning, the individual's offending cycles, and relapse prevention. In addition, module and perpetrator-specific aims and objectives were set. The modules were different from but not more advanced than each other, and so formed a rolling program, which allowed men to enter at any stage. Individual sessions focused primarily on developing sexual fantasy control techniques, therapy relating to survivor issues, restructuring of generalized thinking errors, and development of relapse prevention plans and external networking, including work related to family issues in liaison with specialist staff and the referring agency.

At times the offender's therapist co-worked with other specialist staff and referring professionals to run family meetings. Such meetings ran in parallel with other work that was undertaken with children and family members. These involved couple counseling or other dyadic work and work with whole families. Our knowledge of offender grooming tactics helped us avoid potentially abusive scenarios. Important ground rules for a session that included both the offender and the survivor were that "it does not tap back into grooming or offending behavior ... and is empowering for the survivor" (Eldridge & Still, 1995).

THE LUCY FAITHFULL FOUNDATION'S
NEW RESIDENTIAL PROGRAM

The new program is based on that of Gracewell and has maintained much of its framework, but includes improvements identified through experience as well as information gained from the STEP team's research. An outline of the program is shown in Table 6.1.

The outcome data produced by the external research team (STEP) showed that despite

TABLE 6.1
**The Lucy Faithfull Foundation Residential
Program: An Outline**

4-week assessment
  Psychological tests (used by the STEP team)
  Group exercises
  Individual exercises
  Observation in formal and informal settings
  Introduction to the concept of relapse prevention
  Family-related work and interagency liaison begin
Preintervention phase
  Overcoming the blocks to effective intervention
  In-depth identification of offending pattern
  Beginning to identify a relapse prevention plan
  Family-related work and interagency liaison continue
Intervention/relapse prevention program
  Structured rolling program
  Individual therapy
  Evening skills-based program
  Informal evening and weekend activities
  Family-related work and interagency liaison continue
Monitoring and evaluation throughout
  Videotaped recording system
  Measures and reviews for pre- and post-intervention
  Observation in formal and informal settings
  Monitoring the relapse prevention plan in action

---

the fact that the majority of the men in the Gracewell sample fell into the high deviancy, high risk of reoffending category, improvements were achieved across specific offense-related areas, reducing justifications and distorted thinking and improving victim empathy. However, as in the other programs in the study, a minority developed more distorted attitudes to their victims posttreatment, and hence we subjected our victim empathy work to a major rethink.

The men in the sample showed improved levels of social adequacy; that is, improved self-esteem, reduced emotional loneliness, and reduced underassertiveness posttreatment. This result was particularly pleasing given that the men's pretreatment scores deviated greatly from the normal sample. Marshall (1989) emphasizes the need to include a focus on these areas to reduce the likelihood of reoffending.

THE IMPROVEMENTS

Psychometric Testing

The battery of personality and offense-related measures, which include measures used by the STEP team, arc employed pre- and postintervention (see Table 6.2).

Preintervention Phase: Working with Blocks to Receptivity

We had been concerned for some time that many of the higher deviancy offenders appeared blocked from making progress. As a consequence, we developed the "preintervention" phase for the Lucy Faithfull Foundation's program. After 4 weeks in residential

Table 6.2
Battery of Personality and Offensive-Related Measures

Pre- and posttreatment
  Offense focused
    Children and sex cognitions scale: Emotional congruence and cognitive distortions (Beckett, unpublished)
    Sex offense attitudes questionnaire (Proctor, 1994)
    Relapse prevention (Beckett, & Fisher, unpublished)
  Personal history
    Database. NOTA (National Association for the Development of Work with Sex Offenders)
  Intelligence
    Ammons Quick Test (Ammons, & Ammons, 1962)
  Self image
    Self esteem (Thornton, unpublished)
    Special Hospitals Assessment of Personality and Socialisation (Blackburn 1982)
    Intimacy: UCLA Emotional Loneliness Scale (Russell et al., 1980)
    Fear of negative evaluation (Watson, & Friend, 1969)
    Inventory of interpersonal problems (Horowitz, Rosenberg, Baer, Ureno, & Villasenor, 1988)
  Victim awareness/empathy
    Victim empathy scales (Beckett and Fisher unpublished)
    Empathy scale (Hanson, & Scott, 1995)
  Perspective taking
    Social desirability scale (based on Greenwald & Satow, 1970)
    Empathy: Interpersonal Reactivity Index (Davis, 1980)
  Sexual attitudes and arousal pattern
    Multiphasic Sex Inventory (Nichols & Molinder, 1984)
    Sexual fantasies questionnaire (Fisher, unpublished)
  Self-control
    Michigan Alcoholism Screening test (Selzer, 1971)
    Locus of control (Nowicki, 1976)
    Anger questionnaire (Buss & Perry, 1992)
    Rumination of anger questionnaire "Indicators of Aggression" (Caprara, 1986)
    Assertiveness: Social response inventory (Marshall, unpublished)
    Impulsivity questionnaire (Eysenck & Eysenck, 1978)
Measures and exercises for use at regular intervals throughout the program
  Group environment scale (Moos, 1986)
  Residential checklist. Prison core sex offender treatment program (unpublished)
  Individual clinical rating form (Hogue, 1982)
  Offenses, effects and who is to blame (videotaped exercise) (Eldridge & Wyre, unpublished)
  Breaking the cycle: Offense description and matching relapse prevention plan (videotaped exercise) (Eldridge, 1998b)

assessment, we have a clear view of the individual blocks that prevent a man from being receptive to the program. During preintervention, we focus on a more in-depth analysis of the offending cycle, including the part played by thoughts, feelings, and the senses—sights, sounds, smells, taste, and touch. This helps offenders identify some of their less conscious blocks to change. Blocks commonly include low self-esteem and profoundly negative thinking patterns leading to an expectation of negative evaluation. Extreme vulnerability makes it very difficult for such individuals to accept criticism from others or to engage in self-challenge. During this period we begin work specifically aimed at producing change in these areas, especially on the development of realistic positive thinking.

Another major block to change, especially in the area of victim empathy, relates to childhood experiences as victims of sexual abuse. Those offenders who were clearly sexually victimized as children but deny they were victims, saying "I liked it, I enjoyed it, I consented—in fact it wasn't abuse at all," need early work on this issue. The probable reality is that they tried to take some power back as children by believing they were in control of the abuser and were also encouraged to believe this by their abuser. The problem is that now they are using the same beliefs to say that their victims were willing partners who gave consent. So long as offenders believe this, it is unlikely they will stop abusing. Such men may be blocked from developing victim empathy because to do so puts them in touch not only with their victim's pain, but also the pain of their own sexual victimization. They may have to look at their own childhood in a new and painful way and the sense of loss experienced can be great. Demonstrating empathy with a man's pain, while maintaining clarity about adult responsibility for offending, is an important stance for the therapist to take. By modeling empathy in this way, therapists also begin to help offenders learn to empathize with themselves as children and with their own victims.

Behavioral Techniques for Fantasy Control

At Gracewell, work in this area was part of the structured group work program and as such applied to everyone. However, this work needs timing to suit individuals and is not appropriate for all offenders. Hence, we transferred the work to individual sessions, preferring to use the groups to focus more clearly on the broader role of fantasy and imagination in the offending cycle.

Victim Empathy

The STEP team identified that the men categorized as being high deviancy, who were the most likely to reoffend, often suffered from high levels of emotional loneliness, poor self-esteem, and lack of assertiveness. They suggested that programs should seek to improve these areas before victim empathy training is given. They commented:

> Failure to enhance coping skills and self-esteem may leave some offenders feeling bombarded with the consequences of their sexually abusive behavior but without the emotional resources to cope. As a result some offenders may intensify their cognitive distortions and justifications and become hardened in their attitudes to their victim as a defence strategy. (Beckett et al., 1994, p. 139)

As a consequence, we made two improvements to the new program. First, we began working in the newly developed preintervention phase on the potential blocks to empathy development. Second, we developed a new model for working directly with victim empathy.

There is a lack of clarity in the literature regarding whether sexual offenders have a generalized empathy deficit or whether this is person or target group specific. Some studies (e.g., Hudson et al., 1993) showed that sexual offenders displayed poor skill at recognizing the emotions displayed by both adults and children. Marshall, Fernandez, Lightbody, and O'Sullivan (1994) found in their study that the child molesters were markedly deficient at discerning the emotions their own victims experienced. Our own experience is that some offenders have such marked generalized empathy deficits that work beginning with basic emotional recognition training is required. We begin this work in the new-skills-based evening sessions for those residents who demonstrate a need for it. However, lack of empathy specifically with their own victims is a common theme in the majority of the residents. While some develop empathy for other people's victims, they move quickly into blaming and minimizing harm done when talking about their own victims.

Victim empathy–awareness is one of the core elements of the structured rolling (i.e., open-ended) program. We run an alternative to these modules that is designed for men who have done sufficient preparatory work. This is still in development but essentially focuses on offenders' own victims, culminating in role-play on similar lines to that described by Pithers (1994).

Assertiveness, Anger Management, and the Skills-Based Program

Repeated unassertive behavior can lead to feelings of injustice, frustration, resentment, depression, and vulnerability; all the kinds of emotions that often precede offending and start the relapse process in those offenders who had promised themselves to "never do it again." In order to be effective, release prevention plans require assertive behavior on the part of the offender. Remaining unassertive provides one of the best excuses for reoffending: "I didn't intend to baby-sit; I just didn't like to say 'no!'" Teaching assertiveness skills removes part of the excuse mechanism. In remodeling the Gracewell program for the Lucy Faithfull Foundation, we linked the assertiveness–anger management core element with a new skills-based evening program in which skills are taught according to identified need. In the evening program, assertiveness skills are taught and applied to everyday life. A link with sexual offending is not made directly, as it is important for the men to be encouraged to recognize that they are not just sexual offenders; they are people who can engage in interpersonal relationships of all types. Learning how to be assertive in the world is a key part of developing a lifestyle where the offender feels equal to others and empowered to make choices and take positive opportunities. Being appropriately assertive requires the other skills taught in the evening program: emotional recognition, social skills, problem-solving skills, decision-making skills, realistic positive thinking, and in some cases specific anger management work, as well as direct training in how to become more assertive. It is important to give sufficient opportunity for these skills to be learned by breaking down the skills into their component parts and practicing them.

The daytime assertiveness–anger management core element is directly offense related. In this context, the men are expected to make clear links between what they have learned about assertiveness and positive self-talk generally and their offending cycles and relapse prevention.

Relapse Prevention as an Integral Part of the Program

At Gracewell, work had begun on a detailed relapse prevention program with an accompanying workbook for residents (Eldridge, 1998a), but this was not implemented until the opening of the Lucy Faithfull Foundation's new clinic in 1995. Relapse prevention has become the core of the program with all work explicitly linked to it. Staff and residents are expected to start thinking in relapse prevention terms from the outset of each man's stay. The emphasis on this increases as men progress, and the staff and residents' manuals and workbooks reflect this. For example, the checklists staff complete before and after each session in the interests of program integrity include direct questions about links to relapse prevention. Residents use the new workbook, *Maintaining Change*, which is based on relapse prevention principles, throughout their stay and thereafter. It is introduced to them at the preintervention phase between leaving assessment and starting the long-term intervention program.

Part of each group work module is dedicated to how new learning relates to relapse

TABLE 6.3
The Rolling Groupwork Program and Relapse Prevention

Core element	Module	Length
Victim awareness/empathy	1	8 days + 2 relapse prevention focused
Fantasy in offending	1	8 days + 2 relapse prevention focused
Sexuality and relationships	1	8 days + 2 relapse prevention focused
Assertiveness and anger management	1	8 days + 2 relapse prevention focused
Videotaped monitoring exercise identifying cycle and revising relapse prevention plan		
Victim awareness/empathy	2	8 days + 2 relapse prevention focused
Fantasy in offending	2	8 days + 2 relapse prevention focused
Sexuality and relationships	2	8 days + 2 relapse prevention focused
Assertiveness and anger management	2	8 days + 2 relapse prevention focused
Videotaped monitoring exercise identifying cycle and revising relapse prevention plan		
Victim awareness/empathy	3	8 days + 2 relapse prevention focused
Fantasy in offending	3	8 days + 2 relapse prevention focused
Sexuality and relationships	3	8 days + 2 relapse prevention focused
Assertiveness and anger management	3	8 days + 2 relapse prevention focused
Videotaped monitoring exercise identifying cycle and revising relapse prevention plan		
Victim awareness/empathy	4	8 days + 2 relapse prevention focused
Fantasy in offending	4	8 days + 2 relapse prevention focused
Sexuality and relationships	4	8 days + 2 relapse prevention focused
Assertiveness and anger management	4	8 days + 2 relapse prevention focused
Videotaped monitoring exercise identifying cycle and revising relapse prevention plan		

prevention (see Table 6.3). The ongoing monitoring system includes exercises focusing specifically on the cycle and the development of a linked relapse prevention plan. The "Breaking the Cycle" videotaped exercise (Eldridge, 1998b, p. 16) is repeated after each group of modules and helps build the relapse prevention plan based on increased knowledge of personal cycles and risk factors. The entire program is about the development of an offense-free lifestyle built from self-knowledge and awareness of individual risk factors. Behavioral observation plays a key role in challenging mismatches between words and actions and developing "live" relapse prevention plans.

In addition to structured groups, there are unstructured groups and individual sessions, which provide an opportunity for discussion of self-monitoring. Routes to relapse and thinking, feeling, and behavioral cues to individual risk patterns are discussed and coping strategies are identified. By these means it becomes possible to determine which of a man's emotional needs and wants were being met in his offending. The presence of seemingly innocent and unrelated thoughts, feelings, or scenarios in the cycle, especially in its early stages, help the offender to pick up early warning signals and control his behavior in the future.

Perpetrator Monitoring: Congruency between Words and Behavior

This takes place in the context of the measures described earlier and regular reviews, where possible involving referring professionals and taking account of the views of family members.

In order to measure progress, staff take account of the goals set and achieved and the level of congruency between what the offender says, how he thinks, what he believes, how he expresses feelings, and above all, how he behaves. Linked to this, and of equal importance, are the views of staff who are working with him in both formal and informal settings. If, for example, a staff member examines the facts and recognizes progress but still feels uneasy, this may suggest that the perpetrator is giving incongruent messages.

Regular meetings take place between the referring professionals and our own staff to ensure that knowledge is shared appropriately and that the referrer will be in a position to monitor the offender on the basis of good quality information after his discharge from the program. Opportunity can be negotiated for ongoing contact by Lucy Faithfull Foundation staff with the offender and the professionals working with him postdischarge. Wherever possible, we encourage the setting-up and implementation of long-term monitoring networks. Separate ongoing contact can be made available for the perpetrator's family, through our child and family specialists, regardless of whether or not family reconstruction or contact is being considered.

Program Effectiveness

As the new program has been running for just 1 year and the length of stay in our program is usually 12 months, we do not yet have treatment outcome data on a significant number of men. However, the effectiveness of the overall program and of its discrete components is the subject of ongoing monitoring by both the Home Office and ourselves. The relapse prevention questionnaire has been run at an interim stage, and "the group is performing quite differently to untreated sexual offenders and distinctly better than the Gracewell sample" (D. Thornton, personal communication, 1996). The program and the techniques used are in constant development, being updated with current research findings.

Summary

Our residential program has relapse prevention as its core. It provides 24-hour supervision. Offenders progress through a 4-week assessment plus preintervention work to prepare them for the 12-month intervention program. This includes structured relapse prevention-linked group therapy 5 days a week, individual work, family work, a formal evening skills-based program, and informal relapse prevention-linked work at evenings and weekends. Ongoing monitoring includes observation, case reviews, psychological testing, clinical interviews, relapse prevention plan presentation, and program monitoring.

Problems and Solutions

Despite our emphasis on the importance of using information about how offenders manipulated families to help in the survival process of family members and child victims, it remains difficult to access adequate funding for specialist work with them. Child protection agencies often assume that because the offender is physically away from the family, children are now safe and intervention is unnecessary. This leaves nonoffending parents to deal with the family dynamics the offender has created. This is rather like trying to piece together a jigsaw without having the complete picture as a guide. Work with families needs to access information from offenders from assessment onward, regardless of whether family reconstruction is being considered. In fact, this kind of information can help nonoffending parents make informed choices about the future without the legacy of guilt and responsibility that has been placed on them by the offender. Currently, we are trying to access new sources of funding for this important work.

Long-term follow-up studies will be required to demonstrate how effective we are in preventing reoffending. However, program effectiveness studies will need to take account of the fact that our offenders fall primarily into the high-deviancy group as defined by Beckett et al. (1994). Hence, we cannot sensibly compare their reconviction rates against average deviancy untreated sexual offenders; we will need to control for high deviancy.

If relapse prevention is to be effective, we need much longer-term monitoring and program callback facilities. Currently, the agencies that take over offender monitoring postdischarge do this in the context of relatively short statutory orders. New government proposals should help to lengthen contact, but agencies are underresourced to cope with this. Indeterminate treatment orders within the criminal justice system need to be considered if sexual offender treatment is to be taken seriously.

Sexual offenders need external as well as internal monitoring. To do this properly, we need effective communication and information sharing between criminal justice and child care agencies and we need public education that empowers rather than frightens people. Agency information sharing could be facilitated by the development of a database for sharing information about offender patterns and relapse prevention plans. It would include type of offender, previous convictions and alleged offenses, targeting and grooming tactics, detailed risk factors, and the relapse prevention plan including external monitoring networks. This would be shared by police, offender treatment agencies, and the main child protection agencies. Inclusion in the database could be a condition of program attendance.

We also need to involve the community in offender monitoring. The media portrayal of offenders is usually a monster image linked to child murderers. Most offenders are respected citizens who appear ordinary to others and to themselves. Without consciousness raising about sexual offending, panic and witch hunting can lead to offenders moving from place to place. In order for relapse prevention to be effective, sexual offenders need to be able to engage in a social life that is safe in the context of their individual pattern of offending. This requires an aware culture in which the offender is not an outcast but neither is he the subject of naive trust. The Lucy Faithfull Foundation is committed to working to develop such a culture.

REFERENCES

Ammons, R. B., & Ammons, C. H. (1962). *Ammons Quick Test*. Missoula, MT: Psychological Test Specialists.

Beckett, R., Beech, A., Fisher, D., & Fordham, A. S. (1994). *Community-based treatment for sexual offenders: An evaluation of seven treatment programs*. London: Home Office Publications Unit.

Beckett, R. (1987). Children and Sex Questionnaire: Cognitive distortions: Emotional congruence. Unpublished description in R. Beckett, A. Beech, D. Fisher, & A. S. Fordham (1994). *Community-based treatment for sexual offenders: An evaluation of seven treatment programs*. London: Home Office Publications Unit.

Beckett, R., & Fisher, D. (1994). Victim Empathy Scale. Unpublished Description in R. Beckett, A. Beech, D. Fisher, & A. S. Fordham (1994). *Community-based treatment for sexual offenders: An evaluation of seven treatment programs*. London: Home Office Publications Unit.

Beckett, R., & Fisher, D. (1994). Relapse Prevention Questionnaire, Unpublished. Description in R. Beckett, A. Beech, D. Fisher, & A. S. Fordham (1994). *Community-based treatment for sex offenders: An evaluation of seven treatment programs*. London: Home Office Publications Unit.

Blackburn, R. (1982). Special Hospitals Assessment of Personality and Socialisation. Unpublished. Ashworth Hospital, Liverpool, England.

Buss, A. H., & Perry, M. (1992). The Aggression Questionnaire. *Journal of Personality and Social Psychology*, *63*, 3, 452–459.

Caprara, G. V. (1986). Indicators of aggression: The dissipation–rumination scale. *Personality and Individual Differences*, *7*, 763–769.

Davis, M. H. (1980). A multi-dimensional approach to individual differences in empathy. JSAS Catalogue of Selected Documents in Psychology, 10, 85. Reproduced in A. C. Salter (1988). *Treatment child sex offenders and their victims: A practical guide* (pp. 291–293). Newbury Park, CA.

Eldridge, Hilary (1998a). *Therapist guide for maintaining change: Relapse prevention for adult male perpetrators of child sexual abuse*. Thousand Oaks, CA: Sage.

Eldridge, Hilary (1998b). Breaking the cycle videos. In Hilary Eldridge (1998a). *Therapist guide for maintaining change: Relapse prevention for adult male perpetrators of child sexual abuse* (pp. 16–17). Thousand Oaks, CA: Sage.

Eldridge, Hilary (1998c). *Maintaining Change: A personal relapse prevention manual*. Thousand Oaks, CA: Sage.

Eldridge, H. J., & Still, J. (1995). Apology and forgiveness in the context of the cycles of adult male sexual offenders who abuse children. In *Transforming trauma* (pp. 131–158). Thousand Oaks, CA: Sage.

Eysenck, S. B. G., & Eysenck, H. J. (1978). Impulsiveness and venturesomeness: Their position in a dimensional system of personality description. *Psychological Reports*, *43*, 1247–1255.

Fisher, D., & Thornton, D. (1993). Assessing risk of re-offending in sexual offenders. *Journal of Mental Health*, *2*, 105–117.

Greenwald, H. J., & Satow, Y. (1970). A Short Social Desirability Scale. *Psychological Reports*, *27*, 131–135.

Hanson, R. K., & Scott, H. (1995). Assessing perspective taking among sexual offenders, non-sexual criminals and non-offenders. *Sexual Abuse: A Journal of Research and Treatment*, *7*, 259–277.

Hedderman, C., & Sugg, D. (1996). Does treating sex offenders reduce reoffending? *Research Findings, No. 45*. London: Home Office.

Horowitz, L. M., Rosenberg, S. E., Baer, B. A., Ureno, G., & Villasener, V. S. (1988). Inventory of interpersonal problems: Psychometric properties and clinical applications. *Journal of Consulting and Clinical Psychology*, *56*, 885–892.

Hudson, S. M., Marshall, W. L.,Wales, D., McDonald, E., Bakker, L., & McLean, A. (1993). Emotion recognition in sexual offenders. *Annals of Sex Research*, *6*, 199–211.

Keltner, A., Marshall, P. G., & Marshall, W. L. (1981). Measurement and correlation of assertiveness and social fear in a prison population. *Corrective and Social Psychiatry*, *27*, 41–47.

Marshall, W. L. (1989). Intimacy, loneliness and sexual offending. *Behavioral Research and Therapy*, *17*(5), 491–503.

Marshall, W. L., Hudson, S. M., Jones, R., & Fernandez, Y. M. (1995). Empathy in sex offenders. *Clinical Psychology Review*, *15*(2), 99–113.

Marshall, W. L., Fernandez, Y. M., Lightbody, S., & O'Sullivan, C. (1994). The assessment of person specific empathy deficits in child molesters. Submitted for publication.

Moos, R. H. (1986). *Group Environment Scale Manual, 2nd Edition*. Palo Alto, CA: Consulting Psychologist Press.

Nichols, H. R., & Molinder, I. (1984). *Multiphasic Sex Inventory Manual*. Tacoma, WA: Nichols & Molinder.

Nowicki, S. (1976). Adult Nowicki–Strickland Internal–External Locus of Control Scale. Test manual available from S. N. Nowicki, Jr., Department of Psychology, Emory University, Atlanta, GA.

Pithers, W. D. (1994). Process evaluation of a group therapy component designed to enhance sex offenders' empathy for sexual abuse survivors. *Behavior Research and Therapy*, *32*(5), 565–570.

Russell, D., Peplau, L. A., & Cutrona, C. A. (1980). The revised UCLA loneliness scale: Concurrent and discriminant validity evidence. *Journal of Personality and Social Psychology*, *39*, 472–480.

Selzer, M. L. (1971). The quest for a new diagnostic instrument. *American Journal of Psychiatry*, *127*, 1653–1658.

Thornton, D., & Travers, R. (1991). *A Longitudinal Study of the Criminal Behavior of Convicted Sexual Offenders*. Proceedings of the Prison Psychologists' Conference. London: HM Prison Service.

Thornton, D. (1994). Self-esteem Questionnaire. Unpublished. Description in R. Beckett, A. Beech, D. Fisher, & A. S. Fordham (1994). *Community-based treatment for sex offenders: An evaluation of seven treatment programs*. London: Home Office Publications Unit.

Watson, D., & Friend, R. (1969). *Measurement of Social–Evaluative Anxiety. Journal of Consulting and Clinical Psychology*, *33*(4), 448–457.

Wyre, R. K. (1996). *Conference papers*. Birmingham, England: The Lucy Faithfull Foundation.

Wyre, R. K., & Tate, T. (1995). *The murder of childhood*. London: Penguin.

7

B. Community Settings

Community-Based Treatment with Sexual Offenders

Anthony Eccles and William Walker

The Forensic Behavior Services run a community-based clinic for the assessment and treatment of sexual offenders. The following chapter will describe the assessment and treatment procedures employed by the clinic and will stress particular problems or issues associated with running such a clinic in the community.

PROBLEMS

Funding Issues

The clinic is primarily funded through probation and parole services at both the provincial and federal levels. In addition, the clinic provides services to child welfare agencies, lawyers, and the courts. It is discreetly located in the commercial part of the city, set apart from any schools or residential neighborhoods.

As noted above, the clinic is largely dependent on correctional services for the funding that keeps it operational. This funding is expensive and difficult to obtain. In general, to acquire the funding in the first place, upper management generally has to be convinced that: (1) there is a need that has to be addressed; (2) that the proposed assessment and treatment services can effectively address this need; (3) that they can do so in a cost-effective manner; and (4) that it is the responsibility of that ministry or department to meet the cost of these services. As the number of convicted sexual offenders continues to rise, there is generally little difficulty with (1) and for (2) and (3); there is sufficient research evidence to warrant some optimism about treatment outcome and cost effectiveness (e.g., Marshall & Barbaree, 1990). When it comes to negotiating a budget, agencies always want more for less. The nature of the client population makes it important, however, that in the push to be more efficient with taxpayers' money (as we all should be), the integrity of the program is not compromised in the bargaining process. For example, we have turned down contract offers in which a funding agency wished to put a cap of six sessions per client. With many clients,

Anthony Eccles and William Walker • Forensic Behaviour Services, Kingston, Ontario, Canada K7L 1A8.
Sourcebook of Treatment Programs for Sexual Offenders, edited by Marshall et al. Plenum Press, New York, 1998.

nothing meaningful can be achieved in this time and the net result would have simply been the appearance and not the practice of treatment.

We have received funding from the provincial ministry for the past 10 years. We attribute the longevity of this relationship to the strong support we receive from probation–parole officers, who have recognized the role and value of treatment in the supervision of offenders in the community. The contracts we have enable us to see clients on probation or parole at no cost to the offenders themselves. Referrals from all other sources are charged on a fee-for-service basis. In our opinion, ideally the offenders themselves would be responsible for meeting the costs of their own assessments and treatments, "paying for their crimes" in a literal sense. The reality of the situation, however, is that the majority of offenders attending the clinic have few financial resources. Many are unemployed and live in a meager fashion on welfare payments. We have, in the past, endeavored to have offenders pay a nominal fee ($10) for each visit. However, it was our experience that the time involved in keeping track of these payments and attempting to get the funds from those who fell behind was a poor use of our resources. Nonetheless, when opportunities present themselves, we encourage referring agencies such as the Children's Aid Society to recoup from offenders some of the fee we charge the agency, and in many cases the costs are split between the agency and the individual being referred.

Security Issues

One less apparent disadvantage of running a small community clinic versus running a program within an institution is that security is a greater concern in the community. Offenders can be challenged and confronted within the prisons where there are guards nearby and where the offenders can be monitored closely. Guards can serve as deterrents to unruly behavior or can intervene if necessary and can closely monitor the offenders after group. While this does not altogether eliminate the risks involved in this work, it certainly reduces them. Furthermore, imprisoned offenders are made aware that negative reports that affect the offender (e.g., by taking away his chances of a successful parole application) generally appear within the contents of reports from case managers rather than from the therapists themselves. In the community, however, there is not the same level of security either during or after meetings. Furthermore, negative reports can have the effect of preventing an offender from having access to his children or may cause a spouse to leave her husband. These reports are more likely than institutional reports to be "stand alone" reports, making clinicians more vulnerable when offenders are angered, particularly if they are vindictive in nature and feel that they have nothing left to lose. Concerns of this kind over the years have led us to consider all referrals carefully and to refuse any offender whom we feel poses too much of a risk to be appropriate for a community-based clinic.

Support Issues

It is essential to have the strong support and backing of probation and parole officers in order to run an effective clinic in the community. These officers must make it clear that they expect the offenders to attend and participate, that they will not be flexible on this matter, and that they will lay breach of probation charges if necessary. Having the probation officers be the "enforcers" avoids complicating the role of the therapist in a manner that is countertherapeutic. We believe that the closer the probation and parole officers work with the clinic, the better is the overall service provided. We have been involved in training probation officers in regard to the work we do at the clinic. As such, they are familiar with the concepts and terminology of the relapse prevention portion of the program. This helps them to understand reports from the clinic and assists them in their supervision of the offender. Likewise, the feedback we get from the officers is invaluable in our work with the offenders. Through our discussions with other treatment professionals, we have come to believe that the role of probation and parole officers is generally underestimated and underutilized in many programs. We have used probation officers as cofacilitators in group sessions for several years now and we have found this to be an extremely successful partnership.

In addition to the above, it is also essential that community clinics have the support of the community in which they are based. Members of the public may be extremely concerned about some of the offenders attending the treatment program, on occasion with very good reason. While most treatment programs are responsible and make offenders accountable for their actions, on occasion we have encountered a misperception among community members that treatment program providers are uncritical advocates for offenders. Community support can evaporate in the face of such a perception, replaced by a climate of mistrust that can make it extremely difficult for a clinic to function. It is therefore essential that community clinics for sexual offenders make a strong effort to establish ties with other agencies and groups, particularly those that work with survivors of sexual abuse. Many survivors' therapists have encountered professionals who are working with offenders despite having a poor understanding of sexual abuse issues in general and survivor issues in particular. Understandably, this can make survivor therapists cautious about clinicians they do not know working with offenders. Therefore, ties need to be established to build trust and acceptance, in turn providing for better interagency cooperation and enhanced service provision. It is important to be open about what work is being done with the offenders, to seek the input of therapists who work with survivors on matters relating to victim impact issues, and to include them and/or survivors directly by having them talk to offenders in group meetings.

Finally, an issue that may be of more relevance to clinics in small cities like ours is that because there are relatively few community-based programs for sexual offenders, our clinic gets a great deal of requests from inmates in the many prisons in southern Ontario seeking acceptance into our program, acceptance they hope to use as part of their release plans in applications to the parole board. However, many communities are understandably very sensitive to an influx of high-risk sexual offenders, and a community program that is perceived to be attracting such offenders—who do not come from that community and who would not otherwise go there—will meet with a lot of opposition. Every community has its sexual offenders and therefore must reabsorb some upon release, like it or not. However, this absorption must be appropriate for the size of the community. For this reason, we have a policy of not accepting anyone who applies to the clinic while still incarcerated. If they are paroled to this area and if their parole officer refers them to us, then we will see them. We will not give this guarantee of acceptance beforehand, however. This undoubtedly complicates matters for offenders who are trying to establish release plans, but it helps to ensure that those offenders who do get paroled here are from the community or who otherwise have supports sufficient to convince a parole board that their coming to this community makes sense. This both increases the offenders' ultimate chances of success and helps to maintain support for the clinic in the community.

ASSESSMENT

Assessment Process

There are essentially three phases to the assessment process. Over a period of two to three half days, each offender undergoes interviews, responds to standardized questionnaires, and completes phallometric testing. From this information, we conduct a risk assessment and an evaluation of treatment needs and suitability, as well as making any other recommendations that are pertinent. For example, if the assessment is being conducted for a sentencing hearing, recommendations may be made regarding the kinds of conditions that might be appropriately attached to a probation order. The content of the risk assessment itself is beyond the scope of this chapter. Suffice it to say that a combination of offense, actuarial, and clinical factors are used in aggregation to determine an overall level of risk. Extremely high-risk offenders may be recommended for an institutional program rather than for community-based treatment where the intensity and supervision required is not available. Very low-risk offenders may be passed over in favor of allocating our limited resources to those who are at greater risk. In general, we find that candidates in the moderate-risk range are the most suitable, along with high-risk offenders who have received prior institutional programming.

Assessment Limitations

Because we are a community clinic, we get referrals from a very broad range of individuals and agencies. The most problematic referrals come from individuals (or their legal representatives) whose cases are still before the courts at the trial stage, or before Family Court as part of a custody and access dispute. In our experience, this is the area in which most community-based clinicians are likely to have problems. For this reason, it is an area that we will discuss in some depth.

It is not unusual to get a referral from the accused or his legal counsel, seeking an assessment to indicate that he does not fit the "profile" of a child sexual abuser and therefore is unlikely to have committed the offense. We take the view that no clinician should ever take on such a referral in which the issue is to establish likely guilt or innocence. There is absolutely no test, phallometric or otherwise, that is capable of establishing an individual's potential guilt or innocence (Marshall, 1996). Thus, while there may be *group* differences between offenders and nonoffenders on a certain test, there is so much overlap between the groups that it is not possible to reliably identify a given individual as being a member of one group or the other. It is helpful to consider the following analogy to illustrate the absurdity of using relatively small group differences to make such decisions: A person of unknown gender is measured to establish their height (our "test" in this case). Having completed this test, Dr. X looks at height norms and discovers that the average height for males is 175 cm and the average height for females is 163 cm. Dr. X then confidently concludes that because the height of the person measured approximates the higher of these values, the person clearly does not fit the "profile" of a female and therefore must be male.

With respect to sexual offenders, this kind of faulty reasoning is seen most frequently with phallometric testing. All too often we see cases in which a clinician conducts such a test, finds that the accused responds to consenting adults and not at all to children, then asserts in the report that the accused does not fit the profile of a child molester and is unlikely to have committed the offense. Not only do groups of offenders and nonoffenders overlap considerably, in fact many convicted and admitting offenders show no evidence at all of deviant sexual arousal. Furthermore, among familial offenders, deviant sexual arousal is the exception rather than the rule (Barbaree & Marshall, 1989). This is significant, as we find that most referral requests of this kind are cases of alleged intrafamilial sexual abuse.

It is indeed regrettable that some clinicians still go to court on behalf of an accused to argue that he "could not" or "likely did not" commit a given offense. (In general, such clinicians tend to be arguing the case for the defense. However, it clearly would be just as untenable for the clinician to argue the converse, namely, that an accused likely did commit the offense based on his test results.) In our opinion, this practice represents a blatant misuse of a sexual behaviors assessment. We routinely turn down such requests for our services. Occasionally we do accept certain requests from Family Court to assist in a matter where no criminal charges have been laid despite serious allegations (e.g., because the child may be too young to testify). Even when we accept such cases, however, we make it quite clear that the determination of whether the allegations are founded or not is the court's jurisdiction. Our reports in these instances simply remark on the accused's relative risk to reoffend and the implications of this in the event that the court believes the allegations have merit. However, we discourage even these assessments on the grounds that they are not particularly useful.

TREATMENT

Treatment Process

Involvement in treatment for most participants begins in a group. Exceptions to this are female offenders, offenders with intellectual limitations, and adolescent offenders (i.e., under 18 years of age). For each of these types of sexual offenders, we typically do not have sufficient numbers at any one time to run a group. Treatment with these clients is done on an individual basis. Hereafter, we will speak of our clients as though they were all adult males, but we expect the reader to infer that the same issues are relevant to treating other offenders, except, of course, the group process.

At the man's first group treatment session we have him read over and sign a treatment contract and consent form. If a client refuses to sign this form, we consider him to have declined to participate, and we will not take him into our treatment program. The matter is then referred back to his probation or parole officer.

We run two types of treatment groups at the clinic, both of which meet once per week for 2 hours at a time. The first type of group is a "closed" group, in which all group members start at the same time and finish 15 to 20 weeks later. All participants in a closed group address the same topics at the same pace. In a closed group, we place individuals who have not participated in treatment before and occasionally individuals who have not done the work in an open group and who we feel need the structure of a closed group.

The second type of group is an "open" group, an ongoing group that runs continuously with no common start or end. Individual participants enter when a spot becomes available and they leave when they have completed the requirements of the program and have benefited as much as necessary or to the extent that they are likely to. In the open group, we place offenders who have been through treatment before (most commonly in provincial or federal institutions) and are continuing, as well as individuals whom we consider not to need the full closed group program. We have had high-risk offenders involved in the open group for periods of 2 years or more and we have had some low-risk individuals involved for as little as six sessions.

Each man's involvement in treatment begins with him presenting a complete history of his sexual offending, with group members and the therapist(s) asking him questions. Questions depend on what the man has to say about his crime(s). Men who accept responsibility are asked to discuss further the various factors involved in their offending. Men who deny or minimize their sexually abusive behavior are asked questions about the discrepancies between what they say and what others have said and are given feedback by the group. They are asked to think about this, with particular emphasis on the importance of accepting responsibility. It is explained that not only will this benefit him, it can also help those others he has affected and continues to affect. These men are asked to present their disclosure a second time to the group. Individuals who continue to deny or significantly minimize committing their offenses after this second or sometimes a third presentation are terminated from the group. The curriculum beyond presentation of disclosures is directed at those who have admitted committing a sexual offense; it would be a sham to have deniers remain in group following disclosures to have them discuss, for instance, the impact of their (non)offense on others, the chain of events leading up to their (non)offense, or their strategies for avoiding a (non)reoffense.

Following acceptance of responsibility, we generally work to have the man identify and understand a number of aspects about himself and about his offending. Our treatment program takes a cognitive–behavioral perspective and a relapse prevention approach. We want the man to address who he is—his general characteristics (e.g., underassertive, dominating, impulsive, etc.) and attitudes. We want him to address what was going on in his life during the time leading up to the offense (e.g., relationship difficulties, work pressures, financial pressures) and how he responded, operating from the general premise that men commit sexual offenses when things in their lives are not going particularly well. We want him to address the specifically sexual preoffense elements in his thinking and behavior that must have been present for him to choose to act in a sexually abusive manner. In standard relapse prevention fashion, we have the man develop plans to address the precipitating factors established through analysis of these issues.

To provide a structure for this work, we have developed a workbook with a number of exercises in it addressing:

1. Acceptance of responsibility for all sexual offending
2. Clarification of the impact of their offending on the victim and others
3. The man's offense chain
4. Thinking errors associated with the offending
5. Warning signs along the road to reoffense
6. Table of consequences associated with decisions to reoffend or not to reoffend
7. Building a support network
8. Developing relapse prevention plans

We have individuals complete these exercises and other relevant exercises as we see fit, and we have the men present their work to the group over the course of treatment.

Following the completion of the group, we meet with each participant for a number of individual sessions (usually between 6 and 10) to revise and refine work done over the course of the group. For some individuals we also remain in contact with them to provide ongoing maintenance.

Treatment Suitability Issues

We offer places in treatment to all individuals who have been determined to need it. We present involvement in treatment as a unique opportunity for participants to learn about themselves and plan for the future. We emphasize that they are unlikely to find themselves with a similar forum in which to discuss these difficult subjects in a nonjudgmental atmosphere.

We consider involvement in treatment to be voluntary, and it is the man's choice to attend or not. If a man decides not to attend, we certainly will not "make" him. However, almost all offenders come to us with a court-imposed condition to participate in treatment. Judges in this area now order offenders to *participate* in treatment rather than simply a requirement to *attend* or *enter*. This took some time to establish, but the distinction is an important one that has greatly facilitated our efforts. Thus, the client must choose between participating in treatment or facing the consequences of not participating (e.g., being charged with breach of probation, possible return to jail, loss of access to children). Many men do not eagerly embrace either of these choices and, not surprisingly, feel that they are being "forced" to participate by people who hold sway over them. As noted earlier, in our experience it is better to have the probation or parole officer do the "enforcing" and have the therapist simply lay out the choices. If a client indicates that he is unwilling to attend, we will not expend a lot of energy convincing him to do so; that is the probation officer's job, and one they tend to do very effectively.

We offer treatment to (almost) all we think need it, including individuals who deny committing their offenses. We adhere to the principle that higher-risk individuals (among others, those who deny their offenses) warrant the allocation of more treatment resources.

There are two exceptions to this general rule. The first is the group of offenders who are very high risk and who have had no prior involvement with institutional programming. We do not consider that the level of treatment service we can provide (generally a maximum of one group or individual session per week) is sufficient to meet the treatment needs of these offenders.

The second group are the long-term absolute deniers who are extremely unlikely to change. These intransigent deniers characteristically enjoy considerable support for this denial from family and friends; they have maintained their innocence throughout the court process (e.g., pleaded not guilty, made the victims testify); they have already completed the full term of their sentence; and their victim(s), if family members, are ostracized by the rest of the family. While these men's perspective on their offending raises their risk to reoffend, and in theory we should therefore devote more treatment resources to these individuals, we consider it very unlikely that individuals in this particular situation will see it as being in their best interests to change their position on their offending. Because our treatment resources are limited, we generally do not take these individuals into treatment. We instead have them write (to our satisfaction) a number of 10-page educational essays on, for instance, the effects of sexual abuse on victims and others, why most sexual abusers are male, and excuses used by sexual offenders. We do not consider working on these essays to constitute participation in treatment. We do leave the door to our treatment program open to these offenders by telling them that we will take them into the program if they change their perspective on their offending and wish to participate. Such turnaround is rare; more commonly, if these individuals do reappear at the clinic for treatment, it is because they have reoffended and have become a little more open-minded about the possible benefits of treatment.

Outreach Issues

Our clinic covers a large catchment area, an approximately semicircular area with a radius of 125 km bordered on the south by Lake Ontario and the St. Lawrence River. Since this is a large area, our clients often have difficulty with transportation; to make things a little easier we run treatment groups in Kingston and Belleville, a small city 75 km west of Kingston. We also often hold individual treatment sessions at the various probation offices we serve and we meet with clients at other agency offices (e.g., Children's Aid offices). This serves two functions for us: permitting clients easier access to our services, and allowing us to get to know face-to-face the various probation officers and other staff from whom our clients receive service.

Attendance Issues

Sexual offenders are considered to be a fairly difficult, resistant clinical population. In institutional settings it is generally not hard to track down treatment participants, and the implications for participating versus not participating in treatment while incarcerated can be weighty (e.g., parole vs. no parole).

In the community, however, problems with compliance can arise without a coordinated approach among treatment providers, probation and parole services, and other involved agencies. In the first place, it is essential that at sentencing the courts put in place conditions that require the offender to attend assessment and to participate in treatment. Second, without the support of the probation and parole service who must enforce these conditions, treatment programs themselves have little or no ability to get offenders to attend. Attendance rates can be expected to be low if there are no consequences associated with not participating in treatment. With the support of local probation officers, attendance by offenders with a court order to do so is in excess of 95%. Of those who attend, approximately 4% are asked to leave by us for poor participation, approximately another 2% leave because they are charged with another offense, and about 1% of group members drop out.

We have encountered treatment providers from other jurisdictions who are unable to achieve a high rate of client participation; we give all credit for our success in this respect to the probation officers and managers. In our jurisdiction, offenders who refuse to participate in court-ordered treatment are routinely charged with failure to comply or breach of probation, and we have seen probationers sent to jail for noncompliance. Though this could make for an overall less-enthusiastic group of participants, in fact, this does not appear to happen. What does happen is that these responses underscore the seriousness with which society views these crimes and the need to address the issues that led to them in the first place, and it puts people in treatment chairs so they *can* address these issues.

Adaptability Issues

Institutional relapse prevention efforts, valuable as they are, are somewhat hampered by the fact that they are developed to address a situation to be faced in theory, not one being faced in practice. Men in treatment at our clinic often remark that their lives in the community are quite different from what they had anticipated during incarceration, and that as a result the relapse prevention plans they made while inside require (sometimes extensive) revision. For this reason, we stress the necessity of adaptability in relapse prevention plans, incorporating and addressing unanticipated difficulties and working to develop and broaden the man's scope of alternatives to offending. As well, relapse prevention plans developed in prison often mention employing abilities and opportunities not demonstrated in the community and intentions not yet pursued. We stress to clients the need to regularly analyze their situations, modifying their plans to take into account things they thought would work out but did not, and to include new interests.

Community Support for the Offender

We consider it vital to have the man develop a support network in the community, a network of people who are not only aware of the man's offenses but who are knowledgeable about the work he has done over the course of treatment and to whom he can turn in times of difficulty. When possible, we ask the man's partner to attend the clinic with him to review the man's offending and the work he did over the course of the group, including his identification of risk factors and his plans for avoiding trouble. On occasion, our discussions with the partner about the man's crimes are the first time she has heard the details of the offenses from someone other than the man himself (the partners are most often women). Though we tell the man that we will talk with his partner about our understanding of his offenses, giving him a chance to tell her himself what she is likely to hear from us, the details we present may differ, sometimes markedly so, from what she has been told by him. This can cause friction between the man and his surprised partner, but we consider it important that she knows the truth and that we know she knows the truth. We review with her his warning signs and relapse prevention plans, discussing how she can be of assistance to him in his efforts, but emphasizing that preventing a reoffense is his responsibility, not hers, and that it should not be her role to act as the enforcement person.

We also have offenders identify other sources of community support apart from partners, therapists, and supervision personnel. These commonly include parents, siblings, friends, employers, religious supports, Alcoholics Anonymous sponsors, and other professionals involved with the man and his family.

Family Reunification Issues

As a result of his crime, the offender is commonly separated from his partner and children by order of the Children's Aid or by a condition of probation. Not infrequently, the man and his family desire to reunite. In these cases our first priority is to determine if we think reunification should even be contemplated (i.e., is this risk at all manageable). We base our evaluations here on our estimates of the man's risk to reoffend, the partner's belief in the man's guilt and perspective on reoffending, the victim's vulnerability, and so forth. There have been occasions when we have considered the man's risk simply too high for us to feel confident under any circumstances; in those instances we support the maintenance of conditions prohibiting contact with the children until they reach age 16 years, after which time children's protection agencies and probation services typically have no authority over the man.

More often, however, the family will get back together at some point in the not too distant future. Our aim in these cases is to help the family make the transition with as clear an understanding as possible about who was responsible for the abuse (the offender), what changes must be made and safeguards implemented to minimize the possibility of a reoffense, and who is responsible for making those changes (again, the offender).

We coordinate our efforts in this respect with the agency providing service to the child. Once the man has been through our treatment program and we are satisfied with the quality of his work and his understanding, we have the man prepare an apology to the child and to the family. This apology typically contains the man's acceptance of responsibility for the offending, acknowledgment of the harm he has done, and commitment never to reoffend again. It is presented to the victim when the victim is ready to hear from the offender, a determination made by the victim and his or her therapist.

Beyond Completion of Treatment

Once we are satisfied that the man has gotten as much out of treatment as he is likely to get, we bring our formal involvement with him to an end. We have a wrap-up session involving the man and his probation officer in which the probation officer asks the man questions about the work he did over the course of his involvement with us. We expect the man to be able to answer these questions knowledgeably, without referring to his written work. We also write a report about his progress in treatment including our revised assessment of his risk to reoffend, taking into account his participation with us.

After the end of our formal involvement with the man, we may continue to meet with him periodically for follow-up sessions. As a rule, we continue to have contact with moderate–high- and high-risk cases every 2–3 months, this risk level being determined by our posttreatment assessment of risk. Our limited resources are such that we do not schedule these sessions for moderate- and lower-risk cases. However, if any client asks for them, they are of course scheduled. We like to meet with the man at his residence when possible, as we feel this provides a better, more ground-level picture of how the man is living. These sessions reflect not only the long-term perspective of the relapse prevention philosophy, but also the conclusions of follow-up research (Hanson, Steffy, & Gauthier, 1992). Even after the end of follow-up sessions, we will still make ourselves available as a source of support; essentially, "once a client, always a client," though most men prefer not to think of their involvement with us in this way.

Treatment Evaluation

The efficacy of treatment has been extensively reviewed elsewhere (Marshall & Barbaree, 1990), and it is beyond the scope of this chapter to summarize all this work. Suffice it to say that there is sufficient evidence to provide optimism that sexual offenders, particularly child sexual abusers, can receive treatment that lowers their risk to reoffend. We will refer to two studies in particular, however, as they reflect the work conducted at the Kingston Sexual Behaviour Clinic from which the current program was established. Marshall and Barbaree (1988) published a study that followed child sexual offenders treated at the clinic for an average of approximately 4 years. They found that recidivism rates were markedly lower for treated than for untreated groups. Specifically, the comparisons of recidivism rates for treated versus untreated groups were 18% versus 43% for molesters of nonfamilial female children, 13% versus 43% for molesters of nonfamilial male children, and 8% versus 22% for incest offenders. Similarly, in a study that examined treatment outcome for exhibitionists, Marshall, Eccles, and Barbaree (1991) reported that there also were treatment effects for exhibitionists with treated–untreated recidivism rates of 24% and 57%, respectively. Thus, while there is clearly room for improvement, there is also evidence to support the efficacy of community-based treatment for sexual offenders on probation and parole.

REFERENCES

Barbaree, H. E., & Marshall, W. L. (1989). Erectile responses amongst heterosexual child molesters, father–daughter incest offenders and matched non-offenders: Five distinct age preference profiles. *Canadian Journal of Behavioral Science, 21,* 70–82.

Hanson, R. K., Steffy, R. A., & Gauthier, R. (1992). *Long-term follow-up of child molesters: Risk predictors and treatment outcome.* (User Report No. 1992-02.) Ottawa: Corrections Branch, Ministry of the Solicitor General of Canada.

Marshall, W. L. (1996). Psychological evaluation in sexual offence cases. *Queen's Law Journal, 21,* 499–514.

Marshall, W. L., & Barbaree, H. E. (1988). The long-term evaluation of a behavioral treatment program for child molesters. *Behaviour Research and Therapy, 26,* 499–511.

Marshall, W. L., & Barbaree, H. E. (1990). Outcome of comprehensive cognitive–behavioral treatment programs. In W. L. Marshall, D. R. Laws, & H. E. Barbaree (Eds.), *Handbook of sexual assault: Issues, theories, and treatment of the offender* (pp. 363–385). New York: Plenum.

Marshall, W. L., Eccles, A., & Barbaree, H. E. (1991). The treatment of exhibitionists: A focus on sexual deviance versus cognitive and relationship features. *Behaviour Research & Therapy, 29,* 129–135.

8

B. Community Settings

The Portland Sexual Abuse Clinic

Barry M. Maletzky and Cynthia Steinhauser

AN OUTLINE OF THE CLINIC

Despite the almost magical advances in the physical sciences over the past quarter century, it still seems that the most interesting disciplines are those that address the roots of human behavior. At least so it seemed to those of us participating in the early 1970s in what we naively thought to be a grand experiment in applying principles of behaviorism to the treatment of maladaptive behaviors, such as overeating or sexual compulsions. Skinner had explained it all and it was simply left to us to prove clinical utility.

Fortunately, throughout the years, a broader understanding has developed of what it means to treat sexual offenders. After 25 years, we continue to retreat and begin the experiment again. From what we have learned, we hope to share our attempts to solve problems large and mundane, which will undoubtedly continue to contribute partly cloudy weather to the climate of community-based sexual offender programs into the coming millennium.

PERSONNEL

There should have been no problem in applying behavioral principles to the treatment of sexual offenders. In 1973, in an era of clinical optimism, we began to treat offenders, using aversive conditioning. More than two decades later, we still do, but, hopefully, with somewhat more sophistication and understanding and with the added benefit of cognitive techniques. At first, the methods and the population in which we were interested were enough to garner attention. There were few therapists interested in treating sexual offenders then; it is not yet a crowded field.

Of 27 therapists working for the sexual abuse clinic through these years, 20 have had doctoral-level degrees; the remainder have had MSW, LCSW, MS, or MA degrees. Just six have been women, but the best judge of who will succeed is still the level of interest and energy therapists display in and devote to their work, rather than their gender or the degree after their names.

But it is a difficult field, and therapist turnover is common. Still many of the clinic's therapists have been happily involved for over a decade. Some sustaining features in these

Barry M. Maletzky and Cynthia Steinhauser • The Sexual Abuse Clinic, Portland, Oregon 97202.
Sourcebook of Treatment Programs for Sexual Offenders, edited by Marshall et al. Plenum Press, New York, 1998.

tasks may have been the involvement of all personnel in research and teaching and in sharing clinical responsibilities within a multidisciplinary treatment team. Moreover, some therapists have chosen to subspecialize, enjoying what they do best, for example, in providing aversive therapy, social skills training, family therapy, or group therapy. It has proven helpful to have a medical doctor associated with the clinic for diagnosis and possible treatment of any concomitant medical or psychiatric conditions and for the rare cases when a medication, such as depo-Provera or Prozac, might aid in treating the sexual offender.

There is little hierarchal structure within the clinic, although the senior author serves as director and performs all evaluations, referring clients to individual therapists based on what each needs first, whether group (often an orientation group) or individual therapy (often after an orientation group), family therapy, social skills training, aversive conditioning, relapse prevention, and so forth. All therapists are truly created equal in this semi-democracy; indeed, the clinic has no employees. Its therapists are independent professionals operating their own practices (often *not* exclusively involving sexual offender work, even for the director), banded together to share clients, techniques, knowledge, and support. It has worked well thus far, but assuredly, it is not the only way.

FACILITIES

Although the Sexual Abuse Clinic began in a cramped 10-feet by 10-feet suite, staff now enjoy a number of locations throughout the Northwest, most with more spacious quarters. Despite the addition of cognitive therapy elements, relapse prevention, empathy training, and social skills components over the years, much behaviorally based treatment is still provided. Hence, a laboratory has been essential in each location.

At a minimum, a clinic should have available a plethysmograph, a ready supply of penile gauges, a slide projector, videotape equipment, and the capacity to present audiotaped stimuli. Garnishes over the years have included multicolored biofeedback lights automatically linked to the plethysmograph, vicarious sensitization videotapes (Maletzky & McFarland, 1996), automatic odor pumps, and odor delivery systems employing oxygen cannulae, and the ubiquitous anatomically correct dolls so useful for aversive behavior rehearsal (Wolfe, 1984). With modern-day, elaborated practical technologies, the list will undoubtedly grow; by the time of this text's publication computer-aided design (CAD) software to present visual stimuli and to coordinate novel assessment techniques may be commonplace (Osborn, Abel, & Warberg, 1995).

In the laboratory, the client is linked to nasal cannulae, a penile gauge, and earphones and is presented with diverse and peculiar stimuli; this truly places the offender in the hot seat. Despite this artificial environment, we *do* see penile responses in a surprising number of offenders. Habituation to the laboratory and trust building have both played a role. The offender sits in the same chair to talk to the therapist and to build trust. He comes to realize that he will not be harmed; this is the same chair he sits in for a plethysmograph or to receive aversive conditioning. Attempts to make the offender feel respected may be as important as the technical feats all this equipment can perform (Marshall, 1996).

MARKETING PROBLEMS

Clinic referrals have come largely from corrections officers (65%), usually after sentencing. A substantial number, nonetheless, have been referred by children's agencies

(15%). Many of these latter men have molested children in their own homes. Another 10% have been referred by their attorneys, usually before sentencing. The remaining 10% come from other professionals or enter the clinic under pressure from family, victims, or, rarely, their own consciences. Approximately 55% of offenders treated have molested young girls and the majority of these (70%) have been situational familial offenders, underscoring the outpatient nature of this clinic. However, 35% of clinic patients have either committed crimes against strangers and/or raped, some serially. Of all offenders against girls, 25% have been predatory; among all offenders against boys, 40% have been so. Clinic therapists are thus no strangers to managing risk.

In a simpler age, word of mouth was sufficient to generate more patients than we could treat. In more competitive times, we have attempted to maintain market presence primarily by palpably demonstrating twin concerns: foremost, concern to prevent further victims, but also concern to regard the offender as a member of our own species. Simple human kindness in the face of heinous acts has been rewarded, not only by more referrals, but by the unexpected gratitude of the community, other professionals working with the offender, corrections officials, attorneys, families, and the press. A rigid accusatory manner toward the offender may reap only temporary benefit; professional and concerned are attitudes that can be combined.

Among other devices to bring positive attention to our clinic, our staff has learned that educational efforts are priceless. We provide free seminars to corrections officers, children's agencies and other professionals involved with offenders, and the general public. Topics have included updates on assessment and treatment techniques, reviews of clinical and academic topics, and interesting case histories, especially those presenting novel problems for supervision. From time to time, we have included offenders presenting their own stories—some self-serving, some heroic; sometimes putting a human face on a monster helps.

We have been able to extend educational efforts to the professional community by presenting elective seminars for psychiatric residents at the local medical school and on grand rounds as well. Some residents have accepted an offer to "intern" in our clinic, with actual patient contact. Presentations are given at schools, churches, and clubs. Interviews with the press, often tricky, can still provide value in educating the public about the harm that sexual abuse can cause and about some of its origins; most importantly, they deliver the message that it can be treated.

Beyond formal educational efforts, clinic personnel have been tireless in arranging and attending quarterly meetings with probation and parole officers and other referral sources. A conference is generally arranged with corrections specialists at their offices at their convenience. Corrections personnel may want to discuss individual problem cases under treatment, but inevitably, general topics also arise. The face-to-face meetings have immense value in demonstrating therapists' dedication. Clinic staff have been instrumental in formulating and implementing an area-wide plan to assign and train sexual offender specialists in corrections. Several staff members have even served on regional corrections advisory committees.

After a quarter century of working with sexual offenders, and working with others who do, we have learned that the most important approach to generating goodwill is communication. Every month each referral source receives a typed update of that offender's program in group or individual therapy. Every quarter, that official also will have received a call or visit from the therapist. Any time an offender is in trouble (lapsing, missing appointments, drinking), the referral source will hear from us. We will lean in favor of notification as opposed to confidentiality if there is any hint of risk. We have learned well the lessons of building a support and monitoring system.

It is less clear what, if anything, our commitment to a quarterly newsletter has wrought. While general opinion among marketing experts is negative, at least a newsletter has kept our names known in the community. Recent topics have included brief descriptions of treatment techniques, abstracts of scholarly journal articles touching upon topics of treatment and supervision and new clinic policies (e.g., an updated list of graduation criteria or a new exit test). Frequent mailings serve a similar purpose, for example, a brochure notifying referral sources of a new therapist's qualifications or of an upcoming seminar.

Based on our experiences, a clinic would do well to expand geographically by opening satellite offices if at all possible. Besides visibility, presence in a local community brings therapists closer to a source of concern and facilitates communication with regional authorities, as well as eases the burden of transportation for offenders who do not live in the metropolitan area.

Perhaps the largest potential source for referrals and greatest boon to community presence is also the most overlooked: participation in research. We have been privileged to have treated over 7500 sexual offenders in 25 years. We have met this good fortune with a research program designed to inform us and the communities we serve whether or not our treatments, undoubtedly similar to many cognitive–behavioral programs in North America, have been effective. As an outpatient clinic, this has been no small obligation; but it also has been a pleasure, even when statistics do not go our way. Table 8.1 presents the barest bones of our outcome data, although based on strict criteria (specified in the table), and with

TABLE 8.1
Treatment Outcome for Paraphilias[a]

Category	n	Percentage meeting criteria for success[b-d]
Situational pedophilia, heterosexual	3,012	95.6
Predatory pedophilia, heterosexual	864	88.3
Situational pedophilia, homosexual	717	91.8
Predatory pedophilia, homosexual	596	80.1
Exhibitionism	1,130	95.4
Rape	543	75.5
Voyeurism	83	93.9
Public masturbation	77	94.8
Frotteurism	65	89.3
Fetishism	33	94.0
Transvestic fetishism	14	78.6
Telephone scatologia	29	93.1
Zoophilia	23	95.6

[a] $N = 7156$.
[b] A treatment success was defined as an offender who:
  1. Completed all treatment sessions.
  2. Reported no covert or overt deviant sexual behavior at the end of treatment or at any follow-up session.
  3. Demonstrated no deviant sexual arousal, defined as greater than 20% of maximum erection on the penile plethysmograph, at the end of treatment or at any follow-up session.
  4. Had no repeat legal charges for *any* sexual crime at the end of treatment or at any follow-up session.
[c] Any offender who dropped out of treatment, even if he met other criteria for success, was counted as a treatment failure.
[d] Follow-up sessions occurred at 6, 12, 24, 36, 48, and 60 months after the end of active treatment.

follow-up periods of one to 23 years. Additional references may interest the inquisitive reader (Maletzky, 1993).

We cannot be smug about published results, not when 25% of our rapists will rape again; 5% of child molesters who remolest is 5% too many. Nonetheless, we should be proud of the advances our field has made and should not shrink from publicizing them. It is a remarkable story, first told in this decade. Although mature, this tale is not yet finished.

Not every clinic has had as much experience as we, but each clinic has something to teach: a series of offenders perhaps treated somewhat differently, an interesting case, a tough problem uniquely solved, or an idea of how to proceed in tricky waters. Information hidden in case files or a therapist's memory has perhaps helped just one patient; information shared could help legions.

SPECIAL PROBLEMS IN A COMMUNITY-BASED CLINIC

Safety

Risk to the community must be of the utmost concern when treating sexual offenders, especially because currently, many dangerous offenders reside in neighborhoods, not institutions. While debate swirls about whether community notification lessens risk, clinics still need to demonstrate their commitment to safety and can do so in a number of ways, some well-proven, others novel and experimental; some may need to be unique, depending upon local conditions.

One approach that our clinic has taken is to promote offender accountability. Should an offender miss an appointment, a supervising officer is notified immediately. While not every lapse is reported, any serious situation or probation violation is, as for example, drinking, moving near a school, or starting to date a woman with children. Because gaps have often occurred between initial referrals to the clinic and the first evaluation session, it has helped to have two or more professionals accessible to perform evaluations so this delay can be avoided. In addition, data entry has been established in such a way that a greater than 2-week delay without an offender being seen automatically triggers an alarm and a call or letter to the supervising officer. Concern is not solely (although mostly) for safety, but for clinic and corrections' liabilities as well.

Researchers have been active in trying to predict which offenders are at most risk to be at large (Maletzky, 1993; Proulx et al., 1997). Armed with outcome data, we have participated with the state Department of Corrections in devising an assessment-of-risk scale to help corrections officers keep track of their caseloads. We have strongly advised officers, for example, to increase surveillance and reporting requirements for offenders who have shown predatory patterns, tend to isolate from other adults, or show persistence of high deviant arousal.

To begin treatment, each offender must sign a safety contract, although the term *agreement* is preferred. While most clinics have patients sign some type of treatment consent, these particular agreements should include clauses specific for sexual offending and should vary based on an individual's patterns of offending. Table 8.2 gives examples of typical items from an offender's contract. While many items are standard, each agreement contains some unique items, for example, the type of community service, whether or not maintaining employment is included, or living conditions. While some clinics have broadened these strictures to include many nonsexual areas, such as injunctions to lose weight,

TABLE 8.2
Typical Items from an Offender's Treatment Contract

1. I agree to be honest and assume full responsibility for my sexual offenses and behavior.
2. I agree to sign all releases of information necessary to obtain information about my offenses.
3. I will attend group and individual sessions on time
4. I understand that the only excuse for missing a group or individual session is a verifiable emergency. I will make up any missed group session in individual treatment prior to the next group.
5. I will not disclose any information regarding another group member outside of group, except in a life-threatening emergency. If this occurs, I will report first to the group therapist or, if unavailable, The Sexual Abuse Clinic Director.
6. I will actively participate in group and individual sessions.
7. I will not attend any group or individual session under the influence of alcohol or drugs.
8. I will not become verbally threatening or assaultive toward the therapist or other group members inside or outside the office.
9. I will not commit any criminal offenses.
10. I will do all homework assigned prior to the next session.

keep a cleaner house, or attend church regularly, we believe the requirements should not be so overreaching or punitive and generally should be limited to areas affecting sexual offending.

While contracts are generally thought of as starting points, we also employ a termination agreement in which the offender identifies situations that increase his risk to reoffend and vows to avoid them. A paper-and-pencil exit exam for each offender is in the planning stages. As part of the termination agreement, each offender should be clear that he is free to call or return if troubles recur, sexual or otherwise. We try to reassure the offender that most such problems will not be reportable unless a new crime has occurred or a new danger lurks. To facilitate return and follow-up, all such visits are free.

Efficacy and safety data can prove invaluable in providing reassurance to the community. In our research program, we locate, interview, and test offenders annually to learn if what we are doing works. All follow-up visits, necessary booster sessions, plethysmograph tests, and group visits after the end of active treatment are entirely without charge. When we learn, through the above means or through our routine searches of computerized national police files, that one of our offenders has been charged with (not necessarily convicted of) a new sexual crime, even one for which he was not treated by us (for example, an exhibitionist charged with molesting a child), he is counted as a failure and two procedures are enacted:

1. If appropriate, we offer free treatment for the crime committed (we believe we should have known of the possibility and done something about it)
2. We pay that county's victims' compensation fund the exact amount that offender paid us for his entire treatment

Community Reactions

The community knows sexual offenders not by any sense of personal familiarity, but by a single group of deeds. Neighbors and the families of potential victims are apprehensive about such offenders living in proximity to them, but friends and family members of offenders usually are not. This occurs not just from alliance, but with familiarity as well.

With increasing contact, one learns that offenders have largely the same set of emotional reactions as do most people; they have committed the same types of good deeds and bad (save one) as most of us. If members of a nervous community get to know an offender, the level of apprehension usually falls.

One way to accomplish this is with disclosure. We not only encourage the offender to tell others, where appropriate, about his crimes, we also ask the offender to participate in community seminars about offending, both specific and general. As part of community service, offenders are asked to speak at churches, town meetings, and schools (to parents and teachers) to describe their modes of operating, what offending has meant to them, how it has altered their lives, what penalties they have paid, what treatment is like, and what parents, teachers, administrators, child protection workers, legislators, Boy Scout leaders, camp counselors, and the like can do to prevent it. Offenders who have gone through treatment can even train older children in scrutiny and prevention procedures and, in turn, those children can train the youngest. It does only a little good to treat an offender and bottle up that information; a wider task is undertaken when that offender can share what he has learned.

In a similar fashion, we try not to hide our own identity as well. "The Sexual Abuse Clinic" is displayed on buildings, offices, stationery, and publications. We try not to operate in a spirit of secrecy, as if what we do is so confidential that its very mention might cause unease. Not unlike the practice of psychiatry and psychology 30 years ago, the treatment of the sexual offender should not be demoted to the unmarked basement floors of nondescript institutional buildings, practiced by disadvantaged semiprofessionals who did not aspire to higher treatment callings. Our subdiscipline is an esteemed specialty requiring skill, nerve, and patience. Therapists who are proud of what they do impart that to their patients and, of equal importance, enhance the community's reactions to their efforts.

A number of issues can arise within a community that can determine reactions to outpatient programs. Community notification has engendered heated controversy within the legal and treatment communities (Berliner, 1996; Freeman-Longo, 1996). Of greater impact, frankly, has been the possession and use of pornography to present as stimulus material. Many in our communities misunderstand its use, while a few are more thoughtfully concerned about revictimization. Public education has been more helpful here than attempts to justify our work in the media. We ask offenders to explain not so much why, but how pornographic material is used; listeners are increasingly sophisticated in this area and we have received gratifyingly positive responses thus far. We have also received written acknowledgment (but not approval) to possess these materials from the state Attorney General, a blessing and reassurance. Hopefully, with the advent of CAD images and perhaps nonpornographic testing, these objectionable materials may prove unnecessary in the near future (Card & Olsen, 1996; Laws, 1996).

There is cause for optimism: Community rejection should not be assumed. We have learned that many people alien to notions of psychological treatment are still sympathetic to the task of those treating sexual offenders: to reduce the risk of another victim being harmed.

Visitation and Reunification

An outpatient clinic treating men who have molested children must deal with the reality of some clients' constant pleas to see their children and eventually move back home. No general rules are sufficient in this regard. We have found it best to ensure that an offender is well ensconced in the treatment program and has demonstrated good application and cooperation before visitation begins. Of course, coordination must occur with any therapists involved with the offender's partner or those treating any children in the family. The partner must agree to any arrangements and the children must not object. However, if one or more of the victims is at home, this decision becomes complicated. To avoid splitting the family, it has proven helpful to have the services of a family therapist within the clinic. In some clinics, this therapist might be the one also treating the offender, but we have avoided that arrangement, preferring to have trained specialists carrying out those separate functions. A spouses' group can achieve some of these same purposes.

Supervised visitations are often best approved initially for public places such as restaurants, public playgrounds, carnivals, and the like. As confidence grows, if things are going well, the offender can begin supervised visits at home during the day, eventually spending a night and weekends. During these phases, routine monitoring in treatment and polygraph and plethysmograph testing should occur to make certain visitation is not producing unwanted results. Should all go well, reunification, with family therapy ongoing, may proceed. Each step must be recommended to a supervising official, usually a corrections officer or a children's agency worker, as a clinic should never act as an approving body or, as importantly, never appear to act in such fashion. We have never requested, as a condition of going back home, that all child contact be supervised. Such supervision in a live-in setting is probably impossible and to do so possibly encourages disregard of the law.

Requests by the offender to be allowed to return home are so frequent that therapists regularly report this as one of their biggest burdens. This issue can often prove an impediment to trust building as well. Although evasive, an action we have used has proved helpful: We make each such decision in a team meeting and therapists are given license to blame the team, and especially the director, for being so cruel, obstinate, and distrusting as to block visitations. Some clinics may see value in having the primary therapist take this responsibility. Our way has seemed to work, but it surely is not right for all clinics in every situation. It also sometimes helps to tell the offender to proceed more slowly in this area, since those who rush into family reunification may risk a greater chance of discord later on.

A set of conditions and guidelines should be established for the initiation of visitation and eventual return home. Rather than providing the offender with arbitrary criteria, we initiate a discussion about these guidelines. Usually, over a period of months, this leads to a progression from initial public contact through supervised home visitation to eventual placement back within the family. When this proceeds gradually as a well-prepared process, most families become both well-protected and grateful that the offender can return to his house, home, and normal familial relationships.

Funding

No single issue, save safety, outweighs economics as a headache for community-based programs. Since most programs will, in reality, be private clinics, they and we depend on the following three sources of income to provide services.

Third-Party Payments

Insurance companies and Medicare and Medicaid most often do not pay for services to sexual offenders, nor are they likely to in the near future. The same statement, however, was made two decades ago about services for drug and alcohol treatment, which are now funded, so there is future hope. Clinics and individual therapists should bring pressure to bear in every possible way for coverage, not for each client, but in a general manner. Through lobbying efforts, the Association for the Treatment of Sexual Abusers can strengthen efforts in this direction as well, perhaps by calling attention, both locally and nationally, to the costs of offending as opposed to the costs of treating offenders. Often published, the cost differences are still striking (Marshall & Barbaree, 1991).

Government Contracts

Recognizing the scarcity of services for treating sexual offenders, county, state, and federal corrections and children's agencies have funded treatment directly for the most indigent of their offender caseloads. While the qualifying forms ("Requests for Proposals") have proved formidable, the numbers of new referrals low, and the reimbursement rate abysmal, the effort to obtain these contracts has been more than worthwhile. Our clinic has enjoyed ongoing contracts with five counties, two states, and the federal government. Benefits have included public and agency goodwill, the opportunity to interact more closely with other professionals supervising offenders, and the opportunity to become better known. In a competitive environment, these advantages have been substantial. A clinic would be well-advised to learn from local corrections divisions whether any existing contracts will be expiring and how to submit bids to provide assessment and treatment services.

Fee for Services

Greater than three quarters of our clients have needed to pay for services from their own pockets or those of their families. Treatment adds a considerable financial burden to offenders at a time in their lives when fees to attorneys and courts and possible losses of jobs have all strained their budgets. Moreover, although clients come from all walks of life, many fit the lowest two definable social classes. How can we help clients with this dilemma?

One way some clinics have helped is with sliding fee scales. However, a problem we have encountered with this is lack of consistency and concomitant client hostility if some learn of lower costs for others. Our approach has been a program of long-term payments (we charge no interest on these) to allow an offender to pay a small amount weekly or monthly even if those payments must extend beyond active treatment. Are most offenders to be thus trusted? Although we lack data from our early days, recent experience has shown that the majority of clients honor their commitments to pay; just 21% of offenders now out of treatment have stopped paying or refused to pay, or are unable to be located. Forming a respectful relationship with the offender and continuing good communication with him and his family have been the best indicators that he will honor his obligations.

Offenders often begin treatment amid a chaotic, pressured jumble of legal, financial, and family stresses. Easy access into treatment has been a challenge, and one way our clinic has tried to help is with an orientation group (Maletzky & Prueitt, 1996). Offenders can be referred immediately to this low-cost, 12-session group, hence eliminating the waiting period common between evaluation and definitive treatment. These groups are didactic and interactional, with topics ranging from denial, cognitive restructuring, relapse prevention, and empathy training, to visits to prisons. During some sessions, vicarious sensitization videotapes are shown; during others, probation and parole officers participate and describe the basics of the supervision process; a family therapist joins group for a session on visitation and reunification. These groups provide a basic introduction to sexual offender treatment without a high initial fee and allow offenders, particularly those released from an institution, to marshall the financial resources for treatment that will be needed in the coming months. Some will appreciate this time to search for work; others will need to arrange loans or obtain help from family members.

Funding considerations aside, we still consider one-to-one therapy the gold standard in treatment for the sexual offender. The process of building trust with an offender is delicate, and this, combined with an offender's innate defensiveness and embarrassed hesitance to share private sexual material, makes individual therapy more powerful than group alone. This is especially true in dealing with each offender's idiosyncratic preferences in sexual arousal. Techniques such as aversive conditioning (using foul odors), aversive behavior rehearsal, plethysmographic biofeedback, and masturbatory reconditioning require individual sessions to be fully effective.

However, certain elements of treatment can be effectively presented in a group, and indeed others, particularly relapse prevention and minimization and denial, might be best addressed in that format. Although the orientation group has afforded opportunities to inform and influence our clients, its value as an assessment tool should not be overlooked. We require a plethysmograph and polygraph test for each offender in the orientation group and these, combined with observations in group about the level of participation (both in the group itself and with homework assignments), help us make initial judgments about amenability for treatment following graduation from this group. At that time, each offender is assigned to the therapist and type of therapy that we believe best suits his treatment needs.

While not all of our clients start in the orientation group (some may have had extensive group experience in other programs or are deemed too dangerous to forego immediate individual treatment), those who do have required fewer individual sessions; hence, the total cost of treatment has been reduced. To help further, we ask each participant to consider adding one twelfth the cost of his polygraph and plethysmograph to each session's fees so the entire amounts have been contributed by the time he graduates from group.

Money is a powerful reinforcer; it can be used to advantage in encouraging praiseworthy ends by returning it to a client who has done well. Some of our therapists have devised schemes in which an offender receives rebates contingent on performance, for example, completing homework thoughtfully, showing reductions in deviant sexual arousal (or increases in appropriate arousal), or completing community service assignments. We should not shrink from any novel approach in helping offenders afford treatment. Their positive responses and that of the community at large will more than overcome any minor financial sacrifice. In our experience, the perception among potential referral sources that money is the prime motivator in providing services has been the chief factor in the withdrawal of community support.

ANTICIPATED FUTURE PROBLEMS

Since we have not yet solved everything connected with treating sexual offenders, there should be no shortage of problems to entertain 21st-century clinicians. One basic challenge remains to find a reasonable assessment package for sexual offenders that will help us know whom we are treating, who will respond to treatment, and, most importantly, who will not. It appears that a combination of techniques, including a polygraph, plethysmograph, and perhaps newer instruments such as the Abel Screen II (Osborn et al., 1995) will be necessary. Less likely will be our competent participation in legal proceedings; it now seems improbable that any instruments in the near future will enable us to determine if any client had a high probability of committing any particular past act, although we will improve our ability to predict who may offend again without treatment. We therefore need to continue to be honestly cautious when providing testimony.

A further difficult area will involve the treatment of offenders in denial. Originally impressed that sexual offenders mandated into treatment did as well as those who entered voluntarily (Maletzky, 1980), we began to collect data on treatment outcome for those who maintained denial throughout treatment and those who denied, then admitted, to some culpability. (Contrary to the practice of some clinics, not only do we include deniers in treatment, we also permit them to complete treatment, although we provide them with reports indicating only partial success.) We were surprised that, although, as expected, men who maintained denial were less successful overall, the majority of those not admitting any involvement in the crime yet completing a treatment program have largely been successful at not reoffending (Maletzky, 1991): It was overwhelmingly safer for these men to be at large than a matched cohort of those who admitted complicity yet never completed treatment (Maletzky & McFarland, 1996). In the present political climate, we may be increasingly required to treat those who deny. In our experience, such treatment is possible using behavioral and cognitive techniques, both individually and in group; it is effective in reducing risks, and hence, it is a necessary and vital service to the community. In our opinion, to deny a crime is natural; to deny treatment to those who deny is a crime itself.

Another challenge that a community-based clinic faces daily is the conundrum of whether sexual offenders deserve treatment. Many otherwise sophisticated and sensitive individuals in a community may question why sexual offenders are afforded treatment for breaking the law, while burglars or bank robbers are simply punished. Because some tax dollars are spent on treatment, for example, in public mental health clinics or in government contracts with private providers, citizens have a right to question the expense.

These questions are reasonable and lead to discussions, heated at times, of whether sexual offenders have a legal right to treatment. There is concern for whether an offender should be regarded as having a discrete illness or rather that he (or she) simply exerts a choice to offend. Our view, perhaps simplistic yet also pragmatic, has been that if our efforts can diminish risks, we should present these efforts as treatment of an illness. Certainly others have disagreed, and some call for us to more properly label what we do as offender management and harm reduction (Laws, 1996b). Peering into the murky future waters of offender treatment, we see a danger lurking underneath this glimmering surface by selling ourselves and our services too short. Perhaps what we see here is only a flattering self-reflection, but it still seems that even one victim is one too many, and that our goals (if not our present results) should be set high.

Unfortunately, the majority of sexual offenders in the United States will in all likelihood never be treated, even if their crimes are disclosed, because of lack of funding. Tragically, many may be incarcerated and then released, never to test how effective treatment might have been. To counter this dangerous neglect, a clinic can gain stature by providing education to a variety of audiences to recognize the many faces of offending, and hence, reduce the damages it can cause. Chief among these is the real trauma suffered by a victim, trauma often regarded lightly even in public discourse. In addition, we should address the prevention of offending as thoroughly as we advocate its treatment. While public education is not a panacea, it could inform potential offenders and victims of the harm offending causes, document the number of otherwise law-abiding individuals who carry it out, and explain the potential of treatment to reduce its likelihood. Perhaps this will improve the motivation of some offenders to obtain treatment who otherwise may have been too afraid or too ashamed, or who wished they could stop offending but sadly could not. We hope some of the suggestions in this chapter can assist in achieving those goals.

REFERENCES

Berliner, L. (1996). Community notification: Neither a panacea nor a calamity. *Sexual Abuse: A Journal of Research and Treatment, 8*, 101–103.

Card, R. D., & Olsen, S. E. (1996). Visual plethysmograph stimuli involving children: Rethinking some quasi-logical issues. *Sexual Abuse: A Journal of Research and Treatment, 8*, 267–271.

Freeman-Longo, R. E. (1996). Prevention or problem? *Sexual Abuse: A Journal of Research and Treatment, 8*, 91–100.

Laws, D. R. (1996a). Marching into the past: A critique of Card and Olsen. *Sexual Abuse: A Journal of Research and Treatment, 8*, 273–278.

Laws, D. R. (1996b). Relapse prevention or harm reduction? *Sexual Abuse: A Journal of Research and Treatment, 8*, 243–247.

Maletzky, B. M. (1980). Self-referred versus court-referred sexually deviant patients: Success with assisted covert sensitization. *Behavior Therapy, 11*, 306–314.

Maletzky, B. M. (1991). *Treating the sexual offender*. Newbury Park, CA: Sage.

Maletzky, B. M. (1993). Factors associated with success and failure in the behavioral and cognitive treatment of sexual offenders. *Annals of Sex Research, 6*, 241–258.

Maletzky, B. M. (1996). Evolution, psychopathology, and sexual offending: Aping our ancestors. *Aggression and Violent Behavior: A Review Journal, 1*, 369–373.

Maletzky, B.M., & McFarland, B. (1996). *Vicarious sensitization in the treatment of paraphilic sexual offenders: A pilot study*. Manuscript submitted for publication.

Maletzky, B. M., & Prueitt, M. (1996). A sexual offender orientation group. Paper presented at the annual conference of the Association for the Treatment of Sexual Abusers, Chicago, IL.

Marshall, W. L. (1996). The sexual offender: Monster, victim or everyman? *Sexual Abuse: A Journal of Research and Treatment, 8*, 317–335.

Marshall, W. L., & Barbaree, H. E. (1991). Outcome of comprehensive cognitive–behavioral treatment programs. In W. L. Marshall, D. R. Laws, & H. E. Barbaree (Eds.), *Handbook of sexual assault: Issues, theories, and treatment of the offender* (pp. 363–385). New York: Plenum.

Osborn, C., Abel, G. G., & Warberg, B. W. (1995, October). *The Abel Assessment: Its comparison to plethysmography and resistance to falsification*. Paper presented at the annual conference of the Association for the Treatment of Sexual Abusers, New Orleans, LA.

Proulx, J., Pellerin, B., Paradis, Y., McKibben, A., Aubut, J., & Ouimet, M. (1997). Static and dynamic predictors of recidivism in sexual aggressors. *Sexual Abuse: A Journal of Research and Treatment, 9*, 7–27.

Wolfe, R. (1984). Northwest Treatment Associates: A comprehensive, community-based evaluation and treatment program for adult sex offenders. In F. H. Knopp (Ed.), *Retraining adult sex offenders: Methods and models* (pp. 85–101). Syracuse, NY: Safer Society Press.

9

B. Community Settings

Joseph J. Peters Institute Intervention Programs for Adult Sexual Offenders

Darlene Pessein, Joseph Maher, Enny Cramer, and Robert Prentky

The Joseph J. Peters Institute (JJPI) is a Philadelphia-based nonprofit, licensed, outpatient psychiatric clinic that provides clinical services to victims of sexual abuse and to perpetrators of sexual abuse. The program at JJPI was started in 1955 by Dr. Joseph J. Peters, a psychiatrist at Philadelphia General Hospital. Dr. Peters initially began by treating only offenders, and in 1965, expanded his practice to include the treatment of victims. At the time of his death in 1975, at the age of 52, Dr. Peters had established a national reputation through his clinical practice, his grant-funded research, and his many publications. Indeed, Dr. Peters was the first recipient, in 1966, of a research grant from the National Institute of Mental Health to conduct an experimental treatment outcome study on sexual offenders. After Dr. Peters died, his staff, under the guidance of Dr. Linda Meyer Williams, continued his work, and in 1977, the agency was incorporated.

To the best of our knowledge, JJPI continues to be the only licensed agency in the United States that is devoted exclusively to the full spectrum of sexual violence by providing clinical and forensic services to victims and perpetrators of all ages. From its inception, JJPI has been victim-focused and its primary mission remains the reduction in victimization. As a practical aside, we rely on public funds to support most of our treatment programs. We justify the use of those funds to treat offenders by maintaining that treatment will reduce the risk of reoffense, thereby reducing the number of new victims. That is, offender treatment is one form of secondary intervention that may reduce the likelihood of reoffense, and thus further victimization. One important consequence of our public-funding support is that the offenders we treat are, for the most part, of lower socioeconomic status. The modal adult offender that is referred to JJPI by a parole agent or probation officer usually falls at the bottom of the sliding fee scale and pays nothing for treatment, or is required to make a medical assistance copayment of $3 per session.

Darlene Pessein, Joseph Maher, Enny Cramer, and Robert Prentky • Joseph J. Peters Institute, Philadelphia, Pennsylvania 19102.

Sourcebook of Treatment Programs for Sexual Offenders, edited by Marshall et al. Plenum Press, New York, 1998.

OVERVIEW OF CURRENT SERVICES

The clinical program includes service provision to (1) child victims, ranging in age from 2 to 17 years, (2) adult victims, (3) juvenile offenders, ranging in age from 11 to 18 years, and abuse-reactive children, (4) adult offenders in prison, (5) adult offenders in the community, and (6) impaired professionals. At the present time, the 28 clinical staff at JJPI treat approximately 100 child and adult victims and 200 juvenile and adult offenders per month. These figures represent individuals and not "units of service" (i.e., each victim and offender may be seen 4–12 times per month). The average number of units of service during 1995 was 2763 treatment sessions/month. The clinical program is supported and enriched by the services of social work interns, psychology interns, and psychiatric residents. Referrals for treatment come from the public sector (e.g., child welfare system, criminal justice system, the school system) and the private sector (e.g., hospitals, mental health centers, physicians, attorneys, churches, clergy, employers, and parents). Only a small percentage of clients are self-referred.

In addition, the forensic program, consisting of three staff, a laboratory technician, and student interns/residents, provides specialized evaluations for all facets of the criminal justice system on child and adult victims and offenders. Although most of these referrals come from criminal defense lawyers, the district attorney's office, the public defender's office, or directly from the court, some referrals come from probation or parole, or from private and other public agencies.

Last, the research program, consisting of four staff, currently executes federal grants from the National Institute of Justice and the National Center for Child Abuse and Neglect. The research program addresses issues pertinent both to victims and offenders and actively collaborates with colleagues at Boston University (Professor Austin Lee), Brandeis University (Professor Raymond Knight), University of Pennsylvania (Professors Ann Burgess and Marvin Wolfgang), University of Medicine and Dentistry of New Jersey (Dr. Esther Deblinger), and many others.

Although the mission of this chapter is to focus only on our outpatient adult offender program, we have included our prison-based program as well. We consider our outpatient program to be the second phase of a "step-down" model that begins with treatment in prison. Thus, the two programs are linked conceptually as well as clinically. It is our resolute conviction that the most effective treatment program for sexual offenders provides continuity of care after release from prison and constitutes only one component of a more elaborate aftercare plan that addresses all facets of the offender's needs.

ADULT SEXUAL OFFENDERS: PRISON PROGRAM

Program Overview

The state correctional institution at Graterford, Pennsylvania, constructed between 1929 and 1934, is located 30 miles west of Center City Philadelphia. The walled, maximum-security facility, originally built to house 1800 inmates, encompasses 63 acres inside the wall and thousands of acres of woods and farmland outside. It is the largest prison in the Commonwealth, and the fourth or fifth largest in the country. Although there are roughly 300 men at Graterford with a governing sexual offense, representing about 8% of the 3700 men currently housed there, this figure is quite misleading. The number of "legally identified" sexual offenders clearly underestimates the number of men who committed sexual offenses, primarily due to: (1) plea bargaining to lesser charges (e.g., simple assault), or (2) overriding nonsexual offenses (i.e., the sexual offense is subordinated in importance to other serious charges, such as kidnap and assault and battery).

In the spring of 1986, a modest JJPI sexual offender treatment program became operational at Graterford. The program has since grown from five small groups and one therapist per group, to four short-term psychoeducation groups, two intermediate groups, and four long-term "admitters" or treatment groups. The current groups offered at Graterford include:

1. *Stress and anger management group.* This group focuses on symptoms and unhealthy consequences of stress and anger, and teaches specific counteracting skills.
2. *Sex education group.* This group offers accurate information on male and female anatomy and physiology, healthy sexual choices, acquired immunodeficiency syndrome (AIDS) and other sexually transmitted diseases (STDs), use of condoms, and so forth.
3. *Human sexuality group.* This group examines emotional, spiritual, and sexual aspects of relationships, including the development of attitudes and beliefs, trust, perceptions and expectations of others, and power and control issues.
4. *Human development group.* This group covers long-term effects of early childhood experiences, including physical, emotional, and sexual abuse, on adult coping styles, self-esteem, sexual consent, and entitlement.
5. *Drugs, alcohol, and sexual offending.* This is a 6-month group that explores the effects of drugs and alcohol on both brain chemistry and sexual aggression. Relapse prevention techniques are introduced to cope with substance abuse and sexual offending cycles.
6. *Reentry group.* This group, open to all sexual offenders who are within 12 to 18 months of release, is a composite psychoeducational–process group. Community notification and registration laws, employment-seeking skills, parole board expectations, vocational alternatives, and appropriate work place interactions are explored.
7. *Treatment groups.* These are open-ended, long-term, offense-specific groups for offenders who accept some degree of responsibility for their offense. Offenders who maintain their innocence are not admitted. Treatment groups offer a mix of relapse prevention training, empathy building, and group process. Group relationships are developed to build interpersonal honesty and to work through issues of anger, authority, and shame that act as barriers to growth.

All groups are presently led by a primary therapist and a cotherapist. In total, there are four male and four female therapists that make up the necessary ten dyads. The program is contracted to treat, on average, 75 inmates monthly and to provide 6600 hours of treatment service annually. In the contract year just completed (March 1995–February 1996), the program provided an average of 89 inmates per month with a total of 6520 hours of treatment.

Problems and Solutions

Start-up, Administrative, and Institutional Problems

Start-up problems were plentiful. We had to develop a practical treatment model and administrative forms for documenting and tracking service provisions, establish working relationships with key prison staff to support the program, and locate and hire part-time therapists willing to work with sexual offenders in, at first glance, an overwhelmingly oppressive environment. The contract originally awarded by the Department of Corrections was a fee-for-service agreement, which meant that JJPI could not invoice until inmates were actually receiving treatment. JJPI absorbed all start-up costs for staffing, training, curriculum development, and administrative overhead, with the obvious result that, in the first 2 years, the agency lost money. A major problem contributing to the fiscal loss (and morale) was the percentage of no-shows (i.e., inmates scheduled for evaluations or group treatment who failed to show). Visits, illness, misconducts, resistance, lockdowns, and episodic failure of the inmate pass system were among the many reasons for no-shows.

The physical layout of the prison likewise impeded treatment efforts. The main corridor, 900 feet long, is the length of three football fields from which branch five huge, original cell blocks housing up to 600 inmates each. Since then, new smaller, modular cell blocks have been built, and in the past 2 years the population increased to 4500 inmates, 150% over capacity. At the present time, the population is 3700. The original cell blocks were typically staffed by five to six corrections officers each. Given the officer's obvious first priority of maintaining security in such a volatile environment, ensuring that inmates kept treatment appointments was, to say the least, a low priority. Establishing a willingness by a prison staff to make the sexual offender program "work" by reducing resistance among inmates and increasing cooperativeness among all prison staff became a critical task in the first year and an essential goal in succeeding years. Clearly, the keys to success are developing an effective public relations effort that seeks to build relationships with prison staff and maintaining a stubborn consistency in delivering promised services.

Certificates with an attached "rider" were awarded to inmates for an 80% group attendance rate. The rider explained that the certificate was "not to be interpreted that no further treatment is necessary." This still becomes a point of contention with some inmates who feel the wording sets them up for "games" perpetrated by the prison staff, when the inmates seek parole recommendations. However, it was necessary to structure it this way in order to counter the artifice of inmates, who argued that obtaining a certificate was equivalent to completing the program.

Because of severe space limitations, all groups have been conducted in the evening and on weekends. Indeed, it was the space problems that led to our hiring therapists on a part-time basis. The program director who was full time, without office space, used vacant offices, a hallway bench, or the one group therapy room to conduct interviews. We were eventually given our own office in 1992. For years, however, there literally was no place to put therapists during the day, because all offices were occupied by prison counselors and psychologists. To successfully adapt to the ever-challenging conditions of the prison environment, we found that flexibility and harmony were indispensable, not to mention *de rigueur*.

By 1988, when the third JJPI prison program director was hired, there were 45 inmates active in the program, with each group at 70–80% capacity. The agency was still losing about 25% of potential funds in any given month. This put limits on salaries, staff development, planning, and additional hiring. In 1989, the Department of Corrections agreed with JJPI's request to change the contract to equal monthly installments, thus ensuring 100% draw down of funds during the contract period. The effect of this change in the contract was immediate, with a major shift in focus from the nagging importance of numbers of inmates enrolled to that of quality of care and service.

A major ongoing task has been to try to understand and use positively the prison culture. Understanding how to get things done, identifying who wields power and makes decisions, determining the extent and nature of inmate power, knowing how to keep our role clear and our reputation clean, how to be fair and honest and avoid being absorbed into power struggles within the institution, all have influenced the success and indeed the survival of the program. Recommendations for how to achieve these elusive goals change over time and what helped us once may not apply now. For example, key prison staff who helped us may be promoted or demoted, transferred or retired. It is necessary to walk a very narrow line between being responsive to the needs of prison administrators and retaining sufficient independence and autonomy to preserve credibility in the eyes of both inmates and prison staff.

Life for everyone who works in prison, including vendors, seems to require a seemingly endless avoidance or negotiation of obstacles and pitfalls. One of the necessary strategic responses to "coping" in the prison environment is to maintain a very clear focus on the mission and its limitations. We are a treatment agency contracted to provide a specific treatment program. Even with highly focused objectives, there remain clear and inevitable limits to our sphere of influence.

An example of this involved medication for several inmates who were experiencing highly intrusive sexual thoughts and urges. A separate vendor had the contract for medical and mental health services, and their physicians declined to accept our psychiatrists' recommendations for medication. Although we felt that those inmates were seriously underserved, there was little we could do. One of those inmates was subsequently charged and received additional time for obscene phone calls made from the prison.

There are many other "costs" associated with prison-based treatment. Recently, there has been a major crackdown on parole for sex offenders in Pennsylvania, and inmates have threatened to quit the program or to file suit against JJPI for not doing enough to get them released. Inmates want us to relinquish our neutrality and "take sides" by being a social and political force. It can be very difficult, if not painful at times, to remain neutral when inmates who have made real progress are routinely ignored by prison staff or the parole board.

An additional administrative problem falls under the guise of protection of inmate privacy. In 1993, the new contract (and payment) was delayed by months until it was revealed that the Pennsylvania Law Department was, at its leisure, insisting on a clause requiring our agency to destroy all prison-generated reports for inmates who were paroled and later terminated from outpatient treatment. Once we learned of the requirements, we readily agreed. The delay, however, was costly as monies had to be borrowed in order to meet payroll. Incidents like this help us to be sensitive to the needs, the shortcomings, and the limitations of bureaucracy and to temper unrealistic expectations.

Personnel and Staffing Problems

Over the years, we have learned several valuable coping lessons. Because the JJPI prison staff are part-time, involved in careers that are separate from the prison setting, frequent telephone and in-person staff contact is essential both to keep everyone on track and to keep logistic problems to a minimum. All JJPI prison staff are present as a group only once a month for formal clinical supervision. However, frequent personal contact is necessary so that changes in routine are communicated, problems are aired, and staff input is obtained. In hiring new staff we routinely ask, "Have you ever been arrested?" We routinely seek state police clearance for new therapists before requesting prison clearance, and on several occasions the prison's "clean check" revealed arrest records unknown to us. This resulted in aborting the hiring of otherwise promising candidates.

The program at Graterford was developed and continues to operate against a backdrop of lockdowns caused by inmate upheaval, severe weather and power failure emergencies, changes in the prison and Department of Corrections administrations (including Commissioners of Corrections), serious prison overcrowding, late counts that disrupt or prevent groups from convening, and a host of other problems that are unique to the prison environment. Given these working conditions, staff morale becomes a matter of vital concern. The staff need to be supported not only in terms of the performance of their duties and professional development, but in the larger context of "survival" within the prison (i.e., making the working environment as tolerable as possible). Despite the many potentially aversive experiences in the prison, we have been most fortunate in receiving encouragement and often direct practical assistance from a number of prison administrators, prison treatment staff, and correctional officers. Our therapists have been encouraged to seek and appropriately use the human resources that the prison offers. The positive relationships we have developed over the years have been a sustaining force for our therapists and a crucial factor in the success of the program.

We have been very fortunate in maintaining a low staff turnover rate, all of whom are masters-level clinicians. Their input is sought to make changes in the curriculum. Above all, it has been extremely helpful to develop the program along the lines of staff strengths. Making use of staff strengths and interests has helped us increase the number and variety of group offerings, decrease burnout, and increase staff interest and morale.

As an example, one of our original groups was for inmates who maintained their innocence. Known as "the deniers' group," it eventually wore down the two seasoned therapists to the point that they no longer wanted to facilitate this group. In their regular jobs, they were skilled career vocational rehabilitation counselors, and thus were encouraged to develop a new group that tapped their expertise and that filled a void in the program. This was the origin of the reentry group with its focus on job skills (i.e., seeking, interviewing, and maintaining employment). This group has expanded to include interaction with agents from the state parole board's sex offender unit. Group members learn effective communication skills to improve adaptation in the community, especially in relationships with significant others, family members, employers, and workplace associates. It has been well received by the inmates.

Another staff member, a highly skilled group trainer, has a strong background in treating substance abusers. He developed the drug, alcohol, and sexual abuse group. This group, which is always well-attended, allows inmates to examine their sexual offenses within the more socially acceptable framework of substance abuse. Through intensive homework assignments, they are gradually able to reveal their secrets to him and then to the other members.

Confidentiality

At the point of recruitment into the program, clients are told that our program is *not* a conduit of personal data to the prison records and that much of what they reveal in treatment is *not* shared. They are informed, however, that if they talk of escape, self-injury, plans to injure another person, or details of unsolved sexual offenses, this information will be shared.

Early on, we experienced the problems that arose when detailed treatment summaries were prepared for the parole board. Statements were taken out of context and used to justify parole reversal and were made part of the official reasoning for denial of parole. This one problem had the potential of destroying the program, since it dealt a potentially fatal blow to our credibility. We were labeled as "snitches"; we realized that unless we acted quickly, we could lose whatever trust the inmates had in us. We responded immediately by tailoring reports for the reader. Henceforth, all reports were screened for statements that could be misused or misinterpreted.

A lesson to the wise, however, is that any response to a problem, particularly in a place like a prison, must be moderate. Overreacting to one problem invariably creates an opposing problem. It immediately became apparent that our reports could not truly be free of any potentially damaging statements. Concerns about psychiatric instability, odd or erratic behavior or cognitions, or behavior that was potentially harmful to others had to be addressed in the reports. We sought a compromise that would maintain a high level of confidentiality and still disclose necessary information to protect the safety of prison staff and residents. The compromise that we adopted was tracking forms.

Tracking forms document level of participation and attendance and are prepared for the prison counselors. Unfortunately, some counselors have not always been attuned to the need to maintain confidentiality. On various occasions, they have shared with inmates details of psychopathology that were written exclusively for the counselors. This increased inmate paranoia and resulted in some inmates dropping out. We have had to be sensitive to (1) fears of inmates about being exposed to insensitive prison staff, (2) the potential for JJPI treatment evaluations to be exploited by other agencies, and (3) exploitation of inmate disclosures (and identity) by other inmates and, unfortunately, by a few members of the prison staff. We cannot underestimate the criticality of maintaining the highest level of confidentiality possible under the adverse circumstances of prison-based treatment. The task that we are expecting the inmates to engage in is one of the most difficult and improbable that they face. Indeed, at face value, treatment is absolutely inconsistent with survival in prison. In order to survive in prison, wisdom dictates that you do not reveal yourself "to the man," that you deny committing any sexual offense, and that you employ every coping strategy that you have to recognize danger and avoid it. We ask inmates, however, to leave the jungle once or twice a week, drop all of their defenses, trust the other inmates and the staff, and share the very information that can easily place them at considerable risk in the prison population. Confidentiality, as limited as it may be, is the most powerful tool that we have at our disposal to enable inmates to do the impossible.

In sum, treating sexual offenders in prison raises a unique set of problems and issues not encountered in our other treatment programs. Perhaps the most significant issue is whether effective treatment can be provided at all in a hostile, dangerous, and patently untherapeutic environment. Although there is no easy answer to that question, we do feel reasonably secure in concluding that we can raise the consciousness of many inmates to attitudes, behaviors, relationships, and early life trauma that they took for granted. They become more sensitive to and familiar with treatment process and treatment goals, and this is apparent when we see them on parole in our outpatient program. It has frequently been recognized at our staff meetings that men entering our outpatient therapy groups, who have worked diligently in the prison program, appear to be better candidates for rehabilitation than men coming out of prison who had never been exposed to treatment.

ADULT SEXUAL OFFENDERS: OUTPATIENT

Program Overview

JJPI provides therapy for adult males and females who have been criminally adjudicated as sexual offenders and who are either under parole or probation supervision. Although offenders are referred for treatment primarily from state probation or parole, we also receive referrals from federal parole and other therapists in private practice or in the employ of hospitals or community mental health centers, as well as from managed-care organizations. Under special circumstances, we will accept sexual offenders and noncoercive paraphilics who have not been adjudicated. Typically, these are self-referrals with clear evidence of internal motivation for treatment and no apparent intent to "use" therapy to "modify" a disposition by the criminal justice system or otherwise circumvent responsibility for criminal conduct.

The services that we provide to our adult offenders include: (1) an intake assessment, (2) specialized psychological testing, (3) phallometric assessment (PPG) and/or Abel Assessment (Abel, Lawry, Karlstrom, Osborn, & Gillespie, 1994), (4) psychiatric evaluation, (5) group therapy, (6) psychoeducational groups, (7) time-limited individual therapy, (8) couples therapy, and (9) medication.

Because our two programs that treat juvenile and adult sexual offenders in the community are our highest-risk endeavors, we take extra care to (1) do an in-depth intake evaluation and baseline assessment, (2) closely monitor progress and maintain ongoing communication with the probation officer or parole agent, and (3) gather as much data as possible from a variety of sources at time or discharge.

1. The intake evaluation includes the following components: (1) a clinical interview that covers life history and criminal history and an abbreviated, structured interview that is designed, along with archival data, to yield a score on the Psychopathy Checklist Revised (PCL-R) (Hare, 1991), (2) presenting problem checklist, completed at intake and every 3 months thereafter, and a risk assessment form (Risk Assessment for Adult Sexual Offenders), (3) intake questionnaire that assesses knowledge about sexual offender treatment (e.g., risk factors, understanding sexual assault cycles, cognitive distortions, and victim empathy) is completed by the offender, and (4) a number of psychological inventories are also completed by the offender. The aggregate data collected from the above-mentioned sources provide the baseline assessment.

2. Psychological testing at intake is intended to provide a baseline assessment on those dimensions deemed critical for assessment and treatment of sexual offenders. Our standard protocol, which focuses on such areas of concern as anger, empathy, cognitive distortions, and thoughts, fantasies, and behaviors involving sexual aggression, includes: (1) an inventory that is designed to assess psychological symptom patterns; (2) a multidimensional measure of empathy; (3) the Multidimensional Assessment of Sex and Aggression (MASA), a wide-ranging assessment of sexual and aggressive thoughts, fantasies, and behaviors, as well as a range of other domains, including social competence, early life experiences, history of alcohol and drug use, and exposure to and use of pornography (Knight, Prentky, & Cerce, 1994). In addition, embedded within MASA are a number of attitudinal scales (such as hostility toward women, global anger, and hypermasculinity), behavioral scales (psychopathy and episodic dyscontrol), and sexualization scales (such as compulsivity, preoccupation, guilt, inadequacy, and coercion); (4) the PCL-R, a 20-item

measure of psychopathic behavior (Hare, 1991). A structured 30- to 45-minute interview is administered by the intake clinician. A PCL-R score is derived by the intake clinician based on information from the interview, supplemented by archival information; and (5) a measure of the intensity of anger and how anger is managed and expressed. In addition, other tests are included on a case-by-case basis (e.g., cognitive distortion scales, focal measures of sexual anxiety or sexual compulsivity, neuropsychological tests, or measures of dissociation and posttraumatic stress disorder).

3. We do *not* do routine PPG or Abel Assessments on all offenders who are referred for treatment. We generally only do these assessments as part of a forensic evaluation or when they are specifically requested by an attorney, the court, a therapist, or an institution/ agency. Thus, it has not been our practice to use phallometry for clinical purposes. This decision is dictated primarily by cost. A full laboratory assessment is time-consuming, and thus expensive. Since we treat about 80 offenders per week, the cost of assessing change with the PPG would be prohibitive.

4. Group therapy is cognitive–behavioral and geared toward relapse prevention. Groups include 10–12 offenders and are facilitated by a primary therapist and a co-therapist. The co-therapists typically are student interns or psychiatric residents and are assigned to groups based on their gender (i.e., we try to provide our groups with a female and a male therapist).

5. Psychoeducational groups are intended to complement group therapy. The two most popular psychoeducational groups focus on human sexuality and anger management. In addition, we have a large pretreatment psychoeducational class that focuses on expectations in therapy, and the relapse prevention model.

6. Individual therapy is typically used to prepare an offender for group, to focus more intensively on a specific issue such as childhood victimization, or to do behavior therapy, such as olfactory aversion, covert sensitization, or relaxation training. We also provide individual therapy for offenders whose cognitive deficits might prevent them from benefiting from regular therapy groups.

7. Couples therapy is becoming increasingly requested as more of our offenders are expressing a need for assistance in working through issues with their companion. When the companion is their victim's mother, the issues invariably center around trust and unexpressed or displaced anger. In addition, the health of the sexual relationship is often severely compromised by the man's offenses. In general, we provide couples therapy to assist the offender and his or her partner in improving communication skills, increasing interpersonal skills (e.g., conflict resolution), educating the partner on the offender's offense cycle, and reducing the level of reactivity within the dyad, thereby reducing stress.

We also provide family therapy on limited occasions. When reunification is deemed appropriate, we will provide family therapy, following a lengthy protocol that is designed to facilitate reunification. We also work with newly created family systems to ensure that the children and the couple are aware of risk factors and that the children have safety and refusal skill training.

8. We provide psychiatric evaluations for those offenders who have a history of major mental illness or who, in the course of treatment, have a crisis that necessitates possible inpatient care or medication.

9. We provide routine psychopharmacological services for our clients. In practice, most of our medicated offenders are taking an antidepressant, primarily selective serotonin reuptake inhibitors. We maintain a small number of our offenders on medroxyprogesterone

acetate (Provera, Upjohn). Although we will, if requested, follow clients on antipsychotic medication, we prefer to have psychiatric problems attended to by full-service mental health care providers.

The Review and Discharge Process

Ongoing evaluation consists of the session notes completed after each group, a quarterly progress report, and the quarterly problem checklist. Group attendance is recorded and the probation officers or parole agents for those who fail to attend are notified the next day.

The discharge procedure includes information derived from the following sources: (1) the offender fills out a discharge questionnaire, which assesses acquired knowledge about sexual offense-specific issues; (2) an exit problem checklist, a risk assessment form and a therapist recommendation form are completed by the primary group therapist; (3) two (or more) independent referees who can provide external validation for the offender's community-based adjustment (e.g., employers, parents or caregivers, girlfriend or spouse, etc.) are interviewed and notes recorded; and (4) the offender's probation officer or parole agent is interviewed over the telephone and a form is completed.

The discharge committee includes at least three senior clinicians who are *not* involved with the offender's therapy. This same discharge process is followed for *all* offenders who leave treatment at JJPI, whether they leave at the expiration of supervision or as a result of a review that is initiated prior to the end of their supervision. There are essentially three circumstances leading to consideration for discharge: (1) clinical assessment that optimum benefit from treatment has been achieved, (2) offender decides to leave at the expiration of his probation or parole, or (3) offender remains in denial for 90 days.

Problems and Solutions

Confidentiality

The assumption of confidentiality lies at the heart of the therapist–client relationship. When the client is an offender, confidentiality is limited, and those limits may go well beyond the normal mandatory reporting requirements in the case of suspected child abuse or the "duty to warn" in the case of suspected harm to an identified individual. When offenders are treated in the community, confidentiality may have to be broken if the therapist becomes aware that the offender has violated a condition of probation or parole or if the therapist has good reason to believe that the offender is at high risk to reoffend. In addition, treatment records, not to mention the therapist, can be subpoenaed, providing another potential breach of confidentiality.

We ask the offender to engage in treatment with the caveat that there are limits to what will be held confidential. The only ethical way to address this dilemma is to make it a part of the informed consent process before beginning treatment and to make it an open issue for discussion in treatment. We are very clear with our offenders about our obligations and our duties with respect to communicating with their probation officer or parole agent. A policy of complete, open communication with the offenders is essential. Although they may not like the limits imposed on confidentiality, they hopefully will understand the reason for the limits and, at the very least, they will know the ground rules. It is fair to conclude that knowing when to violate confidentiality and when there is a duty of warn pose the greatest challenge for the therapist. It poses a challenge not only to provide effective treatment services under conditions of limited confidentiality, but it also presents the greatest risk for legal liability (Weiner, 1985).

Informed Consent

A second major issue that we face is acquiring informed consent. Informed consent requires that the offender fully understands what he is being asked to consent to (i.e., what participation in treatment will involve and what the potential benefits and risks are. We often assume, without justification, that offenders *know* what treatment entails and what will be expected of them. An offender may have no acquaintance with therapy and have no idea what treatment involves. Moreover, if we are treating adolescent sex offenders, they may be minors, in which case they are not legally competent (i.e., they cannot give voluntary, informed consent) and a caregiver or guardian must given substituted consent. If we are treating adult sexual offenders with major mental illnesses or very low intelligence, they may be clinically incompetent. Last, we must keep in mind that some informed consent is more difficult to obtain, depending on the intended intervention (i.e., some interventions require more information for the client to be adequately informed). Informed consent is relatively easy to obtain if the client is an adult of average intelligence and is being asked to participate in a psychotherapy group. If that same adult is being asked to consent to olfactory aversion, the informed aspect of the consent is more complicated. If that same adult is being asked to consent to phallometric assessment, the informed part of the consent is even more complicated. The most complicated consent process may come about when we ask the offender to take antiandrogenic medication.

In addition to the aforementioned competency issues related to obtaining informed consent, there always remains the problem of voluntariness. Consent that is not given voluntarily is consent that is not valid. The question of whether an incarcerated offender can give voluntary consent has been the subject of much debate. Precisely the same issues arise, however, when treatment is stipulated as a condition of probation or parole. In what manner can it be construed that consent is voluntary when the price of nonconsent is violation of probation or parole and possible incarceration? The matter of concern is whether the offender is truly "volunteering" to be in treatment. There is no optimal solution to this problem, other than to address it candidly with the offender, both at intake and, if necessary, in therapy.

During intake, the treatment process is discussed with the offender and our expectations of him are spelled out (e.g., attendance, timeliness, participation, acceptance of responsibility for the governing criminal offense, limits of confidentiality, and responsibility for payment). The offender is asked to sign three forms: a consent for treatment, an agreement or contract that delineates our expectations, and a release that permits us to speak with his probation officer or parole agent as well as other individuals (e.g., spouse/companion, relative, physician, etc.).

Legal Liability and Security Issues

Areas of legal liability in outpatient offender treatment are legion. In addition to the many potential areas of liability confronting clinicians in general practice (i.e., those not working with offenders) (cf. Appelbaum, 1993), there are problems unique to the population that we serve (i.e., sexual offenders). Sexual offenders have demonstrated their capacity for harming others, and their potential for reoffending presents obvious liability and security issues. The best way to properly protect against law suits is to keep impeccable treatment records, insure that all communications with third parties are protected by releases, and be scrupulously careful about informing the offender in writing about all aspects of the treatment and discharge process.

Staff and client security is of very considerable concern to us. We never have our adult offenders on site at the same time as our victims, which is why all offender groups are scheduled in the evenings. We have adopted a very strict protocol for safety of our staff: (1) the building that our agency is in has good 24-hour internal security, and building personnel know about the clients that we treat and assist us in monitoring their entry and exit from the building, (2) staff are not allowed on-site during off hours alone, (3) staff generally leave the office together after hours, (4) we practice a "buddy system" in the office, in which one staff person will "keep an eye out" for another staff person who is working in a closed office with someone who might be highly agitated or dangerous, (5) staff are supplied with a body alarm when working with particularly volatile or dangerous clients, or simply if they feel the need to have one, and (6) we have hired, on occasion, a plain-clothes security guard to sit in an adjacent room during large group sessions with juveniles when one or more of the youths appears to be particularly volatile. To the best of our knowledge, in JJPI's forty year history no staff member has ever been physically assaulted.

The potential for reoffense in the community remains a major concern, however, and we are ever-vigilant for signs that our offenders may be at increased risk. In our experience, the vast majority of men who are revoked and return to prison fail early in their offense cycle (i.e., before committing a sexual offense). Although most of the men are revoked for contaminated urine samples (substances, primarily marijuana and cocaine), some of the men are revoked for verbal or physical (nonsexual) assaults, or chronically failing to keep appointments with their probation officer or parole agent. The latter problem is invariably a symptom of another problem, such as substance use.

Community stability and adjustment often is very fragile for the men we treat, particularly those who have returned to society after release from prison. The roots that provide stability are often shallow and easily perturbed. One of the critical tasks of "reentry" is to provide sufficient support and supervision to permit deeper roots to take hold. In addition to the once weekly contact for treatment, we are in communication with the probation officer or parole agent, and we request permission to speak with the offender's spouse or companion, family members, employer and so forth. We are aware, moreover, of the potential for treatment itself to place men at increased risk. Thus, we do not allow men who are highly agitated in group to return directly to the street. After the group, we go for a "therapeutic walk" or simply remain with them until they appear safe to leave. Last, we have a 24-hour emergency call service, so that an offender who is in crisis can reach a therapist.

Clinical and Personnel Issues

Like all of our programs, the treatment of adult sexual offenders makes its own unique demands on therapists. There are those who are drawn to working with sexual offenders for personal reasons (e.g., trying to understand their own history of, or experiences with, abuse). Although it is generally unethical, not to mention illegal, to ask prospective therapists if they have been abused, we do discuss life experiences that make this type of work extremely difficult, even traumatizing. During the initial interview, we also discuss the need to do a criminal background check to insure that we are not hiring former offenders. The inevitable countertransference issues must be addressed vigorously in supervision and ample time is provided after group for therapists to "decompress." Since our groups include a primary and a co-therapist, the postgroup discussion provides time for feedback, teaching, and sharing feelings about how the group session went. We also provide 1 hour of group supervision each week. In this forum, with all therapists together, the focus is on group process issues, problem solving and countertransference problems. In addition, as part of supervision, therapists must be encouraged to pursue outside of work those activities that promote self-care, to be vigilant for signs of burnout, and to protect against burnout by taking time off to pursue restorative leisure activities.

From a clinical standpoint, most conventionally trained therapists are unprepared to tackle the demands of offender therapy. Most of us have grown up in a psychodynamic or Rogerian tradition. Even those of us who received rigorous training in behavior therapy are often hampered by the basic assumptions of treatment that we were taught (e.g., clients seek therapy because they are in distress, and the absence of any distress or discomfort bodes poorly for therapy). Much of our training and many of our assumptions are cast aside when working with offenders, who deny or majorly minimize the very behavior that is supposed to be addressed in therapy. Moreover, these men frequently are not in distress and have no desire to be in therapy. They often present with a long history of manipulativeness, and their sexual offenses are frequently characterized by devious strategies for setting up or grooming their victims. Under these circumstances, the potential value of psychodynamic or Rogerian therapy is severely limited. It is typically necessary to assume a highly proactive, aggressive posture to break through the layers of denial and minimization and get the offender to "come clean." This phase of treatment can be long and fraught with constant struggles and backsliding. This aggressive posture, however, must be tempered with a clear, unambiguous message that the therapists are caring, dedicated, and highly invested. Once an offender has come clean, the most effective tools for modifying behavior and sustaining change are cognitive–behavioral. All of these therapeutic demands may be quite alien to the conventionally trained clinician and may require training as well as intensive supervision. Overall, the three critical personnel issues in sex offender treatment are: (1) a very careful, thoughtful process for recruiting therapists, (2) intensive supervision, and (3) adequate training and ongoing professional development.

CONCLUSION

The Legal and Ethical Burden of Treating Sexual Offenders

There are innumerable legal, social, and ethical problems, some more inscrutable than others, that complicate and often undermine the treatment of sexual offenders. These problems and the issues they raise have been addressed elsewhere (e.g., Aubrey & Dougher, 1990; Berlin, 1989; Gordon & Verdun-Jones, 1983; Grubin & Prentky, 1993; Weiner, 1985) and limitation of space does not permit a thorough discussion here. As Weiner (1985) noted, the criminal justice system has, for at least the past 60 years, treated sexual offenders differently from other criminals. Although the statutory regulation of this one class of offenders has legitimate, occasionally honorable, motives, the consequences of the profusion of laws enacted primarily by state legislatures have served a very limited constructive purpose. Indeed, the phenomenon of enactment and repeal of sexual psychopath laws highlights the reactionary nature of most of these laws. The laws often are a reflex response by politicians to constituent's anguish over a particularly heinous sexual crime (Carter & Prentky, 1993). The explicit intent of the laws is to increase social control over this group of offenders by imposing an indeterminate sentence. Suits filed by (or on behalf of) incarcerated sexual offenders raise both procedural and substantive due process issues. The outcome of many of these suits is the need to justify indeterminate detainment of sexual offenders with due process considerations such as treatment and routine reviews of dangerousness, typically conducted annually. These laws carry an obligation, or burden, to provide some form of intervention that will remedy the problem that led to the indeterminate sentence, thereby permitting the offender reentry to society. The principal form of intervention has been treatment, and inadequate treatment has been the basis for endless procedural challenges on the grounds of equal protection. That is, without sound argument to the contrary, requiring only sexual offenders to submit to treatment until some degree of cure permits their reentry to society appears to violate equal protection.

The issues raised by shining the legal and social spotlight on one class of criminals raises an array of problems for clinicians who, in effect, carry the weight of the statutory burden to assess and treat sexual offenders. Perhaps the most onerous and vexatious problem is mandated treatment of a population that no mandator wants to treat. The net result is, at the very best, half-hearted and highly equivocal social and monetary support for treatment. This is a recipe for failure, and in this case, failure translates to more victims. As we have argued elsewhere, we must overcome our resistance to treating sexual offenders, not for the sake of the offenders but for the sake of the victims (cf. Prentky, 1995; Prentky & Burgess, 1990). It is not enough, however, simply to provide treatment services. To accomplish the only mission that we set for ourselves—reduction in the number of victims—we must set the most rigorous standards for treatment. Lip service support and suboptimal treatment will fail to accomplish the mission.

Impact of Managed Care

A critical concern facing all of our outpatient treatment programs is how to maintain proper standards of care in a time-limited fashion (cf. Appelbaum, 1993). Symptom reduction is easily measured, and health maintenance organizations tend to focus on those presenting problems that can be measured easily and ameliorated. Perpetrators as well as survivors of sexual abuse frequently have numerous other problems, however, that are less easily measured and take much longer to treat (e.g., problems with attachment, impaired self-reference, difficulties in relationships, and numerous intractable cognitive distortions). The reduction of presenting symptoms does not equate with recovery from sexual abuse for survivors or adequate, stable risk reduction for offenders. Most of our clients have experienced multiple losses and numerous traumas by the time they reach our agency, and problems that often took a lifetime to develop cannot be treated in a few sessions. Education and advocacy within the managed-care environment for the needs of these clients is one response.

Crossing the Final Frontier

There has long been disharmony between those who treat victims and those who treat offenders. As both clinical subspecialties have grown in size and sophistication, the gulf between them seems only to have widened. Rather than working together on the common problem of sexual violence, they often appear to be adversaries. From our vantage, the source of the conflict appears to be hostility for the offender that is displaced onto those who treat offenders, coupled with, or perhaps resulting from, the overidentification of therapists with their clients (victim therapists with victims and offender therapists with offenders). Whatever the sum and substance of this hostility, it does a major disservice to our collective efforts to combat sexual violence.

At JJPI, where victim and offender therapists work together, we have struggled to achieve the ultimate goal, not just accommodation and harmony among our therapists but crossover in caseloads. At the present time, half of our full-time clinicians work with victims as well as offenders. We have consistently found that they glean from their experience a unique and richer perspective on the problem of sexual violence. The complexity of the problems that we face and the reductionistic myopia of grouping all clients into one of two categories—victim or offender—is illustrated by a very recent case of a male survivor in his early 30s who was screened for our male survivors group. During the course of the interview, he revealed that he had seven victims, though none within the past 2 years. He reported numerous distal effects of childhood sexual abuse, one of which was the recapitulative sexual abuse of others. Given his complex symptom picture, however, it was difficult to classify him as an adult survivor or as a child molester, and thus to determine whether he should be placed in the group for survivors or in a group for child molesters. He, like many of the children and adolescents that we see, was both. We eventually decided to place him in a time-limited male survivors group, allow him to work on his own abuse, and then move him into an offender group and have him work on his abuse of others.

In summary, the tasks that we face demand nothing less than social activism. We must move beyond responding after the fact to traumatized children and work for the right of children to grow up in a nonviolent community with nonabusive caregivers. We must move beyond responding after the fact to traumatized adults and work for the right of women to enjoy their lives unencumbered by the interminable fear of sexual assault. If primary prevention does not become our resolute goal, then secondary intervention will be our unremitting burden. Only by harnessing our collective energies, pulling in a common direction, and speaking with a single, strong voice can we muster the authority that is needed to effect genuine social change.

REFERENCES

Abel, G.G., Lawry, S. S., Karlstrom, E., Osborn, C.A., & Gillespie, C.F. (1994). Screening tests for pedophilia. *Criminal Justice and Behavior, 21*, 115–131.

Appelbaum, P. S. (1993). legal liability and managed care. *American Psychologist, 48*, 251–257.

Aubrey, M., & Dougher, M. J. (1990). Ethical issues in outpatient group therapy with sex offenders. *The Journal for Specialists in Group Work, 15*, 75–82.

Berlin, F. S. (1989). The paraphilias and depo-Provera: Some medical, ethical and legal considerations. *Bulletin of the American Academy of Psychiatry and the Law, 17*, 233–239.

Carter, D. L., & Prentky, R. A. (1993). Forensic treatment in the United States: A survey of selected forensic hospitals. Massachusetts Treatment Center. *International Journal of Law and Psychiatry, 16*, 117–132.

Gordon, R., & Verdun-Jones, S. N. (1983). Ethics and ethical dilemmas in the treatment of sex offenders. In S. N. Verdun-Jones & A. A. Keltner (Eds.), *Sexual aggression and the law* (pp. 75–96). Burnaby, British Columbia: Criminology Research Centre, Simon Fraser University.

Grubin, D., & Prentky, R. A. (1993). Sexual psychopathy laws. *Criminal Behaviour and Mental Health, 3*, 381–392.

Hare, R. D. (1991). *The Hare Psychopathy Checklist–Revised.* Toronto, Canada: Multi-Health Systems.

Knight, R. A., Prentky, R. A., & Cerce, D. C. (1994). The development, reliability, and validity of an Inventory for the Multidimensional Assessment of Sex and Aggression. *Criminal Justice and Behavior, 21,* 72–94.

Prentky, R. A. (1995). A rationale for the treatment of sex offenders: Pro Bono Publico. In J. McGuire (Ed.), *What works: Reducing reoffending guidelines from research and practice* (pp. 153–170). Sussex, England: John Wiley.

Prentky, R. A., & Burgess, A. W. (1990). Rehabilitation of child molesters: A cost-benefit analysis. *American Journal of Orthopsychiatry, 60,* 108–117.

Weiner, B. A. (1985). Legal issues raised in treating sex offenders. *Behavioral Sciences & the Law, 3,* 325–340.

10

B. Community Settings

Community Treatment in the United Kingdom

Richard Beckett

INTRODUCTION

The 1990s has seen a rapid expansion in the provision of community sex offender treatment programs in the United Kingdom. A number of factors—societal, professional, and legislative—contributed to this expansion. At a societal level, as in North America, the women's movement had raised cultural awareness as to the role of women and challenged the economic, social, and personal disadvantages and discriminations that flowed from this. As this awareness developed, so increasingly did the focus encompass the physical and sexual victimization of women and children and society's response to it. In 1986, Childline, the national, confidential counseling and advice telephone service was opened. This followed a television program focused on the hidden nature of child abuse. It invited viewers' responses and jammed the British Broadcasting Corporation telephone lines with calls from children, many of whom had been sexually abused and had never disclosed before. The 1980s also saw increasing public and professional concern highlighted by high-profile child abuse enquiries (e.g., Butler-Schloss, 1988), which exposed high levels of pervasive hidden child sexual abuse within communities. These, together with evidence emerging from North American studies as to the prevalence of child sexual abuse (e.g., Russell, 1983) and rape (e.g., Koss, 1989), provided the impetus for changes in both professional and judicial responses to sexual assault. In 1979, 20% of convicted sex offenders received immediate custodial sentences. By 1989, this figure had risen to 33%. As a consequence, the number of male prisoners in custody convicted of sexual offenses rose from 4.7% in 1980 to 7.5% in 1989. The increased likelihood of receiving a prison sentence or extended probation order for a sexual offense received greater impetus under the Criminal Justice Act of 1991, where special provision was made for the sentencing and management of sex offenders. Prior to this act, automatic parole for sex offenders was commonplace and often involved minimal supervision. However, changes within the legislation placed much greater emphasis on sex offenders addressing their offending behavior as a condition of probation or parole. Provisions were made within the act that

Richard Beckett • Department of Forensic Psychology, Fair Mile Hospital, Wallingford, Oxfordshire, England OX10 9HH.

Sourcebook of Treatment Programs for Sexual Offenders, edited by Marshall et al. Plenum Press, New York, 1998.

allowed the courts to make orders for offenders to be closely supervised right through until the end of their parole. In practice, the likelihood that a sex offender would receive a probation order or that more serious offenders would be released on parole became increasingly dependent on whether a suitable community-based treatment program was available for the offender.

Prior to the late-1980s, the provision of sex offender treatment was sparse and largely confined to that carried out within maximum security special hospitals, the newly established medium security Regional Forensic Services and specialized hospitals such as the London Tavistock and Portman Clinics and the Maudsley Hospital. Historically, much of the treatment provided for sex offenders had been conducted by psychodynamic and psychanalytic therapists; where this was not the case, therapeutic interventions focused predominantly on reconditioning sexual arousal and social heterosexual skills training (e.g., Perkins, 1982). In the late 1980s, a new style of treatment program developed. These new treatment programs were almost exclusively cognitive–behavioral in their approach and were delivered by practitioners who espoused a common philosophy and value base. These values placed child protection and multiagency working at their core, and many programs made explicit their stance on nonsexist values and attitudes, empowerment to women and children, and the need to challenge the abuse of male power. In order to achieve this, treatment programs laid particular emphasis on female and male therapists co-working and trying to ensure that therapists related to each other in ways that did not reflect cultural stereotypes: for example, where the male might be expected to be the active leader with the female taking the more passive role. Female co-leadership was also seen as particularly valuable in helping maintain a sensitivity to victim issues and to help ensure that male therapists did not get inadvertently drawn into collusive attitudes with their male clients. The structure and content of these therapeutic programs were strongly influenced by a small number of North American practitioners. David Finkelhor's four-factor model of sexual abuse (Finkelhor, 1984) and Stephen Wolfe's cycle of offending (Wolfe, 1984) were particularly influential and provided practitioners with frameworks around which they developed their therapeutic programs. Practical books and manuals, particularly those of Anna Salter (1988), and Abel et al. (1984), were especially influential in providing intervention strategies to challenge denial and cognitive distortions and for enhancing victim empathy.

THE FIRST NATIONAL SURVEY OF UNITED KINGDOM PRACTICE

In 1991, Barker and Morgan undertook a national survey of community-based treatment programs run by the probation service, who, by this time, were emerging as the lead providers of such services. Barker and Morgan's report (1993) graphically illustrated the rapid increase that had taken place in the development of community-based treatment programs and also raised a number of areas of concern. Of the 55 probation services surveyed in England and Wales, only 13 claimed not to be running some type of treatment program for sex offenders; of those 13, 7 said they were planning to run programs in the near future. Overall, a total of 63 probation-run sex offender treatment programs were identified of which 37% have been running for 2 years or less and a further 31% had been started within the previous 5 years. The vast majority of treatment was offered in a group work context by probation officers frequently working outside their normal working hours and without work load relief. This level of commitment and enthusiasm, however, was not always reflected by the support individual practitioners received within their probation services. The majority of treatment programs drew on specialist advice and consultation, typically from forensic psychologists. Probation managers, however, varied considerably in their support for such programs. For example, only 2% of the services studied were found to have a formal policy on how their sex offender treatment program might be resourced, managed, and supported. From a practitioner perspective, this lack of organizational support at times created resentment and frustration and, over the longer term, raised the possibility of practitioner burnout and program collapse. Probation management also had its concerns. Sex offenders accounted for only approximately 5% of the overall probation caseload, yet this small group was absorbing a disproportionate amount of practitioner time and generating an increasing demand for resources. Moreover, because the impetus to develop treatment programs had been practitioner-led, many managers lacked the skills and confidence to supervise this area of work. The final concern was that of program evaluation and treatment effectiveness. Despite Furby, Weinrott, and Blackshaw's (1989) pessimistic review of treatment outcome for sex offenders and subsequent critiques of outcome methodology (e.g., Quinsey, Harris, Rice, & Lalumiere, 1993), the overwhelming mood was of treatment optimism. This was underpinned by a conviction that effective treatment and management of sex offenders needed to be developed if the high rate of sexual victimization was to be reduced.

British practitioners' optimism and drive to improve therapeutic effectiveness drew support from a number of North American and British researchers and practitioners. Marshall, Ward, Johnston, Jones, and Barbaree's "Optimistic Evaluation of Treatment Outcome with Sex Offenders" (1991) and the results emerging from the California Sex Offender Treatment Evaluation Project (Marques, Day, Welson, Milner, & West, 1991; Marques, Welson, West, & Day, 1994), together with British reviews (e.g., Thornton, 1992), all contributed to this momentum. Increasingly, and particularly under the auspices of the National Association for the Development of Work with Sex Offenders (NOTA; see below), high-profile North American practitioners (Bill Marshall, Anna Salter, Richard Laws, and Bill Pithers) traveled to the United Kingdom to deliver workshops and academic papers. The question remained, however, as to the effectiveness of British sex offender treatment programs. As Barker and Morgan (1993) described, not only had many treatment programs only recently been established, but they varied along a number of dimensions. Group treatment programs varied in their intensity and duration. Some probation services offered 2-week intensive group treatment programs, while others met weekly or even fortnightly. While some programs were of fixed duration, others were rolling programs admitting offenders at different points throughout their treatment cycle. As a consequence, time in treatment could vary from 50 hours to upwards of 150 hours depending on the program available. Programs also varied in who they treated. While the majority of programs were, in principle, open to child abusers, rapists, and exhibitionists, the majority in practice treated only child abusers. As well as being less available for treatment, rapists (frequently young men often with extensive criminal backgrounds) were generally less motivated for treatment. It was also suspected that practitioners themselves felt less confident in treating rapists, not only because of the difficulty in engaging such men in a therapeutic dialogue, but also because the results of North American studies (e.g., Pithers and Cummings, 1989; Maletztsky, 1991) suggested they were more difficult to treat. Although the vast majority of United Kingdom treatment programs ascribed to the cognitive–behavioral model and described broadly similar therapeutic objectives (breaking down denial by examining an individual's cycle of offending, challenging cognitive distortions, enhancing victim empathy, developing relapse prevention skills), the techniques and strategies used by individual programs to achieve this varied as evinced by the training manuals produced by different treatment programs across the country. Finally, few programs attempted to systematically evaluate their work either in the short or longer term. In the shorter term, group leaders typically used a combination of therapeutic judgments combined with group work exercises to evaluate a man's progress in treatment. The assessment of deviant sexual arousal through penile plethysmography was confined to a small group of forensic psychologists working within the British maximum-security special hospitals and some of the regional forensic services. Such a facility was and indeed remains largely unavailable to those running community-based treatment programs for sex offenders. With regard to longer-term follow-up of offenders treated by community-based programs, no information was available. In part, this reflected the fact that the majority of treatment programs had been in existence for less than 5 years. Where reconviction studies could have been carried out on the more established programs, these had not taken place due to a combination of factors, including lack of time available to practitioners, lack of organizational support and a belief in some parts that because programs were evolving rapidly, reconviction data on previously treated clients would not necessarily and might indeed reflect adversely on current practice.

THE SEX OFFENDER TREATMENT
AND EVALUATION PROJECT (STEP) REPORT

By 1992, the high cost of delivering community-based treatment for relatively small numbers of men raised fundamental questions. Was community-based treatment effective. Did treatment programs vary in their effectiveness depending on their content and style of delivery, duration, and intensity. Were the treatment programs more effective with child abusers as opposed to rapists and, given the heterogeneity of child abusers, were some types benefiting more than others. In response to these questions and to political pressure to finance treatment programs (e.g., the Gracewell Clinic), the British government commissioned the first British systematic evaluation of community-based sex offender treatment programs.

The STEP study (Beckett, Beech, Fisher, & Fordham, 1994) evaluated six representative community-based treatment programs for sex offenders, together with the Gracewell Clinic, a specialist residential treatment program for child abusers. There were several aims of this study. These included examining the impact on clients treated, to identify which elements of the treatment programs were most effective, to make recommendations on how programs might improve their effectiveness and to collect data for a long-term reconviction study. Of the programs selected, two were rolling long-term, open-ended programs and three were short-term, intensive programs offering, on average 54 hours of treatment over approximately 2 weeks. The other was a short-term intensive week program followed through with the client seeing his own probation officer and one of the group leaders as a team. In total, 52 child abusers were systematically assessed before and after 54 hours of community-based treatment and these were compared with clients treated by the residential program who had on average received 462 hours of therapy.

Psychological Measures

These could be divided into three broad categories. The first set of measures assessed offense-specific problems, those areas that were believed to directly relate to offending behavior and typically the targets of cognitive–behavioral treatment. These included denial of offense planning and deviant fantasy, cognitive distortions and justifications, empathy for victims, and relapse prevention knowledge and skills. The second set of measures assessed those areas of personality functioning that had been previously described in the literature as of relevance to sex offenders. Such areas included self-esteem, assertiveness, general empathy, locus of control, and emotional loneliness. Finally, three validity scales were included to assess the extent to which offenders were biased toward producing socially desirable responses, had insight into their general thoughts and feelings, and were prepared to be open about their sexual behavior. In a number of key areas, for example, victim empathy, emotional congruence, cognitive distortions, and relapse prevention, appropriate measures did not exist and therefore had to be developed and standardized during the preliminary stages of the research. For comparison purposes, the majority of scales used were standardized on 81 nonoffending British men. In addition to these measures, the therapeutic climate of the treatment programs was assessed by means of the Group Environment Scale (Moos, 1986), which was completed by both leaders and clients and provided a measure of group process: leadership style, client self-actualization, and group organization and structure.

Deviancy and Risk

The normal, nonoffending sample of men provided a standard against which the child abusers entering treatment could be compared. Using a statistical procedure–cluster analysis—it was possible to describe the child abusers entering treatment in terms of the extent to which they deviated from normal men (Beech, in press). It was found that those child abusers who differed very highly from the normal sample of nonabusing men also had profiles of high-risk child abusers. They typically had high numbers of victims, had committed offenses inside and outside the family, against male and female victims, and had high statistical risk of further sexual reoffending (Thornton & Travers, 1991; Fisher & Thornton, 1993). In contrast, some child abusers were found, on assessment, to have personality profiles that differed relatively little from that found in the nonoffending male sample. They did, however, differ on the offense-specific measures. They typically showed patterns of denial and minimization, justifications for their offending, poor victim empathy, and lack of relapse prevention knowledge and skills. Such men were most commonly incest abusers against female children, were not recidivists, and had low statistical rates of reconviction.

Nature of Treatment

To a greater or lesser extent, all the community-based treatment programs studied used the same group treatment methods. These included group discussion, working in small groups or pairs on selected topics. The therapeutic exercises included (see Beckett, 1994, for further details):

- Reducing denial through working in detail on the client's offense, its antecedents and consequences. Such exercises emphasized the client taking responsibility for his actions and served as a vehicle for investigating the offender's motivation, offense planning and fantasies, and how he groomed the victim and overcame their resistance and attempted to ensure the child's silence.

- Challenging the offender's self-justifications for their behavior and the distorted thinking they employed to help overcome their inhibitions to abuse. Opportunities to focus on these areas often arose naturally during the course of the offense analysis work, though programs often also used other group exercises to examine how clients misinterpreted children's behavior and convinced themselves that the victim was consenting and was not harmed by the abuse.

- Lack of victim empathy was seen as a major cause of sexual abuse. Consequently, enhancing victim empathy was seen as a core component of all treatment groups. During treatment, offenders were typically shown videotapes of victims describing their own abuse and the impact it had on them, both immediately and in the longer term. Reading material was often provided and some programs invited outside speakers to describe problems victims experienced as a result of the abuse. Most programs asked offenders to write victim apology letters that were not sent to the victim but were used as a vehicle to help clients accept responsibility for their behavior and the damage it had caused.

- Education as to the relationship between deviant fantasy, arousal, and offending was also commonly undertaken. Such discussions emphasized the importance of not masturbating to thoughts of children, what strategies clients might employ to reduce the frequency of their deviate sexual fantasies, and what constituted appropriate sexual fantasies. However, programs studied did not undertake individual fantasy modification such as masturbatory reconditioning or covert sensitization (Laws & Marshall, 1991).

- Eleven programs said they undertook relapse prevention work. Drawing on information gathered from the other treatment modules, therapists helped clients identify potential victims and high-risk thoughts, feelings, behaviors, and situations. Emphasis was placed on helping clients accept the possibility of future risk and on developing strategies to recognize, cope with, or escape from risk when it occurred. The longer-term, rolling programs also described themselves as variously offering social skills and anger management training, sex and alcohol education, and work on developing appropriate personal relationships.

Effectiveness of Treatment

Offenders were retested on the personality and offense-specific measures at the end of 54 hours of treatment, though this did not represent all the treatment they would have received in the more extended programs. At the end of treatment, 54% of child abusers had the profiles that fell largely within the nonoffending range. That is, they could not be distinguished from nonoffending men in terms of their levels of assertiveness, ability to empathize with victims, their level of cognitive distortions and emotional congruence, and their sexual obsessiveness. Even though these offenders' scores on some factors, such as self-esteem and emotional loneliness, did not reach normal levels, they still showed very marked and positive changes after treatment. The results also illustrated the relationship between treatment change and length of time in therapy. Highly deviant child abusers needed a considerable longer time in treatment before they reached a nondeviant "successfully treated" profile. Overall, 65% of the men who began treatment with a low deviancy profile were successfully treated, compared with only 42% of men who started treatment with a highly deviant profile. Short-term group work successfully treated 62% of offenders entering treatment with low deviancy profiles. Such men became much more open about their sexual offenses and sexual problems, showed significant reductions in their justification for offending, and considerably reduced levels of cognitive distortions. With highly deviant men, however, short-term programs were largely unsuccessful. Less than 20% of these offenders had treated profiles by the end of treatment. Long-term therapy, averaging 462 hours of treatment, was more successful than short-term treatment in treating low deviancy men (80% compared with 62%), and considerably more successful in treating highly deviant men (60%). In particular, long-term treatment, as well as reducing denial, justifications, and cognitive distortions, was particularly successful in improving the self-esteem, assertiveness, and intimacy skills of these highly deviant child abusers.

Program Deficits

The research also highlighted a number of areas where treatment needed to be improved. In particular, it was found that 25% of the men treated in both the short- and long-term programs had deteriorated in their empathy for victims by the end of treatment. This was a surprising result given the emphasis all programs placed on enhancing victim empathy. It was hypothesized that this deterioration in victim empathy was due to two factors: one related to client characteristics, the other to therapist variables. The results suggested that clients with particularly low levels of self-esteem and an inability to cope with the feelings of others were emotionally ill-equipped to deal with victim empathy modules, which bombarded them with the consequences of their abusive behavior. As a result, their attitudes toward their victims may have become hardened as a defense strategy. Group observations by the researchers also suggested that certain therapists whose personal style was overconfrontational and unsupportive were more likely to produce clients whose empathy for victims deteriorated during the course of treatment. The second main area highlighted for improvement was that of relapse prevention knowledge and course of treatment. The second main area highlighted for improvement was that of relapse prevention knowledge and skills. On a relapse prevention questionnaire only 27% of clients were able to demonstrate some knowledge of relapse prevention strategies at the end of treatment. Where offenders had improved, these improvements tended to reflect offenders becoming more aware of the factors that might put them at further risk rather than the knowledge of how to cope with risk when it occurred. Perhaps not surprisingly, shorter-term programs were less effective than the long-term program in teaching relapse prevention skills.

Therapeutic Environment

Toward the end of treatment, all group members, both therapists and clients, were given a questionnaire designed to measure the therapeutic environment of the treatment program. Considerable variation was found between different treatment programs with regard to the therapeutic climates they created (Beech & Fordham, 1997). The most successful treatment programs appeared to be those that were well-organized and highly cohesive, produced a sense of group responsibility, encouraged open expression of feelings, empowered group members, and instilled in them a sense of hope for the future. Where leaders were overconfrontational, overcontrolling, and strictly enforced group rules, this appeared to have a countertherapeutic effect. Perhaps because of its more extended duration and its residential nature, the long-term program tolerated considerably more open expression and sharing of feelings than the other programs studied. This, in turn, may have contributed to the finding that the long-term program was particularly effective in helping men who started treatment with particularly low self-esteem, emotional loneliness, and problems of assertion.

STEP Recommendations

As a result of the STEP research, a number of recommendations were made for improving sex offender treatment. The STEP research had shown that treatment success depended on how deviant clients were before treatment, treatment length, and the therapeutic environment. In order to improve treatment effectiveness, it was clearly important to systematically assess all men entering treatment and determine the level of their deviancy so that they could be allocated to a treatment program of a suitable length. This, in turn, required an initiative to identify and train psychologists currently involved with treatment programs in the use of the psychometric tests developed during the course of the STEP research. It was recommended that short-term programs could be effective for low deviancy child abusers provided they extended their length to include better relapse prevention training. However, long-term treatment programs were also needed, and consequently it was recommended that a number of residential treatment programs be established for highly deviant child abusers. Furthermore, a significant proportion of highly deviant child abusers had left the long-term treatment program still with a range of personality problems. These personality problems might never resolve themselves but might contribute to long-term risk of reoffending. Consequently it was recommended that maintenance groups should be established to provide long-term monitoring and support for highly deviant child abusers and those who did not achieve a treated profile by the end of treatment. Not only had the study identified problems in the area of victim empathy and relapse prevention training that needed to be addressed, but few programs provided fantasy modification training. It was recommended that some probation officers could be trained by psychologists in fantasy modification techniques so that this approach could be more widely available to those clients who needed it. It was recognized that all these recommendations had resource and organizational implications. Extending short-term programs and employing psychologists to assist in program evaluation would require further funding. It was not clear how funding might be made available to finance longer-term residential programs. Furthermore, although maintenance programs might be relatively inexpensive, probation and parole orders rarely exceeded 3 years; beyond this, even high-risk offenders could not be mandated into maintenance.

Current Practice in the United Kingdom

In 1995, a survey of all probation services in England, Wales, and Northern Ireland was undertaken by the Association of Chief Offices of Probation (ACOP). This survey replicated and developed the previous research undertaken by Barker and Morgan in 1991. The results of this survey were encouraging and illustrated the extent to which probation had developed a core commitment to its work with sex offenders. By 1995, 82% of probation services had issued a specific policy statement regarding the supervision of sex offenders, whereas only 21% of services had such policies in place in 1991. Moreover, more than half of the 56 probation services surveyed had a coherent strategy for supervising sex offenders and a further 43% were in the process of developing such strategies. The most common strategic partners for probation services were child protection organizations such as Social Services, National Society for the Prevention of Cruelty to Children, and health authorities, thus illustrating how probation work with sex offenders had developed as part of a multiagency strategy for the protection of children.

By 1995, 52% of services had created specialist probation posts to manage and deliver treatment for sex offenders, and of these posts there had been a marked increase in the number of senior managers who now held specialized posts in sex offender work. Reflecting the multiagency approach for sex offender work, 44% of programs now involved other professionals such as psychologists and social workers in the delivery of their programs. The funding arrangements also illustrated the multiagency nature of the work. Although 60% of the programs were funded exclusively by the probation service, 40% were now funded through some form of joint partnership with other agencies.

By 1995, 109 programs for sex offenders were being run by the probation service compared with 63 in 1991, an increase of 73%. All programs surveyed accepted both intra- and extrafamilial abusers of children, and 72% in principle also accepted rapists of adult women. A quarter of programs accepted referrals from women who sexually abused children and a third of programs had made special provision for minority groups, such as offenders with learning difficulties. Some services offered individual treatment for offenders who could not be accommodated within the mainstream group treatment programs. These included female offenders, those with disabilities such as hearing impairment, and those too immature to fit within the adult treatment program.

CURRENT TREATMENT APPROACHES

Programs still vary considerably in the number of treatment hours they offer. The amount of time spent in treatment, per offender, can range from 8 to 225 hours per year, with an average of 81 hours. Seventy percent of the programs offer weekly treatment sessions, with 31% offering intensive treatment on a daily basis. Group work remains the most common form of treatment intervention (97%), though in the majority of programs, co-working, ongoing supervision by individual probation officer and the involvement with mental health professionals are also cited as parallel treatment interventions.

With regard to treatment intervention, Fig. 10.1 shows the variety of treatment goals pursued. Increasing victim empathy, controlling sexual arousal, reducing denial, and improving family relationships are the most commonly cited goals. Interestingly, less than half the programs surveyed still cite relapse prevention as an explicit goal.

Research and Evaluation

Whereas Barker and Morgan (1993) found very few services engaged in such work, by 1995, 64% of probation services said they were undertaking research to evaluate the effectiveness of their work. Researchers included not only probation officers, but also psychologists and university researchers. Seventy-eight percent of programs surveyed said

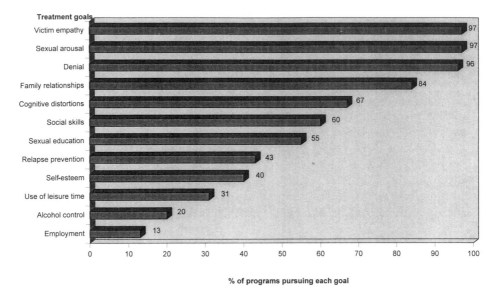

FIGURE 10.1. Treatment goals pursued by sexual offender programs. From Proctor & Flaxington (1996). Reprinted with permission.

they were using psychometric tests, though the nature of such tests were not determined, and 62% were conducting recidivism studies.

National Association for Development of Work with Sex Offenders

The inaugural conference of the National Association for Work with Sex Offenders (NOTA) occurred in 1991. This organization drew together for the first time probation officers, psychologists, social workers, psychiatrists, and other professionals who worked with sex offenders. Through its annual conferences, regional branch meetings, and training workshops, NOTA provides a means by which practitioners can develop and update their knowledge and skills and gain support from others working with sex offenders. NOTA produces a quarterly newsletter that also provides an important vehicle for discussion and debate. In addition to articles on topical issues, the newsletter contains research reviews, conference reports, and digests of the briefing papers produced by the organization and its subcommittees. NOTA has produced a number of briefing papers for practitioners working in the field. These include good practice guidelines for the multiagency management of sex offenders, on the use of sexually explicit material, and on adolescent abusers. A number of subcommittees report to the national executive of NOTA. These include a policy on ethics subcommittee responsible for developing practice standards and guidelines and their research subcommittee, which has developed a national database for adult and adolescent abusers. At a national level, NOTA aims to influence government policy through its submissions to national enquiries on sexual abuse and on proposed legislation. Over the last 2 years, it has developed its international links through affiliation with the American Association for the Treatment of Sexual Abusers and through links with European groups working with sexual abusers. In 1995, NOTA launched the *Journal of Sexual Aggression*, the first British journal devoted to the therapy, research, and dissemination of information on sexual abuse.

The Thames Valley Project—An Illustrative Treatment Program

The three south of England counties of Berkshire, Buckinghamshire, and Oxfordshire cover several major centers of population: Reading, Slough, Oxford, Aylesbury, and Milton Keynes, which together contain a population of 2.3 million people. This area is covered by two probation services, four health authorities responsible for purchasing health service, and four local authority social services departments that carry the lead responsibility for child protection. In 1994, 111 sex offenders were registered with the probation services of the three counties, and a considerably greater number, particularly of child abusers, were known to social services but were beyond any form of statutory supervision such as that provided by the probation service. A long-term treatment group for recidivist child abusers had been established in 1991. This long-term rolling program, however, treated only ten men a year. A probation service also had a 2-week intensive group treatment program, which ran twice or three times a year and treated around 18 offenders a year. These two programs, however, could not deal with the high demand for treatment for even those offenders on probation or parole license. Although some high-risk child abusers known to social services were sometimes admitted to the long-term rolling program, the vast majority of child abusers known to social services received no treatment whatsoever. Where such men attempted to return to family life, social workers typically had to apply to the court for supervision or care orders on the children and had to face the prospect of long-term involvement with the family and the anxiety of trying to protect the children from an untreated sex offender.

Motivating the Organizations

Leading up to the start of the Thames Valley Project, a number of goals had to be achieved to persuade the relevant organizations to provide financial support for the project and to create the conditions necessary for its successful operation. A number of elements contributed to this process. Special interest groups for probation officers working with sex offenders were established. These meetings provided a forum within which practitioners could meet with the local forensic psychologist to discuss problematic cases, to disseminate research, and to gain peer support. In parallel with this development, a sex offender working party designed a strategy to improve the treatment and management of sex offenders. This working party established basic principles on which services were to develop in the future. These principles recognized that working with sex offenders was a specialist task that required a suitable work load relief to enable high-quality work to be undertaken. It also established that all probation officers working with sex offenders should be properly trained and supervised. As a consequence, all probation officers were encouraged to attend workshops on the assessment and treatment of sex offenders. In addition, a series of workshops were also held for probation managers. These workshops helped sensitize managers to the impact sex offender work had, both professionally and personally, on practitioners and focused on developing supervision styles appropriate to this type of work. These developments helped practitioners and managers increase their confidence in working with sex offenders and provided a structure for discussing how the probation services could improve its practice.

Arguing the Case to Improve Treatment Services

A "business case" provided a rationale for why not only the probation service but also health and social services should support the development of a new interagency sex offender treatment program. The business case (Beckett & Goodman, 1994) argued that the health service already dealt, both directly and indirectly, with the consequences of sexual abuse. It recognized that forensic psychologists and psychiatrists faced a heavy demand for assessment of sex offenders but were not resourced to provide a treatment service. It argued that adults who had been sexually abused as children presented, directly or indirectly, to a variety of mental health services. For example, women who had been sexually abused as children were known to be disproportionately represented in psychiatric outpatient admissions and also more likely to experience repeat hospital admissions (Browne & Finkelhor, 1986). Child and adolescent psychiatry services were often asked to become involved in the diagnosis of sexually abused children. A number of research studies had shown that a disproportionate number of young people, referred to such services because of disordered sexual behavior (Fredrich, Urquiza, & Beillke, 1986), running away from home (Herman, 1981), and truancy (Reich & Gutierres, 1979), had been sexually abused. Social services departments argued that successful treatment could reduce the amount of money spent on supervising families where an untreated sex offender had returned home, as well as reducing the incidents of reabuse. Finally, the business case reviewed the rates by which untreated sex offenders are reconvicted and, while acknowledging the problems associated with measuring treatment success (Furby et al., 1989), drew attention to more optimistic outcomes of treatment effectiveness (Marshall et al., 1991) and the recently published Home Office evaluation study (Beckett et al., 1994).

Program Delivery

The Thames Valley Project assesses over 140 sex offenders a year and runs six 2-week intensive group treatment programs, taking up to eight offenders in each group. The structure of the treatment program conformed to the principles of the "what works" literature (Andrews, 1995; Lipsey, 1995). As such, the program is community-based, cognitive–behavioral in its orientation, and selects clients on the basis of risk assessment. It also employed a variety of means in order to ensure program integrity (e.g., Lipsey, 1992; Hollin, 1995): ensuring that the project's clinical effectiveness is systematically assessed; employing trained and experienced practitioners who were initially involved in designing the therapy program; and using treatment manuals and involving managers who are expert in this field of work. Furthermore, the project offers the prospect of improving interagency working, providing an additional training resource, and establishing a systematic database on sex offenders that will assist in the planning of future services.

Staffing and Organizational Support

The Thames Valley Project has four full-time members of staff: A senior probation officer who acts as project coordinator, a forensic psychologist and a probation officer, supported by an administrator and clerical officer. The project team is supported by a small management team consisting of probation managers, a consultant forensic psychologist and consultant child psychiatrist, and child protection coordinators drawn from the participating social services departments. The project also has a multiagency advisory group, which

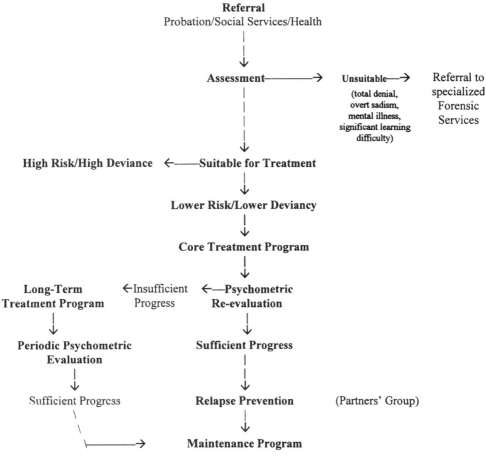

FIGURE 10.2.   The Thames Valley Project structure.

meets biannually, provides the project with political support and guidance, and helps ensure the project's profile within organizations that might have an influence of its future direction and funding.

Program Structure

Figure 10.2 illustrates the structure of the Thames Valley Program and its referral and treatment process. Referrals come from three main sources: probation officers, social workers, and members of the health profession. Clients referred by the probation service may be mandated as part of a probation order or parole license to attend treatment. Alternatively, they may be referred for assessment prior to a criminal sentence. Clients referred by social services departments are most typically men with a history of sexual offending who wish to gain less restricted access their children or return to family life. Whereas most probation clients have offended relatively recently, some social services clients are referred to the project having abused many years ago. The 2-week intensive group treatment program accepts any rapist, child abuser, or exhibitionist who is prepared to acknowledge, albiet minimally, that they have committed some form of sexual assault. Clients with overt psychiatric disorder or who have significant learning difficulties are excluded. Although excluded, nonadmitters are seen by forensic psychologists and probation officers where attempts are made on an individual basis to overcome the client's denial.

The assessment focuses on the client's risk and suitability for treatment and to enhance his motivation to change. At this stage, the client also completes the standard set of psychological measures developed during the course of the STEP research. These measures are used for two main purposes. First, they provide the program leaders with a psychological profile of the client. Since the previous STEP research shows that clients with highly deviant psychological profiles do not change sufficiently during the course of 60 hours treatment, clients who are found to have such profiles may, at this stage, be referred to the long-term rolling treatment program. Alternatively, plans can be made at this stage to refer the client there once they have completed the intensive treatment group. Second, the psychological measures provide a baseline against which to judge treatment change. Clients who successfully reduce their deviant profile during the course of treatment to that similar to a nonoffending group are regarded as having been "successfully" treated. Providing that other appropriate relapse prevention strategies are in place, such clients are recommended as suitable for rehabilitation back into their families. Clients whose psychological profile does not change sufficiently are regarded much more cautiously and may be referred for longer-term treatment.

Core Treatment Program

This consists of 2 weeks of intensive group treatment providing 45 hours of treatment, which is then followed by six more 2-hour groups focused on developing relapse prevention knowledge and skills (Bates & Wilson, 1996). Each group is led by two of the project team, with the third team member acting as a consultant–debriefer. As the project develops, additional probation staff are trained as co-therapists. The initial group session uses a number of therapeutic exercises designed to develop trust and openness between group members and to build group cohesion. The subsequent group sessions have a number of key objectives. These include reducing denial and justification for offending, improving victim empathy, and setting a framework for the relapse prevention model. A detailed cognitive–behavioral analysis of each client's offense provides the main means by which denial is confronted and overcome. Finkelhor's four-factor model (Finkelhor, 1984) provides a structure for examining the offender's motivation: how he justified his abusive behavior, targeted the victim, overcame their resistance, and tried to keep the abuse secret. It is during the course of this exercise that deviant sexual fantasies are often disclosed and these are targeted during subsequent individual treatment sessions. This analysis of the offender's behavior provides a main source of information for constructing the client's relapse prevention plan.

The victim empathy components of the program uses a combination of group work exercises and educational inputs. Group work exercises include having offenders reflect on their own experiences of victimization and its impact on them and the writing of a "victim apology letter." The educational component includes clients watching and discussing videos of victims talking about their experiences and a talk by a member of a local child psychiatry team on their work with sexually victimized children.

Toward the end of the 2-week program, offenders undertake an exercise to assess how they perceive each other's risk of further offending. This helps group leaders assess how needed to develop a consensus as to what should be measured and in standardizing the assessment measures used. It is only through the development of agreed standards in this area that treatment programs can match offenders to the treatment available, measure short-term outcome, and compare relative effectiveness across treatment programs. Moreover, an increasing number of sex offenders are now leaving prison having completed the core treatment program (see Chapter 4, this volume). Given that these offenders will show variable degrees of treatment change, systematic postrelease assessment is needed to identify those in need of further therapeutic intervention. In an effort to address this issue, during the last year, the STEP research team has run a series of training workshops to disseminate the STEP research measures to forensic psychologists involved as consultants to probation programs.

Although there are grounds to be optimistic regarding the short-term effectiveness of British treatment programs for child abusers, their longer-term effectiveness, through British treatment programs has yet to be determined. Proctor (1996) followed up a mixed group of recidivism studies, has yet to be determined. Proctor (1996) followed up a mixed group of sex offenders treated by a well-established cognitive–behavioral program in Oxfordshire, for 52.37 months on average. Their recidivism rate was compared with that of a matched group of sex offenders supervised by the probation service. Unfortunately, because the untreated offenders were observed for significantly longer than the treated group, because the sample size was relatively small and the base rate of reoffending of the untreated group was low, there was no statistically significant treatment effect. The results, however, did show an encouraging trend. Untreated offenders were reconvicted at three times the rate of their treated counterparts. Moreover, none of the treated rapists were reconvicted, compared with five of the ten untreated rapists, albiet that they were followed-up for a longer (29 months) period of time. In another relevant study, Hedderman and Sugg (1996) conducted a 2-year follow-up of 133 sex offenders referred to one of the seven community-based treatment programs studied by the STEP team. These were compared with 191 sex offenders given probation orders but not allocated to an identified treatment program. At the 2-year follow-up, only 4.5% of offenders attending one of the treatment programs had been reconvicted of a sexual offense, compared with 9% of the probation-supervised sample. Furthermore, the probation-supervised group was five times more likely to be reconvicted of a further nonsexual offense than those treated by one of the STEP treatment programs. Interestingly and encouragingly, none of the sexually reconvicted men from the STEP sample had been assessed as "successfully treated" according to the STEP psychological measures. This suggested that the psychological measures used might help predict sexual reconviction as the research team hoped. Clearly, however, a minimum of a 5-year follow-up and an expanded treatment sample are necessary before these results can be considered reliable.

In addition to the above, United Kingdom treatment programs face a number of other future challenges. Over the last 3 years, cuts in public service expenditure has presented the probation service with difficult decisions over how it prioritizes its work. While on one hand there remains considerable public and professional pressure to maintain treatment programs for sex offenders, they remain labor intensive and expensive. Moreover, the National Health Service, a major employer of forensic psychologists, has been reorganized into purchaser and provider units. Consequently, psychological services that are needed, for example, to assist probation in evaluating their programs must now be purchased, which is a further demand on the probation services diminishing budget. In this period of economic stringency, to consolidate the existing programs would be an achievement in itself. However, it is questionable whether resources can be found to fund the development

much clients have understood about the causes of sexual assault and vulnerability to future risk. On the final day of the program, clients present the work—analysis of their offending, victim apology letter, and so on—to their supervising probation officer or social worker. This is used to help identify goals for ongoing therapeutic work. Clients then take the assessment questionnaires, which, when scored, help decide whether sufficient treatment progress has been achieved.

Relapse Prevention

The relapse prevention component of the treatment program starts approximately 6 weeks after offenders have completed the core group work. This module consists of six 2-hour weekly sessions. The main objectives of this module are to provide the offender with a clear understanding of the relapse prevention process, for him to examine his most likely route to a relapse, and to help each individual develop coping and escape strategies to deal with lapses when they occur. By the end of this module, clients are expected to have a clear relapse prevention plan. This involves not only developing their own personal strategies to avoid and cope with risk, but also one that involves plans for a realistic and positive offense-free lifestyle and involves others, both family and professionals, in monitoring agreed-upon behavior. Group work material is retained by the group member and shared with both the group member's family and their individual supervising officer so that there exists a network of appropriate people who can act as external monitors.

The initial relapse prevention session reviews what clients have learned from the core treatment program and reinforces motivation to remain offense free by examining the short- and long-term costs and gains from their offending. Subsequently, clients are educated in the principles of relapse prevention (Pithers, 1990): the differences between "lapse" and "relapse," the role of "seemingly irrelevant decisions," the nature of urges and the components of risk. In the following weeks clients keep a lapse diary as a homework assignment in which they are encouraged to record thoughts, feelings, and behaviors related to their offending and how they coped with these. These diaries are analyzed at each treatment session, and group members help each other develop strategies to cope with or avoid the lapses recorded. Role-play is also used to help group members rehearse behavioral strategies that could be used to cope with risk situations. Toward the end of the program, each client constructs a personalized relapse prevention plan. This is shared with their supervising officer and others, such as partners, who have been identified as a member of the client's external monitoring network.

Partner's Group

The role of a nonabusing parent is considered central to protecting children within a family. Consequently, when offenders are considered for return to their family, a module has been developed to enhance the protective abilities of the nonabusing partner. Run by a member of the project staff and selected social workers, this module runs for six sessions. The main objectives of this module are to consolidate and enhance the effectiveness of the offender's relapse prevention plan by actively developing the role of the nonabusing partner. This is achieved by informing the nonabusing partner of the offender's *modus operandi*, thus giving them greater insight into those thoughts, feelings, and behaviors that are relevant to the individual's offending behavior. The module gives the partner an opportunity to discuss their own reactions to the abuse that has taken place and how this affected them and their family. As such, the module acts as a support group for partners who themselves have suffered as a result of the offender's behavior. Throughout the group the possibility of future risk is emphasized, as is the need for the nonabusing partner to be empowered and confident in challenging behaviors that concern her and on using the support of others around her.

Long-Term Treatment Group

This long-term rolling program runs parallel to and complements the core treatment program. It offers long-term treatment to high-risk sex offenders, predominantly child abusers. As such, the group targets recidivist child abusers or, irrespective of their previous offending history, men with highly deviant psychological profiles as measured on the STEP assessment scales. Unlike the 2-week intensive program, clients are only discharged from the rolling program after having successfully completed all of its modules and who are found on retesting to have a "treated" psychological profile. The majority of offenders attending the program are mandated as part of probation or parole license, though others join the program because without attending they can have no prospect of returning to family life. The structure of the group treatment program closely follows that of the English Prison Service core treatment program (see Chapter 4, this volume), which provides in excess of 120 hours treatment. The program has extended modules focused on reducing denial, detailed analysis of the client's previous offenses, and relapse prevention training. Extensive work is also undertaken on deconstructing often deeply entrenched patterns of distorted thinking regarding children and their sexuality, enhancing victim empathy, and reducing the emotional significance (emotional congruence) children often have for fixated child abusers. Clients attending the program usually present with a sexual preference for children that manifests as deviant sexual arousal to children. Consequently, it is necessary to offer all men attending the program individual fantasy modification sessions that may take several months to complete. In addition, the vast majority of men attending the program have been abused themselves, sometimes extensively. This issue is addressed directly during the course of treatment, though for a substantial number of clients, individual therapeutic sessions have to be provided. The majority of clients who attend the program also suffer from social inadequacy, a history of failure in adult relationships, and social isolation. The problems necessitate not only therapeutic interventions focused on social and relationship-building skills, but also on providing a broader range of support: assisting with work and accommodation and helping introduce clients to appropriate networks of longer-term social support. For gay men who abuse children, the program draws on gay counseling and support networks to aid appropriate social networking and to help them establish gay consenting relationships.

Maintenance Group

Maintenance is seen as particularly important for recidivist sex offenders and men returning to family life. The maintenance group recognizes that for the socially inadequate child abusers and rapists, future risk may remain significant even after they have attended over 2 years of group treatment in the long-term rolling program. Maintenance is also seen as important for sex offenders returning to family life. In such cases social services and the courts are encouraged to grant offenders access to their families or approve family reintegration and the lifting of care and supervision orders on condition that offenders agree to

participate in the long-term maintenance group. The maintenance group is seen as important for these individuals not only in order to regularly review their relapse prevention plan and skills but also to provide longer-term personal and social support. Maintenance sessions take place at appropriately 8-week intervals in the first year after active treatment has finished. Thereafter, clients are encouraged to attend at 3-month intervals. Most clients attend with a detailed relapse prevention plan constructed during the course of previous treatment. Sessions focus on this plan on those specific factors identified during treatment that might indicate the risk of possible relapse. Clients are encouraged to report on their success at dealing with lapses and risk situations, as well as to report on problems and difficulties. Since relapses are often preceded by life events that result in loneliness or depression in child abusers, or anger and resentment in rapists (Pithers et al., 1988), specific questions are asked about the occurrence of life events, personal setbacks, and disappointments that might undermine the client's capacity to cope. Maintenance sessions not only review, but also directly enhance coping skills by, for example, drawing on other group members' advice on how to solve an individual's problems, role-playing problematic situations, or helping to challenge thinking patterns that might contribute to low mood. Clients are also encouraged to look forward, to anticipate potential problems and challenges, and to plan their coping strategies in advance.

CONCLUSION—ISSUES AND FUTURE DIRECTIONS

This chapter has described the rapid expansion of community-based treatment for sex offenders that has taken place over the last 10 years. This expansion was spearheaded particularly by probation officers working with forensic psychologists, often in their own time, and with variable and quite frequently inadequate organizational support. During the early 1990s, probation services started to invest heavily in this area of work, developing policy and practice guidelines for the treatment and management of sex offenders and creating specialist posts at both main grade and senior levels. As these programs have developed, the trend has been toward involving other agencies within the child protection system to share both the funding and the delivery of these services.

With regard to the future development of sex offender treatment in the United Kingdom, a number of issues arise. At the level of program delivery, the majority of probation programs are still relatively short, most offering less than 100 hours of treatment. On the basis of the research described in this chapter, such relatively short programs cannot be expected to effectively treat highly deviant offenders. Moreover, despite the finding that relapse prevention was inadequately addressed in many programs, still less than half the treatment programs recently surveyed identified relapse prevention as a core treatment task. Whereas there can be little doubt that all the treatment components offered within programs do contribute to relapse prevention, the question still remains as to whether programs sufficiently focus on training clients in those specific skills needed to recognize, avoid, or cope with future risk. There also remains a lack of expertise in the area of sexual fantasy modification. While the demand for this work cannot be met by the relatively few available forensic psychologists, there has yet to be any training initiative to help probation officers develop these skills. Consequently, the majority of treatment programs offer education on the role of deviant fantasy rather than interventions to modify them. The assessment of sex offender treatment also continues to be problematic. Although the majority of programs now describe using various psychometric tests to evaluate treatment impact, progress is

of new and needed services. These include groups for rapists, "nonadmitters," for partners of child abusers wishing to return to the family, and learning disabled and female sex offenders. With these latter two groups, the relatively small numbers of such clients coming into contact with the probation service is likely to require initiatives that draw in clients from catchment areas larger than those covered by most single probation services. This may act as a disincentive to the development of such programs. Moreover, with learning disabled offenders, for example, their slower rates of learning may necessitate longer programs, a further disincentive to their development. Another much-needed development is noncustodial, residential treatment programs for highly deviant child abusers. This is especially the case for certain (highly deviant) social services clients who have abused but have not been prosecuted, or who received a prison sentence too short to allow custodial treatment. Increasing demands on social services and health budgets have seriously restricted development in this area.

The prospects of developing maintenance groups, however, are more likely. Not only are such programs relatively inexpensive, newly proposed changes in criminal justice legislation may necessitate their development. The new legislation will enable courts to specify, at the time a sex offender is sentenced, extended periods of supervision that far exceed the current length of probation and parole orders. For some offenders this will be lifetime supervision. In such cases maintenance programs may prove the most cost-efficient way for the probation service to carry out these new responsibilities.

ACKNOWLEDGMENTS. The author expresses thanks and appreciation to Krissi-Hartley-Morris and Rob Bailey for their help in the preparation of this chapter.

REFERENCES

Abel, G., Becker, J. V., Cunningham-Rathner, J., Rouleau, J., Kaplan, M., & Reich, J. (1984). *The treatment of child molesters—A manual.* (Available from SBC-Tm, 722 West 168th Street, Box 17, New York, NY 10032.)

Andrews, D. (1995). The psychology of criminal conduct and effective treatment. In J. McGuire (Ed.), *What works: Reducing reoffending. Guidelines from research and practice* (pp. 35–62). Chichester, England: Wiley.

Barker, M., & Morgan, R. (1993). *Sex offenders: A framework for the evaluation of community-based treatment.* London: Home Office Publishers.

Bates, A., & Wilson, C. (1996). *The Thames Valley project handbook.* (Available from Thames Valley Project, 17 Park Road, Didcot, Oxon, England.)

Beckett, R. C. (1994). Cognitive–behavioural treatment for sex offenders. In T. Morrison, M. Erooga, & R. C. Beckett (Eds.), *Sexual offending against children: Assessment and treatment of male abusers* (pp. 80–101). London: Routledge.

Beckett, R. C., & Goodman, P. (1994). *Business case for the Thames Valley sex offender project.* Oxon, England: Oxford Forensic Service, Fair Mile Hospital.

Beckett, R.C., Beech, A., Fisher, D., & Fordham, A. S. (1994). *Community-based treatment for sex offenders: An evaluation of seven treatment programmes (1994).* London: Home Office Publishers.

Beech, A. R. (in press). A psychometric typology of child abusers. *International Journal of Offender Therapy and Comparative Criminology.*

Beech, A. R., & Fordham, A. S. (1997). Therapeutic climate of sex offender treatment programmes. *Sexual Abuse: A Journal of Research and Treatment, 9,* 219–237.

Browne, A., & Finkelhor, D. (1986). Impact of child sexual abuse: A review of the research. *Psychological Bulletin, 99,* 66–77.

Butler-Sloss, E. (1988). *The report of the inquiry into child abuse in Cleveland, 1987.* London: Her Majesty's Stationary Office.

Finklehor, D. (1984). *Child Sexual Abuse, New Theory and Research.* New York. Free Press.

Fisher, D., & Thornton, D. (1993). Assessing risk of reoffending in sexual offenders. *Journal of Mental Health, 2*, 105–117.

Fredrich, W. N., Urquiza, A. J., & Beillke, R. (1986). Behaviour problems in sexually abused young children. *Journal of Paediatric Psychology, 11*, 47–57.

Furby, L., Weinrott, M. R., & Blackshaw, L. (1989). Sex offender recidivism: A review. *Psychological Bulletin, 105*, 3–30.

Hedderman, C., & Sugg, D. (1996). Does treating sex offenders reduce reoffending? *Home Office Research Findings*, No. 45. London: Home Office.

Herman, J. (1981). *Father–daughter incest*. Cambridge, MA: Harvard University Press.

Hollin, C. (1995). The meaning and implications of 'programme integrity.' In J. McGuire (Ed.), *What works: Reducing reoffending. Guidelines from research and practice* (pp. 195–208). Chichester, England: Wiley.

Koss, M. P. (1989). Hidden rape: Sexual aggression and victimisation in a national sample of college students in higher education. In M. A. Pirog-Godd & J. E. Stets (Eds.), *Violence in dating relationships: Emerging social issues* (pp. 145–168). New York: Prager.

Laws, D. R., & Marshall, W. L. (1991). Masturbatory reconditioning with sex deviates: An empirical review. *Advances in Behavioural Research and Therapy, 13*, 13–25.

Lipsey, M. (1992). Juvenile delinquency treatment. A Meta-analytic inquiry into the variability of effects. In T. Cook, H. Cooper, D. Corday, H. Hartman, L. Hedges, R. Light, T. Louis, & F. Mosteller (Eds.), *Meta-analysis for explanation: A casebook*. New York: Russell Sage Foundation.

Lipsey, M. (1995). What do we learn from 400 research studies on the effectiveness of treatment with juvenile delinquents? In J. McGuire (Ed.), *What works: Reducing reoffending. Guidelines from Research and Practice* (pp. 63–78). Chichester, England: Wiley.

Maletztsky, B. M. (1991). *Treating the sex offender*. Newbury Park, CA: Sage.

Marques, J. K., Day, D. M., Welson, C., Milner, M. H., & West, M. A. (1991). *The sex offender treatment and evaluation project: Fourth report to the Legislature in response to PC 1365*. Sacramento, CA: California State Department of Mental Health.

Marques, J., Welson, C., West, M. A., & Day, D. M. (1994). The relationship between treatment goals and recidivism amongst child molesters. *Behaviour Research and Therapy, 32*, 577–588.

Marshall, W. L., Ward, T., Johnston, P., Jones, R., & Barbaree, H. E. (1991, March). An optimistic evaluation of treatment outcome with sex offenders. *Violence Update*, 1–8.

Moos, R. H. (1986). *Group Environment Scale Manual*, 2nd Edition. Palo Alto, CA: Consulting Psychologists Press.

Perkins, D. (1982). The treatment of sex offenders. In M. P. Feldman (Ed.), *Developments in the study of criminal behaviour, Vol. 1* (pp. 191–214). Chichester, England: Wiley.

Pithers, W. D. (1990). Relapse prevention with sexual aggression: A method for maintaining therapeutic gain and enhancing external supervision. In W. L. Marshall, D. R. Laws, & H. E. Barbaree (Eds.), *Handbook of sexual assault: Issues, theories and treatment of the offender* (pp. 343–361). New York: Plenum.

Pithers, W. D., & Cummings, G. F. (1989). Can relapses be prevented? Initial outcome data from the Vermont Treatment Program for sexual aggressors. In D. R. Laws (Ed.), *Relapse prevention with sex offenders* (pp. 292–310). New York: Guilford.

Pithers, W. D., Kashima, K. M., Cumming, G. F., Beal, L. S., & Buell, M. M. (1988). Relapse prevention of sexual aggression. In Robert A. Prentky & Vernon L. Quinsey (Eds.), *Human sexual aggression: Current perspectives* (pp. 244–260). NY: Annals of the New York Academy of Sciences, Vol. 528.

Proctor, E. (1996). A five-year outcome evaluation of a community-based treatment program for convicted sexual offenders run by the probation service. *Journal of Sexual Aggression, 2*(1), 3–16.

Proctor, E., & Flaxington, F. (1996). *Community-based interventions with sex offenders organised by the probation service: A survey of current practice*. London: Association of Chief Probation Officers.

Quinsey, V. L., Harris, G. T., Rice, M. E., & Lalumiere, M. L. (1993). Assessing treatment efficacy in outcome studies of sex offenders. *Journal of Interpersonal Violence, 8*, 512–523.

Reich, J. W., & Gutierres, S. E. (1979). Escape/aggression incidence in sexually abused juvenile delinquents. *Criminal Justice and Behaviour, 6*, 239–243.

Russell, D. (1983). The incidence and prevalence of intrafamilial and extrafamilial sexual abuse of female children. *Child Abuse and Neglect, 7*, 133–146.

Salter, A. C. (1988). *Treating child sex offenders and their victims—A practical guide*. Newbury Park, CA: Sage.

Thornton, D. (1992). *Long-term outcome of sex offender treatment*. Paper presented at Third European Conference on Psychology and the Law, Oxford, England.

Wolfe, S. C. (1984). *A multi-factor model of sexual deviancy*. Paper presented at Third International Conference on Victimology, Lisbon.

11

B. Community Settings

The Development and Implementation of a Regional Sex Offender Treatment Network

Lloyd G. Sinclair

There are more sexual offenders in need of treatment than there are professionals who are qualified to evaluate and treat them effectively. The lack of treatment providers often results in offenders not obtaining needed services, which can, in turn, contribute to risk for reoffense. Public policy ramifications of this shortfall are potentially severe.

The present chapter presents a model for the development and implementation of a regional organization whose primary purposes are the following: (1) to train mental health clinicians to understand and work effectively with sexual offenders; (2) to promote collegiality and cohesion among the trainees; and (3) to provide ongoing education and support for clinicians who work in a specialty with extraordinary personal and professional demands. In other words, the organization sought not only to offer high-quality training, but also to nurture its graduates in an effort to prevent demoralization and desertion of the field. The model described here was implemented in a state whose population is approximately 5 million persons. Its essential features can be utilized in other jurisdictions where similar needs are identified.

GETTING STARTED

A nonprofit corporation was selected as the organizational structure to encompass both the educational purposes and the need to be available for grant funding. A volunteer board of directors was formed in order to obtain guidance and establish credibility for the new organization. Potential members of the board who might have an interest in the missions of the organization were identified and contacted. Persons were sought who represented geographic (within the state), cultural, and professional diversity and who were widely regarded as successful professionals within their fields. When contacted, these potential board members were informed of the nature and purposes of the organization.

Lloyd G. Sinclair • Wisconsin Sex Offender Treatment Network, Inc., Madison, Wisconsin 53719.
Sourcebook of Treatment Programs for Sexual Offenders, edited by Marshall et al. Plenum Press, New York, 1998.

They were told their involvement would be limited to two 3-hour meetings of the board of directors annually, occasional brief review of materials through the mail, and officer or committee work if desired. In other words, in order to attract suitable candidates for the board, the demands on their time were to be quite limited. Examples of individuals who served on the initial board of directors included a Roman Catholic archbishop, the clinical director of an inpatient prison sex offender treatment program, a prosecuting attorney, a leader in the Native American community, the director of the state department of corrections, a psychiatrist, a psychologist, and the director of a sensitive crimes unit of a metropolitan police department.

STAFF

Two staff persons served initially as volunteers until the first training program was initiated and income was generated; after that time these staff were paid from the organization's budget. One person served as the executive director, whose functions included managing the organizational aspects of the program. The other person served as training coordinator, whose job involved all matters pertaining to the curriculum and delivery of the training program. The executive director applied to revenue authorities for tax-exempt status, established the corporate entity with the relevant government agencies, developed bookkeeping and tax accounting systems, hired and supervised a part-time clerical assistant, and generally performed or supervised all organizational tasks. The training coordinator developed a tentative list and schedule of qualified experts as trainers. A curriculum committee, consisting of members of the board of directors who had expertise in sex offender evaluation and treatment, was convened. Using the training coordinator's draft as a model, the committee discussed and developed the final curriculum. The training curriculum is detailed in Appendix 1.

FACULTY AND CURRICULUM

Potential trainers included a mix of internationally recognized as well as local experts in various aspects of sex offender evaluation and treatment. These selected faculty members were contacted, and after determining their interest and availability, contracts were developed. Contract provisions included the content areas to be covered; the dates, times, and location of the training; the provision by the trainer of continuing education information (educational learning objectives, the curriculum outline, paper copies of slides and overheads to be used, titles of required readings, course content questions and the trainer's curriculum vitae); travel arrangements; and honorarium. Appendix 2 is a sample contract.

The training coordinator oversaw the entire curriculum to ensure that all relevant topic areas were covered while avoiding redundancy, since visiting faculty would have no knowledge of the content of other presentations. The goal was to hire the most qualified presenters for the curriculum. Therefore, topics were occasionally presented out of sequence to accommodate the particular faculty member's schedule and areas of expertise. Since the class attended all 24 days of the training, if materials were slightly out of logical order, the curriculum would be complete by the end of the training program.

Each training episode involved three components. In addition to the 2 days' training, trainees were required to read relevant professional literature in preparation for each module. These readings averaged 150 pages per 2-day session. During the last hour of each module, an examination of the session's content was administered. Successful completion of the program was contingent on attendance and satisfactory performance on examinations. Graduates of the training program were then designated fellows in the Wisconsin Sex Offender Treatment Network.

ENROLLMENT

A letter describing the training program was written and sent to members of the associations of psychologists and social workers in the state approximately 3 months prior to the commencement of the training program. The letter described the nature and purpose of the organization, the curriculum, training calendar, trainers and sites, entry and graduation requirements, and fees. Approximately 5500 letters were mailed, resulting in the enrollment of 55 trainees.

Trainees were required to have a minimum of a master's degree but not necessarily any knowledge or experience with sexual offenders. In the initial training class, about two thirds had master's degrees, with the remaining third possessing doctorates. Most trainees had little or no previous experience in working with sexual offenders, although about ten were quite experienced and elected to participate in the training to upgrade their skills.

Incentives for enrollment stemmed from the three goals of the organization. Potential trainees were offered specialized training in a comprehensive curriculum delivered by experts and fellowship with other practitioners who shared professional interests and experiences. In addition, graduates' names would be included on a list of qualified treatment providers to be forwarded to referring agencies throughout the state who were seeking the services of sex offender treatment specialists.

Since the training program was a comprehensive curriculum, the board of directors decided to require trainees to attend all sessions and, conversely, to deny attendance to any one session for nontrainees. Although some interest was expressed from the professional community to attend selected sessions, the board determined that occasional attendance would be inconsistent with the overall goals of the organization. Also, seminars on particular topics are available from other organizations so that the training program was not essential as a resource for this purpose. It was also believed that the goal of developing a closely knit cadre of experts would likely be diluted if the sessions were attended by a different group of individuals each time.

TRAINING SCHEDULE AND LOCATIONS

Most of the enrolled trainees worked in full-time professional employment. A compromise was needed to accommodate those who wished to have as little time away from their workplaces during the week (typically private practitioners) and those who preferred to have the sessions occur during the work week (typically, public-sector employees who were given time off to attend the training program). Thus, a schedule was arranged that included six Thursday–Friday sessions and six Friday–Saturday sessions. Sessions were conducted for 2 days each month for 1 year. The training days were scheduled from 10:00 AM to 6:00 PM on the first days and from 8:00 AM to 4:00 PM on the second days. This schedule enabled persons who could travel to the training site in a few hours to avoid having to stay overnight before the first day and likewise allowed people to leave relatively early at the end of the second day of training. As noted above, the examination was administered during the last hour of each 2-day training module.

Consideration had been given to having a single location for all sessions, such as in the largest city in the jurisdiction; however, it was believed that to do so risked discouraging potential trainees who resided in more outlying areas. Therefore, training sites were selected throughout the region, thereby sharing the inconvenience of travel fairly. Since sex offender treatment professionals are typically concentrated in the more populous areas, situating the sessions in a wide variety of geographic locales reinforced that part of the organization's mission aimed at training professionals working in underserved areas.

Sessions were located at hotels offering discounted sleeping room rates to trainees and that agreed to provide a meeting room at no charge to the organization. The training facilities were adequate and economical, although not opulent.

BUDGET

Early in the life of the organization, there were no guarantees that supplementary funding would be forthcoming. The initial budget was developed assuming that all revenues would be generated from trainee tuition. In order to meet budgetary requirements, trainees were charged $100 per training day, totaling $2400 for the entire course. Enrollment of approximately 45 trainees was required to generate the necessary revenue for the training program.

The organization was fortunately able to obtain outside financial assistance primarily from two sources. First, the US Department of Justice National Institute of Corrections underwrote a portion of some of the training sessions during the first year, resulting in a stipend of approximately 14% of the first year's budget. The state Department of Corrections contributed photocopying services for handouts and related materials and for examinations through their prison print shop. This assistance resulted in considerable savings to the organization.

ACCOMMODATING EXPERIENCED CLINICIANS

The board of directors addressed the issue of possibly "grandparenting" existing sexual offender treatment providers into fellowship without training, recognizing that some professionals within the region did not need the 24-day training course. After considerable discussion, the board decided that since no suitable mechanism had been developed to evaluate potential experts satisfactorily for this waiver of training requirements, admission to the fellowship without completion of the training program would not be granted.

To deal with this problem, an alternative mechanism was developed that created a category defined as an advanced trainee. This category was designed for persons who desired some training but believed they did not require classes in all the topics offered. In order to become an advanced trainee, a candidate was required to submit two work samples for review by the curriculum committee (which consisted of clinical psychologists with considerable expertise in sexual offender treatment). The first submission was to be a videotape of the candidate working with sexual offenders, wherein the individual demonstrated sex-offender-specific evaluation and/or treatment interventions. The second sample was to be a sex offender evaluation, which included the following areas: (1) a summary of the official description of the offenses; (2) the client's version of the offenses; (3) a summary of the client's life history with particular emphasis on factors that the evaluator identified as contributory to the sex offenses; (4) a sex offender risk assessment; and (5) an overall assessment with treatment recommendations. Candidates were instructed to conceal the identity of their clients. Applications for advanced trainee designation were reviewed by committee members who were not acquainted with the candidate. Approximately half of these applications were accepted, totaling eight advanced trainees, with the others determined to be of unacceptable quality to merit advanced trainee status.

Advanced trainees were allowed to omit training sessions selectively according to their perceived educational needs, but they were not allowed to attend fewer than 4 days of the 24-day training program. As was the case for the regular trainees, however, advanced trainees were required to pass all examinations. When advanced trainees were not in attendance at a training module, they were mailed the examination for completion, return, and grading. Advanced trainees were charged the same tuition as regular trainees for the sessions they attended, and they were assessed half of the training fee for sessions they omitted. This price structure was developed to encourage advanced trainees to attend rather than avoid training sessions, as it was not a great deal more costly to attend sessions than it was to miss them. Of the eight advanced trainees, most elected to attend the vast majority of the sessions, while a few attended closer to the minimum number required.

PROFESSIONAL COMMUNITY REACTION

The overwhelming reaction to the organization and its efforts was positive. However, there were some sex offender treatment professionals who took exception to not being allowed inclusion into the organization with a waiver of the training requirements. These professionals suggested it was unfair for them to be required to pay tuition, obtain training, and be tested in order to be listed as fellows since they were perceived in the community as qualified. They expressed concern that in spite of the organization's claims to the contrary, community perception would be altered toward the belief that only designated fellows would be considered experts in the region. If this alteration in perception occurred, those who were not fellows could be viewed as professionally inferior or unqualified to evaluate and treat sexual offenders. When functioning as an expert in court or when seeking contracts with referring agencies to work with sexual offenders, being perceived as less qualified than a fellow could be detrimental to one's career.

These understandable concerns were discussed by the board of directors at great length. Based on previous reasoning, the board continued to believe that its earlier decision was sound. Nevertheless, the board wished to respond to the concerns voiced by the existing professionals. Another mechanism was developed for entry into fellowship for a limited number of experienced clinicians who could demonstrate their competence without having participated in any aspect of the training program. This mechanism permitted persons to apply for fellowship by submitting for peer review a videotape and evaluation similar to those described above for advanced trainees, and by obtaining a passing grade on an advanced candidate examination set by the curriculum committee for this purpose. This

50-question objective examination covered a breadth of topic areas in the sex offender field, including recent research and relevant empirical findings. Applicants for this procedure were permitted to apply at any time and were charged a nonrefundable processing fee of $500, used to reimburse peer evaluators for their services. Professionals known to treat sexual offenders in the region were notified of the exemption procedure.

CONTINUING EDUCATION

The board of directors recognized that the rapidly evolving field of sex offender evaluation and treatment requires clinicians not only to be well trained but also to be updated in their education. To ensure maintenance of expertise in the field, Fellows are required to attend no fewer than 4 days of continuing education offered by the Wisconsin Sex Offender Treatment Network annually following the initial 24-day training year. These continuing education seminars, termed training updates, are offered in 1-, 2-, and occasionally 3-day segments. This requirement also promotes collegial support and professional consultation, which is thought to be critically important to the survival and success of clinicians in this demanding specialty area. Examples of training update topics have included advanced and specialized training in sex offender reoffense risk prediction; administration of the Hare Psychopathy Checklist (PCL-R); the clinical polygraph's role in sex offender treatment; effective clinical techniques useful in the detection of deception; culturally appropriate interventions with sexual offenders; the development and implementation of an inpatient sex offender treatment program for sexually violent persons; evaluation and treatment of professional sexual misconduct; information about recent legislation that pertains to sex offender supervision, registration, and treatment; and clinical case consultations.

EXPERIENCE TO DATE

The initial training program was presented the first year, during which only two trainees discontinued their participation. During the second year, the organization offered only training updates. There was sufficient interest to enroll another 50 trainees in the 24-day training course the third year; thus, a new group of trainees was identified and the full training program, as well as training updates for fellows, was provided during the third year. Minor modifications were made in the 24-day training curriculum and faculty based on feedback from the first group of fellows.

As of the fourth year of the organization, approximately 15 of the original 53 fellows have become inactive and lost their fellowship status as they have failed to fulfill their training update requirements. When queried about their reasons for discontinuation, these training program graduates most often cited job responsibility changes (such as promotions to supervisory positions where they no longer provided direct services to clients) or a loss of interest in evaluating and treating sexual offenders after learning about the field. By contrast, many fellows indicated significant changes in the nature of their practices. They cited considerable increases in their caseloads as they received many referrals of sex offender clients. They also noted increased job security and satisfaction due to implementing new learning and promoting community safety from sexual assault. Most fellows indicated that they enjoyed and benefited from the collegial interaction with peers, which reduced their feelings of professional isolation. This was particularly the case for clinicians who practice in sparsely populated areas where they are the only sex offender treatment provider in a large geographic region. Additionally, many fellows developed lasting friendships with others in their training group that they report as personally enriching.

VIDEOTAPE TRAINING PROGRAM

The organization was interested in providing an option for training professionals who were not in the immediate geographic region where the live training program took place. Thus, a similar comprehensive training program was produced on videotape. To make the videotapes, most of the live training program was filmed. An attitudes-and-values training that was largely experiential and would not translate well into the videotape training program was omitted. The films were edited to remove extraneous material or content that related exclusively to the local jurisdiction. The edited videotape program was organized into a 22-videotape training program consisting of about 100 hours of training. As an adjunct to the videotapes, 11 examinations were developed to correspond with the content covered. An answer key is provided, making it possible for videotape program trainees to correct their tests or for agencies to administer and score the examinations as a part of staff training. In addition, the handout materials provided by the trainers, which consist of paper copies of slides and overheads and supplementary readings, are included in the videotape training program. The videotape program has been distributed in the United States, Canada, Australia, Belgium, Great Britain, Hong Kong, and elsewhere around the world. After the videotape development costs were met, the sales of the training program have been used to supplement the organization's budget, thereby enabling programming for fellows at fees that are below the actual cost of providing the services.

CLOSING

It has been satisfying to witness the excitement and absorption of trainees engaged with a trainer. The opportunity to observe the development of friendly and supportive relationships has been equally satisfying. After the first day's work in a module, trainees typically gathered to enjoy dinner together, sometimes followed by dancing or a visit to a nearby casino. On some occasions, trainees who resided in the area where the training was held hosted a reception. The rigorous academic work and the social activities enhanced one another and produced a rich experience for all involved.

As of this writing, the organization is in its fourth year, a year of update trainings with the now approximately 90 fellows. The future of the organization is evolving with each years' passage. Thus far, it has met its initial goals and continues to serve clinicians and the region.

APPENDIX 1

Training Curriculum

Presented in 12, 2-day modules held monthly for 1 year:

- Module 1 Evaluation of participants' attitudes and values related to the wide range of human sexual behavior and how those attitudes and values affect their work, normal childhood sexual development, treatment outcomes with sexual offenders.

- Module 2 Prevalence of sexual assault, multiple paraphilias, social and biological factors that contribute to sex offending, screening pedophiles out of volunteer organizations, professional sexual misconduct, supervision of sexual offenders during postacute treatment.
- Module 3 Sex offender assessment: review of background materials, evaluation of previous treatment or other interventions; the assessment interview: outline, techniques, management of denial and resistance, collateral contacts, overview of the evaluation report.
- Module 4 Standardized tests, inventories, and card sorts utilized in the assessment of sexual offenders, typologies, and classification of sexual offenders; the Multidimensional Assessment of Sex and Aggression.
- Module 5 Limits of sex offender assessment, when assessment is not indicated, the sex offender evaluation report: evaluation issues, present and previous offenses, offender history, sex offender reoffense risk assessment, conclusions, and recommendations.
- Module 6 Sex offender treatment interventions: sex offender group management, client selection and mix, closed versus open-ended groups, contracting, treatment of sexual offenders who deny their offenses, order and pacing of interventions, confrontation, autobiography, community management of sexual offenders, intellectually disabled sex offender evaluation and treatment.
- Module 7 Sex offender treatment interventions continued: sex education/sexual values clarification/sexual dysfunction prevention, social skills training, covert sensitization, masturbatory satiation, cognitive restructuring, victimization awareness/ empathy training, working with psychopathic sexual offenders, therapist safety, gender issues in the treatment of sexual offenders.
- Module 8 Racial, cultural, and ethnic issues in sex offender treatment; sexual, emotional, and physical abuse in the history of the sex offender; institutional management of sexual offenders; compulsive sexual behavior; female sexual offenders; pharmacotherapy with sexual offenders; ethics and standards in working with sexual offenders; field trip to inpatient sex offender treatment center.
- Module 9 Sex offender group management, management of resistance, levels of sex offender treatment, anger management, assertiveness skills, impulse control and empathy training, reducing loneliness in sexual offenders, development of a prosocial support network, management of dropouts and treatment failures, criteria for treatment completion, sex offender treatment evaluation.
- Module 10 Youthful sexual offenders, penile plethysmograph, polygraph, sadistic sexual offenders, incest offenders and incest family dynamics and treatment.
- Module 11 Preassault cycle, sexual abuse cycle, treating dysfunctions of childhood in sexual offenders, determining client progress, relapse prevention, systems approach to sex offender treatment, management of confidentiality, informed consent, duty to warn, limits of professional capability, treatment literature, sex offender treatment specialist support and burnout prevention, supervision and consultation, trends in sex offender treatment.
- Module 12 Sexual assault legislation including sexual predator and community notification statutes, understanding the criminal justice system, forensic evaluation expert witness rules of admissibility and expert testimony, managing ethics in the adversarial legal system, evaluator/therapist client privilege, attorney work product privilege, expert witness qualification, skills in court testimony, what judges value in expert witnesses.

APPENDIX 2

Sample Trainer Contract

I, _____, agree to serve as a faculty member by providing training for the Wisconsin Sex Offender Treatment Network, Inc. (WSOTN), on (dates and times) at (training site).

The general topic of my presentation will be _____.

I agree to provide WSOTN with the following: (1) Clear master copies of any handouts I would like participants to obtain related to my training. These include (a) readings to be completed by trainees prior to my presentation, such as journal articles and book chapters, and (b) paper copies suitable for photocopying of slides or overhead transparencies that I anticipate using in my presentation. I understand that WSOTN needs time to obtain copyright permission to reproduce copyrighted material and that these materials must be photocopied and distributed to trainees well in advance of my presentation, and therefore they need to be submitted to the WSOTN office no later than [date]. (2) A copy of my outline with general time delineations for the purpose of WSOTN applying for continuing education credit (CEUs) for my presentation. I understand this outline is to be at the WSOTN office no later than [date]. (3) Also for CEU application purposes, three educational learning objectives related to my training. Educational learning objectives are typically completions of such phrases as "By the completion of this training, trainees will be able to [specific skill and knowledge acquisition.]" These educational learning objectives need to be submitted to the WSOTN office by [date]. (4) A current copy of my curriculum vitae, also for CEU application purposes, due at the WSOTN office by [date]. (5) Objective test questions and answers related to my didactic presentation and the readings I provide to be incorporated into the examination that will be administered to trainees immediately following the training module I present. I will submit approximately [number dependent on the length of that trainer's section] such questions, with answers to guide the person who scores the examination. These questions and answers need to be in the WSOTN office by [date]. (6) Information about my audiovisual equipment needs. WSOTN will provide me with any of the following equipment, provided I request this service: overhead, slide, 16-mm film and/or videotape projectors, videocassette player, easel and markers. WSOTN needs this information by [date].

I will be paid an honorarium of [amount] for my presentation as well as any travel, lodging, and meal expenses I incur in order to provide this training. If I need to travel to the training site by air, WSOTN will arrange my airplane reservations after consulting with me and obtaining my agreement on flight times, and WSOTN will purchase my airplane tickets and forward them to me well in advance of my training. WSOTN will also reserve a sleeping room for me at the training site hotel and pay for that room. I will submit my mileage and any expense receipts for reimbursement following the training, and will be reimbursed promptly.

_____   _____
[trainer name]   [date]

_____   _____
[WSOTN executive director name]   [date]

Trainer please sign one copy of this agreement and return to the WSOTN office; the other copy is for the trainer's records. Thank you.

12

B. Community Settings

Invitations to Responsibility
*Engaging Adolescents and Young
Men Who Have Sexually Abused*

Alan Jenkins

In this chapter, I will describe a model of engagement for working with adolescent boys and young men[1] who have sexually abused. The practice of engagement concerns assisting young men to find motivation to discover their own preferences and capacities for respectful ways of being and relating. It involves processes for inviting adolescents to cease abusive practices by choosing to undertake and invest in a journey toward responsibility and respect of self and others. A detailed description of theory and practice concerning the application of this model to adult men who abuse has been previously documented (Jenkins, 1990). This chapter concerns specific developments and applications of the model for young men.

I will focus on the early stages of engagement that involve establishing *readiness* in young men, to enable them to choose to invest in an intervention program. There is a considerable body of literature concerning intervention models and practices based on concepts such as relapse prevention and psychoeducational theory (Ryan & Lane, 1991). Strategies for confronting young men's resistance and modifying their behavior have been extensively documented. However, little attention has been paid to the important issues of readiness and motivation of young men to make their own choices to address their abusive behaviors.

In this area, the dominant intervention practices can establish a context in which confrontation and coercion are used to enable intervention strategies. Young men are subjected to processes of psychological and physiological assessment and categorization by well-intended workers who then impose strategies for behavior change. Workers appear to have more motivation than their clients, who may resist or acquiesce and accommodate to intervention practices, but take little responsibility for their actions.

The present model of engagement is designed to invite young men to establish their own intervention goals and develop their own motivation to achieve them. The model can provide a context in which many of the excellent ideas that have been developed in relapse prevention and psychoeducational models can be located and applied in a collaborative, rather than confrontative, context.

---

[1]I will use the term "young man" throughout this chapter to refer to my client group of males aged 13–20 years.

Alan Jenkins • NADA Counselling, Consulting, and Training, Stirling, South Australia 5152.
Sourcebook of Treatment Programs for Sexual Offenders, edited by Marshall et al. Plenum Press, New York, 1998.

It requires a shift in focus from dominant intervention practices that involve the cataloguing of individual psychological deficits and limitations, confrontation, and the external imposition of moral choices, desired ways of being, and intervention goals by workers. It is a shift away from practices that constitute the construction and documentation of a dominant story of identity: that of the "sexual offender." I have previously described the ways in which we can inadvertently assist the construction of this identity through well-intended intervention practices (Jenkins, in press). If we co-create the identity of sexual offender, our clients will live out this identity before our very eyes. We can inadvertently assist our clients to reproduce behavior that is manipulative, sneaky, and deviant. The sexual offender is regarded by others, and generally regards himself, as a "loser"; one who cannot control himself and is disrespectful to himself and others. Such an identity informs and is informed by practices of avoidance of responsibility and blame.

A model of engagement by invitation aims to promote the discovery and construction of an alternative story of identity: one that is informed by qualities and practices of responsibility and respect. It proposes that the young man may have preferences and a capacity for responsible, equitable, and respectful behavior; preferences, and a capacity that are likely to have been overlooked or ignored by others and by the young man himself. It proposes that there may be more to the young man than his abusive and irresponsible behavior. Qualities such as honesty, equity, and responsibility may be discovered and developed in an appropriate context, and these can lead to an alternative view of self; that is, an alternative to the dominant story of sexual offender.

It is a model that highlights the concept of choice in intervention. The young man chose to abuse, and therefore he can be assisted to make respectful choices, including the decision to take responsibility for and to cease his abusive behavior. There is no need to invest in psychological explanations that only serve to attribute responsibility to factors and circumstances outside of the young man's sphere of influence and control. He is assisted to separate his actions (what I have done) from his identity (who I am); to recognize that he may have done a terrible thing, but that he is not necessarily a terrible person. There is no place for psychological labels of identity, such as *sexual offender* and *perpetrator*, and no place for any constructs that minimize a sense of responsibility for one's actions, such as *personality disorder*, *impulse control disorder*, and other concepts that define individuals in terms of psychological limitations.

The young man is invited to make his own decisions, based on his own preferences, whether or not to undertake a journey toward responsibility and respect. This is not a journey of accommodation to the wishes of workers or parents, nor is it an adversarial battle centered around resistance to their influence. It must be the young man's journey; one that he has chosen for himself. He chooses to face his own shame as he takes steps toward accepting full responsibility and making maximum restitution for this abusive actions. In this way he is assisted to develop self-respect as he discovers his own sense of justice, courage, and integrity.

This model of engagement is informed by three major principles that relate to notions of:

1. Responsibility: Individuals who abuse are held fully responsible for their abusive behavior.
2. Accountability: Intervention principles and practices must be informed by, and be accountable to, the experiences of those with least power and privilege, particularly those who have been subjected to abuse.
3. Respect: Intervention practices must, at all times, be respectful to those who have abused and must promote and enhance respect of self and others.

Respectful engagement is a concept that poses considerable challenges and dilemmas for workers. We have a responsibility to assess and monitor our own practices of power in intervention—the ways in which we use and abuse power. We must actively address our inevitable tendencies to reproduce abusive behavior and to act in ways that are coercive and controlling. If we are serious about stopping abuse, we cannot afford to justify our own abuses of power in the name of therapeutic intervention, even if in the service of a noble cause.

Engagement concerns assisting young men to discover their own motivation. This model is concerned with alternatives to confrontation, coercion, and popular forms of "benevolent bullying," designed to secure cooperation. It is concerned with respectful intervention that is designed to assist young men to discover their own preferences for respectful behavior and their own motivation to act according to these preferences and desires. Engagement is concerned with maintaining a premium on responsibility and accountability, while ensuring that all interactions in intervention are respectful and just.

Engagement practices should be conducted within a broader context of strong statutory responses to abusive behavior. It is statutory authorities who are empowered to deliver clear and unequivocal messages that abusive behavior is unacceptable, to provide sanctions for violations, and to mandate expectations that individuals will address their abusive behavior. Our responsibilities, as nonstatutory workers, are to work in collaboration with statutory authorities, but not to act as though we were statutory authorities. We must develop respectful and noncoercive means of intervention to assist those who abuse to consider and make their own choices that are based on their own values and preferences.

I work with adolescents and young men who are primarily referred by juvenile justice and statutory child protection agencies as a consequence of sexual offenses against younger children or peers. Most of these young men are known to have sexually assaulted only one other person at the time of referral to my program. Forty-five percent of these young men eventually acknowledge having sexually assaulted three or more individuals. Some acknowledge vast numbers of sexual assaults. When these young men first present, there is little evidence of responsible thinking and behavior in relation to their abusive actions. They demonstrate considerable minimization of the abuse and accept little responsibility for their actions. These young men are often frightened of the likely consequences of their actions, and their avoidant and minimizing behavior masks a profound and pervasive sense of shame. They expect deprecation from others and feel little respect for themselves. Their sexual assaults and subsequent apprehension confirm to themselves that they are "losers" whose only option is to run and hide from what they have done and what they think it says about them.

I see many young men who also have experienced considerable abuse, oppression, and neglect and who have a strong sense of injustice in their own lives. For many of these young men, their own experiences of injustice, abuse, and victimization have not been understood by others. For example, young Australian Aboriginals and economically disadvantaged youth have experiences of oppression and disadvantage that are seldom understood in the context of intervention programs. They may experience a profound sense of injustice and may have been subjected to a range of abuses. Yet, there is an expectation that they will address their own abusive behavior, an expectation that sometimes constitutes a *responsibility overload*, or a set of unreasonable and unrealistic expectations.

Many young men are well-used to hearing others' advice on what they should do and how they should live their lives. Some have wide networks of official and unofficial advisors, including police, welfare workers, parents, courts, counselors, and so on. These well-established patterns of advice-giving often constitute *responsibility underloads*, whereby others appear to work harder in the service of responsibility than the young man himself, who actively resists their attempts to colonize his experience, and he increasingly abdicates initiative and responsibility for his own life.

The consequences of responsibility overload and underload are generally reflected in patterns of resistance to others' ideas, usually at the expense of responsibility and respect. Some young men "shut down" and respond to any attempt at intervention with silence or, "I dunno." Some passively acquiesce and accommodate to what they think others want to hear. Others resist more actively by storming out of the room, slamming doors, or displaying other violent actions.

In these contexts, intervention is experienced as intrusive or unjust. I believe that resistance to injustice is a quality deserving of admiration and respect. Young men typically experience considerable injustice, particularly in Western cultures that sacrifice the interests of youth for the economic goals of adults. Intervention should foster processes and outcomes that are just, and they should support resistance to unjust practices and oppressive circumstances. I am concerned with just interventions that are sensitive to experiences of oppression and victimization and that promote and honor resistance, but not at the expense of responsibility and respect.

ENGAGING CAREGIVERS

Intervention is facilitated with a combination of individual, family, local community, and group work. Effective intervention is located within the context of the various communities of which the young man has membership; a context that is much broader than that provided in a group or residential setting. It then becomes vital to engage the cooperation and active participation of caregivers, who can include parents, foster parents, extended family members, residential care workers, youth workers, teachers, and police.

It is the young man's task to accept full responsibility for his abusive behavior. However, it is the responsibility of caregivers to make this task accessible and to provide the extensive support that young men require to successfully undertake it. Caregivers must assist the young man to discover, name, and attribute meaning to the steps he takes toward responsibility and respect. They provide an invaluable audience that offers respect for each step taken in the young man's journey. Intervention is of limited effectiveness in the absence of appropriate and coordinated caregiver support.

I usually conduct my initial interview with the young man and his caregivers, usually his parents, if they are accessible, and it appears that such a meeting is likely to be safe and respectful for all persons concerned. This can help to avoid a responsibility overload where the young man might feel that he is expected to handle the whole issue on his own and caregivers might feel that there is no job for them to do or that their help is not needed. The inclusion of caregivers also helps to avoid a responsibility underload where we might begin to work much harder than the young man by attempting to motivate him and to encourage his participation in the interview. With caregivers present, I can discuss matters with them and create a context in which the young man contributes when he is ready to do so.

When parents first present, they tend to be highly preoccupied with blame, a construct that is never helpful in promoting responsibility. Most parents are familiar with some popular psychology and they expect to be blamed by professional workers for their children's problems. They expect to have their own feelings of guilt and insufficiency confirmed by workers. Many are ready to defend themselves by identifying external factors to which they can attribute blame; for example, attention deficit disorder, drugs, or the influence of peers. Parents may invite workers to become similarly preoccupied with limitations, deficiencies, and disorders that might explain the abusive behaviors of the young man: "What is wrong with him?"; "Why did he do it?" Alternatively, parents may feel increasingly desperate, lost, and defeated so that they appear paralyzed, having lost hope for themselves and their children.

As I listen to parent's stories, I have two primary foci in mind: (1) what evidence is there of desire, competence, and agency to provide appropriate support and assistance for the young man? and (2) what factors might prevent this caregiver from providing such assistance and support? In order to illustrate these issues and the way problems are approached, let me describe an actual case. The names, of course, have been changed to pseudonyms.

AN ILLUSTRATIVE CASE

Jake's Referral

Jake was one such young man who was 15 years old when mandated to attend the program by the Youth Court. This referral followed his conviction on charges of "indecent assault" of his 8-year-old half sister, Amy. Jake was initially charged with the offense of "rape," following Amy's disclosure that he had penetrated her vagina with his fingers and his penis. In fact, Amy disclosed that Jake molested her using his hands, mouth, and penis, over an 18-month period. She disclosed coercion by Jake, that he had threatened her at times, if she did not comply or if she disclosed the abuse. I later discovered that Jake had also sexually assaulted another 8-year-old girl, one of Amy's friends. However, this abuse had not been disclosed at the time of referral.

Jake's charges were reduced to "indecent assault" through legal negotiations, subsequent to his appearance in court. Jake made a partial acknowledgment to the police. However, he denied the allegations of penetration and oral–genital sexual molestation. Jake also denied that he had coerced Amy in any way. Despite high levels of distress experienced by Amy, Jake tended to minimize the seriousness and impact of his actions: "It's no big deal"; "I didn't hurt her."

Jake's mother, Jill, was shocked and devastated by Jake's abusive actions and particularly by his reaction following Amy's disclosure: "He doesn't seem to care": "He has no remorse"; "He just goes on as though nothing has happened." She worried, "He is becoming like his stepfather." Jill, with her three children, Amy, 8, David, 9, and Jake, left Jake's stepfather, Terry, 3 years prior to the referral, as a result of Terry's violence and abusive behavior.

Jake was now living in a supported youth accommodation group home, following statutory child protection intervention. Jake has been visiting his mother's house regularly and had, following arguments with his mother, damaged her property and threatened her on occasion. Finally, Jill called the police when Jake assaulted her after she refused to give him money. This resulted in a restraining order served on Jake, forbidding him from approaching his family or the family home. Jake had a reputation for violence and "disruptive behavior" at school, and he had shown increasing violence and aggressive behavior toward his mother and siblings over the 2 years prior to referral.

Engaging Jill

Patterns of Concern and Intent

In Jake's case, I was concerned about his recent violence toward his mother and I decided therefore to meet with Jill separately. When I first met Jill, she appeared sad and defeated. I knew very little about her family and background, but she presented as a person who had struggled in the face of considerable letdown and disappointment throughout her life. Jill detailed a long history of concerns and worries about Jake. These included: Jake's apparent lack of remorse regarding his abuse of Amy; Jake's disrespectful and aggressive treatment of family members, both prior to and subsequent to Amy's disclosure; and Jake's reputation for "losing it," both at home and at school, for fighting and disruptive behavior. Jill had experienced Jake as increasingly disrespectful, demanding, and aggressive over the past 2 years. She described damage to her property and bullying of the younger children when "He doesn't get his own way." Most recently, when she refused to give Jake money, he grabbed her and shook her, and then pushed her over, causing her to hit her head, which required medical attention. Jill spoke of her worry that Jake was "Turning out to be just like his stepfather."

I attended closely to Jill's concerns and worries about her son and inquired about her efforts to assist him in his development. As she described extensive efforts over a considerable period of time, throughout which she felt ineffective and inadequate, Jill began to sob. She revealed that she felt "weak" and "guilty" with respect to her parenting of Jake. I inquired:

"Who understands how much you have worried about Jake?"

"Who understands how much you have wanted to help him to get his life on track and how hard you have tried?"

"Who knows how it has felt to have to carry this responsibility on your own?"

"Who knows how much you agonize over the restraint order on Jake?"

"Who understands how important it is and how hard it is for you to stand by and support both Amy and Jake?"

These questions, with their "Who understands?" format, serve to highlight the caregiver's well-intended efforts and caring values, qualities that are easily overlooked and lost sight of in the face of the disappointment and frustration of unattained goals. Caregivers are invited to draw attention to good intent despite actions that may have had limited effectiveness.

A responsibility overload for Jill could begin to be identified, named, and addressed, as she detailed her lone struggle to care for her children against overwhelming odds. Jill's experience must be understood and her good intent and caring qualities affirmed if she is to challenge pervasive feelings of guilt and inadequacy and develop the capacity to assist Jake in his journey.

Patterns of Resistance

Jill was reluctant at first to talk about Jake's biological father or her ex-partner, Terry. She began to describe Terry as having been violent and abusive toward her for the entire 11 years of their relationship. He showed little caring and respect for Jake, either putting him down or ignoring him. This time represented a chapter in Jill's life that was terribly painful for her and one she wanted to leave in the past. Jill was clearly experiencing intense guilt about Jake having been exposed and subjected to Terry's violence and abusive behavior. In many respects, she felt culpable for Jake's current violence and abusive behavior.

I asked Jill's permission to inquire further about her experience with Terry in her family. She related incidents in which she felt trapped, helpless, and humiliated. She spoke of her feelings of hopelessness, defeat, and guilt about her children witnessing and, at times, being subjected to violence and abuse. Jill was intensely self-critical and self-deprecating. While speaking with Jill, I also began to see glimpses of an alternative story about her, which incorporated qualities of caring, strength, and resistance to injustice; an alternative to her dominant experience of herself as weak and insufficient. Stories of concern for her children and resistance to the injustice perpetrated by Terry began to emerge. Certain lines of inquiry were pivotal in facilitating these conversations:

> "Who understands what it felt like to witness your children suffering as a result of Terry's abuse, to feel unable to stop it?"

> "Who knows what it felt like to witness the effects of Terry picking on Jake and favoring Amy and David?"

> "Who understands what you were up against? How, whenever you tried to make a stand, you and the kids were hurt even more?"

In this way, the depth of Jill's concern for her children and her opposition to Terry's injustice and abuse was further identified and named. Jill began to speak of her attempts to resist Terry's unjust and abusive behavior. Each attempt at open resistance resulted in Terry not only punishing Jill, but picking on Jake more. Jill learned subtle ways to deflect Terry's attacks away from Jake and onto herself. She worked out when she needed to "walk on eggshells" and when she could allow the children some freedom. Jill began to plan means of escaping throughout the last 4 years of her relationship with Terry. She was advised by her extended family to try harder to please Terry, while her few friends told her she was wrong to stay with him. Whatever she did, she felt that she was failing. However, Jill continued subtle forms of resistance and continued to develop her escape plan. I inquired:

> "How did you manage to keep planning when, every time you stood up for yourself, you got knocked down?"

> "How did you manage to find what it took to leave Terry?"

> "Who understands what you were up against?"

> "Who understands how hard it was to make such a stand on your own?"

> "How important was it for you to make this stand against violence for your kids and yourself?"

An alternative story of courage, in the face of adversity, began to be told and named. Jill spoke of the hardships of having to cope on her own with three children and no resources. She was harassed and stalked by Terry for 2 years after leaving him. The police provided little help. Terry initiated Family Court proceedings for custody of the two younger children. Jill found the aftermath of leaving Terry more difficult to cope with than learning to dodge, deflect, and tolerate his abusive outbursts. She had, in fact, anticipated that this would be the case before she left him.

Jill also showed honesty, courage, and integrity in recognizing and acknowledging her children's suffering. She was inclined to blame herself for not leaving Terry sooner than she did. I became increasingly curious about how she had managed to leave him under such adverse and unsupportive circumstances.

> "What does it say about you that you kept on planning to leave without any support, and with little hope that you could escape Terry?"

> "What does it say about you as a mother that you know what Terry did to you all, but you don't make any excuses for yourself for not protecting your kids?"

An alternative story of Jill's caring and concern for her children and her courage and extraordinary valor in resisting injustice, against almost impossible odds, was gradually told, given appropriate labels, and owned by Jill. It was this alternative story that provided a foundation for Jill to actively assist Jake in his journey toward responsibility and respect.

Establishing a Solution Focus with Jake

I began to address Jill's concerns about Jake's apparent lack of remorse and caring for Amy. Invitations to speculate about the young man's intent are often helpful in this context:

> "Do you think Jake wanted to hurt Amy and make her suffer, or do you think he only thought about what he wanted and didn't think of Amy's feelings at all?"

> "Is Jake usually cruel? Does he get off on hurting others, or can be he considerate and caring of other people?"

> "Do you think Jake doesn't care about Amy's feelings, or do you think he is having trouble showing his caring?"

In this way, parents are invited to speculate and draw distinctions regarding the young man's intent: Does the abusive behavior reflect cruelty and a desire to harm, or self-centered failure to consider the other's feelings? Such questions invite caregivers to adopt a solution-focused orientation to explain the abusive behavior. The search for psychological deficits and limitations, as explanations, can be interrupted. Characterological explanations, based on notions of cruelty or badness, are contrasted with solution-focused ideas, which suggest that the young man may have a capacity for caring and considerate behavior that was not evident when he sexually abused. If the young man is not bad, but has failed to consider the other's feelings and well-being, then the solution is obvious: He needs now to consider the other's feelings and remedy this lapse in his consideration and caring.

If it is thought that perhaps the young man did want to hurt the child he abused, it may still be possible to explore:

> "Is Jake someone who gets off on hurting others, or is he someone who gets caught up in his own hurt feelings and then takes them out on others?"

> "Does Jake hurt others out of cruelty or meanness, or does he hurt others when he is feeling really hurt himself?"

Jill leaned toward the view that Jake had not considered Amy's feelings and had not intended to cause her harm. I inquired about evidence that might support the notion that Jake has a capacity for caring and considerate behavior, a capacity that was not evident when he sexually abused Amy or when he bullied his siblings and assaulted his mother.

Jill began to identify past situations and circumstances where Jake had acted in caring, protective, and considerate ways. She recalled times when Jake had worried about her and tried to protect her and his younger siblings from Terry's violence. She recalled acts of bravery and self-sacrifice when Jake had risked harm to stand by his mother. A description of Jake's capacity to be loyal, considerate, and protective and to stand up against injustice began to emerge—a story in sharp contrast with Jake's recent abusive, violent, and disrespectful behaviors.

Establishing and Addressing Responsibility Overload for Jake

This alternative story can inform further exploration of solution-focused explanations that are based on notions of restraint (Jenkins, 1990; White, 1986) rather than causality:

> "What do you think might be stopping Jake from taking responsibility for his abusive behavior?"

> "What do you think might be stopping Jake from thinking and feeling about what he has done to Amy?"

> "What do you think might be stopping him from treating Amy respectfully now?"

I reiterated the priority that Jake must accept full responsibility for the abuse of Amy and any other violent or abusive actions, and inquired:

> "What might Jake have on his mind that could be making it hard for him to think about his abuse of Amy?"

> "What might be happening in Jake's life now that makes it hard for him to face up to what he has put Amy and your family through?"

Jill and I began to document a range of injustices, challenges, and difficult circumstances that could preoccupy Jake and prevent him from showing responsibility, caring, and consideration in relation to his abuse of Amy. These included Jake's abandonment by his biological father (Jake's father had not attempted to make any contact with Jake since he left when Jake was a baby); witnessing Terry's abuse of his mother (I invited Jill to speculate about the amount of worry and hurt that Jake might have experienced, and the consequences of his attempts to stand up to and resist Terry's abusive behavior in the family); Jake's experience of being subjected to Terry's violence and humiliation; Jake's experience of Terry's neglect and favoritism toward his biological children; Jake's likely experiences of shame and fear with disclosure of his abuse of Amy; and Jake's having to leave the family and live in supported accommodation.

I invited Jill to speculate further, with the following style of inquiry:

> "How worried do you think Jake has been about ...?"

> "How big do you think Jake's hurt about ... has been?"

> "How unfair do you think he feels ... is?"

Jill had not previously discussed these matters with Jake or anyone else. These recollections and realizations were painful and provoked feelings of guilt and self-doubt. Jill was once again invited to identify and honor her own courage in considering Jake's experience in this context, and to speculate about the usefulness of this course of action in helping Jake to find a responsible direction in his life.

> "Do you think Jake knows that you realize so much about him?"

> "What do you think it would mean to Jake if he knew his mother was thinking about his feelings in this way?"

"What does it say about you as a mother that you are facing these painful feelings about your son?"

"Do you think that understanding and discussing all of this could help you and Jake, or do you think it will just stir up the past and make you both feel worse?"

We considered the likelihood that Jake's experience of his own victimization, injustices, and challenges might feel much bigger, in his mind, than the injustices he had caused to Amy and others in his family.

"What do you think Jake would think was worse, what he did to Amy, or what he has been through himself?"

"Do you think Jake knows how much you have tried to understand the challenges, hurts, and unfairness he has been through?"

Young men are often expected to take responsibility for and appreciate the impact of the abusive behavior they have perpetrated, in the absence of feeling that anyone has attempted to appreciate their own experiences of victimization and oppression. The following invitations can set the scene to address a responsibility overload and provide a basis for realistic expectations, justice, and a solution focus:

"How fair would it be to expect Jake to face his abusive behavior and the effects on Amy, if he felt that no one had understood or acknowledged the things he has been put through himself?"

"If we didn't understand and talk about what Jake has been through, would it be fair to expect him to talk about and understand what he has put Amy through?"

"What would Jake be likely to do, in these circumstances?"

Jill is invited to consider providing the same thing for Jake that she expects of him in relation to his sister. However, it is vital that such restraints to Jake taking responsibility are not considered as causal in relation to his abusive behavior. This point was highlighted in conversation with Jill:

"If we begin to understand and acknowledge what Jake has been through, do you think it will help him face what he did to Amy, or do you think he will use it as an excuse?"

"How do you think it could help Jake to avoid following in Terry's footsteps?"

This priority of Jake accepting responsibility for his abusive behavior must be kept in the foreground at all times, as Jill is invited to address the overload.

"What will it take to talk about this with Jake?"

"What will it say about you as a mother?"

In this way, Jill was assisted in preparing for a meeting with Jake that was designed to foster mutual respect in their relationship and to support him in his journey toward responsibility and respect.

Engaging Jake

Initial Meeting with Jake

I try to meet adolescents with one or more of their caregivers, for reasons previously stated. I decided to meet with Jake with his support worker from the youth accommodation service. This worker appeared to be supportive of Jake and ready to adopt a solution focus in his work.

Jake initially presented as surly and uncooperative. His physical posture and gestures suggested resentment and contempt. He fluctuated between appearing agitated and combative and then resigned, sullen, and withdrawn. It would not have been difficult to take offense at Jake's attitude and lack of cooperation, and to engage in an adversarial dispute that would most likely culminate in Jake's swearing, storming out of the room, and slamming the door. Jake appeared to be inviting a fight. This is an invitation I always decline. An adversarial dispute would only confirm and add to Jake's sense of injustice and lack of belonging in the world. An adversarial dispute also sets the context for responsibility underload, whereby workers are regarded, and regard themselves, as needing to take increasing responsibility on behalf of their clients, who in turn take less responsibility for themselves.

Early in the interview, I stated the reason for the meeting and attempted to establish an initial focus on Jake's abusive behavior. I explained that Jake was mandated to attend the program by the Youth Court as a result of his conviction for sexually assaulting his younger sister, Amy. This context (that Jake is responsible for and is here to address his abusive behavior toward Amy) must be kept in the foreground in all meetings with Jake. However, Jake cannot be coerced into adopting this priority. He can only be invited to consider it for himself. I need to set a context where such consideration is possible.

Addressing the Experience of Injustice

This requires a focus on understanding Jake's experience:

"I know what the court and your mother want, but I don't know what is important for you."

"I don't know where all this has left you, or what you think needs to happen."

"Can you help me understand …?"

Jake's response was to raise his eyebrows, turn away, and mutter, "This sucks." It is, of course, unlikely that Jake will begin to respond to these inquiries by telling his story in a cooperative way. However, by his response Jake had already begun to help me to understand his pervasive sense of injustice, as well as his capacity for resistance to external invasion.

I continued to pursue my interest in Jake's experience while externalizing[2] factors that may be restraining Jake from participation. These seemed likely to be: a sense of injustice and disqualification by others; shame about his abusive actions; and fear of further consequences. The issue of injustice appeared to be most prominent.

"I don't want to push anything on to you. I don't want to tell you to do anything. That would be unfair and I guess you've probably had enough unfair things pushed on to you already."

"I don't even want to talk about what you did to Amy until I understand what you think is important."

---

[2]To externalize is to make a restraining idea or practice accessible to address and challenge. For a detailed account of this, see White (1995).

"I have a hunch that, for a lot of your life, it has felt like you have had other people trying to push you around or tell you what to do and not listening to what you think or what you want?"

Jake became animated and responded:

"Yeah, the courts, the whole lot of you. I just want to be out of here."

I responded:

"I guess it feels like you have had a lot of unfair things pushed on to you and nobody listens to what you think or cares about how you feel?"

"This feels like another thing that's unfair and that has been pushed on to you?"

Jake nodded and acknowledged that this was his experience. I continued:

"How much of your life have you had other people pushing you around and trying to tell you what to do and not listening to you and how you feel?"

Jake initially responded with an air of defensive bravado: "Well, shit happens." He then looked extremely sad, vulnerable, and helpless.

I proposed a deal to Jake. The deal was based on these understandings:

"You have to come here. You've got no choice in that. But you don't have to put up with being pushed around or made to do things that are unfair."

"I need to listen to and understand what is important to you and where you stand before I even think about talking to you about Amy."

"You have the right to speak out or refuse anything that I do or say that feels unfair and I will respect this and back off. You should not have to put up with anything that is unfair in here."

Jake tentatively began to tell, for the first time, the story of his experience of injustices, abuse, and challenges. This story would eventually, over several discussions, include his experiences of abandonment by his father; Terry's abusive behavior toward his mother and himself; Terry's favoritism with his biological children; his mother's decision to leave Terry, by moving the family out of the house, and Terry's subsequent harassment and the custody battle; problems at school, including harassment by other students and Jake's learning difficulties; Amy's disclosure of the abuse, and the subsequent police and court action and other's reactions; having to leave the family and moving into supported accommodation; the current restraint order; and, finally, Jake's feelings that he does not fit in or belong anywhere.

Identifying Resistance

Jake's story concerns many events outside his control and a sense of being picked on and disqualified, of invasion, attack, and attempted colonization by others, particularly by those in authority. Extreme challenges and injustices were identified, named, and highlighted through inquires about Jake's capacity for survival:

"That's very unfair. That must have seemed impossible."

"How did you manage to keep going? How did you get by?"

"What is it about you that stopped you from giving up?"

Throughout this story of injustice and victimization, an alternative story of survival, loyalty, and resistance to injustice began to emerge. Jake acknowledged that he worried about his mother's safety when his stepfather was abusive. As a little boy he stayed awake at nights, listening and worrying. He attempted to intervene when Terry was hurting his mother, sometimes getting hurt himself in the process. He helped his mother to clean up the mess when his stepfather damaged her possessions. Jake took his younger siblings to a safe hiding place when his stepfather was abusive and they were frightened. On several occasions he had encouraged his mother to leave and supported her when she made the decision to go.

As Jake began to describe his experiences of unfairness and tell his stories of resistance, I frequently checked to ensure that my questions were not intrusive or inappropriate, and I sought permission to continue our conversation:

"Is it OK? Can you handle me asking about this?"

In this way, speaking out about matters that are painful and that remind the young man of past hurts is defined as evidence of inner strength and courage. This provides a new context for defining strength that contrasts with traditional definitions concerning physical attributes. It must be borne in mind that Jake had not told these stories and had learned to deal with his experience by trying not to think about it.

"Is this the first time you have spoken out about ...?"

"How much guts does it take to speak out like you are doing?"

I became increasingly preoccupied with the stands against injustice that Jake had taken throughout his life; stands taken in the face of extreme adversity. It is generally helpful to externalize such stances:

"Jake, are you a person who believes in standing up against things that are unfair or putting up with things that are unfair?"

This invitation led to an earnest conversation about the importance of resistance to injustice and the difficulties involved in enacting such resistance. Jake expressed clear preferences for resistance and an identification with the concept of justice. We discussed his preference for Afro-American rap music in this context. I made it clear that I also believe in standing up against things that are unfair and invited Jake to discover and appreciate his own capacity for resistance, even as a little boy:

"When did you first start to realize how unfairly Terry was treating your family?"

"When did you first start to worry about your mother and your brother and sister?"

"When did you first try to stand up to the unfairness?"

"When did you first try to stand up for your mother and your brother and sister?"

Amazing stories of resistance began to emerge. Jake's preference and capacity for resistance assumed increasing significance when considered in the light of the differences in power and resources between Terry and other family members. Ingenious and subtly creative ways of solving problems could be discovered and appreciated. For example, Jake found safe places where Terry could not get to but from which he could still monitor his mother's safety. He hid Terry's alcohol and the bullets for his gun at critical times. Jake learned clever ways to deflect Terry's attention and disrupt his abusive behavior. On one occasion, he made his younger brother hide and screamed out to his parents that David had run away, in order to disrupt Terry's behavior.

I am constantly amazed by the cleverness in these stories of resistance. One young man learned to voluntarily bring on asthma symptoms, which enabled him and his mother to make timely escapes to hospital. These "David and Goliath" stories of resistance can help to establish a context for counteracting the common experiences of worthlessness and culpability that are so prevalent among those who have been victimized.

"How did you manage to think up such amazing ideas when you were only nine?"

"What were you up against?"

"What does that say about you?"

Jake had been told many times, by his mother, that he acted "just like his stepfather." I invited Jake to consider ways in which he might *connect through difference*, rather than identify similarities, with Terry. These connections became quite pivotal in assisting Jake to clarify his own preferred ways of being.

"How much bigger and stronger was Terry compared to you and your mother?"

"Did he ever stop to think about what he was doing to people smaller than him?"

"Did he think more about himself or others in the family?"

"Is he a guy who could face up to his own problems, or did he just blame others?"

"In what ways are you different to Terry?"

"How are your ways of doing things different from Terry's ways?"

This sets the scene for further deconstruction of Jake's experience of victimization in later interviews where he was assisted to challenge the attributions of blame and worthlessness:

"Whose job was it to worry about your mother?"

"What was Terry's job in the family?"

"Did Terry face his problems or blame other people?"

"Do you think Terry thought he was strong or weak?"

I inquired further about Jake's preferences and practices regarding justice and respectful behavior:

"Are there other times that you have stood up against things that are unfair?"

"Are there other times you have stood up for other people who have been treated unfairly?"

"Are you a person who will try to help someone when they are in trouble, or are you someone who is more likely to kick the other person when they are down?"

"How important is it to stand up for people who are smaller or weaker who are being treated unfairly?"

At first Jake was unaware of other examples of his resistance to injustice. However, he began to discover and recall situations where he stood up for and helped friends who were in trouble. Jake spoke of situations at school where older kids had been bullying younger children and he had stepped in to protect the younger children. He spoke of a situation at school where a teacher had attempted to discipline a student in a way that he believed was violent and unjust. Jake intervened and tried to stop the teacher from continuing this course of action. Jake had, on many occasions, got into fights when he felt treated unjustly by other students. I maintained a focus on Jake's preference for justice and desire to resist injustice, despite the fact that his means of resistance may have, at times, been inappropriate or unjust.

The process of Jake speaking about his beliefs concerning justice and his responses to injustice was highlighted and examined in terms of its meaning:

"Have you spoken about this before?"

"Is it right to speak out or is it better to put up with it in silence?"

"Would Terry want you to be speaking out or would he prefer you to hide behind your silence?"

"How hard is it, and what does it take to speak out and be reminded on the unfairness and hurt in the past?"

"What does it say about you as a guy that you are speaking about what you believe in?"

"Are you being yourself in doing this or are you going along with other people's ideas?"

Jake was invited to consider and evaluate his beliefs and practices regarding fairness and justice, in the context of his own history of experience of injustice and adversity:

"What does it say about you that you believe in standing up for fairness even though you have had a lot of unfairness in your life?"

I drew Jake's attention to examples of his resistance, when he had tried to stand up against injustice, in ways that were fair and just:

"It is so easy to take out hurt feelings on other people. Do you realize you stood up for yourself without being unfair to yourself?"

"You were feeling really hurt when …; how did you manage to stand up for yourself without hurting them back and without being unfair yourself?"

I invited Jake to consider other people he knew who took out their feelings of unfairness and hurt upon others, and to compare this with his own beliefs and preferences.

It is important at this time to maintain a focus on Jake's unjust behaviors: his abuse of Amy and his violence toward his mother. However, these behaviors are presented as exceptions to Jake's preferred ways of being, as "out of character," rather than as reflections of Jake's true values and beliefs. At this point, many young men are mindful of the inconsistency between their preferences and their abusive actions, and some are ready to acknowledge a strong sense of shame and remorse and begin to show unprecedented levels of honesty in addressing their abusive behavior. While Jake was aware of this inconsistency, I felt he was not yet ready to address his abusive behavior in a responsible manner.

However, it was important to acknowledge Jake's active and responsible contributions in the interview:

"How are you managing to speak out for yourself here today?"

"The court can make you come here but they can't make you speak."

"At the beginning, you looked like you weren't going to last even 10 minutes, let alone speak out. How did you manage it?"

"What does it say about you?"

Jake was invited to discover and document personal qualities that he may not have thought about before. These included: resistance to injustice; loyalty; caring and consideration for others; and creative problem solving in situations of adversity. Throughout the interview, Jake's key worker was invited to contribute to these discussions and to witness and provide feedback to Jake:

> "What are you discovering about Jake in the way that he is handling responsibilities at the house?"

> "How do you think he is handling being here today?"

> "What do you think it says about Jake that he ...?"

Addressing Responsibility Overload

The scene is now set to create a just context for discussing Jake's abusive behavior. As workers, we contribute to a responsibility overload if we expect more of Jake than has been provided to him. If we expect Jake to face responsibility and understand the impact of his abusive actions, when this responsibility and understanding has never been provided for him in relation to his experience of victimization, we are acting unjustly. Not surprisingly, Jake will resist this injustice.

I initially encouraged Jake to name and attempt to quantify some of his experience of victimization:

> "Who understands how big the unfairness is that you had to face in your family?"

> "Who understands how big your worry about your mother was?"

> "Who understands how much Terry hurt you and your mother?"

Jake was invited to rate aspects of his experience on a 10-point scale. He scored both the unfairness and his worry at 10. Jake was also invited to rate his current experience:

> "How much does it still feel unfair when you think back?"

> "How big is the hurt when you look back?"

A context was created to consider other people's knowledge and understanding of Jake's experience and to name the overload:

> "People expect you to face up to what you have done to Amy, but who has taken the time to stop and think about what you have been put through?"

> "Do you think Terry ever took the time to stop and think about what he put you through?"

> "Do you think your mother knows how worried you were and how unfair it felt for you?"

> "Do you think the police, or your teachers, or the judge have any idea what you have been through?"

> "Who knows how hard it is to face what you did to Amy when you have been through extreme unfairness and worry yourself?"

> "Who understands how hard this makes it to face what you did to Amy?"

An opportunity is created for the worker to state a clear position about justice and equity that is, in fact, consistent with the young man's stated preferences by saying something like the following:

> "I believe that people should face up to unfair stuff that they have done and do something to try to put it right, but I also believe it should be fair for them too. I believe in fairness. It would be unfair for anyone to expect you to face up to anything you have done that has hurt others until they understand things you have been put through that have hurt you."

> "How fair would it be to expect you to face up to what you had done to Amy and try to understand what you might have put her through, if nobody understands or has thought about what you have been through?"

A Context for Addressing Abusive Behavior

I endeavor to create a context of justice and fairness, principles that accord with the young man's own preferences, within which he can be invited to address his abusive behavior. Processes of respectful engagement can enable his preference and capacity to be just to be highlighted, along with other honorable and respectful qualities. This constitutes a foundation for the discovery of respect of self and others.

Intervention can now be directed toward encouraging the young man to face and take responsibility for his abusive behavior. In this context, it is possible to prevent the telling of irresponsible and minimizing stories and to avoid adversarial interactions and unhelpful confrontation. In a context of justice and fairness, Jake could be invited to discover and consider his own motivation for taking responsibility for his abuse of Amy. I attempted to initiate conversations about taking responsibility and what this would mean for Jake and others: a process of "talking about talking about abuse." Engagement in this context involves three strategies: *invitation*, *declination*, and *acknowledgment*.

Invitation constitutes inquiry directed toward providing opportunities for the young man to consider respectful and responsible positions in relation to his abusive behavior that accord with his stated preferences and values. Invitation is usually accompanied by acknowledgment, which involves assisting the young man to notice respectful and responsible positions, including the steps he has already taken, and to examine their meaning in the light of his goals and preferences.

I generally allow the young man privacy to begin to talk about his abusive behavior. For example, I asked Jake's permission to speak with him on his own and requested that the key worker leave the room. I began to inquire:

> "Can you handle me asking about something that has puzzled me about what you did to Amy?"

It is vital that we ask permission to address abusive behavior. It is akin to the courtesy of knocking on doors and waiting to be invited in, rather that barging in uninvited. If I am hoping to assist Jake to develop respectful relationship boundaries, then it is vital to respect Jake's personal boundaries and privacy. Such an invitation also points to the strength and courage required to talk about such difficult matters.

I continued by inquiring about Jake's (partial) acknowledgment of his abuse of Amy, which he made to his mother and the police after an initial period of total denial:

> "How did you manage to begin to face up to what you did to Amy?"

"How did you find the guts to start to own up?"

"You must have felt like running away from it—how did you begin to own up to it?"

Jake was invited to consider his own internal resources: his inner strength and courage, which were required to face his own feelings of shame and fear of consequences. Jake's acknowledgment is labeled as a "beginning." For virtually all young men, initial acknowledgments are never complete; there is always more to be faced, but only when they are ready to do so. Facing up is an ongoing process, which Jake has just begun. These beginnings must be recognized and honored:

"What does it say about you that you did begin to face up?"

"Have you started to handle this in Terry's way, or in your ways?"

"What does it say about how your ways are different from Terry's ways?"

"In what ways do you think you have begun to be true to yourself?"

In subsequent interviews, Jake's caregivers could also be invited to consider:

"What do you think it took for Jake to begin to face up to his abuse of Amy?"

"What do you think he was up against?"

"How do you think he managed to avoid running away from it altogether?"

"What do you think that says about Jake?"

Jake was invited to consider his (partial) acknowledgment in the light of Amy's experience:

"What would it have said to Amy if you had copped out and never began to own up to what you did to her?"

"How would it have affected her if you had gone on saying that you didn't do anything and calling her a complete liar?"

"What would it say about you as a person if you had never begun to face up?"

"What does it say about you that you have begun to face up to what you did?"

"What do you think it says to Amy about you?"

I invited Jake to consider his intent in relation to his abuse of Amy:

"Do you reckon that you set out to try to hurt Amy, or do you think it was more that you just went after what you wanted and didn't think of her feelings?"

Jake aligned himself with the latter position but began to protest that he had not harmed Amy and that she had made some allegations that were not true. The strategy of declination is helpful to prevent further telling of an irresponsible and self-righteous story of minimization or external attribution of responsibility. Declination involves interruption of the story but without affirming or confronting its content. Both adversarial confrontation and unwitting collusion through silent listening are avoided. The irresponsible story is interrupted by inquiry that shifts the focus from self-righteous preoccupation to a previously established factual matter or responsible position that Jake has taken. Further inquiry enables this position to be developed and restraints to responsibility to be externalized.

"You have made it really clear that you didn't want to hurt Amy, that you don't get off on making people suffer."

"You know what it is like to be let down and hurt yourself."

"How shocked were you when you heard that Amy had told someone?"

"How much would it upset you if Amy was hurt, in a big way, by what you did to her?"

As we began to discuss Amy's disclosure and Jake's dilemmas in facing responsibility for his actions, Jake, like many other young men, began to experience increasing feelings of shame and fear. These experiences are more often reflected in the young man's posture and physical expressions than in his words.

I noticed at one point that Jake's eyes began to look watery and he looked down. I guessed that he was experiencing shame. I inquired:

"It takes a lot of guts to come here and talk honestly. I have a hunch right now you are feeling pretty bad about what you did to Amy. Is this right? What are you realizing about what you did to her?"

Jake nodded and acknowledged that what he did to Amy was wrong because she was his little sister. He agreed that he was feeling very ashamed. It is vital to assist Jake to acknowledge and attribute meaning to this experience. Facing responsibility must foster self-respect rather than self-deprecation:

"What does it say about you that you feel bad and ashamed about what you did to Amy?"

"What would it say about you if you could think about what you did without feeling ashamed?"

"Does anyone else know that you feel ashamed? Does your mother know?"

"Do you think other people realize that you feel bad about what you did or could they think that you don't care?"

"What would it say to them if they knew how badly and how ashamed you do feel?"

"How much courage is it taking to think about what you did to Amy?"

"Is this the first time you have talked about how it affects you in an honest way?"

"Can you respect the courage in yourself or would you respect it more if you were running away from the truth?"

"How scary is it to begin to face the truth?"

Facing responsibility and shame gradually become identified as both signs and determinants of inner strength and integrity, rather than being interpreted in terms of weakness and self-disgust. Jake was, once again, invited to draw connections through difference between himself and Terry:

"Do you think that Terry ever took the time to think and feel about what he did to you and your family, like you are starting to do now for Amy?"

"Do you realize that you are doing something that he never had the guts to do? What does that say about you?"

These invitations were extended to assist Jake to begin to consider his position more fully, in light of his sister's experience. Jake was invited to consider goals and reasons for facing responsibility, in order to make some form of restitution to his sister:

"If your abuse has hurt Amy, would you want to try and do something to help her or would you be prepared to leave it for her to worry about?"

"Can you handle facing up to what you did to your sister and carry it on your shoulders, or would you be prepared to leave it for her to carry on her shoulders?"

"How fair would it be to leave it to Amy to have to sort it out?"

Jake was invited to take a stand on this issue and to consider its meaning in terms of self-respect and respect from others:

"Will this make your shoulders stronger or weaker?"

"What would it say about you if you could handle facing up to your abuse and carry the responsibility on your own shoulders?"

"What would it say if you wimped out and left it for your little sister to have to carry and sort it out for herself?"

"What would you respect most in yourself?"

"What do you think others would respect most in you?"

The significance of Jake beginning to address his abuse of Amy in the face of his own experiences of victimization should never be overlooked or underestimated. In this context, Jake was invited to consider the importance of considering and understanding the potential impact of his abusive actions upon Amy:

"What does it say about you that you are beginning to face up to your abuse of Amy even though you are hurting a lot from the abuse that was done to you?"

"If you carry the responsibility on your shoulders, how different would this be to the way that Terry handled things?"

"Did Terry ever stop and think about how you felt?"

"What difference would it have made if he did?"

"Do you think that you will need to understand how it made Amy feel?"

"If you just tried to say 'sorry,' but didn't really understand how you had affected Amy, would this be enough? What would it say to Amy? How fair would it be?"

"What would it say about you if you had the guts to really think hard about what you might have put Amy through?"

Jake was invited to consider his readiness for embracing this journey toward responsibility and respect:

"This will mean taking a much tougher path than Terry chose."

"It will mean spending time with me talking and thinking about how your abuse might affect Amy."

"Are you sure you can handle this?"

"What would you prove to yourself if you could handle it?"

In this way, Jake was also being invited to consider a vital goal and reason for facing up: the development of self-respect. Most young men experience considerable shame when they think about their abusive actions. This shame is usually experienced only as self-deprecation and a sense that they are deficient or deviant individuals. It is vital to create a context whereby facing shame becomes a part of a healing journey toward the development of self-respect rather than self-deprecation:

"When you think about your abuse of Amy, how does it make you feel about yourself?"

"What would it say about you if you didn't feel ashamed?"

"What do you think you would respect most, facing up to it or running away from it?"

"Which do you think others would respect most in you?"

"Do you think facing up to it will make you stronger or weaker on the inside?"

"Do you think running away from it will make you stronger or weaker on the inside?"

"What are you proving about yourself and to yourself as you face up to it here?"

In this way, Jake was encouraged to consider and develop new definitions of strength, courage, and integrity, and to explore them and incorporate them into an alternate identity. Jake was continually encouraged to consider whether facing up to his abusive actions was consistent with his own goals, values, and preferences:

"Does facing up to this fit with the kind of guy you are and the kind of guy you want to be? Are you being true to yourself?"

"How does facing up fit with your ways of doing things?"

"Could you live with yourself if you copped out and hid behind your little sister?"

"Which direction will help you make sure you never abuse again: facing up or running away from the truth?"

"What steps have you already taken to face up to and take responsibility for what you have done?"

"What would it say about you if you could continue to face up even though you still feel a lot of hurt and unfairness about the things you have been put through?"

"Can you feel any strength or courage as a result of the gutsy steps you have taken here today?"

"Who do you think would be surprised at the steps you have taken here today?"

The reasons and goals for facing up are kept in the foreground throughout intervention. They include: making restitution to those who have been hurt; earning self-respect and respect from others; and preventing further abuse.

Broadening the Context

Involving Caregivers

Caregivers are invited to participate in interviews with the young man in order to prevent responsibility overloads and to provide an audience to witness and respond to his steps toward responsible and respectful behavior. Jake's residential caregivers were invited to appreciate and respect Jake's courage in facing his abusive actions. They also provided opportunities for conversation about justice and maintaining vigilance for evidence of responsibility and respectful behavior outside of the context of sexual abuse. In this way, caregivers were invited to assist Jake in evaluating and attributing meaning to his own behavior and thinking and in developing a respectful identity.

I usually endeavor to establish a respectful family context in which parents provide support for and witness evidence of the young man taking responsibility for his actions. My initial separate meetings with Jake and his mother were partly aimed at establishing readiness for a joint meeting. In my initial meeting with Jill, she demonstrated readiness to meet with Jake to discuss his experience within the family, in order to assist him to take responsibility for his abusive actions. In my initial two meetings with Jake, he recognized that there were aspects of his experience of victimization that his mother might not understand. Jake also acknowledged that his mother had not witnessed any evidence of his shame or remorse about his abuse of Amy. I was mindful of Jake's violence toward his mother, and sought his permission to inquire further about this. At first, he indicated that he "didn't feel proud" on the way he hurt his mother, but tended to justify his actions by suggesting that his mother's behavior was provocative. Jake acknowledged a mutual loss of respect between himself and his mother over the past 2 years. He acknowledged that he hated his mother comparing him with Terry and that he had felt somewhat neglected and let down by her during the custody dispute. Jake clearly experienced a sense of disappointment and letdown in relation to his mother, which had been overshadowed by his experience of Terry's violence and abuse in the family. Jake also conceded that his violence toward his mother and her property and his abuse of Amy had considerably and justifiably weakened her respect for him. He recognized that his mother had not heard him acknowledge shame and remorse about any of these actions. I inquired:

> "Do you think your mother was right in standing up against violence and deciding to leave Terry?"

Jake added that he wished she had taken this stand sooner and went on to tell me about the violence he would do to Terry now if he encountered him in the street. I acknowledged Jake's disappointment with his mother and his sense of entrapment when Terry was in the family. I went on to inquire:

> "What would you think if someone else went into your mother's house, pushed her around and smashed her things?"

> "Do you think your mother has a right to be safe and not have her property destroyed in her own home?"

> "Do you think your mother should ever put up with violence again?"

> "Do you think she is right in refusing to put up with violence from you?"

Jake impressed me with his maturity in these conversations and we speculated about how Jake's feelings and realizations about what he had done to his mother and younger siblings might surprise her if she knew. I reaffirmed my belief in fairness and justice and pointed out that Jake did have a responsibility to his mother and siblings. However, it would be extremely unfair for Jake's mother to expect him to acknowledge ways that he had hurt her and his siblings unless she also was prepared to understand and acknowledge his feelings and his experience of feeling let down and hurt.

I facilitated three meetings with Jill and Jake that were extremely moving. Stories of entrapment along with stories of resistance were exchanged, many for the first time. Toward the end of the second meeting, Jill was extremely distressed and courageously acknowledged to Jake that she felt she had let him down, that he had tried to look after her when it was really her job to protect him. After Jill and Jake held each other and cried, we considered the strength and courage in Jill's acknowledgment to Jake. I raised the question:

> "Do you think that Jake will follow your example and face up more to what he has done to Amy, or do you think he will blame you and use what you have said as an excuse for what he has done?"

Jake responded before Jill had an opportunity to answer. He began to apologize and made a commitment to share some of his realizations about his actions at the next meeting with Jill. I invited Jake and Jill to review and document the evidence of each other's strength, courage, honesty, and caring demonstrated in their meetings together.

Facing Up to Abusive Behavior

Another two individual meetings with Jake were carried out concurrently with a meeting that included his mother. These individual meetings focused on assisting Jake to develop and enact an agenda for facing up to the details and impact of his abuse of Amy. Once a young man is actively engaged in the process of facing responsibility and is demonstrating some self-motivation, then he may be ready to enter a group intervention program.

Further Intervention Processes

A facing-up agenda initially requires a commitment to full acknowledgment of abusive behavior and proceeds through to complex and sophisticated matters, such as appreciating the potential impact of abusive behavior (Jenkins, 1990). However, these levels of responsibility do not necessarily follow a linear sequence, as each area is continually developed and enhanced over time according to the readiness of the young man. The processes involved in "talking about talking about abuse" are employed to establish self-motivation to focus on specific details of the responsibility agenda. These processes are continued throughout the intervention to assist the young man to make sense of and further invest in the steps he is taking.

I initially establish a context that provides permission and support for full acknowledgment of abusive actions. At this stage, Jake had made what appeared to be only a partial acknowledgment of his abuse of Amy. He told this story to family, police, and lawyers and had, to some extent, painted himself into a corner from which it could be hard to emerge without a significant loss of face. I generally explain that no one ever faces up fully to all details of abuse at first meetings. I understand this and do not expect them to make full acknowledgment. I speak in the third person, while externalizing restraints to facing responsibility:

> "When guys abuse, and it comes out in the open, they generally panic; they worry about what is going to happen to them and what other people will think of them if they tell the whole truth. Most guys feel deep shame and they worry about what it might say about them. People might think they are really sick or weird. Some bits are easier to face up to but other bits just feel too hard. They try to push it to the back of their minds and not think about it and hope that it won't have to come out. Guys need to gradually check out that it is safe to talk about it and that they will be treated respectfully, otherwise they would be crazy to face up more."

I attempt to normalize the process of minimization and explore the consequences of facing up for the young man himself and for others. I invite the young man to consider his own readiness. I let him know that I expect there will be more to be disclosed, but that it is important to do this at his own pace. I make it clear that I always stand by and support people who have the courage to face up to the harder bits. I relate examples of this regarding other clients. Group meetings also provide another source of such experiences. I explain that many young men who I see have also abused other persons and have not yet disclosed their abuse. I propose face-saving ways for making further disclosures by speaking about the tendency to push details to the back of the mind and even temporarily to forget them. I explain that these details always emerge as memories and these experiences are examined.

A context is gradually established where acknowledgment is respected and permission is given for the young man to take his time to find the trust and courage required to search his mind and make complete acknowledgment, at his pace, not his worker's pace. I explain the principle of limited confidentiality and the need to notify unreported incidents of abuse along with the likely consequences of such notifications. The young man has a right to confidentiality and privacy, but any matters that could affect the safety or well-being of others are not kept confidential. The young man is informed of the processes by which I establish lines of communication with those who have been abused and their advocates, and with statutory authorities, to ensure that intervention is accountable.

When inviting a young man, such as Jake, to tell the story of his abusive behavior, I structure the intervention context to prevent, as much as possible, the telling of irresponsible stories of denial and minimization. I try to prevent the telling of irresponsible stories in order to avoid having to take on an adversarial or confrontative position. I invite the young man to tell the story within certain constraints that tend to maximize responsibility and integrity. A context is constructed for "telling it like it is" rather than allowing the story to be told through the lens of the young man's justifications and wishful, self-centered thinking about how it might have been. This requires a specific focus on the power differential between the young man and those he has abused and opportunities for the experience and interpretation of feelings of shame. Stories told outside of this context are inevitably minimized, self-centered, and emotionally detached.

I invited Jake to tell me about Amy and their relationship prior to his abuse of her. I asked quite specific details about Amy, about Jake, and about their relationship. Jake described a 7-year-old girl whom he had protected from Terry's violence but about whom he felt resentful because her father favored her and treated her more respectfully than himself. He detailed ways in which he had protected her and ways in which he had picked on her and bullied her. We began to focus on Amy's likely needs and experiences. Jake began to describe how vulnerable and needy Amy appeared to be. She had clung to him and looked to him "like a father." She followed him around, which he found to be a nuisance at times. Jake pointed out that Amy would have done anything be told her to. I inquired, in specific detail, about differences in age, size, and knowledge between Jake and Amy. As I made these inquires, I noticed that Jake looked down with watery eyes and appeared to be experiencing shame.

It is important to highlight Jake's experience of shame and invite consideration of its meaning in terms of a journey toward responsibility and respect:

"What are you realizing about Amy and what you did to her?"

"What are the differences you see between yourself and Amy?"

"Can you handle thinking about it in a more real way?"

"How does thinking about this affect you?"

"How are you thinking about your abuse of Amy now that is different to how you were thinking about it before?"

"What difference does it make as you start to see it like it really is, rather than pretending it wasn't so bad?"

"What does it take to start to see it like it really is and tell it like it really is?"

"Is this the right way for you to go or would it be better to pretend?"

"Will this make you a stronger or a weaker as a person?"

"What do you respect more?"

I invite young men, such as Jake, to consider appropriate labels for their actions:

"Can you handle calling what you did to Amy by its proper name, sexual abuse?"

"What makes it sexual abuse?"

"How hard is it to use the name, sexual abuse?"

"What difference does it make when you call it sexual abuse?"

Jake was encouraged to relate specific details of his abuse of Amy and was assisted to locate his account of his abusive behavior within an appropriate and realistic context that was sensitive to the imbalance of power and Amy's experience. He was invited to discover and identify his own strength, honesty, and integrity as he told the story. As Jake gradually began to tell his account, within a structure that highlighted the dynamics of abuse and the potential impact on Amy, he could engage in self-confrontation and self-acknowledgment. The need for external confrontation and challenge was then greatly reduced. Some questions that are helpful in creating this context are as follows:

"Whose idea was it?"

"How old were you; how old was Amy?"

"How did Amy feel about you beforehand?"

"What are the differences between you and Amy?"

"What did you notice about Amy that led you to choose her?"

"What were you thinking in the lead up to the abuse?"

"What were you telling yourself about it?"

"How did you first set Amy up and trick her into sexual abuse?"

"How did you get her trust?"

"How did you give her the message that what you were doing was OK?"

"How did you train Amy to get more involved in the abuse?"

"How did you plan opportunities to abuse her?"

"How did you try to get Amy to keep it secret?"

"Whose feelings were you thinking of, yours or hers?"

"Who did you block out Amy's feelings?"

"What would have happened if Amy hadn't told someone when she did?"

Jake was asked to relate specific details about what he did to Amy and what he got Amy to do to him within this context. When Jake made new disclosures or important realizations (e.g., "I did it to Amy because it was easy to do it to her"; "I didn't think she would tell anyone"), he was invited to consider the full meaning and implication of what he was realizing:

"What make it easy for you to sexually abuse Amy?"

"How does it affect you to think about:

- how you set Amy up?
- how Amy really trusted you, looked up to you, and relied on you?
- how you put what you wanted onto her and didn't think about her feelings?
- how you took advantage of the fact that she didn't know any better?
- how you used her to get off on, like she was just a magazine?"

Over the course of the intervention, in individual and group meetings, Jake was invited to extend these realizations, to consider more about Amy's likely experience at the time of the abuse and in the future. Jake was encouraged to consider and contrast his own experience in situations and circumstances where he had felt betrayed, trapped, and powerless or used. This fostered empathy through a set of emotional responses, rather than a set of detached, intellectual responses.

On all occasions, Jake must be invited to consider the meaning of these challenging and shameful realizations in the context of his stated goals and preferences; that is, his true identity:

"What does it take to be seeing it more and more like it really is?"

"How does it affect you to think and feel about it in a real way?"

"How is this different from what you were telling yourself about it before?"

"What does it say about you that you are starting to feel it and tell it like it really is?"

"What ways are you catching yourself out now?"

"What does it say about you that you are working it out rather than needing me to point things out to you?"

"Is this the direction you want to go? Even though it hurts?"

"How does this fit with the kind of guy you are?"

In this context, which is maintained in group and individual settings, honesty and disclosure are honored as reflections of the young man's identity and preferred ways of being. Self-confrontation is preferred over external confrontation, which is rarely used. When a young man discloses new information, it is not to placate the worker, but reflects his readiness to extend his journey toward responsibility and respect. It fits with what is right for him and his view of himself. We are fortunate in South Australia to have a juvenile justice system that also takes account of and respects honesty and responsibility.

I allowed Jake opportunities to consider what it would mean, for Amy and for himself, if there were truth to her allegations of penetration and coercion and he had the courage to face it. Jake could then own his eventual disclosures as his own, rather than confessions that had been extracted from him under duress. The process of disclosure then represents a victory for self-respect: a moment of honor, rather than an experience of defeat or accommodation.

Over time, Jake's account of his abuse gradually became more detailed than Amy's One day, as I routinely inquired about the possibility of other abuses, Jake informed me that there was something he had not talked about. He then acknowledged having sexually abused one of Amy's friends on several occasions when she had slept over with Amy. Jake was aware that this abuse would be notified to child protection authorities. His disclosure, however, while shocking, became a testament to Jake's integrity and earned him considerable respect from others, including police and juvenile justice authorities. Amy's friend was now able to be helped and a further burden had been lifted from Amy who knew of Jake's abuse of her friend but had not wanted to disclose and get Jake into any more trouble.

WHERE TO FROM HERE

I have focused on initial engagement and detailed some aspects of a model that I have found helpful to set a context for inviting young men to undertake a journey toward responsibility and respect. This context, whereby young men find their own motivation and develop practices of self-confrontation, rather than relying on external confrontation, can be a helpful one within which many of the more traditional concepts and strategies in intervention can be applied and used more effectively. At this point, the young man is in a position to learn, benefit from, and contribute to psychoeducational and relapse prevention strategies.

Jake continued to address and document details of his abusive actions and his realizations about them in terms of their potential impact on Amy and others. He gradually found courage to share these realizations with his mother and eventually with Amy herself. Jake did eventually reunite with his family after working out and enacting some specific ways to make appropriate restitution to Amy, David, and his mother. Family reconciliation must, of course, be informed by appropriate and responsible goal attainment. I have previously published details of strategies, relating to various levels of responsibility, designed to assist goal attainment and to set a context in which relapse prevention strategies can be utilized (Jenkins, 1990).

Intervention with Jake concerned several other foci, including his relationships with peers and his ability to argue and disagree with his mother without hurting her or damaging her property. Jake's behavior at school and with teachers was also addressed. In group settings, young men are invited to locate and understand abusive behavior within the context of dominant masculine practices and ways of being. The group provides an opportunity to externalize and challenge these practices. Sexually abusive behavior should always be addressed within the broader context of the young man's life and experiences and never considered in isolation. However, as is the case with most young men, when Jake began to take responsibility for his sexual abuse of Amy and her friend, and began to experience a sense of integrity and self-respect through this process, he found other challenges and responsibilities in his life more accessible and easier to address. When a young man develops his own path to take responsibility for sexual abuse of another, he invariably applies the maturity and confidence that he develops to other areas of his life and relationships.

REFERENCES

Jenkins, A. (1990). *Invitations to responsibility*. Adelaide, Australia: Dulwich Centre Publications.

Jenkins, A. (in press). Facilitating a journey towards responsibility and respect. In D. Fisher, M. Cardgo, & B. Print (Eds.), *Sex offenders: Toward improved practice*. London: Whiting & Birch.

Ryan, G., & Lane, S. (1991). *Juvenile sexual offending: Causes, consequences and correction*. Boston: Lexington Books.

White, M. (1986). Negative explanation, restraint and double description: A template for family therapy. *Family Process, 22,* 255–273.

White, M. (1995). *Re-authoring lives*. Adelaide, Australia: Dulwich Centre Publications.

13

C. Psychiatric Settings

Working with Sexual Offenders in Psychiatric Settings in England and Wales

Dawn Fisher, Don Grubin, and Derek Perkins

Sexual offenders in England and Wales are dealt with by psychiatric services when they are deemed to be mentally disordered as defined by the Mental Health Act of 1983, or are referred as outpatients for assessment and treatment. They are generally dealt with by forensic psychiatric services, which are divided into regional forensic units and the special hospitals. The special hospitals are maximum-security hospitals for mentally disordered offenders and the regional secure units are regionally based medium-security units for mentally disordered offenders. The types of sexual offenders seen and the particular problems posed within each of these settings will be discussed separately, as they operate in quite distinct ways. The role of psychiatry in dealing with sexual offenders will also be discussed, as those offenders who are detained under the Mental Health Act have to be under the control of a "responsible medical officer," which in most circumstances will be a psychiatrist.

THE ROLE OF PSYCHIATRY WITH SEXUAL OFFENDERS

The Mental Health Act of 1983 provided the framework for the involuntary detection and compulsory treatment of patients in psychiatric hospitals in England and Wales (Scotland has its own slightly different Mental Health Act). To be detained under the act, patients have to suffer from mental disorder (defined as mental illness, psychopathic disorder, mental impairment, or severe mental impairment) and require detention in hospital either for their own health or safety or for the protection of others. In the case of psychopathic disorder, patients must also be "treatable."

Dawn Fisher • Psychology Department, Llanarth Court Psychiatric Hospital, Llanarth, Nr. Raglan, Gwent, Wales NP5 2YD. **Don Grubin** • Department of Forensic Psychiatry, St. Nicholas' Hospital, Gosforth, Newcastle-upon-Tyne, England NE3 3XT. **Derek Perkins** • Psychology Department, Broadmoor Hospital, Crowthorne, Berkshire, England RG45 7EG.

Sourcebook of Treatment Programs for Sexual Offenders, edited by Marshall et al. Plenum Press, New York, 1998.

Patients can either be detained under civil provisions contained in part II of the act or criminal provisions contained in part III. Additionally, those sent to hospitals by the courts can have a "restriction order" placed on them which involves the Home Office in their management; such patients cannot be granted leave from hospital or discharged without the approval of Home Office ministers. Discharge in such cases can be conditional, with recall to hospital following a breach of these conditions. Whether civilly or criminally detained, patients can appeal to mental health review tribunals for release, and in the case of restriction orders they can apply for an absolute discharge.

The Mental Health Act also governs the way in which medication can be prescribed for involuntary patients. In most cases this either requires the patient's consent or the approval of a second, independent physician appointed by the Mental Health Act Commission where consent is lacking. In the case of injected hormone treatment, however, as might be considered for sexual offenders, consent and the approval of a second physician are necessary. The use of orally administered drugs like cyproterone acetate, however, does not require this additional process, nor does the use of injected hormones in patients who are not detained under the provisions of the act.

Psychiatrists in Britain typically display a good deal of ambivalence in relation to sexual offenders. At one level, they show little reluctance to provide reports to the courts in which they assess risk in individual cases, and on occasions they will recommend that an offender should be dealt with by way of a hospital order rather than a prison sentence. They are also frequently involved in assessing suitability for release from prison when sexual offenders come up for parole and they sit on the national boards that make the parole decisions. Similarly, they assess and make recommendations about the relatively small group of sexual offenders who are compulsorily detained in hospital for treatment; they always sit on mental health review tribunals, which determine whether such offenders are treatable and whether they are safe enough to be released. However, when it comes to actually providing treatment for sexual offenders, psychiatrists are often much more reticent, particularly when treatment is associated with compulsory admission to hospital. Sexual offenders can be detained against their will in hospital under the provisions of the Mental Health Act of 1983 under the category of psychopathic disorder, which is defined as "a persistent disorder or disability of mind ... which results in abnormally aggressive or seriously irresponsible conduct." The paragraph of the act that immediately follows this definition, however, states that a determination of mental disorder can not be made "by reason only of ... sexual deviancy." This rider, meant to protect homosexuals from compulsory treatment, is sometimes used by psychiatrists as a reason to exclude pedophiles and rapists from the act. Of course, there is a legitimate concern that too judicious a use of mental health legislation in relation to sexual offenders may lead to the risk of detaining obviously dangerous men in hospital for whom treatment is either inappropriate or ineffective. In addition, if and when the release takes place of compulsorily treated sexual offenders, many psychiatrists feel particularly vulnerable to criticism should their patients then reoffend.

The need to avoid one extreme, however, has led many psychiatrists to argue that, since sexual offenders are not usually mentally ill or mentally disordered, there is little that psychiatry can offer these men. Unfortunately, this conclusion is based on a generally poor understanding that British psychiatrists have of sexual offenders. Not only does this mean that treatment that could be offered is not, but also that the basic assessment or risk is often faulty. Psychiatric training in the United Kingdom focuses on mental illness and, to some extent, dysfunctional behaviors that lead to personal distress. The assessment and treatment of sexual offenders does not fit easily into this framework, with the exception of those psychiatrists who have a particular attraction to psychoanalysis. Consequently, many psychiatrists are simply unaware of modern notions about the etiology of sexual offending and do not understand the components that are necessary for a treatment program to be effective.

It is also relevant that psychiatrists who are most interested in sexual behavior usually have little experience with serious sexual offenders. Their practice focuses on sex therapy, and they tend to see couples with sexual difficulties or patients who indecently expose themselves, are voyeurs, or who have disturbing sexual fantasies but who on the whole do not sexually assault others. Forensic psychiatrists, on the other hand, see offender patients, but they do not have much experience of "normal" sexuality. Their assumptions about abnormal sexual fantasy and behavior are based on a population with extreme sexual deviance and on a few articles in the psychiatric literature of questionable validity. Indeed, two particularly influential articles in Britain are frequently referred to by psychiatrists. Brittain's (1970) description of the "sadistic murderer" as an introverted, timid, over-controlled, and socially isolated man, overdependent on his mother, sexually prudish and inexperienced, but with a rich, sexually deviant sadistic fantasy life was based wholly on clinical anecdote and experience rather than research of any formal kind; it is now, however, part of the British psychiatric folklore. MacCulloch, Snowden, Wood, and Mills' (1983) account of the importance of fantasy in sadistic offending was based on 13 special hospital patients and has not been shown to be applicable to clients in other settings, but nonetheless it forms the psychiatric basis for assessing the risk represented by fantasy.

Although sexual offenders can be found in hospitals of all levels of security in Britain, it is in the special (high security) hospitals where they are most common; indeed, it is estimated that nearly half of all offender patients in the special hospitals have a sexual component to their offending. While psychiatrists have responsibility for these patients in terms of their management and eventual release, they are not usually involved in treatment, delegating this instead to psychologists or nursing staff. The exception is the psychotic sexual offender, where the psychiatrist will take an interest in the treatment of the psychosis. Even here, however, the behavior associated with the sexual offending will either be ascribed to the psychosis and effectively ignored, on the assumption that the risk disappears with the symptoms of the mental illness, or dealt with by another member of the clinical team.

In this respect, a recent study of treatment outcome for personality-disordered patients discharged from Broadmoor Hospital is of interest (Reiss, Meux, & Grubin, 1996). Approximately half of the patients in the study had a sexual motivation associated with their offending. Although the majority of these patients were treated on a ward specially tailored for personality-disordered patients that offered a range of psychotherapeutic treatments, both individually and in groups, treatment in relation to sexual offending consisted either of nonspecific psychotherapy or sex education. Of those released, five patients (20% of those discharged) reoffended. All of these reoffenses were sexual in nature: two sexual killings, two serious sexual offenses, and one less serious sexual offense. It was concluded that perhaps a more cognitive–behavioral treatment program for sexual offenders should be introduced to the hospital regime.

Medication, the type of treatment that is often associated with psychiatrists, is used sparingly in Britain. Cyproterone acetate is prescribed by very few psychiatrists with any regularity, although neuroleptics are sometimes used for their antilibidinal effects. It is not really clear why this should be the case, but it probably reflects a general lack of experience in prescribing the medication and a misperception of the risks associated with it. There can be little doubt that this treatment modality is currently underused in Britain.

REGIONAL SECURE UNITS

Regional secure units (RSUs) were established throughout each of the 14 health authority regions in England and Wales in the 1970s, in response to two influential reports. The Glancy Report commented on the need for secure provision for mentally ill patients, whose behavior was such that they could not be contained safely in psychiatric hospitals. The Butler Report highlighted the need for some form of secure psychiatric accommodation for patients leaving highly secure, long-term special hospitals that could offer the opportunity for gradual rehabilitation into the community in the patient's area of origin. RSUs were seen as the answer for these patients and were established accordingly. They offer a limited number of inpatient beds (ranging from 15 to 100) based on estimates of need according to the size of the population served and are run along multidisciplinary lines with nursing, psychiatry, psychology, social work, and occupational therapy tending to be the main disciplines represented. The majority of RSUs also offer some form of outpatient service, the level of which depends on the staffing available.

Sexual offenders are eligible for admission to RSUs only if they are mentally disordered. Generally they are of two types: those who have been diagnosed as having a psychopathic personality disorder, and those suffering from mental illness, such as schizophrenia. Those who are not mentally disordered are referred to outpatient services and generally are seen by both psychiatrists and psychologists for assessment and treatment. This population may account for up to a third of all referrals to outpatient services. These patients place a huge demand on resources. In a survey of the work undertaken with sexual offenders by clinical psychologists working in forensic settings such as RSUs and special hospitals, Houston, Thomson, and Wragg (1994) found that all RSU psychologists undertook a substantial amount of work with sexual offenders as outpatients and almost a quarter of these psychologists were involved in running groups. In some establishments, the huge demand for work with sexual offenders has led to discussion of whether or not sexual offenders should be seen, the argument being that those who are not mentally disordered should not be dealt with by the health services but should be more properly seen as clients of the probation service. However, as yet there has been no move to stop such referrals.

The number of inpatient sexual offenders tends to be relatively low in most RSUs. Those with a psychotic illness tend to be referred from the court for assessment for having committed an offense while mentally ill. Such sexual offenders are regarded more sympathetically by staff, who often take the view that the individual would not have offended if they had not been ill and that controlling the mental illness will prevent further sexual offending. While this may be true in some cases, there are certainly a number for whom sexual offending is not contingent on their psychotic mental state. The other group of sexual offenders seen as inpatients are those with psychopathic personality disorders. These offenders are generally referred from special hospitals for rehabilitation into the community and are frequently regarded as being difficult if not impossible to treat. Given that such offenders are overrepresented in the small number of serious reoffenses that have occurred in RSUs, there is often a great reluctance to admit them. Indeed, there have been periods when certain RSUs refused to admit such patients owing to the fear of them reoffending and the difficulty in establishing when it is safe to discharge them into the community. Changes in the Mental Health Act of 1983 resulted in fewer sexual offenders with the diagnosis of psychopathic personality disorder being admitted to forensic psychiatric establishments because of the current requirement for admission that "such treatment is likely to alleviate or prevent a deterioration of his condition."

Inpatients

Due to the fact that there are usually only a few inpatient sexual offenders within each RSU at any one time and the likelihood being that they will be mentally ill, the type of work that can be undertaken with them is restricted. It is not usual for RSU staff to run group therapy for inpatient sexual offenders, although, as described above, a number of staff (usually clinical psychologists) are involved in running or consulting to outpatient groups. In order to illustrate the type of work undertaken with inpatient sexual offenders and the issues surrounding this work a number of cases will be described.

Case 1 is a mentally ill man in his 30s who has a long-standing history of schizophrenia. He has committed several sexual offenses including indecently assaulting a child and raping a fellow adult inpatient at a local psychiatric hospital. While it is acknowledged that the offenses were committed when he was mentally ill, it has not been possible to ascertain whether or not he is likely to offend when relatively stable on medication. He is not willing to discuss his offenses and becomes distressed and angry if any attempt is made to do this; he also refuses to complete any questionnaires. Attempts have been made to engage him in work with both male and female staff with no success. His mental illness has resulted in him being very poorly motivated; he has no wish to leave the RSU, so there is no motivating factor to obtain his cooperation. In the absence of any psychological work being possible, it was suggested to him that he be prescribed an antilibidinal drug, but he has also refused this. In summary, he is a frustrating case since it has not been possible to carry out a full assessment of his offending, he is not amenable to any therapeutic work, and he cannot move to a less secure setting until there can be some degree of confidence that he is not likely to reoffend.

Case 2 is a man in his late 20s who was admitted to the RSU following violent assaults upon staff in his former psychiatric hospital. He also becomes very aggressive and sexually disinhibited when acutely psychotic. He makes sexually inappropriate remarks to female staff and attempts to touch them sexually. There is no doubt that if he were back in the community in this disturbed state, he would commit a sexual offense. When acutely ill he has no insight and it is not possible to work with him. However, when he responds to medication, he settles well and the aggression and inappropriate sexual behavior resolve and are not a problem. The treatment strategy with his man is to ensure that he is stabilized on medication, and when discharged from the RSU, he will be followed up in the community to supervise and monitor his taking of medication.

Case 3 is a man in his 50s who committed a serious rape while mentally ill. However, there is also a suggestion that he may have sexually abused one of his daughters over a period of time when there was no suggestion he was mentally ill. Soon after starting antipsychotic medication, a rapid improvement in his mental state was seen and an assessment of his sexual offending was attempted. He was not keen to cooperate and initially used the excuse that he could not understand what was being said, since English was not his first language. It was noted that he did not seem to have any difficulty conversing on nonsexual topics, but he continued to maintain he could not understand. This effectively prevented any further work being done with him until the arrival of a staff member who spoke the same language and was available to undertake joint sessions with the psychologist. Using a cognitive–behavioral approach, it was possible to obtain a full picture of the factors surrounding his offending and the accompanying cognitive distortions and victim-blaming attitudes. He maintained for some time that he had not raped his victim and that she was a willing participant. Through the work undertaken with him, he was able to admit that he had been attracted to the girl and had planned how he could manage to be in a situation where he could be alone and undisturbed with his victim. Although the work could be said to be successful in getting him to admit his responsibility for the rape, he remained entirely lacking in any remorse for his victim and he would not admit to abusing his daughter. It would have been useful at this point to have been able to put him into a group setting, since this may have exerted more influence over him, but the language problem precluded this possibility.

Case 4 was a man in his early 20s who was referred for an assessment by the court as to the most suitable disposal for him. He had committed an attempted rape on a young girl while he was psychotic. He responded very quickly to medication, but he was defensive and victim blaming and unwilling to discuss his offenses. There had been previous allegations against him of a sexual nature and he had a long history of offending generally, including violent offenses. He presented as having a psychopathic personality disorder in addition to mental illness and was regarded as being unmotivated for treatment and at high risk of reoffending. In view of the fact that he would be difficult to treat, and thus impossible to discharge because of the possibility of him reoffending, it was felt that he would be best dealt with in the penal system where he would be given a definite sentence. Should he become mentally ill again while in prison, he could then be transferred to the RSU until he was stable enough to return to prison.

The above cases illustrate the difficulties associated with working with mentally ill sexual offenders in RSU settings. Such patients are frequently poorly motivated and will not cooperate with completing questionnaires (the results of which may be dubious anyway, given the clients' mental state). These patients also have difficulties discussing their offenses and in some cases of even getting out of bed to attend a session. Because of their general level of apathy, it is difficult to motivate them, since often they do not care whether or not they remain within the RSU indefinitely. With the psychopathic personality-disordered individuals the issues are more about treatability. RSUs are not intended to be long-stay institutions, and if it is thought that an individual will require treatment beyond approximately 2 years, they are likely to be deemed unsuitable for admission. Additionally, the structure of the multidisciplinary team is such that a psychiatrist is the responsible medical officer (RMO) and therefore the person who will take the responsibility should something go wrong. The situation can thus arise where the psychologist, who is the most likely professional to be carrying out the treatment, may be willing to work with the patient but the psychiatrist who is the RMO has the ultimate sanction and may veto the admission.

Outpatient Groups

The majority of sexual offenders seen by RSU psychologists are referred as outpatients for assessment and treatment. The survey carried out by Houston et al. (1994) demonstrated that while a large percentage (95%) of forensic psychologists in RSUs were involved in carrying out a variety of assessments and individual treatment of sexual offenders, only 25% were involved in group treatment. Most of the group treatment, directly run by psychologists, was time limited. Only 3 of 18 groups were long term. All groups were cognitive–behavioral in orientation and involved co-therapists from a range of professional backgrounds.

As outpatient programs are being described elsewhere, this account will limit itself to a brief overview of a service set up and run for outpatient sexual offenders in one RSU. Prior to setting up the treatment group, outpatient sexual offenders had been worked with (on an individual basis) by a small number of clinical psychologists. As numbers grew and more was written in the literature about group work with sexual offenders, it was decided to set up a group program. Initially a local multidisciplinary interest group for professionals involved in working with sexual offenders was set up as a way of both identifying a potential group of therapists and also providing a forum for training. While individual practitioners were very enthusiastic about being involved in running groups, management personnel in some agencies were very wary and initially refused to allow their staff to become involved. One of the reasons for this was that the sexual offenders often came from geographic locations outside the usual catchment areas, and thus were seen as "not being their clients." Given that this issue was taking an interminable amount of time to resolve, it was decided to go ahead and set up the first group using those individuals who were available. Once the first group was underway, this acted as a catalyst for those agencies who had been reluctant to allow their staff to become involved, perhaps because they did not want to be perceived as being left behind in a new development.

The first group operated as a long-term open-ended group that met once a week for 2 hours. The group was run along cognitive–behavioral lines by two psychologists from the RSU, a psychologist from a special hospital, and a freelance social worker. The group was held in the evenings in a therapy room at a local family center run by Barnados, a voluntary agency for children and their families. The four group leaders operated a rota system, so that two staff (where possible, one male and one female) would run the group and a third staff member would observe through a one-way mirror. Working in this way meant that staff absences did not affect the running of the group. The group is still in operation, and over the years that it has been running, new staff have been introduced with little disruption. As a staff training aid, observation of the group has been allowed for interested professionals with the provision that they observe three groups in succession to avoid the problem of "professional voyeurism." Numbers of observers have been limited to two per session, and they are required to abide by the rules of confidentiality of the group. Group members are aware that they are observed from time to time, as a training method, and they sign a contract agreeing to this.

In addition to the original group, a further long-term group has been set up and a short-term introductory group was tried for 10 weeks. The purpose of the short-term group was to accustom clients to being in a group and to assess how motivated they were to take part in the longer-term program and how disruptive they were likely to be. While this made sense in theory, it did not work out in practice, and the group was abandoned after a couple of trial runs. The main problem with this group was that clients became attached to the group and were then reluctant to leave and join a new group and seemed more disruptive as a result. Additionally, places in the long-term groups rarely became available when needed, and clients were then subject to long delays before joining the next group, which heightened their anxiety and decreased their motivation.

For a period of time the RSU was able to operate a range of services for sexual offenders, with two long-term groups plus an adolescent group program. Indeed, one of the group members from the initial long-term group was used as an "assistant" in another group, which proved highly effective.

Unfortunately, one of the main agencies that had been allowing their staff to run groups decided to set up their own program, which led to a decrease in the number of programs that could be sustained with the available staff. As a consequence, the service for sexual offenders in the area became fragmented. Due to the loss of key staff members at the RSU, much of the momentum was lost and it was not possible to rebuild the service to the level it had been previously. This illustrates how vulnerable such programs can be to the loss of key personnel and indicates the need for managers to recognize the value of the work being done and to ensure that the work is an integral part of the whole service and not just something that interested staff set up in addition to their other duties.

SPECIAL HOSPITALS

There are three special hospitals that provide care, treatment, and containment for mentally disordered patients requiring maximum security in England and Wales. There is also a single Scottish special hospital that performs similar functions for that population, but that will not be included in this survey.

Most special hospital patients are suffering from a major mental illness (notably schizophrenia) and most have been hospitalized following court appearances under sections 37/41 of the Mental Health Act of 1983. Most have index offenses (i.e., offenses that have led to their admission) of homicide (30.2%) or other serious physical violence (37.3%). Over 80% of special hospital patients are male. Many of these patients have histories of profoundly disturbed early experiences and have been traumatized through emotional, physical, or sexual abuse in ways that are implicated in their subsequent antisocial behavior.

Approximately 13% of the male population in the special hospitals have index offenses that are legally classifiable as sexual offenses. This proportion increases to about one third if previous sexual offenses plus sexual motives or features of the index offense are included. The picture for female patients is less clear, due in part to the relative dearth of research with this group. While less than 0.5% of female patients have a legally defined sexual index offense, a number have manifested either past or current sexually motivated aggression as part of their reasons for entering hospital (Coid, 1993). Each patient entering a special hospital has an individualized multidisciplinary treatment plan that is prepared by the patient's clinical team in consultation with the patient and is aimed at identifying and addressing the patient's therapeutic and security needs.

The task of the special hospitals, particularly through the work of the multidisciplinary team, is to ameliorate the patient's mental disorder, meet the patient's therapeutic needs, and reduce his or her propensity to engage in dangerous behavior outside the conditions of maximum security. Additionally, staff are expected to behave in ways that will "respect the rights of individuals and the needs of the community" and "recognize the emotional, spiritual, physical, material and cultural needs of individual patients" (Broadmoor Hospital Strategic Direction, 1995/96).

Sexual offender patients are among the most challenging to the mental health system. The evidence on treatment efficacy within therapy programs in sparse (Furby, Weinrott, & Blackshaw, 1989), although there was evidence of a small but robust overall treatment effect in a more recent meta-analysis (Hall, 1995). The challenge within the special hospitals is to achieve the best match between the patient's individual therapeutic and security needs and the available clinical and physical resources to meet these needs. This generates challenges to the formulation of sexually offending behavior and challenges to the effective collaborative working of the multidisciplinary team.

Design, Development, and Evaluation

Among the ways of meeting this challenge are, at the one extreme, the setting up of totally individualized, multidisiciplinary treatment programs that might in practice prove difficult to coordinate and deliver within the available regime and resources. At the other extreme are standardized treatment programs or packages that, while addressing significant needs for the majority of patients, would fail to address every treatment need for each patient at the ideal time. What is needed, therefore, is the best compromise between these two positions (standard treatment packages and individualized therapy) that takes into account the available human, environmental, and financial resources available to the hospital. Clearly, this is a very complex task. The breadth and complexity of individual patient's needs and problems, together with the fact that these should be addressed as soon as possible after the patient's admission, means that the skills and knowledge of all members of the multidisciplinary team need to be drawn on to maximum effect.

The therapies provided for sexual offenders need to address as far as possible all major aspects of their treatment needs and likely future risk factors, linked to an individual formulation of the patients' sexual offending behavior, which draws from developmental, historical, and contemporary factors. Treatment ideally should be multifaceted and multimodal as well as multidisciplinary in nature. This is particularly important within special hospitals that, because of the initial risks posed by the patients, place constraints on the extent to which patients can be exposed to opportunities for freedom of movement and freedom to interact with others, especially in the early part of their hospitalization. On the other hand, one thing that is available in abundance for the treatment of special hospital patients is time. The average length of stay in special hospitals being about 8 years.

At the developmental level, many patients will have experienced emotional, physical, and sexual abuse. These issues need to be explored, clarified, and resolved so that they do not present as risk factors for future offending. Unresolved anger at being a victim of abuse as a child needs to be confronted and resolved, while taking care not to feed into denial mechanisms that distance the patient from responsibility for his own, subsequent actions. This is particularly challenging in a psychiatric setting where mental disorder has, at a medicolegal level, encouraged the client to think that they have a disease that is beyond their control and for which they therefore have no responsibility.

At the offense-maintenance level, the relationship between the individual's personal circumstances, their level of functioning and social adequacy, and the offense itself needs to be explored. The extent to which a patient is able to recognize and control deviant sexual fantasies, urges, and cognitive distortions, engage in socially appropriate and skillful behavior, be able to control emotional responses such as depression and anger, and recognize and avoid future risk factors will all need to be taken into account in therapy. Similarly, different aspects of the patient's functioning need to be brought together into the therapeutic equation, including behavioral observation, psychometric assessment, psychophysiological assessment, interview data, and responses in group situations.

A patient's progress through special hospital is marked by gradual steps toward meeting treatment and security needs as the patient's risk to others and his or her mental disorder are gradually reduced. Dangers lie in any assumption that a reduction in mental disorder automatically implies reduced risk to others. For some sexual offenders an amelioration in mental disorder will bring correspondingly reduced risk, while for others the two issues may be quite independent or even in some cases inversely related. Progress is assessed initially by the patient's multidisciplinary team with input from the patient, but subsequently rests on the opinions and advice of clinical staff at the facility where the patient is intended to move (usually a regional secure unit) as well as from the Home Office, which has a specific role in monitoring and advising on public risk in the case of restricted patients. This means that a patient's departure from a special hospital, which is generally an expressed goal for most patients, is contingent on recorded progress in relevant treatment programs and the acknowledgment within and outside the hospital that sufficient progress has been made. Hospitalization is to that extent indeterminate. This indeterminacy has an impact on the patient's motivation to engage in therapy and there can be tensions for the patient between: (1) an intrinsic desire to participate in treatment; (2) an inclination to avoid uncomfortable issues raised in therapy, and hence avoid effective treatment; and (3) a desire to participate in treatment in order to achieve the goal of transfer or discharge from the special hospital.

This process is further complicated by its interaction with the patient's legal rights to have his or her case regularly reviewed by an independent mental health review tribunal. This tribunal has the power to rule on the patient's legal detention in hospital and to discharge the patient if his or her detention is found to be no longer necessary. The tribunal also has a right to give advice regarding further assessments or treatments that seem to it to be relevant, although there is no requirement of the hospital or clinical team to act on this advice. The patient's engagement in therapy is thus a complex interaction between: (1) the patient's perception of the effects of engaging in treatment; and (2) the external contingencies operating on the patient, including the clinical team case reviews, decisions of the mental health review tribunal, and advice from the Home Office.

External contingencies such as those described above cannot be ignored in therapy, since they directly affect the patient's thoughts and feelings about his or her sexual offending. They are, therefore, either consciously separated from therapy or else, more usefully, integrated within the therapeutic interaction. Particularly in the case of sexual offenders, this might mean, for example, having to work through with the patient the consequences for their decision to participate or not in particular assessments or treatments as they progress through the hospital, and then negotiating this with the offender and the receiving unit.

CONCLUSIONS

Mentally disordered sexual offenders present a number of areas of difficulty for those involved in their assessment and treatment. Those who are suffering from mental illness, such as schizophrenia, tend to present both communication and motivational difficulties. There may also be differences of professional opinion over the role the mental illness plays in the sexual offending. Where the belief is that the mental illness led to the offending, there may be a tendency to discharge the patient once the mental illness has been treated without fully assessing the patient's offending behavior and attitudes. Due to concerns over treatability and fears of patients reoffending, psychiatrists may be wary of becoming involved in cases of personality-disordered sexual offenders and reluctant to admit them for treatment. Thus, in many settings, the focus of work with sexual offenders has been on an outpatient basis, with patients being seen largely for assessment and to a lesser extent for treatment, particularly individual treatment. The mentally disordered sexual offenders have to some extent been a neglected group, but recently there has been some interest in attempting to develop treatment programs specifically geared to their needs, and such work is currently being planned in the special hospitals. It is to be hoped that such work will be developed and researched, and that by so doing, the reluctance of professionals to become involved in such cases will be gradually overcome.

REFERENCES

Brittain, R. P. (1970). The sadistic murderer. *Medicine, Science and the Law, 10,* 198–207.

Coid, J. (1993). Personality disorder and self-report questionnaire. *British Journal of Psychiatry, 162,* 265–270.

Furby, L., Weinrott, M. R., & Blackshaw, L. (1989). Sex offender recidivism: A review. *Psychological Bulletin, 105,* 3–30.

Hall, G. C. N. (1995). Sexual offender recidivism revisited: A meta-analysis of recent treatment studies. *Journal of Consulting and Clinical Psychology, 63,* 802–809.

Houston, J. C., Thomson, P., & Wragg, J. (1994). A survey of forensic psychologists' work with sex offenders in England and Wales. *Criminal Behaviour and Mental Health, 4,* 118–129.

MacCulloch, M. J., Snowden, P. R., Wood, P. J. W., & Mills, H. E. (1983). Sadistic fantasy, sadistic behavior and offending. *British Journal of Psychiatry, 143,* 20–29.

Reiss, D., Meux, C., & Grubin, D. (1996). Young psychopaths in special hospital: Treatment and outcome. *British Journal of Psychiatry, 168,* 99–104.

14

C. Psychiatric Settings

The Treatment of Sexually Aggressive Offenders in the Dr. Henri van der Hoeven Kliniek

A Forensic Psychiatric Institute in the Netherlands

Daan van Beek and Jules Mulder

INTRODUCTION

Since the early 1980s, a number of members of staff of the Dr. Henri van der Hoeven Kliniek have been paying special attention to sexually aggressive patients. They have introduced diagnostic instruments and methods of treatment that have been specially developed for this category of patient and have been gradually integrated into the total program of treatment of the clinic.

The first part of this chapter will deal with the type of patients attending the clinic, the general principles for treatment at the Dr. Henri van der Hoeven Kliniek, the reasons for paying special attention to sexually aggressive delinquents, and to the specific methods of diagnosis and treatment for those sexually aggressive delinquents who have been admitted for treatment at the clinic. Finally, factors will be discussed that have had a beneficial or detrimental affect on the process of implementation of these specific interventions as part of the whole range of treatment available.

The second part of this chapter deals with the way the day treatment in the clinic is put into practice. This special facility has existed since the early 1990s, and offers patients a short-term, highly structured cognitive–behavioral therapeutic program of treatment.

THE DR. HENRI VAN DER HOEVEN KLINIEK

The Dr. Henri van der Hoeven Kliniek is a forensic psychiatric hospital in Utrecht, the Netherlands. The clinic treats patients with various psychiatric problems and offense

Daan van Beek and Jules Mulder • Dr. Henri van der Hoeven Kliniek, Forensic Psychiatric Institute, 3500 AD Utrecht, The Netherlands.

Sourcebook of Treatment Programs for Sexual Offenders, edited by Marshall et al. Plenum Press, New York, 1998.

backgrounds. All patients have committed serious offenses and have been declared to be unaccountable, or to exhibit diminished responsibility, for their offenses owing to psychiatric disturbance. After their arrest, they undergo a psychological and psychiatric examination. The judge will take the results of this examination into account when sentencing and determining the necessity of treatment in a forensic psychiatric clinic. The judge also decides what chances there are of a repetition of the offense. In the case of unaccountability and of diminished responsibility, the judge will impose a TBS measure, which in effect makes staying at the clinic involuntary. After a period of 2 years, the judge will decide whether to prolong the measure for a further 2 years or to remove the TBS measure. In doing so, the judge makes use of the evaluative treatment report submitted by the clinic.

The Patients

At any one time there are approximately 90 patients at the clinic, 10% of whom are women. Patients are mostly in their 20s or 30s and are of average intelligence.

Almost every patient has a problematic life history. Discontinuity of upbringing, serious neglect during early childhood, and physical and/or sexual abuse have often been part of the picture. Many patients exhibited behavioral disturbances at an early age. Outpatient or clinical treatment often has been stopped too early, which means that it has had no chance of having effect. Incomplete education and frequent changes of working environment are the rule rather than the exception. Patients often have a conflict-filled relationship with their immediate environment. They find it difficult to relate to people and maintain relationships. They have learned to make use of survival strategies such as passivity, the denial of their problems, or blaming others for their difficulties. Addiction, aggression, and criminal behavior often crop up at an early age.

The offense background of the patients consists of nonsexual violence such as grievous bodily harm, manslaughter, or murder (44%); sexually aggressive offenses (35%) of which three quarters involve assault or rape of women; child sexual offenses (25%); arson with danger to life (14%); and nonviolent offenses to property (7%).

The psychiatric problems are of a complex nature. Most patients suffer from one or more personality disorders. Combinations of a number of antisocial, narcissistic, borderline, paranoid, passive–aggressive, and evasive personality disorders occur frequently. These problems are further increased in some patients by complicated disturbances of mood, fear, impulse control, or one of a sexual (paraphiliac) nature. A small group (15%) also have a pronounced tendency toward psychosis. If such psychotic problems are in remission, personality problems come to the fore. Seventy percent of the total population of the clinic have a history of abusing psychoactive drugs, and in the case of 30% there is a question of actual addiction.

The Principles of the Treatment

In the case of patients with psychotic problems, who have mainly committed their offense(s) during period of psychosis, psychosis relapse is the central issue. The main ingredients of such treatment involve the acquisition of insight into the illness, a course of medication, and learning to derive benefits from a regular, structured life. Another aim is to develop any potential that the patient may possess. Since these patients constitute a small proportion of our patients, there will be no further discussion of this issue during the rest of this chapter.

For patients with personality disorders, the curbing of a career of delinquency stands high on the agenda. Though they will have to learn to live with limitations to relationships, repairing deficits in development is one major goal of treatment.

Patients live in groups of nine. High priority is given to collective responsibility during daily life and to their relations to counselors and to one another. In their living groups, patients can gain experience of living together to enable them to further develop social skills. In principle, each patient is treated in and by way of the living group. A team of five group counselors stimulates patients to concentrate on developing their positive qualities. Old, inadequate behavioral patterns are discouraged through setting clearly defined limits. Together with the head of treatment and a social worker, the counselors form a treatment team that is responsible for the planning, continuity, and evaluation of treatment.

Patients also participate in an activities program that is tailor-made to suit their type of problem. This consists of various kinds of instruction, vocational training, sport, creative subjects, and different forms of individual and group psychotherapy.

Approximately two thirds of the patients have had problems with work. It is the policy of the clinic that patients are given work training. The average patient works for half the working week, the other half being taken up by the various activities in his program. Entering or reentering the labor market is of great importance if resocialization is to succeed. The clinic offers a broad range of opportunities for work, including workshops for woodwork and metalwork, a department for painting and assembly, the kitchen, the garden, the administration, the facilitatory service, and the store.

The great majority of patients have reached a lower level of school education than their intellectual capacities would, under the right circumstances, allow them to achieve. Clinic policy is to reduce discrepancies between previous attainments and the potential of patients, by means of instruction. Patients are able, according to their capacities, to attend courses at primary, secondary, vocational, and tertiary educational level. Such education may also take place outside of the clinic insofar as it is safe to do so. Patients who are educationally subnormal cannot attend courses that would lead to a certificate. The main aim with such patients is to improve their language and arithmetic skills and to help them accept the limitations of their intellect.

The following opportunities are provided by the clinic to help patients develop their creative skills: handicrafts, drawing, photography, textiles, drama, mime, music, sculpture, and modeling. The average patient spends some 4 hours a week on one or more activities of this kind. Patients are given the chance to practice various kinds of technical, psychological, and social skills, for example, reading music, learning to cope with frustration, overcoming their fear of failure, and learning to ask for help when needed.

Sport and physical training are popular among patients. The clinic has a well-equipped sports hall, swimming baths, a sauna, a judo hall, a fitness hall, and an outdoor sports field. Patients can develop their skills in such sports as football, volleyball, badminton, judo, and tennis. A large proportion of patients are out of condition when they arrive at the clinic and sports provide a basis for all patients to develop social contacts still further.

The psychotherapy department is a hive of activity: While in former years this department concentrated on psychodynamic and interactional activities, recent years have seen the growth of cognitive–behavioral therapy. Now, individual psychotherapy is mostly directive and problem-oriented. During the first phase of treatment, the psychotherapists support the patients and try to find solutions for their problems in daily life. They also act as a go-between for patients and group counselors. When this relationship has become established, psychotherapy then focuses on attempting to gain an understanding of their personality problems and to develop alternative behavioral patterns. Intervention is typically derived from cognitive–behavioral therapy (Beck, Freeman et al., 1990). At a later phase, attention is focused on the situations that led to the patients' offenses. Finally, the psychotherapist, in conjunction with the patients and group counselors, draws up relapse prevention plans based on the everyday experiences of the patients during therapy. These same psychotherapists also conduct group therapy courses. These sessions consist of a limited number of psychoeducative group sessions, each devoted to a particular theme such as addiction, social skills, aggression control, and sexuality. There is also a separate group for women patients.

Psychotherapists attend staff meetings and are not bound by confidentiality during therapy. Patients are, of course, made aware of this fact. Many patients derive support from their psychotherapy, in part because they know that they can make their voice heard at staff meetings via the psychotherapist, since it is at staff meetings where important decisions affecting the patients are made.

Apart from the types of therapy mentioned above, patients also have access to psychotherapists who work on a consultative basis and who do not belong to the staff of the clinic. These psychotherapists play a more investigative role and what is said to them by patients remains confidential.

Therapists try to liaise with the family and other persons important to the lives of patients inasmuch as such contacts further strengthen and promote the therapy itself. Here, social workers play a significant role. They contact everyone who belongs to the social network of the patient. They inform such people of the work carried out at the clinic, the problems the patients are confronted with, their demands, and their prospects. Where possible, family and friends also actively participate in the treatment itself. Sometimes contacts are limited to providing support to the patient's partner and in some cases there is a question of family therapy. Finally, this approach greatly reduces the risk of the patient and his network "ganging up" against the clinic.

FOCUS ON THE SEXUALLY AGGRESSIVE DELINQUENT

In 1985, one extremely problematic patient was admitted to the Dr. Henri van der Hoeven Kliniek. He was completely preoccupied with sexually aggressive thoughts and feelings that led to behavior to which he constantly subjected fellow patients and members of staff.

The structural group approach to patients who have little self-control offered no solution. The patient in question was unable to function in a group. As a result of a number of incidents, he stayed for a longer period of time in separate quarters intended for intensive individual care where it was tried, by means of a program involving rewards, to get his dangerous behavior under control. When he had relapses even there, the staff decided that the patient should come up for reselection and consequently he was transferred to a forensic psychiatric hospital where security was more rigorous. This case made a number of members of staff involved take a greater interest in sexually aggressive patients. They first took a closer look at the literature available and then they contacted the University of Utrecht and other colleagues dealing with the same problem area in order to gain more knowledge and compare notes.

Colleagues from other institutions also found sexually aggressive patients an extremely difficult group to deal with, often regarding contact with such patients as fraught with difficulties. Such patients often appear to have a very low motivation for treatment.

Denial and trivializing their condition are major factors, making it difficult to influence such patients. Serious relapses, both inside and outside of institutions, are a fairly frequent occurrence and give rise to deeply emotional reactions by society and the institutions involved.

The average length of inpatient treatment of this category of patients is 6 years, which is significantly longer than for all other categories of patients admitted to such institutions for whom inpatient treatment lasts 4 years. Relapse is high: 25% have relapses involving sexual offenses. Only the perpetrators of offenses to property have a worse relapse record. A significant proportion of forensic patients who are likely to have chronic relapses are offenders with a history of sexually sadistic or child sexual offenses.

The number of sexually aggressive delinquents who come into consideration for a TBS measure is on the increase. According to a policy document issued by the Dutch Ministry of Justice, there were estimated to be 200 such offenders in 1994. This is approximately 30% of the total number of people to whom a TBS measure is applied. These figures led to closer attention also being paid by other forensic psychiatric institutions to sexually aggressive delinquents, which produced significant cooperation between institutions.

From an examination of the literature available, it emerged that large discrepancies existed between treatment in North America and that taking place in Europe. Table 14.1 illustrates this. One interesting treatment phenomenon at the Dr. Henri van der Hoeven Kliniek and other forensic clinics in the Netherlands was the lack of attention paid to the behavioral pattern of the offense itself and that of its immediate antecedents. There are a number of possible explanations for this fact. First, when approaching a problem in a psychodynamic manner, the offense itself is not given very high priority. It is supposed that the symptom, i.e., the offensive behavior, will disappear once the underlying problem is solved. Second, both therapists and patients are rather reluctant to speak about the actual sexual offense. Therapists project their own diffidence in this matter onto the patients themselves, who "aren't yet ready for it." Patients do not discuss the subject, since they have learned their lesson. And they have, after all, resolved that they will not commit the offense again.

Being able to discuss an offense and the events leading up to it appeared to be an important expansion of the treatment package. The psychotherapists decided to tackle this problem. They developed a procedure to motivate the patient to talk about his or her offenses and termed this the "offense script procedure."

The Offense Script Procedure

This procedure consists of a semistructured interview that attempts to map out the cognitive, emotional, behavioral, and situational factors involved before, during, and after

TABLE 14.1
Differences between North American and European Programs

North America: Problem-oriented	Europe: Person-oriented
Approach mainly cognitive behavioral therapeutic	Approach mainly psychodynamic
Sphere of activity for psychologists	Sphere of activity for psychiatrists
Treatment by category	Noncategory treatment
Emphasis on "control" (internal and external)	Emphasis on "healing"
Offense-oriented (risk factors)	Patient-oriented (interactional model)
Long tradition of research (university clinic)	Lack of research

the offense was committed; that is, the "script" of the offense (van Beek & Mulder, 1992). This is a means by which patients, who are sometimes very defensive and ready to deny matters, are offered the opportunity to discuss their offense behavior and to learn how to keep these factors under control. The procedure leads to the offense script, which is a chain of risk factors. Inspiration for this work came from the relapse prevention model discussed in Pithers, Marques, Gibat, and Marlatt (1983) and the sexual abuse cycle discussed in Ryan and Lane (1991).

The offense script provides concrete information about the way in which the patient reacts in tense situations, how he tackles conflict in himself and with others, the role that sexuality and aggression play in his offense, and his offense pattern. It also gives information about the attitude adopted by the patient vis-á-vis his offenses. Does he deny them? Does he trivialize them? Do (serious) cognitive distortions occur? Does he feel responsible for his actions? Or guilty? Does he possess the capacity to empathize with his victim(s)?

The offense script affords insight into factors that can be directly related to the offense itself or to "triggers" that set it off, as well as into the personality of the offender. Clues to problems that are to be expected and to the positive and negative forces at play during the therapeutic process and in the therapeutic relationship itself, therefore can be deduced. Knowledge of the offense and the situational and personality factors involved is important when assessing the chances of relapse and potential dangerous behavior. By systematically describing how he feels, thinks, and acts before, during, and after an offense the offender will be presented with another cognitive framework: An offense is not something that simply happens to him, and thus he is able to gain insights into his behavior in an offense situation. He learns to gain control over his tendency to commit offenses by being obliged to draw conclusions from this information. Both the concrete descriptive work and the actively structuring attitude of the therapist dovetail well with the attitude of passive expectancy the offender tends to adopt when confronted with a difficult task. He is not entirely left to his own devices when attempting to tackle problems, but the therapist leads him by the hand, so to speak, so that satisfactory results are arrived at through a process of cooperation. The offense script provides the building blocks when choosing specific methods of treatment, especially in the area of relapse prevention programs (Laws, 1989). Some examples of treatment methods are self-control techniques, training in coping with aggression, social skills training, sex education, and empathy training.

The Four Phases of the Offense Script Procedure

If a sexually aggressive patient has sufficient understanding of his personality problems so that he can function reasonably well in a living group, he is sent on recommendation of his treatment team to a psychotherapist to work out his offense script. The treatment team will have already informed him of the aims and working methods of this course of action. The psychotherapist first assesses the patient's chances of bringing this aspect of the treatment to a successful conclusion: Patients who totally deny having committed offenses and those who act very much on impulse are temporarily filtered out, and patients who still have difficulties in distinguishing between fact and fantasy are advised to wait a little longer, while psychotics are denied access to this aspect of treatment.

The procedure consists of four phases. Differences depend on the content, the attitude of the therapist, and the expectations of the patient.

The procedure commences with an educative phase. Important goals here are motivating and instructing the offender. The importance of the offense script is explained to him, as is the working method. In this phase, the therapist adopts the attitude of an expert or lecturer but at the same time acts as someone who has an empathetic understanding of the problems the patient is facing. The therapist explains the importance of drawing up the offense script in an active, structured, and expressive manner, makes use of the blackboard, sketches the basic outline of the method, and illustrates it by means of analogies. He invites the offender to make comments and critical remarks. The therapist makes clear the difficulties involved: chiefly, the painful confrontation of the patient with himself, his feelings of shame, and the tendency to evade or cover up the problem at hand. He also accentuates, however, the great benefits to be derived from drawing up the script: more insight into the offense and into the workings of his own mind and the reduced chances of relapse, as well as the opportunities to be released on probationary leave or the withdrawal of the application of a TBS measure.

During the practice phase, the offender must familiarize himself with the working method to such an extent that he can distinguish between the various components and put them into practice. Here, the therapist supplements the skills of patient, filling in where inadequacies arise on the part of the patient. He also confronts the patient with the first signs of evasive behavior such as not being able to remember something, failing to do his homework, and nonattendance. He invites the offender to call to mind his latest offense and to think back 6 hours before the offense took place. This is the point at which the offense script begins. The therapist then proceeds to ask the offender about the first hour: Where was he; what was he feeling, thinking, and doing? The patient must present the information in such detail that the therapist can imagine the situations and events. This could be termed a guided exercise in imagination. During this phase, the therapist restricts himself to asking "where" and "who" type questions and deliberately avoids asking "why" questions. It is this approach that will bring the patient memories back to the present. The present tense is used and the therapist makes sure that important themes are brought up. When the offender has managed to reconstruct the first hour, with the help of the therapist, he is given homework that entails working out what happened during the second hour. This homework is carefully evaluated by the therapist. Weaknesses in the skills of the offender are compensated by practice or by being added to the homework. In this way, some offenders restrict themselves to the description of facts, while others concentrate on thoughts. Still others concentrate exclusively on their emotions or lose themselves in justifications for their behavior.

What are termed "memory problems" (e.g., "I can't remember what happened") are not as yet dealt with in any detail by the therapist. The usual explanation given to the patient is that putting together an offense script is comparable to doing a jigsaw puzzle: each new piece increases the chance of obtaining a complete picture. Pieces can also be missing, which will inevitably increase the risk of obtaining a false picture with all the consequences of this for the offender. The therapist also reassures the patient and leaves room for a "recovery of memory": "We'll see how far we get, and if we're lucky, the missing pieces will turn up in the end."

At each of the following sessions, 1 hour of the offense script is dealt with. The offense itself usually takes up two sessions. Working speed, of course, does depend on the cooperation of the offender. At this stage no efforts are made to obtain a complete picture of events. The chief aim is to develop the skills necessary to work with the procedure as a whole and to familiarize the offender with talking about events, feelings, and thoughts. The therapist does not yet tackle evasive behavior forcefully; at most, he expresses his doubts about the behavior of the patient with phrases such as "Is that so? There's something missing here. I can't quite picture what was happening there." He praises the efforts made by the offender and, if homework has not been completed, he makes comments such as, "Still rather difficult, isn't it?" And he asks the patient not to give up or even offers to help complete the homework with the patient. Sometimes he challenges the patient with, "Perhaps you are not ready for it yet?" If none of this helps, the therapist is obliged to conclude that drawing up the offense script is still too difficult a task. This phase is concluded when a skeleton version of the offense script has been committed to paper. The time taken to complete this phase can vary considerably.

The aim of the confrontation phase is to fill out the contents of the script in as great a detail as possible, attempting to reduce any remaining resistance to a minimum, while at the same time increasing the emotional charge of the script and allowing the offender to take a greater responsibility for his actions. The therapist now compares the information offered by the patient with that from other sources such as the courts and previous psychiatric reports. He challenges the patient on any inconsistencies. Important themes are examined. The therapist looks closely at the sexually aggressive fantasies of the patient and reminds him constantly of his responsibilities vis-á-vis his thoughts, feelings, and actions. The offense itself is examined in detail. Confrontation, even when coupled with shame, fear, or rage, is of utmost importance. The therapeutic relationship is maintained by the therapist showing that he accepts the patient, even if his behavior as such is unacceptable.

In cases where several offenses have been committed, the therapist and patient look at a few of the offenses at random, though always including the first one, since this will mark the beginning of the pattern that the other offenses have taken. This is followed by the procedure described above in a shortened version. The offenses are compared in order to highlight similarities and differences, and hypotheses are made as to factors that have played a significant role in the offenses.

Up to this point, the procedure is mainly restricted to cooperation between the patient and a psychotherapist, and only general information is passed on to the treatment team. The patient may, of course, submit more detailed information should he so desire.

The treatment phase consists of informing people around the patient of the results of the offense script procedure: the treatment team, family, the probationary officer, and other important people involved are invited to attend a meeting where the patient presents and explains the offense script. The aim of this meeting is to enable the patient to take a greater measure of responsibility for his actions, now that he has gained further insights into the events leading up to the offense, although he may in fact not yet be entirely able or prepared to shoulder this responsibility. It is therefore desirable that a network exists that can support him in maintaining the progress he has so far made. At this juncture, the relapse prevention program plays an important role at the end of the offense script. In this session, taking responsibility is linked to the seriousness with which the patient regards the relapse prevention program. The relapse prevention program can be dovetailed with the regular program at the clinic.

Involving members of the patient's family in the procedure has a number of further aims. First, the family may go along with consistent denials by the patient and even stimulate such behavior: "Our son cannot have done such a thing," or "He'll never do it again." If the patient himself ceases to deny what he has done, this makes it all the more difficult for his family to continue to do so. Second, the family may have had a clear role in the development of sexually aggressive attitudes and behavior by being unclear about values and norms, by exposing children to hard-core pornography at an early age, and by sexual aggression in the family. Third, the family can be "excused" for the delinquent behavior of the patient. Often, members of the family harbor guilt regarding their relations to the patient (e.g., "He did it, because we didn't bring him up properly"). Even if upbringing has not been optimal, the patient must not hide behind this fact as a means of avoiding personal responsibility for his actions. Finally, it is important that the family receive adequate information about the delinquent behavior of the offender and the factors leading up to it. Sometimes families are (partially) ignorant of such matters, while on other occasions they can furnish extra information themselves. And information can make it possible to more easily identify the (delinquent) behavior of the patient and make a coordinated effort to put a stop to it.

The offense script and the relapse prevention connected with it have been expanded during the past decade to become the core of the special treatment for sexually aggressive patients at the Dr. Henri van der Hoeven Kliniek. The psychosexual background of sexually aggressive patients is also more accurately mapped out with the help of a psychosexual anamnesis list and the Multiphasic Sex Inventory (MSI) with which various aspects of deviant sexuality can be measured. While drafting offense scripts, a profile typical for offenders gradually emerged, demonstrating close affinities with the classification system set out in Knight and Prentky (1990). These systems have been made available for use by the clinic. At first, a psychoeducative group dealing with aspects of sexuality and one dealing with aggression control were created especially for this type of patient. Later, these became mixed groups in which patients with a different history of delinquency could participate. Finally, techniques that originated with behavioral therapy are now applied, such as sensitization to discourage patients from allowing themselves to be dominated by deviant fantasies, plus directed masturbation to stimulate the development of nondeviant fantasies.

The Implementation Process

The directive, problem-oriented approach to sexually aggressive patients has gradually come to play a significant role in the integrated treatment offered by the Dr. Henri van der Hoeven Kliniek. The model has been given a specific place in the treatment plan: It plays an important role in the formulation of the core problems of patients and gives an insight as to the degree of internal and external control of the patient and contributes to risk assessment. The model also forms part of the information provided to the courts. The application of this model has also been expanded in scope to include patients with a variety of backgrounds in delinquency. Finally, it has provided the basis for the day treatment where the program is cognitive–behavioral. The process of integration took place under circumstances that can be described as being mainly positive. A number of factors have influenced this.

For a long while, sexually aggressive patients had been regarded as a problematic category in the field of forensic psychology. Serious relapses and the concomitant social unease put this theme on the political agenda. Direct confrontations with sexually aggressive patients in the clinic led staff to look for other methods of treatment. These highly motivated members of staff were afforded the opportunity to travel abroad to, for instance, the United Kingdom, the United States, and Canada in order to acquaint themselves with new forms of treatment. Along with a number of other colleagues in the field, they founded the Nederlands Vereniging voor Forensische Seksuologie (VFS; The Netherlands Forensic Sexological Association) and fostered contacts with similar organizations in the United States (ATSA) and the United Kingdom (NOTA). The began to treat patients according to these new principles.

The problem-oriented approach was linked to the ambivalence of patients who, at first, only cooperated reluctantly in drawing up the offense script. They found it difficult but were obliged to admit that it helped with the problems that brought them to the clinic. Hesitation in cooperation was further reduced by the fact that noncooperative attitudes would be included in the progress report submitted to the courts, a report to which judges attached a good deal of importance. Patients began to encourage one another to take part in the procedure. On several occasions, patients even came voluntarily to ask.

Finally, this problem-oriented approach was linked with the draft for treatment at the clinic, with emphasis being placed on living groups and cooperation with the family. The relapse prevention model, first in conjunction with the group leadership during the clinical phase and later with the probation office and networks such as the family and halfway facilities, provides a framework whereby a guarantee can be given for external monitoring. Not all patients, however, have sufficient opportunities to develop self-control skills, and thus remain dependent on external monitoring.

The implementation process was not, of course, entirely problem free. The status of a problem-oriented psychotherapist differs from that of the insight-oriented psychotherapist. Insight-oriented therapists remain more on the sidelines regarding the daily functioning of the clinic. Problem-oriented therapists make a point of bringing everyday life into their therapy, giving instructions to group counselors and trying out possibilities for patients to experiment with their new behavior outside the clinic. This approach was something those treating the patients had to get used to. Problems increased when patients began to put pressure on group counselors via their offense script procedure. Patients began to demand more freedom of movement outside the clinic on the basis of their cooperation with the drafting of the offense script. This led to considerable tension between the treatment team and the psychotherapist. Sometimes these contradictions could be bridged by close liaison with other treatment teams.

Expectations ran too high, which led to a further increase in tension. Patients found it difficult to link the necessary behavioral consequences to the "insights" gained from examining the approach phase of their offense, especially during the relapse prevention phase. Denials of actions previously admitted to and serious relapses reduced these expectations, sometimes even creating the impression that the program was of little value.

This led to a reconsideration of the place of the offense script within the whole range of treatment offered by the clinic. The heads of treatment have now made agreements with the psychotherapists, and their respective responsibilities have been clarified. As a result, it has been decided that the heads of treatment remain responsible for the phasing of treatment, but also that specific treatment plays an important role in this.

In conclusion, the specific program for the treatment of sexually aggressive patients has been firmly anchored to that of the Dr. Henri van der Hoeven Kliniek as a whole. After a positive trial period, the program has found its true place among the wide range of treatment offered by the clinic. It has not proven to be a panacea for all problems that crop up when treating sexually aggressive patients. A survey of 20 rapists classified according to Knight and Prentky (1990) as MTC: 3R (Massachusetts Treatment Center, typology for rapists: version 3) profited from the sexual type of this treatment as regards reduction and denial. Of a group of eight patients, seven denied less after the program concluded. The opportunistic type of patient (6) and the vindictive type (6) also benefited, but to a significantly lesser extent. It was noticeable that married patients of the vindictive type fared particularly badly. They continued to categorically deny their actions. Owing to the impulsive nature of sexual offenses committed by the vindictive type of patient, detailed attention should be paid to the whole of the (criminal) lifestyle aspect of the relapse prevention approach, since this is of greater importance than an analysis of the 6 hours prior to when the offense was committed. At present, research is being conducted at the clinic into the various application aspects of the offense script procedure.

THE DAY TREATMENT PROGRAM

The forensic day center was opened in February 1992. It started as an experiment, and there were places for ten patients. The rationale behind this was that there existed in the Netherlands a large group of offenders who had committed serious offenses and who needed treatment that they were not receiving. Day treatment appeared to be the solution. A polyclinic was also started to cope with intake and aftercare. People were admitted to the day treatment center mostly via the probation office. Clients have a variety of legal constraints put on them such as special conditions attached to a particular part of their sentence, or after being dismissed from preventive detention, or while waiting for the results of an appeal. A smaller number come voluntarily.

Clients attend the day center from 9 AM to 3 PM, five days a week, for 6 months. In the afternoons, individual activities take place as well as discussions concerning relationships and family. Evenings and weekends are spent at home. The history of offenses committed varies from client to client: assault, arson, and sexual offenses with adults and children. Both men and women attend the center, but in practice clients are predominantly male. Clients often suffer from antisocial personality disorders, the late consequences of early traumas, sexual disorders, and disorders in the area of impulse control. Severely addicted persons are not considered as day treatment clients, nor are psychotics. One general rule is that forensic psychiatric problems, where behavioral changes can be achieved within a period of 6 months, should be present and these changes should be of the type that the risk of relapse is so low that aftercare at a polyclinic is regarded as providing sufficient safeguards for the prevention of any repetition of the offense. Clients must not be so impulsive that the treatment offered cannot provide sufficient structure to prevent relapse during the actual treatment itself.

In order to participate in day treatment, a client must exhibit sufficient motivation, preferably backed up by the "stick-and-carrot" approach of a suspended sentence. These external forms of motivation are sometimes vital to enable the client to continue to attend to what can be a painful and wearying treatment. The external pressure supplied by the threat of punishment is relatively modest, considering the duration of the sentence involved, and only works for the first few months of treatment. After that, the client must become self-motivated.

The theoretical basis of the treatment is the relapse prevention model. While working with the clinic, it became logical to fit the treatment to the prevailing circumstances of a day center. Although the day treatment was originally intended for sexual offenders, the model has been further developed so that it can be used to prevent all kinds of offenses.

Treatment of Groups with Homogeneous or Mixed Composition

At the start of day treatment, the decision to work with a mixed (sexual and nonsexual offenders) offender group was a simple one. In the hospital, there were only mixed groups; since the day treatment center had only one treatment group, it had to accommodate all referrals. Most of the time, this worked fine. Sometimes, however, it did not. It is clear that mixing sexual offenders and aggressive offenders can produce tension. This tension can be very productive but can also become destructive. Child molesters especially can sometimes have a difficult time, particularly when they rationalize their offense or deny their behavior in other ways. One problem is that denial is more or less encouraged by the group situation in which the sexual offender finds himself. The less the child molester has done wrong, the less he will be condemned. Clients who have committed impulsive aggressive offenses also have problems in mixed group situations. They sometimes find it difficult to restrain themselves, especially if there has been some form of sexual abuse in their past or in their immediate environment. In that case, their constant state of anger interferes with the therapeutic process.

When the day treatment program started with ten clients, it was very important to try to use the positive aspects of heterogeneity in the treatment program and compensate for the positive aspects of homogeneity. According to Yalom (1975), the positive aspects of heterogeneous groups are that such groups can in many ways be seen as a representation of the world at large. This means that the transfer of training is optimized. It also invalidates the potential growth of a group culture, where the group is regarded as being a safe and convenient place to escape from the "cruel" world outside. A mixed group produces tension. People gravitate toward the reduction of tension. Tension can be reduced by working hard, by accepting others, and by changing. In an atmosphere of different ideas and different norms, a climate of confrontation stimulates people to learn more quickly. On the other hand, in a homogeneous group there is a greater cohesion. Clients are more prepared to accept one another. They will support each other more, feel safer, and therefore will have fewer inhibitions when talking about their offenses. We concluded that it would be wise to work with heterogeneous groups, unless the group in question raised more problems than it solved.

When the day center expanded to treat 24 clients, it was concluded that one group of offenders would be helped with a specialized group. Child molesters did not fit well within the mixed offense structure. Quite a few child molesters who are referred to the center deny a good deal of the responsibility for their offenses. Almost all claim to have done less than they in fact did, and less than what they have been charged with. As long as they admit to having committed a part of the offense and have a sincere wish to stop offending, this denial is not an unsolvable problem. The rest will emerge during the course of treatment. The desire to stop offending will earn them respect. But when offenses are rationalized, when the responsibility is passed onto the child, and when the offender complains of being seduced or tricked by their young victim, then he will inevitably awake the hostility of a mixed offense group. These kinds of rationalizations are not accepted, and the level of tension and aggression can mount so highly that a climate of constructive and relatively safe treatment cannot be maintained. In the last few years this has happened on a number of occasions. As a consequence, when the day center expanded in August 1994, three treatment groups were formed and it was decided to start one group of clients by offense. By putting child molesters in one group, a special program could be developed with a great deal of emphasis placed on breaking down all forms of denial, on sexual education, and on victim empathy, as well as on developing insight into the offense cycle and the grooming process.

Work with the group proved very successful. There is high cohesion, less tension, no dropouts, and much openness. By starting this group, the advantages of the heterogeneous group risked being lost. It is the task of staff to compensate for this gap. Staff must confront these clients a great deal in order to challenge all forms of denial and the avoidance of responsibility for their behavior. They have to take on the role of society at large and set norms condemning delinquent behavior. They have to challenge clients and reduce the safety of the isolation of being in a group with co-offenders. The therapist must preserve a climate of action and a diversity of experience.

The experience of the last year and a half has been positive. Taking responsibility and accepting the consequences thereof are the main objectives of the treatment program for all clients. With these clients this means that members of staff have to work quite hard, and they are frequently frustrated by the shared secrets of clients, the tenacity of behavior patterns, and the evasive actions of the clients to prevent real change from occurring. The step that must be taken from talking about oneself to acting on the insights gained is a large one. There is also external control provided by the contact with partners, family, and probation officers. On the other hand, staff do not have to worry about attendance. Clients come every day without fail. They talk quite openly about their offenses, sexual fantasies, of feeling attracted to children in the street, and how to act in such circumstances. Although the child molesters are unlikely to tell everything, they do tell a good deal more than they would in a mixed group.

The Treatment Elements

The structure lacking in the personality constellation must be compensated for by the day treatment. There is question of "horizontal programming." Each day begins with a morning interview where the events of the previous evening and the plans for the coming evening are discussed. Every fifth week the treatment is evaluated in the group after a report is prepared in writing by the client on the basis of a number of questions. The components of the program are linked to the various components of the relapse prevention chain. Each client is taught to recognize his own offense chain and learns how to intervene at each link in the chain.

In general, the treatment program is followed jointly by the group as a whole. The group constitutes the backbone of treatment. Individual support or psychotherapy takes place where necessary. Family and partners are involved as much as possible. When choosing what is to be offered in the program, methods are sought that will strike a chord with these clients. A good deal of attention is paid to motivating clients and keeping them motivated.

The weekly schedule of the day center is filled with activities similar to those of other (clinical) programs: attempts are made to improve lifestyle balance, there is a relapse prevention group, and social and sexual skills training, anger management, and victim empathy are addressed. What is special about the day treatment program is that everything occurs in one group and that the client can talk each evening with the people around him about what he has experienced that day.

The Implementation Process

The day center and the polyclinic were created because of the difficulties experienced when treating sexual offenders at the clinic. It was thought that more specific methods of treatment specifically suited to these types of offenders were needed. To be able to qualify for a TBS measure the offender must have committed very serious offenses within the Netherlands, such as violent rape involving adults or children, often committed on more than one occasion. It struck us that if such clients underwent treatment at an earlier stage, chances for success would be greater, and the creation of new victims could be prevented. One form of day treatment, implemented for a long period of time within the framework of the sentence, seemed to be a necessary supplement to the preexisting range of options for forensic clients. The authorities also approved the idea. The Netherlands is experiencing a shortage of cell space, and certainly one way of tackling this problem is the introduction of alternative sanctions. Day treatment for a period of 6 months seemed an attractive form of "sentencing" from the point of view of the Ministry of Justice, since it did not involve the use of cells.

A period of 6 months was chosen for a variety of reasons. It is a period during which a real process of change can begin to occur, and it gives clients, who in most cases lack any previous experience of being helped, the chance to see whether they can remain motivated. A period of 6 months also concurs with the attitudes of the courts, since it is a tough sentence (by Dutch standards) but not yet a TBS measure.

One last factor that helped was that the central government encouraged the ministries of justice and of health to cooperate more. This had never occurred up to that point. The day center seemed the perfect project to achieve such cooperation without costs rising too high. By beginning as an "experiment," the cost aspect became even less important. It was possible to curtail the project at any time.

As stated, the experiment began in February 1992, with ten clients. At this initial stage, a model for treatment had to be chosen. Owing to developments in North America, it seemed natural to choose the relapse prevention model. The treatment is problem-oriented; each client knows why he has to undergo each specific aspect of treatment. This is extremely important for clients who lack experience of therapy. Furthermore, the treatment is based on the principle of constant care to prevent relapses from occurring: there is no cure. This is a reality principle that offers both clients and staff clarity and requires follow-up treatment after day care in the polyclinic. The decision to set up a day center based on a specific model had the advantage that the model could be consistently applied, something which has proved much harder to do in a clinic.

Great demands are placed on the center. The clients, some of whom are dangerous, go home every day and are out of contact at weekends (no electronic tagging exists in the Netherlands) and could relapse at any time. Living with this uncertainty places heavy demands on the staff, especially on the daily counselors. It proved possible to bring a number of sociotherapists, who were very experienced in working with forensic patients, from the clinic to start off this unique project. The clinic psychiatrist and the psychologist led the project. Creative teachers and sports teachers were approached to help clients structure their leisure hours.

By beginning with a small staff and a small group of clients, the relapse prevention model was developed as the project proceeded. Development still continues, 4 years after the commencement of the project.

When taking a completely new treatment model as a starting point, things do not always run smoothly. Problems come from various quarters: referrers must know that opportunities to undergo such treatment exist, they must have faith in it, and they must know who they should refer. The first step that had to be undertaken was to develop good public relations. This meant writing a good, well-documented, and clear brochure for referrers, phoning and making appointments with potential referrers, as well as holding lectures and inviting guests. Three activities prior to the commencement of the course were of great help: the appointment of what is termed a counselors' committee for the experimental phase of the day treatment. Representatives of the probation service, regular medicare and the health insurance field, the Ministry of Justice, and the courts were invited to sit on the committee. By allowing them to take part in the process of development, their involvement and commitment to the day center were increased. This led to the development of a positive atmosphere within a number of the organizations involved. Second, external conditions had to be made especially attractive, such as the appearance of the brochure and the premises in which the treatment was to take place. The idea of treatment according to the relapse prevention model also fit here: the client was not viewed as someone suffering and unable to express his problems in a suitable manner. During the day treatment, the prevention of offenses was focused on and the client was required to take responsibility for his behavior and for the prevention of offenses in the future. A third important principle was that the requests made by referrers were reacted to swiftly and efficiently. Intake took place within a week. During the course of one interview a judgment was made as to whether the client could be admitted to the day treatment program. A low threshold was set; the point of departure was that clients would stand a good chance of being accepted, but that once they had started to participate, then they would have to work at it. The inability to keep promises would mean the termination of treatment. This way of viewing treatment also prevailed against another frequently raised objection to treatment: people often regard such treatment as a soft option, an easy way out. Attendance 5 days a week for 6 months, taking responsibility, and the motto of "no cure but control" is attractive to the clients themselves, the probation service, and the courts. The day center was soon inundated by referrals and a 6-month waiting list resulted, a fact that led to the expansion of the clinic from 10 to 24 clients.

In the Netherlands, making prison the consequence of removal from the course can only be put into practice to a very limited degree. This presents problems for the day center. Sentences are already much shorter than in the United States and the consequences of the termination of treatment are often very limited. The onus is therefore on the client himself to maintain and heighten motivation. A treatment contract is drawn up and signed. Family and counselors from outside the day center are invited at an early stage and are also involved with the treatment at subsequent stages. While treatment mainly occurs in the group, support interviews with a mentor are given a place on the schedule. Considering the way the day treatment is structured, clients often tend at first to be ambivalent. Such clients must be given a higher degree of motivation right from the start to enable their behavior to be tackled successfully. This motivation is one of the most important aims for counselors. Clients are motivated in every imaginable way.

The external motivation is increased by explicitly and expansively playing on the threat of sanctions: treatment or prison. The threat of prison is often less powerful than the risk of losing a partner or of having children who are ashamed of their father. Increasing empathy for victims is also a powerful means of stimulating the client to fight against relapse. In the treatment itself, the expectations of the group help the client to persist during difficult periods. Finally, motivation is increased by creating a structure for the way the treatment is to proceed, setting realistic and concrete goals in the treatment contract, by rewarding positive developments, monitoring the keeping of promises and even the threat of removal, plus instilling in the client the belief that the treatment actually works. Internal motivation is further strengthened by group interaction and personal counseling. Here, contact with members of the group and with counselors is most important. Both short-term and long-term goals are set up, facilitating success. Clients are thus given the hope that starting a new life remains an option for them.

One last difficulty, which has not been dealt with up to now, is the fact that starting day treatment according to the relapse prevention model presupposes a good deal of ability in translation and improvisation. Since the Netherlands had not worked before with the model, exercises had to be translated and adapted, and a workable and effective form had to be found. Starting with a small group afforded the opportunity to try out exercises and for the course tutors to also familiarize themselves with the techniques used. Visits to conferences and to other institutions where treatment takes place in the United States during 1991 provided support. Another potential problem that has in fact never occurred in practice is the initial reaction of local residents to the presence of the day center where a large variety of different types of offenders are present. The fact that local residents have not reacted negatively, although the center is situated right in the middle of a housing district, is presumably due to the fact that the day center is located next to the clinic itself. The clinic maintains good contacts with local residents, hires out halls for parties and to the dance school, and makes the swimming baths available to a pensioners' association. People have grown used to the presence of a clinic for dangerous offenders. Since the day center was started, street lighting in the area has been improved, which was greatly appreciated. It appears that residents, once they are used to the building and to deriving benefits from the facilities, will not raise objections. There have not been any incidents in the vicinity of the day center.

Since the start of our day center, three other day centers and four polyclinics have been opened in the Netherlands. The policy staff from these various outpatient departments meet every 4 months to discuss "growing pains."

CLOSING REMARKS

When looking back over 4 years of day treatment of sexual and other offenders using the relapse prevention model, the following can be noted. It is concrete, goal-oriented, and linked to the often limited motivations of clients by focusing on offense prevention. All treatment activities are derived from the prevention model. This also fits with current views on the treatment of serious personality disorders: the symptom is treated in the first instance and a structure for daily life is built up. Not until the client is at ease and the risk of relapse is reduced is there scope for working with underlying causes. The second phase of the treatment can take the form of individual psychotherapeutic interviews, which can be started during the day center phase and continued during the follow-up treatment at the polyclinic. A straightforward organization and a small professional treatment team fit in with the aims of the day treatment. Research is of vital importance. This research is self-evaluative and the public is shown the importance of the treatment. The results have been promising. During the 6 months of their treatment, a reduction of problems can be seen to have taken place among sexual offenders, denial has decreased, and more responsibility is shouldered for the offenses themselves. Virtually all sexual offenders stay for at least 6 months and participate in the follow-up treatment. Telephone contact is maintained for a long while afterward. Research has also been conducted into relapse during 1 and 5 years after leaving the day center. Over the years, the group of sexual offenders who have left the day center on completion of the course of treatment is still too small to be able to provide accurate relapse data, but the survey is ongoing.

REFERENCES

Beck, A. T., Freeman A., et al. (1990). *Cognitive therapy of personality disorders*. New York: Guilford.

Knight, R. A., & Prentky, R. A. (1990). Classifying sexual offenders: The development and corroboration of taxonomic models. In W. L. Marshall, D. R. Laws, & H. E. Barbaree (Eds.), *Handbook of sexual assault: Issues, theories, and treatment of the offender* (pp. 23–52). New York: Plenum.

Laws, D. R. (Ed.). (1989). *Relapse prevention with sex offenders*. New York: Guilford.

Pithers, W. D., Marques, J., Gibat, C. C., & Marlatt, G. A. (1983). Relapse prevention with sexual aggressives: A self-control model of treatment and maintenance of change. In J. G. Greer & I. R. Stuart (Eds.), *The sexual aggressor: Current perspectives on treatment* (pp. 214–239). New York: Van Nostrand Reinhold.

Ryan, G., & Lane, S. (1991). *Juvenile sexual offending: Causes, consequences, and corrections*. New York: Lexington Books.

van Beek, D. J., & Mulder, J. R. (1992). The offense script: A motivational tool and treatment method for sex offenders in a Dutch forensic clinic. *International Journal of Offender Therapy and Comparative Criminology*, *36*, 155–167.

Yalom, I. D. (1975). *The theory and practice of group psychotherapy*. New York: Basic Books.

15

C. Psychiatric Settings

Sexual Offenders' Treatment Program of the Philippe Pinel Institute of Montréal

Jocelyn Aubut, Jean Proulx, Bernadette Lamoureux, and André McKibben

The Philippe Pinel Institute of Montreal (PPIM) is a maximum-security psychiatric hospital, founded in 1970, whose specific function since its inception has been to take charge of mentally disordered offenders. These include offenders diagnosed with a variety of conditions, from personality disorders to psychoses, who are sentenced under provincial jurisdiction (less than 2 years and 1 day) or under federal jurisdiction (more than 2 years), and under the lieutenant governor's warrant (indefinite period of detention for subjects found not guilty due to insanity). Therapeutic management used to be based on current non-specialized psychiatric models. It was soon realized, however, that more specialization was required. Fortunately, this necessity was fully recognized by the clinicians and researchers as well as the administrators of PPIM.

On the social plane, the issue of sexual aggression emerged, involving problems related to both the victims and the aggressors. In the past, this issue was rarely discussed in the media; certain persons, however, knowledgeable in various social domains, foresaw the necessity of creating a specialized task force to take care of sexual aggressors. This foresight instigated the founding of a special unit for sexual aggressors at the PPIM in partnership with the Correctional Services of Canada, Québec region. Consequently, a service contract was negotiated between the PPIM and Corrections Canada.

INITIATION PHASE

In the beginning, we had to carry out a major reorganization of all the hospital units. Specialization of several units necessitated a major upheaval for the patients as well as the

Jocelyn Aubut and Jean Proulx • University of Montréal and Philippe Pinel Institute of Montréal, Montréal, Quebec, Canada H1C 1H1. **Bernadette Lamoureux and André McKibben** • Philippe Pinel Institute of Montréal, Montréal, Quebec, Canada H1C 1H1.

Sourcebook of Treatment Programs for Sexual Offenders, edited by Marshall et al. Plenum Press, New York, 1998.

clinical staff. A number of patients, who had been staying in the same unit for a long time, were forced to be transferred into another unit, causing them some anxiety. The nonprofessional staff of the PPIM (nurses, psychoeducational workers) were not forced to participate in the specialization programs of their units. Thus, some of them decided to remain with the unit for the treatment of sexual aggressors, while others preferred to transfer to units where more conventional treatment programs were carried out. This, naturally, caused great commotion and "bumping" at the hospital. Fortunately, the administration's determination remained steadfast to implement the specialized programs and a cooperative spirit became manifest among the interested parties including the unions.

The professional staff's (psychiatrist, psychologist, criminologist, and sexologist) mandate was to develop specialized treatment programs for criminal personalities, as defined by Yochelson and Samenov (1976) and for sexual aggressors. Consequently, the authors of this chapter, in association with other members of the clinical staff at PPIM, developed a specialized treatment program for sexual aggressors on the basis of experience gained from such cases in the past as well as from studies of the current scientific literature.

Before preparing a treatment program, two of the authors (JA and AM) visited several East Coast centers of the United States whose programs had already been described in the literature. There, we found a wide discrepancy between the official programs and what actually happened. Thus, whatever the basic treatment model may be, difficulties were associated with most of these programs, such as insufficient staff to cope with the treatment needs of the patients, strong patient resistance to treatment, low patient compliance with prescribed treatments, chronicity, even untreatable conditions of certain aggressors, and, finally, lack of assessment strategies to measure treatment efficacy.

All these facts, as well as thorough deliberations by our founding group, resulted in a vision of how our future treatment unit should be established. Three branches were originally defined, and which we have upheld ever since: clinical practice, teaching, and research. It became apparent, right from the start, that one unit of 21 beds would not suffice to take care of all the sexual aggressors in the province of Québec. Our unit had to become a model of its kind for the whole province, and we had to serve as a research and teaching center. This enlarged role encouraged the launching of other treatment programs.

In our opinion, since the beginning and up to the present time, no theoretical model has yet been shown to be superior to the others. The special cultural status of Québec amid the Anglo-Saxon North American and European French cultures has proved to be particularly useful. It became evident from the start, however, that the basic theoretical concepts were weak and that only a rigorously clinical and scientific approach would finally arrive at a better knowledge of the causes of sexual aggression.

The former behavioral approach aimed primarily to control the cardinal symptoms such as deviant sexual arousal. The psychoanalytical approach at one time was little concerned with the cardinal symptoms but mostly with repressed affective experiences. Thus, two opposite theoretical models existed, each with advantages and disadvantages, each explaining only partly the phenomenon of sexual aggression, and each being incomplete and insufficient to develop a valid therapeutic regimen. The originality of the program at the PPIM was due to the fact that our therapeutic approach included past and current factors; that is, integrating behavioral, cognitive, and affective aspects with some psychodynamic factors. For example, humiliation is an important feature of the sexual preferences of numerous rapists and can be measured phallometrically (Proulx, Aubut, McKibben, & Côté, 1994). The role of anger and other negative emotions in the genesis of deviant sexual fantasies could be identified using a specific instrument such as the "Rapport d'Activités Fantasmatiques" (Fantasy Report) produced by McKibben, Proulx, and Lusignan (1994).

The model developed at the PPIM has been undergoing a constant evolutionary process deriving from our own research as well as from empirical findings by various North American and European research. This model always seeks to link the diverse components of the sexual aggressor's personality to the nature of his crimes. The different aspects of each aggressor's life are taken into account: biological, psychological, and social. In the psychological sphere, we are assessing behavioral, cognitive, and affective aspects. Furthermore, experiences in the aggressor's past (e.g., sexual abuse) and at the present time (e.g., marital dissatisfaction) are analyzed as to their possible impact on the subject's criminal activities.

Consolidation Phase

The first year was certainly a period of exploration and experimentation. Quickly, however, typical characteristics of sexual aggressors emerged that increasingly permitted us to direct our management approach to specific targets. Some of the key elements that we have established for the treatment program as it has developed over time include: (1) sexual aggressors constitute a heterogeneous group as to the committed crimes, their personality types, ability of abstraction, representation, and motivations for treatment; (2) the relational mode of most sexual aggressors is significantly disturbed either by an excessive desire to attach themselves to others or by an inability to live intimately with somebody; (3) the resort to deviant sexual behavior appears to be the usual way to resolve daily conflictual situations or negative affects; (4) deviant sexual fantasies are frequently aroused by daily life conflicts (e.g., clash with an authority; disappointment in love); (5) daily life conflicts at the treatment unit generally consist of conflicts similar to those experienced by the patient in the community; (6) although no sexual crime has occurred in the treatment unit itself, several situations experienced by the patients are precursors of such crimes (e.g., rape fantasies about women in authority); and (7) the chain of events, thoughts, or affects leading to deviant sexual fantasies and to the act of carrying them out follow a fixed pattern in most sexual aggressors.

However, we had to adapt our treatment program to the patient and not the reverse, and we have adopted a credo: "The right treatment, for the right patient, at the right time." It has taken several years to arrive at an eclectic management approach that answers more appropriately the specific needs of sexual aggressors. Each therapist may not be eclectic in the strict sense of the term. In fact, a therapist may not be at the same time competent in applying both cognitive–behavioral and psychoanalytic techniques. It is not the therapist himself who is eclectic but his vision of the patients. Patients having different needs and different psychological characteristics, thus cannot all be treated in the same fashion.

Initiation of a new treatment program does not always run smoothly. The clinical staff had to go through several crises arising primarily from leadership problems, recognition of the specific competencies of each staff member, and splitting induced by the patients. We should point out that for some time several research investigators have been describing deep-seated personality disorders in sexual aggressors. These basic personality structures seem to determine the characteristics of variables associated with criminal acts (e.g., degree of violence), patients' treatability, and recidivism (Proulx, Aubut, Perron, & McKibben, 1994).

The nonprofessional staff had to adapt to a class of patients with personality disorders, and therefore had to abandon their usual way of dealing with psychotic patients. Traditionally, management of psychotics is more paternalistic, demanding little responsibility of the patients. The psychotic patient is taken charge of and does not openly contest the authority of a member of the staff. It is quite different, however, when dealing with sexual aggressors who are not shy about contesting a staff member's authority. At first, this created a moralizing stance by the staff. It also took them some time to deal with the combative attitude of the patients. They had to bear in mind that the patients' hostility reflects the personality disorders that play a role in their daily lives, and that also underlie their crimes.

In our opinion, personality disorders affected not only the patients' behaviors in the treatment unit but also their life in the community. In fact, several dimensions were affected by personality disorders such as difficulty in establishing and maintaining stable intimate relationships, criminality, toxicomania, and so on. Once these problems were identified, it was recognized that these are among the causes of sexual aggressive behavior. For example, the difficulty in establishing intimate relationships, as described by Marshall (1989), has been included in our clinical analysis of sexual aggressors as a contributory factor in the genesis of sexual aggression. The difficulty of coping with anger and other negative affects and its impact on deviant fantasies also has been included in our clinical analysis. Moreover, this latter point served as a cornerstone in the concept of "conflict sexualization," a concept related to the relapse prevention model. The inability of many sexual aggressors to cope with their conflictual daily life situations and the conversion of these conflicts and unresolved malaise into deviant fantasies and masturbatory activities have become our central focus in the analysis of sexual aggressors' problems.

The principal observation during the consolidation phase was that conflictual situations generating deviant sexual fantasies occur daily in the treatment unit. The rapists openly expressed their anger against women in a position of authority (the nurses), in whose presence they felt particularly humiliated. The pedophiles, most having poor social skills, could only express their anger indirectly, but also felt humiliated in the presence of an adult in a position of authority. Children appear to them to be less menacing.

The treatment unit served not only as a place for treatment and leisure time but also became a place for the clinical staff to observe aspects of the patients' interpersonal problems related to sexual aggression. Consequently, the treatment unit became a place for the patients to experience new relationship modalities that they tried to acquire throughout the treatment course. The unit also became a place for the therapists to assess the patients' progress. For example, a patient who is learning how to control his anger in group therapy is bombarded with many daily situations to test his control ability. The new skills acquired by the patients in the treatment unit permit them to cope with situations they may face in the community. Special attention is also given to helping the patient to link conflictual situations occurring in the treatment unit with those in his past life in the community.

Obviously, all this did not proceed smoothly. Many times clashes caused by patients who seemed to progress faster in the therapists' offices than in the treatment unit had to be ironed out. Furthermore, the staff had to cope many times with the patients' anger. Although no major acting out occurred in the unit, there was a tendency for the clinical staff, confronted with the patient's rage, to question the staff's actions, especially since this rage more often was directed against women than men. We had to engage in constant communication as to the phenomenon of countertransference. We also always had to look out for the security of the staff—proactively rather than retroactively.

Furthermore, the program had to be adapted to the constant and rapid development of clinical and scientific models in the field of sexual aggression. Attendance at congresses by the professional staff and the transfer of the newly acquired knowledge to the rest of the clinical staff permits us to keep our program up to date with recent developments in diagnostics and treatments. Moreover, the program is constantly renewed through staff discussions and by listening to the patients during and after their hospitalization. Since hospitals today are expected to ensure the satisfaction of their patients, for the past years we have been soliciting the opinions of the patients who have returned to the community in order to discover what features they had found best while they were in the treatment unit. Naturally, we are not going to base the directions or evaluations of our programs solely on these opinions. These opinions, however, have been a useful tool, permitting us to readjust our treatment targets. We believe that it is important for us to know what coping strategy the patients use to be able to function in the community without relapsing.

After several years, the program was firmly established, clinically as well as administratively. The conceptual framework has passed from a psychodynamic beginning to today's biopsychosocial model. For each aggressor we carry out an analysis of factors associated with the development and persistence of the problem: biological (alcoholism, drugs, brain damage causing impulsive behavior), psychological (former abuse, inappropriate expression of anger, cognitive distortions, personality disorders, deviant sexual preference), and social factors (marital discord, use of pornography, inappropriate leisure activities, etc.). Of course, the treatment plan has to be individualized to respond to the specific needs of each patient, but always according to a biopsychosocial model. On the biological plane, medication is rarely used and only when a definitive pathological condition is diagnosed, e.g., the use of an antiepileptic drug for patients with strong impulsiveness associated with frontal lobe dysfunction, demonstrated radiologically and by neuropsychological evaluation. Antilibidinous drugs such as medroxyprogesterone or cyproterone are rarely used except for patients at the end of their hospital treatment who still feel a certain sexual impulsiveness.

For psychological aspects, several psychotherapeutics are available for patients, again as specifically needed. These include individual and group psychotherapy, a relapse prevention program, fantasy reconditioning, aversive therapy, social skills training, stress management training, anger management training, and prevention of drug and alcohol abuse.

On the social plane, special attention is given to the families and mainly to the patients' partners who are asked to participate. Communication difficulties and sexual dissatisfaction between couples, responsibilities heaped upon the female partner, and the possible support role of the female partner are systematically explored. The families are continuously informed about our therapeutic objectives, the therapeutic process, and about resistance to treatment.

Inappropriate functioning at work or leisure is systematically treated because in many cases this is a significant element in the sequence ending in a crime. For example, many rapists spend a large part of their free time drinking in erotic dance bars. Many child molesters spend a good part of their time at playgrounds where they can be in direct contact with children.

On the administrative plane, we had to establish specific admission criteria acceptable to our partners in Corrections Canada. In the beginning, offenders were often referred to us because of their difficulties in adapting to life in prison, not because they wanted to be treated. Sex murderers and those with life sentences with eligibility for conditional release in the distant future were the first to be referred to our program. Therefore, a close liaison had to be established with the case management officers and the psychologists of the penitentiary to explain our admission criteria. This is necessary to prepare the prisoners for the transfer to the treatment program and to assure adequate transmission of information when the prisoners are returned to the penitentiary at the end of the treatment course. We also had to make sure that the prisoners would continue working toward their objectives inside the prison and later when permitted out on conditional release. All essential information is given to the personnel in charge of the release in the form of a resumé file as well as through personal contacts. The concept of continuity of treatment has always been at the center of our concerns.

EXPANSION PHASE

Now that the clinical and the administrative bases of the program are established, we focus on teaching and research projects. It has been apparent from the start that an inpatient treatment program is only the first stage in the therapeutic course for sexual aggressors. They are in the grip of a chronic problem of several years' duration and often have undergone unsuccessful treatment trials. Moreover, conditions in the treatment unit do not completely reflect those the aggressors will be facing in the community. Therefore, we arranged for a follow-up system for patients outside the hospital to monitor the continuity and effectiveness of the treatment and we established an outpatient program. Since it is not in the scope of this chapter to describe our outpatient treatment program, we only wish to point out here that the outpatient treatment is based on the same treatment philosophy as the inpatient program. At the start, the transition proceeded directly from the hospital. This was not simple, because several patients overestimated their ability to function in the community and stopped their treatment. During the past years, and mainly for administrative reasons, the transition to the outside has been taking place from the prison where the prisoner was originally incarcerated. There, our patients were able to note that they had modified their relationship with others, which were no longer based on force as is so often the case in the cultural environment of a prison. On the other hand, they had to face a certain mourning period as with a separation. They were no longer surrounded by a clinical staff 24 hours a day. They had to be responsible for the quality of their life and to ask for help when needed.

Over the years, teaching has become a priority. All the program's clinical staff have voluntarily shared their knowledge with trainees and students. We had to draw up a special teaching program because no program related to sexual aggressors exists at the universities. On the other hand, the students and trainees are eager to question our operational methods, and thereby encourage us to remain competent. Thus, students of various disciplines and at different stages of their training periods have studied at our treatment unit: students in psychology, criminology, psychiatry, sexology, and nursing.

The special cultural position of Québec has provided us with the opportunity to receive a large number of students from European francophone countries. Clearly, the language dimension plays a significant role in attracting these students, but most of all they are interested in our program that links the traditional European psychoanalytic approach with the North American cognitive–behavioral concepts. Thus, students from France, Belgium, Switzerland, and Spain have come to our unit and these links have been maintained.

As our program has developed over the years, we are focusing especially on its research aspects. The administration of PPIM has strongly supported us in permitting us to engage a researcher (JP), who has become a member of our team. Our research activities are described in a separate section of this chapter. We should emphasize here, however, that there is a very close collaboration between the researcher and the clinical staff. The research program has always focused on clinical preoccupations and concepts. In humiliation research, for example, humiliation rape preference as part of the phallometric evaluation stems from the clinical observations of rapists under treatment. On the other hand, the clinical staff have always been inspired by the results of research, in particular on the topic of recidivism and the optimal duration of treatment (Pellerin et al., 1996; Proulx et al., 1997).

SELECTION PROCESS

Most patients admitted to the program come from Corrections Canada. A small number of patients are directly admitted from the community either by the patient himself or are referred by a professional health care worker. This type of admission is generally associated with a fear of a sexual acting out or of self-mutilation.

With most of the patients sent to us from Corrections Canada, we insist beforehand on establishing a liaison mechanism to assure a better transition of the patients to the PPIM, and back to Corrections Canada. As for the administrative part, the Corrections Canada administration and the general managers of the PPIM are ultimately responsible for admissions and transfers of patients. Actually, this task is given to certain members of the staff of both institutions who have worked out a satisfactory liaison system.

In the beginning, certain admission criteria were set down and accepted by both parties, such as: (1) the prisoner has to admit the crime for which he has been sentenced; (2) the prisoner is not mentally retarded, of medium or severe magnitude; and (3) the prisoner has not committed a sexual murder. Owing to only a few reports in the scientific literature as to treatment and the release from prison of this latter type of patient, we have no guidelines on how to take care of them. As further outlined below, these criteria were modified to the extent that we now admit mentally retarded prisoners and sexual murderers into our treatment program. We have to acknowledge that putting these criteria into practice was difficult. First, these criteria were too imprecise. Thus, certain aggressors admitted to having had sexual contact with the victim, but denied that the type of contact was of a criminal kind, pleading that the victim—adult or child—had enticed them. Some admitted the crime but declared themselves entirely "cured," having no deviant fantasies and no risk of a relapse. Others firmly refused any evaluation of their problem and any treatment.

Second, the case management officers and Corrections Canada psychologists are confronted with much pressure associated with the behavioral problems of certain prisoners in their establishment. Sometimes a case management officer will refer an inmate not only because he needs treatment, but rather because he needs protection or is a troublemaker. The administration imperatives of an institution are not always the same as those of a treatment program. On the other hand, limited resources, only 21 beds for several hundred sexual aggressors, forced us to assign these few places with great care for treatability and efficacy.

To avoid unnecessary friction between the Corrections Canada case management officer and the clinical staff of the PPIM and to assure a better transition mechanism of prisoners from one institution to the other, we had to set up a system of consultation and close liaison. Several steps were undertaken. First, we arranged a general tour of Corrections Canada institutions to clarify not only our selection criteria but their underlying reasons. Following this tour, several case management officers came to visit our treatment unit for sexual aggressors at the PPIM to show them how our program is operating and to become better acquainted with how the prisoners are functioning under our treatment program. Finally, the selection process was modified to permit the case management officer responsible for the prisoners to participate jointly in the selection with a clinical representative of PPIM.

The prisoner himself is invited to discuss his sexuality problem and his motivation to participate in a treatment program. After the interview, the case management officer and the PPIM clinician arrive at a decision together and then advise the prisoner. Prisoners who are not ready to enter the treatment program are given an opportunity for a number of intermediate objectives (e.g., to lessen the intensity of their denial of the crime). A joint interview is also arranged after the treatment course, when the prisoner is returned to the prison, to assure a better exchange of information (apart from the resumé file) and to establish certain objectives to be continued in prison (e.g., anger control).

Over time, a more precise protocol was designed for clarification of the concepts, better collaboration, and, above all, a draft of a common language. This protocol allows us to evaluate each sexual aggressor on the basis of five aspects: (1) recognition of the crime; (2) effects on the victim; (3) deviant sexual fantasies; (4) recognition of other problems in his life; and (5) the need for treatment. Clarification of these aspects permits better comprehension of how the aggressor faces his sexual problem, its adverse effects on his life, and his need for treatment.

PROGRAM IN PROGRESS

In the beginning, the duration of the treatment program was over 2 years. As time went on, however, the duration was considerably shortened, owing to administrative and clinical considerations. Budgetary constraints have forced us to cut the length of the treatment to 12 months. Based on a recent study (Pellerin et al., 1996), the treatment should last at least 12 months to permit the patients to assimilate the principal components of the treatment and to reduce the risk of recidivism. It should also be noted that the cases have since become more difficult: more violent crimes, sexual murders, multiple recidivism, drug abuse, and severe personality disorders. The treatment program therefore has been adapted to the specific characteristics of those types of offenders.

The treatment program at the PPIM can be described as a close connection among a series of specific therapeutic modalities and an environment permitting systematic observation of inappropriate behaviors as well as application of acquired skills by the patients. The therapeutic management team in our treatment consists of professional and nonprofessional staff. The nonprofessional staff consists of a coordinator, male or female psychoeducational worker, and nurses, who are with the patients 24 hours a day, 7 days a week. Their principal tasks are to observe the patients closely and to assess how they use the skills they have learned during the specific therapeutic activities. For example, a patient who is learning to control his anger in group therapy is subjected to different kinds of daily frustrations, allowing the experienced nonprofessional staff to assess the patient's ability to control his anger and to communicate this information to the professional staff. The multidisciplinary professional staff is responsible for the supervision of the nonprofessionals and the operations of the specific therapeutic activities such as social skills training, sexual education, and relapse prevention.

The programs consist of four standardized stages, although they may vary from one patient to another. It must be emphasized that the treatment for each patient is individualized. Even if the same modalities are used for all the patients, they are adapted to the individual needs of each. Moreover, during personal interviews or group meetings, the patient learns to link the factors inducing his negative affects, deviant sexual fantasies, and the risk of recidivism.

First Stage

This involves a clinical evaluation and phallometric and psychometric testing, as well as systematic observation of behavior in the treatment unit. This typically takes from 4 to 6 weeks. At the end of this period, there is a discussion of the case, acceptance or refusal of the patient into the treatment program, and a determination of the objectives and the treatment plan. The patient is present at the discussions to motivate him to take more responsibility for his treatment.

Second Stage

At this stage there is integration into the treatment program. Within the integration process certain specific activities are started that are aimed at getting the patient used to the diverse therapeutic modalities, their objectives, and their necessities. At this stage, we also introduce less intrusive therapeutic activities such as sex education. At the end of this stage, the patient has to fill out a fantasy report every 2 days for 2 months. This report is a self-administered computerized questionnaire. Thus, the patient records conflicts he has with his current environment and normal and deviant sexual fantasies. As a result, the patient begins to realize that his deviant sexual fantasies are not entirely accidental, but are often precipitated by unresolved conflictual situations. For example, an aggressor often feels humiliated by his contacts with the female nurses in the unit. He will soon realize, however, that almost each time he feels he is being humiliated by one of the nurses, he gets mad, followed by a marked outbreak of his deviant sexual fantasies. Eventually, the patient realizes that this reaction of humiliation is not caused by the nurse but reflects his usual reaction to women, as has been manifested several times in his life in the community.

Third Stage

It is here that the intensive program begins. The patient participates in all the activities of group therapies, such as anger control training, social skills training, relapse prevention, prevention of abuse and dependance on alcohol and drugs, and modification of sexual preferences.

The patient is also involved with the individual activities (e.g., orgasmic reconditioning and covert sensitization) and the fantasy reports. From these latter reports the linkage of conflict–emotion–fantasies is established and the patient is asked to evaluate his strategies to cope with these situations. In fact, from the experience acquired from the fantasy report, a new tool was created—the Coping Strategy Report (McKibben & Proulx, 1998). This is another self-administered computerized questionnaire that permits the patient to record the strategies he uses to cope with his negative affects, his deviant sexual fantasies, and his interpersonal conflicts. Furthermore, the patient evaluates subjectively the efficacy of the strategies he uses. These may have been learned spontaneously or through specific therapeutic modalities. What is important, however, is to know the nature of the strategy used and to recognize its effectiveness.

It is also important to understand why certain strategies are not being used. For example, certain pedophiles do not use covert sensitization, fearing that as a result they will be unable to feel any kind of sexual pleasure. During individual interviews or in group therapy, these patients indicate their preferred strategies, their effectiveness, and their resistance, and finally they are led to accept new strategies to break the cycle of conflicts– negative affects—deviant sexual behavior.

On the whole, relative to these therapeutic modalities, a link is always established between the learning involved in each modality, the actual experiences in the treatment unit, past experiences, and the experiences preceding the crime. The third stage takes on average from 4 to 6 months.

Fourth Stage

This stage does not last more than 2–3 months, but it is crucial in integrating what has been learned. At this stage, the integration of learned skills is being tested during daily lifestyle functioning. Such integration is essential, otherwise the patient will rapidly forget what he learned during treatment and not use it in other settings. Most of the sexual offenders are able to acquire the content of what they have learned, but they must integrate this into all aspects of their lifestyle (affective, behavioral, and social). The changes should not be superficial; they should become an intrinsic part of the offender's personality and be reflected in the kind of lifestyle he chooses. This is now the crucial role of the nonprofessional staff who will validate these lifestyle choices of the patient in his attempt to manage his conflicts, stress, anger, and low self-esteem.

Special attention is given to the family during the treatment period but more so during this fourth stage. To render the therapeutic objectives as closely as possible to the patient's living conditions and to assess the generalization of his learning in the context of his community life, it is important to meet regularly with the patient's family. They are made to understand the meaning of the crime and to identify risk situations and the forewarnings of relapse. They are asked to cooperate in the prevention of recidivism once the patient returns to the community. The family is also asked to help in overcoming the strong resistance by some patients to undergoing treatment. At the start, most patients resist attempts to modify their attitudes. They cling to a few strategies to solve conflicts in their daily life. It is not easy, however, for the patient to develop new strategies, to abandon strategies that seemed to be useful in the past, and, above all, to give up the pleasant feelings associated with deviant fantasies and behavior.

Resistance to treatment appears in different forms—from conformity to open revolt against everything proposed by the clinical staff and a refusal to accept treatment. It must be remembered that treatment is provided if accepted voluntarily; there is no legal compulsion to undergo treatment. There is, however, an incentive to be treated in order to have a favorable report presented to the National Parole Board. Nevertheless, the patient is free at any time to stop treatment for whatever reason and to return to the penitentiary.

Obviously, treatment must continue after the patients leave the hospital. Patients who have benefited from the hospital treatment are followed up in the community at the Forensic Psychiatric Center of Montreal (Centre de Psychiatrie Légale de Montréal), in most cases on conditional release terms. The follow-up is then carried out in close collaboration with the staff of the halfway house, with the parole officer, and with the offender's family. Such collaboration in the follow-up procedures is essential to prevent recidivism. The patient has been made aware of the risk situations and the warning signs that may lead to a sexual crime. He has been taught to lead a better quality personal life. Above all, he has been taught to be able to ask for help, when necessary, before a relapse occurs.

RESEARCH

Since the beginning, we have endeavored to integrate our research activities into the clinical operations. Research and clinical activities, however, do not always work in harmony. In our institution the researcher and the clinicians work independently but find areas of common concern. The search for factors underlying sexual aggression and for factors associated with recidivism has been at the center of clinicians' and the researcher's preoccupations in our team. A climate of mutual cross-fertilization thus has developed, with research influencing clinical activities and vice versa.

Cooperation and complementarity between the researcher and the clinicians have permitted us to develop certain theoretical and clinical concepts. For example, it was believed by the clinicians that there was a relationship between the type of personality disorders and the type of crime committed. The results of an investigative study (Proulx, Aubut, Perron, & McKibben, 1994) have demonstrated that the most violent rapes are usually committed by a sexual aggressor with an antisocial personality disorder and the less violent rapes by men having an avoidant personality disorder.

We soon became interested in the affective variables associated with sexual aggression. Cognitive variables, especially cognitive distortions, have been extensively investigated (Segal & Stermac, 1990). However, the affective components, which seem to us crucial factors in sexual aggression proclivity, have been largely neglected. Therefore, we have developed a strategy, the "Fantasy Report," that permits us to assess the aggressor's daily activities, the conflicting situations they face, their associated negative affects, and their deviant sexual behaviors. A research project we have carried out with the Fantasy Report has shown that a link exists between negative affects and deviant sexual behavior (McKibben et al., 1994). We, therefore, hypothesized that negative affects are important constituents in the chain leading to sexual aggression.

Research findings also have permitted us to refine certain diagnostic tools. We were surprised to discover that some aggressors, who recognized their use of rape fantasies during masturbatory activities, did not react to rape stimuli involving sexual activities and physical violence during phallometric assessment. Interviews with these aggressors revealed that their rape fantasies involved sexual activities and humiliation of the victim. We therefore developed rape stimuli in which the coercive dimension was humiliation rather than physical violence. The use of two types of rape stimuli permits better discrimination between rapists and nonrapists (Proulx, Aubut, McKibben, & Côté, 1994).

Research investigations of recidivism are difficult and entail numerous methodological problems but are essential (Marques, Day, Nelson, & West, 1994). We have become especially interested in the factors associated with recidivism in our population and have studied the static factors (part criminality, age, relationship, and legal status) and dynamic factors (sexual preferences and personality characteristics) in rapists and pedophiles (Proulx et al., 1997).

The impact of treatment on recidivism has also been measured (Pellerin et al., 1996), showing that various treatment components have a different effect, depending on the types of patient. One factor stands out, however, and that is the influence of the length of the treatment. We (Pellerin et al., 1996) have found that treatment of less than 1 year has little effect on pedophiles, whereas treatment of more than 2 years is necessary for rapists. This is not surprising when one considers the early emergence of deviant behavior in sexual offenders, the multiplicity of their deficiencies, their initial denial of their crime, and their resistance to treatment.

Our future research activity will concentrate on the efficacy of the coping strategy used by sexual offenders to prevent recidivism. We plan to have sexual offenders fill out the coping strategy report after they return to the community. Our future research activities will also concentrate on the factors that could improve patients' compliance with treatment, in particular the effect of personality variables in adhering to a treatment program.

CONCLUSION

The major elements of our approach to treatment have been described elsewhere (Aubut, 1993). As we have emphasized before, our approach is of a global nature, addressing a diversity of components, including present and past events, as well as the biological psychological, and social aspects. The key factors are continuity of treatment from the treatment unit to the community, generalization of learning, and the aggressor's responsibility for his life quality and for avoiding recidivism.

Obviously, numerous clinical and theoretical dimensions still need to be developed, refined, and validated. These points have been dealt with by Marshall (1996). However, certain problems need special attention. For example, it is important to offer continuous clinical and scientific support to the clinical staff because motivation to deal with difficult patients on a long-term basis is very trying. Moreover, replacing clinical staff is facilitated by our close links with different university departments (criminology, psychology, psychiatry, etc.).

REFERENCES

Aubut, J. (1993). *Les agresseurs sexuels: Théorie, évaluation et traitement.* Montréal: Les Editions de la Chenelière.

Marques, J. K., Day, D. M., Nelson, C., & West, M. A. (1994). Effects of cognitive–behavioral treatment on sex offender recidivism: Preliminary results of a longitudinal study. *Criminal Justice and Behavior, 21,* 28–54.

Marshall, W. L. (1989). Intimacy, loneliness, and sexual offenders. *Behaviour Research and Therapy, 27,* 491–503.

Marshall, W. L. (1996). Assessment, treatment, and theorizing about sex offenders: Developments during the past twenty years and future directions. *Criminal Justice and Behavior, 23,* 162–199.

McKibben, A., & Proulx, J. (1998). *Sexual aggressors' perception of effectiveness regarding strategies to cope with negative emotions and deviant sexual fantasies.* Manuscript submitted for publication.

McKibben, A., Proulx, J., & Lusignan, R. (1994). Relationship between affective components and deviant sexual behaviours in rapists and pedophiles. *Behaviour Research and Therapy, 32,* 295–310.

Pellerin, B., Proulx, J., Ouimet, M., Paradis, Y., McKibben, A., & Aubut, J. (1996). Etude de la récidive post-traitement chez des agresseurs sexuels judiciarisés. *Criminologie, 29,* 85–108.

Proulx, J., Aubut, J., McKibben, A., & Côté, M. (1994). Penile responses of rapists and nonrapists to rape stimuli involving violence or humiliation. *Archives of Sexual Behavior, 23,* 295–310.

Proulx, J., Aubut, J., Perron, L., & McKibben, A. (1994). Troubles de la personnalité et viol: Implications théoriques et cliniques. *Criminologie, 27,* 33–53.

Proulx, J., Pellerin, B., Paradis, Y., McKibben, A., Aubut, J., & Ouimet, M. (1997). Static and dynamic predictors of recidivism in sexual aggressors. *Sexual Abuse: A Journal of Research and Treatment, 9*, 7–27.

Segal, Z. V., & Stermac, L. E. (1990). The role of cognition in sexual assault. In W. L. Marshall, D. R. Laws, & H. E. Barbaree (Eds.), *Handbook of sexual assault: Issues theories and treatment of the offender* (pp. 161–174). New York: Plenum.

Yochelson, S., & Samenov, S. E. (1976). *The criminal personality: A profile for change.* New York: Aronson.

16

C. Psychiatric Settings

Treating the "Sexually Dangerous Person"
The Massachusetts Treatment Center

Barbara K. Schwartz and Gregory M.S. Canfield

The Massachusetts Treatment Center for Sexually Dangerous Persons is a remnant of an outdated concept of human behavior. It is one of the last of the original sexual psychopath programs. Unfortunately, the trend is starting to spread across the country again, beginning in 1990, with the opening of the Special Commitment Center in Monroe, Washington, where sex offenders are civilly committed until such time as they can prove that they are no longer "sexually dangerous predators." This chapter will explore not only the history of the Massachusetts Treatment Center (MTC) and the civil commitment of sex offenders but the authors' experiences in providing sex-offender-specific treatment first under the Massachusetts Department of Mental and then the Department of Corrections.

HISTORY OF SEXUAL PSYCHOPATH LAWS

The theoretical foundation for the civil commitment of sex offenders dates back to Caesar Lombroso (1911), a physician working in French prisons. He believed that antisocial individuals were "atavists," genetic "throwbacks" who could be identified by definite physical characteristics. As ludicrous as that may seem, it inspired a whole approach to problem behavior in the early part of this century. Defective delinquent laws were instituted on the presumption that certain persons are born with a proclivity to commit crimes. Because they are genetically programmed to behave in an antisocial manner, they could not be considered to be criminally responsible, yet they are a menace to society. Therefore, they needed to be placed in a facility that would confine but not punish them. These laws existed until the middle of this century, and indeed there are residents at the MTC who were originally institutionalized under these laws. During the period from 1900 to 1931, these laws were used to confine political dissidents (Cohen, 1995). Consequently, they were abolished, but their philosophy lived on through the mentally disordered sex offender

Barbara K. Schwartz and Gregory M.S. Canfield • Justice Resource Institute, Bridgewater, Massachusetts 02324.

Sourcebook of Treatment Programs for Sexual Offenders, edited by Marshall et al. Plenum Press, New York, 1998.

(MDSO) statutes, which assumed that some sex offenders are mentally ill and could respond to traditional mental health treatment versus other sex offenders who are not mentally ill and were rarely offered treatment within the prison environment.

The first such law was established Michigan in 1937, and the individual who inspired the passage of that law is still confined in the forensic mental health system there. The Massachusetts Sexually Dangerous Person Law was passed in 1947. However, the treatment center authorized by that legislation did not open until 1957, following a notorious crime in which a sex offender who had been out of prison for 2 months murdered two young boys.

In Massachusetts, a sexually dangerous person is defined by Chapter 123A of the Massachusetts General Laws as anyone

> … whose misconduct in sexual matters indicates a general lack of power to control his sexual impulses, as evidenced by repetitive or compulsive behavior and either violence, or aggression by an adult against a victim under the age of sixteen, and who as a result is likely to attack or otherwise inflict injury on the objects of his uncontrolled or uncontrollable desires.

In 1979, a report prepared by the MTC reported that of 4000 men who were screened by the MTC 1300 wee referred for intensive evaluation and 390 were committed to the 1 day-to-life sentence as a sexually dangerous person (Boucher, 1979).

Controversies over MDSO Laws

Only during the year 1989 was the country unified in believing that MDSO laws were a bad idea. In 1990, the state of Washington, which in 1988 had closed their Sexual Psychopath Program and opened a voluntary treatment program in the Department of Corrections, reinstituted civil commitment for "sexually violent predators." While the district federal court has ruled this particular law unconstitutional, Washington State is appealing and it is anticipated that this matter will eventually go the Supreme Court (in re Young).

The controversy over civil commitment involves a number of basic questions. Are these men mentally ill? Can they be treated? Can they only be treated if they have a mental illness? Can they be treated in a prison or do they need to be in a mental hospital? Do these programs represent incarceration mascarading as treatment? What types of treatment, if any, are most effective with this population?

In 1984, the American Bar Association's *Criminal Justice Mental Health Standards* stated that MDSO legislation is based on six assumptions:

> … 1) there is a specific mental disability called sexual psychopathy, psychopathy, or defective delinquency; 2) persons suffering from such a disability are more likely to commit serious crimes, especially dangerous sex offenses, than normal criminals; 3) such persons are easily identified by mental health professionals; 4) the dangerousness of these offenders can be predicted by mental health professionals; 5) treatment is available for the condition; and 6) large numbers of sexually dangerous persons afflicted with the designated disabilities can be cured (1984, p. 15)

Whether sex offenders are suffering from a mental illness is a topic of considerable disagreement. While one might argue that pedophilia is included in the listing of mental illnesses found in the American Psychiatric Association's (1994) *Diagnostic and Statistical Manual of Mental Disorders*, 4th edition (DSM-IV), under "paraphilia," rape, unless it is sadistic, is not included. This has been an area of much political contention, with proponents for including rapists in the DSM-IV pointing out how this behavior is comparable to all the other paraphilia and opponents arguing that this would be tantamount to turning a violent crime into an illness. Additionally, there are many conditions that are included in the DSM-IV that would never be considered to be mental illnesses, such as nicotine addiction or alcoholism. There is no reference in this manual to "Mentally Disordered Sex Offenders," "Sexual Psychopaths," or "Violent Sexual Predators." These are legal, not clinical, terms. The federal court in Young ruled that politicians cannot invent mental illnesses to justify commitments. Because these conditions are impossible to define in objective terms, it is a challenge to identify which people belong in these categories and even more difficult to identify when someone no longer fits the definition so that they can then be released from confinement.

However, behavior does not have to be considered a mental illness to be changed. Drug abuse is not considered to be a mental illness (even though it is included in the DSM-IV), but this does not lead to the conclusion that drug abusers cannot be helped to change their behavior. The MDSO laws referred to "curing" sex offenders as one might cure someone with appendicitis. The concept of "cure" is not a realistic goal for sex offender treatment. The term itself is absolute and not relevant when discussing complex human behavior problems. Many behavior problems can be changed, controlled, or modified but not cured. However, sex offenders, like drug addicts or like individuals with diabetes, can be taught to the techniques to manage their deviant urges.

History of the MTC

As previously noted, the MTC was opened after a horrendous crime committed by a newly released sex offender. It was originally placed at the Massachusetts Corrections Institution-Concord and the residents were referred to as "prisoners." However, in 1972, a federal law suit, *Williams v. Lesiak*, greatly increased the role of the Department of Mental Health and mandated that the term and philosophical approach to the residents be changed from "prisoners" to "patients." The MTC remained housed in an antiquated prison but was administered by the Department of Mental Health.

In 1979, a proposal for enhanced staffing reported that there were 171 individuals civilly committed to the MTC. Furthermore,

> ... there were only the equivalent of seven full time clinicians to supply therapy services to the entire Treatment Center population. While varying mixes of behavioral, individual, group, and couple or family therapies may be indicated, our present capability is limited to an offering of one or two of these treatment modalities to any given patient. (Boucher, 1979, p. 27)

The *Williams v. Lesiak* consent decree also mandated the establishment of a new treatment center, which was completed in 1986. Upon moving into the new building, the Department of Corrections began joint operation with the Department of Mental Health. In 1989, the Governor appointed the Special Advisory Panel on Forensic Mental Health to evaluate the MTC. Their resulting report began with a quote from the American Psychiatry Association (1977), Which stated, "We see special sex offender legislation as an approach to sex psychopaths that has failed, and consequently we feel that these statutes should be repealed" (p. 1). This report challenged the idea that sex offenders suffer from a mental illness: "Sexual violence is clearly not a mental illness ... it is a criminal behavior" (Petrella, Richardson, & Burney, 1989). They also concluded that "The treatment industry that has developed following the 'sexual psychopath' laws has been innovative, but has effected little in the way of demonstrably successful long-term interventions" (Petrella, Richardson, & Burney, 1989, p. 61). This conclusion was particularly interesting given that the panel referenced at least three articles that quoted a variety of efficacy studies showing that treatment of sex offenders lowered recidivism rates. Among the panel's recommendations were that the civil commitment of "sexually dangerous persons" be abolished, that certain individuals in the MTC be transferred back to prisons, and that the Department of Corrections establish its own sex offender treatment program (Petrella et al., 1989).

Shortly thereafter, civil commitments were abolished. A long battle then ensued to transfer the program to corrections. Legislation was repeatedly introduced and then stalled or defeated until 1994, when the transfer legislation finally passed. The transfer was then delayed for a year while the court wrestled with a legal standard that states that a consent decree can only be modified if there is a substantial change in the situation. Was the new legislation to be regarded as a substantial change in the situation? The federal district court said, "no," but the federal court of appears sand "yes." In 1995, the court authorized the transfer to corrections but has staid many of the specific changes proposed by the transfer.

In 1990, in a series of budget cutbacks to the Department of Mental Health, rapid staff changes impacted the MTC so that many long-term clinicians were laid off or were "bumped" by other mental health employees with no experience in treating sex offenders. Some men at the MTC had 15 therapists in a 2-year period. This occurred in a population that due to their early histories, had trouble establishing trust, and their experience in an environment that always had had a major identity crisis did not improve their ability to bond to staff. This compounded an ongoing problem that was documented in 1979 by Cohen and Boucher (1979):

> Involuntary commitment … creates an opposition between those who work in the system and those who are placed within the system. With rare exceptions, the patients at the Center did not seek such an indeterminate sentence or treatment. Since a characteristic of such patients is to externalize the sources of their life difficulties, they see the law, the Center and the staff as the opposition and further evidence of the uncaring, hostile society. The clinical staff, trained to deliver therapeutic services to those in need who seek assistance, are overwhelmed by the anger and rejection of the offer to help. They are distressed at being perceived as judges and jailers (p. 3).

The problems at the center were further compounded by a series of escapes by men in the Community Access Program, which led to the cancellation of a program that was a primary motivator for the patients. Men who had been on community release programs, working in local towns and spending considerable amounts of time with their families, were suddenly recalled back into the center. This obviously engendered considerable frustration and anger. In May 1992, a man who had been declared by the court to be "no longer sexually dangerous" and returned to prison was paroled and shortly thereafter murdered two women.

It was onto this scene, in July 1992, that Justice Resource Institute (JRI), a private, nonprofit corporation, came to take over the treatment, rehabilitation, and medical programs of the MTC. Although the state was undergoing extensive privatization at that time, the introduction of JRI into the MTC was more centered around the agency's expertise in program management than in any cost-saving or political agenda. At the bidder's conference in 1992, JRI was told that although the contract was being let by the Department of Mental Health, the program and the whole facility would "soon" be transferring to the Department of Corrections: "soon" ended up being September 1995.

TREATMENT PHILOSOPHY

The Sex Offender Treatment Program at the MTC is based on the integrative model (Schwartz & Cellini, 1995). Over the years, a number of treatment techniques have been developed, starting with group therapy, then adding various behavioral techniques, with the later development of cognitive–behavioral techniques, including relapse prevention. However, in the past several years, experts in the field have stressed the need to add affective, physiological, familial, and spiritual components to the treatment regimen (Bernard, Fuller, Robbins, & Shaw, 1989; Pithers, 1993; Knopp, 1994; Marques, 1995; Schwartz, 1995).

Each of these issues has been systematically incorporated into the integrative model, which views sexual deviancy as the product of the interplay between physiological, cognitive, affective, behavioral, interpersonal, familial, societal, and spiritual issues. Of course, not every individual has problems in each of these areas that impacts their sexuality. The combination differs for each person, but a comprehensive sex offender treatment program should be prepared to address the full range of issues.

The emphasis in this theoretical approach is on the dynamic, holistic relationship of these factors. This has been inspired by basic paradigm changes in the physical sciences that stress a move away from mechanistic, single-factor theories to complex, relationship-based approaches and has motivated changes in almost every aspect of human endeavor from medicine and management to politics and spirituality. In applying this new paradigm to the treatment of sex offenders, it becomes apparent that a simple method or technique is not sufficient to change something as basic as the quality of one's interpersonal and sexual relations with others.

Treatment Issues

At the MTC, eight issues are dealt with through a multimodel approach:

1. *Physiological*: Sex offenders may have a number of physiological issues that impact their behavior. They may have inherited a genetic predisposition for certain types of pathology such as mood disorders, attention-deficit disorders, substance abuse, or depression, which, while certainly not directly responsible for sexual acting out, can contribute by disinhibiting behavioral controls. Disruption of the biochemical balance of the brain (Prentky & Burgess, 1991), early trauma (Van der Koch, 1995), or brain damage may predispose an individual to violence. The MTC utilizes psychiatric consultants with not only an expertise in treating the more common psychiatric problems that some of the residents manifest but who also have an interest and expertise in treating the conditions that might contribute to sexual deviance. This might include selective serotonin reuptake inhibitors, which appear to be particularly useful in treating intrusive sexual fantasies, or anticonvulsants, which might be related to explosive rage. The program also has the capability of conducting neuropsychological testing to identify deficit areas that might need cognitive rehabilitation.

2. *Cognitive*: Sex offender treatment specialists have long recognized the extraordinary cognitive distortions used by sex offenders to excuse, justify, minimize, and rationalize their behavior. Yochelson and Samenow (1976) have identified basic "criminal thinking patterns" that sex offenders may share with their fellow convicts and Alcoholics Anonymous has discussed the "stinkin' thinkin'" of substance abusers for decades. Furthermore, many offenders seem to have very basic problems in just how to think. They have difficulty

with understanding the consequences of their behavior or considering alternatives when making decisions. Group therapy at the MTC is particularly beneficial in identifying and confronting cognitive errors. Classes in problem-solving and thinking strategies, such as T3 Associates' "Reasoning and Rehabilitation" curriculum, help residents learn to make better decisions.

Relapse prevention is a cognitive technique that is designed to help the offender identify his offense cycle and develop appropriate interventions. At the MTC, this is done through three 12-week classes that culminate in the preparation of a comprehensive relapse prevention plan. The final class focuses on a role-playing game called "Lifting the Weight," which was developed by the Geese Theater to teach relapse prevention.

3. *Affective*: Pithers (1993), Knopp (1994), and Marques (1995), along with Bernard et al. (1989) and Schwartz (1995) have pointed out the need to supplement cognitive–behavioral treatment with affective work, primarily to enhance motivation. Developing empathy for the victim as well as for others in their life is a prime method of motivating sex offenders. They must truly appreciate the devastating consequences of their behavior. Sex offenders may have difficulty empathizing with others because they are emotionally numb or because they are afraid of the guilt and shame that facing their behavior will cause them. They may also be afraid of facing their own history of trauma, and thus they seal both themselves and their victims in a cocoon of denial. Breaking into that cocoon can be a formidable task. Affective work is begun in psychoeducational classes and continued in group therapy. Experiential therapies are particularly useful in enhancing motivation and allowing the offender to begin to feel real emotions.

4. *Behavioral*: Deviant sexual arousal is assumed to have been at least reinforced, if not initially developed, through the reinforcement of linking a deviant fantasy with orgasm. A variety of techniques have been developed to break that positive linkage. Covert sensitization pairs the deviant fantasy with an aversive mental image. Assisted covert sensitization adds some type of noxious odor to the repellent scene. Individuals are encouraged to develop positive sexual fantasies through orgasmic reconditioning.

Final approval for use of phallometric assessment has just been received. This had been considered highly controversial in Massachusetts, and in 1984, a laboratory was established and then almost immediately shut down. Reopening of the behavioral laboratory will allow for the identification of those individuals needing behavioral interventions as well as the monitoring of progress in reducing deviant arousal.

5. *Interpersonal*: In institutional drug treatment programs, drugs may continue to be available in the larger prison environment, and thus there is an opportunity to relapse. Progress in treatment can be monitored through urine tests. However, sex offenders are not presented with the same types of temptations. Nevertheless, their behavior may reflect the start of the deviant cycle through inappropriate interpersonal relations. The participant may begin to abuse power or project his anger on innocent bystanders. This behavior can be observed with the therapeutic community. The Jesness Behavioral Checklist (Jesness, 1984) is used to assess daily interactions with others. The ratings on 16 behaviors by the correctional officer, the therapist, and the offender are compared.

Various coping skills are taught to enhance interpersonal relations. Psychoeducational classes, including social skills, effective communication, communicating with women, and human sexuality, are taught.

Empathy is a crucial component of all interpersonal relations. It is perhaps the most vital component of sex offender treatment. If one can learn to appreciate and care about the harm one has done to another human, this appreciation can provide the motivation to engage in the difficult process of therapy. At the MTC classes are taught in victim empathy, which present readings and films on the impact of sexual assault on victims. Drama therapy using offense reenactments and exploration of the sex offender's personal victimization evokes powerful emotional identification. Survivors of sexual assault volunteer to share their experiences with the MTC residents. This has been a transformative experience for both the offenders and the survivors.

6. *Familial*: The distorted personal relations that are the basis of sexual assault are almost always developed in childhood. The offender usually comes to treatment with either deep-rooted anger toward or fear of others. Exploration of early experiences and intra-familial dynamics can provide an understanding of why adult relations are so disturbed. At the MTC, participants are introduced to an understanding of their early experiences through psychoeducational courses in family dynamics, and this is further investigated in experiential therapies.

7. *Societal*: Males in this society are socialized into a culture that has contributed to their need to exercise power over others, to repress their emotions, and to value competition over cooperation. Distorted ideas about what it means to be a "man" have contributed to their aggressiveness in the case of some offenders and to their isolation in the case of others. At MTC, *Men's Work* (Kivel, 1993), a curriculum developed by the Oakland's Men's Project, is used to acquaint the men with unrealistic gender role expectations and destructive attitudes toward aggression and violence. This is a particularly popular program among the residents. Psychoeducational classes also point out how the media objectifies others and presents distorted ideas about sex roles as well as sexual assault.

8. *Spiritual*: The integrative model conceptualizes spirituality as an integral part of a holistic view of human behavior. One need only read the papers for a week to see the extent to which sex offenders have distorted their spirituality (e.g., the minister who sexually assaults members of his congregation). Rarely does one see this degree of conflict between one's behavior and one's beliefs in other crimes. It is the aim of the treatment program at the MTC to help sex offenders integrate their spirituality, whatever it may be, into their overall recovery so that it becomes a positive force. This is done with courses such as spirituality and recovery. Twelve Step groups including Alcoholics Anonymous, Narcotics Anonymous, Sex and Love Addicts Anonymous, and A Way of Life meet weekly.

Cognitive Levels of Treatment

Not only must a variety of different dimensions of the problem of sexual deviancy be evaluated and treated, but they need to be addressed on increasingly complex cognitive levels. The mastery of any skill depends on it being integrated into one's behavioral repertoire at a gradually increasing level of sophistication. This has been summarized in Table 16.1. Participants are initially introduced to concepts through psychoeducational classes. These are basically classroom presentations of fundamental knowledge of concepts designed to allow the participant to identify, match, define, and select the basic information needed to progress to a higher level of understanding. The content of these classes will be elaborated upon later in this chapter.

The next level is comprehension where an individual can understand, summarize, and generalize the information mastered at a knowledge level. This is done in advanced classes and in group therapy where a participant brings the information obtained in a psychoeducational class into his primary group to discuss how this might apply to his own life. Next, the participant begins to use his ability to apply what he has learned to actually change his own

TABLE 16.1
Bloom's Taxonomy Applied to Sex Offender Treatment Techniques

Stages of learning	Characteristics	Treatment techniques
Evaluation	Students make judgements, appraise, judge, justify, critique information	Utilizing relapse prevention, transition to community
Synthesis	Students can produce something original, create, design, devise, formulate, generate, rearrange, reconstruct	Drama therapy, art therapy, therapeutic community
Analysis	Students can break information into parts and identify relationships between parts, can compare, identify, infer, relate	Relapse prevention, insight-oriented groups, victim empathy work
Application	Students can solve problems, use rules, laws and methods, change, discover, modify, and relate	Groups, therapeutic community, social activities
Comprehension	Students can understand facts, explain, generalize, paraphrase, demonstrate and summarize	Psychoeducational classes and groups
Knowledge	Students can remember facts, choose, define, describe, label, list, match, select	Psychoeducational classes

behavior. At this point it is important that the participant in an institutional program be placed in a therapeutic community so that his daily interactions with others can be monitored. At this stage the participant begins to analyze situations by breaking down a situation into its component parts so that the appropriate therapeutic intervention can be applied. After this the individual can begin to synthesize the material at a level where he can create something new and original based on his experience. At this stage the experiential therapies such as art and drama therapy offer opportunities to practice this stage of cognition. Finally, the participant is ready for reintegration into the community. This must be a slow and highly structured process that allows the individual to experience different situations, try out the interventions and responses he has learned in therapy, and then analyze with his group and therapist the results of these behaviors. Community integration is provided through the pretransition program where men can live in a residence on the grounds and begin to wean themselves away from the institution. Men who have finished their criminal sentence are eligible for the transition program. While living in the residence, they can begin to go out into the community for therapy and eventually for work or school.

TREATMENT CENTER OR PRISON?

As previously stressed, the MTC is a hybrid. Under the Department of Mental Health, the center was administered by a state agency that was not comfortable with servicing this population. Because of the need to maintain a low profile during the transfer process, which has gone on for over a decade, few major decisions were made for fear of creating controversy. For example, the Department of Mental Health would never approve the plethysmograph laboratory. Simultaneously, the Department of Corrections has always conceived of the institution as at least a medium-security prison. Due to these two conflicting visions, the two agencies could not agree to written policies. Up until 1996, the facility had less than ten mutually agreed on policies, which were kept locked in a filed cabinet to which no one would admit to having a key. Further confusion existed around the consent decrees and what they meant. The persons who negotiated the decrees were no longer involved with the center. This left the decrees open to interpretation based on oral history. One example of the vagaries of this system is the approach to infractions. To this date, there are no clear disciplinary policies that set forth infractions and sanctions. This was the result of the *King v. Greenblatt* consent decree, which mandated that punishment could not be used to manage residents. Unfortunately, this produced a system that can be almost totally subjective. One individual might be placed in the minimum custody unit for an infraction for which another inmate might receive a verbal reprimand. Every sanction had to be "therapeutic" in nature, which put quite a strain on the creativity of the staff and was probably more aversive to the resident than having to mop the floor. The Department of Corrections has proposed a disciplinary system that would be more objective, but the court must decide whether it is punitive.

There were other policies that, while applicable to mental patients, were unusual in sex offender treatment programs. Sexual liaisons were rampant and had for years been ignored, if not encouraged. One recommendation handed down by the board that evaluates the men as to their sexual dangerousness was for a particular resident to establish a sexual relationship with another resident to demonstrate that he could relate in that manner to an adult.

Whether the MTC is a "prison" or a "treatment center" assumes that those terms have clear definitions. Many treatment centers are more restrictive than prisons. Prisons around the country have conjugal visits. Some have animal training programs. At least one has had a traveling street theater group. They typically have a systematic way of moving inmates through lower security facilities. Treatment centers, particularly in forensic settings, often have to set policies to protect highly volatile and unpredictable mental patients and those who are more stable may have their privileges limited as a consequence. A more appropriate question might be, "What is necessary for the residential treatment of civilly committed sex offenders?"

TREATING THE CIVILLY COMMITTED SEX OFFENDER

The civilly committed sex offender is a treatment challenge. These individuals are not voluntarily in treatment. They have been singled out for a variety of reasons as supposedly being the "worst of the worst," but even a cursory investigation suggests that they are probably no different from many offenders who did not receive the "sexually dangerous" label. They are serving a day-to-life sentence, which can engender hopelessness. They have great difficulties adapting as their many therapists come and go in their lives.

The contrast between this population and sex offenders in a prison program is particularly dramatic, since 50 Department of Corrections inmates in the statewide sex offender treatment program managed by JRI were transferred to the MTC. In the prison program, men are treated for a maximum of 4 years and do most of their intensive work in the 18 months they spend in a therapeutic community. They can be terminated from the program if their participation is unsatisfactory or their behavior disruptive.

The challenge to treating those who are civilly committed is to arouse and maintain motivation. One way of doing this is to establish clear and objective treatment goals. JRI's program has eight overall goals that are broken down into five to eight subgoals. Currently, men in the MTC program are beginning to complete those goals and are beginning to be cleared by the Community Access Board and the courts.

Another challenge to treating this population is to continually update and develop new and interesting methods that can motivate men who have been in "treatment" for up to 20 years. This should be done in a way that does not make it seem that the rules are always being changed.

But perhaps the greatest challenge is to be able to balance the provision of treatment with the provision of security. This must be a cooperative task in which both the therapy staff and the custody staff share a common vision of recovery and work together to provide an atmosphere in which this can be achieved. Whether this is an achievable goal remains to be seen.

CONCLUSION

The MTC is the product of a controversial philosophy that states that some sex offenders are suffering from some type of mental condition that sets them apart from other sex offenders, making them "sexual predators," "sexual psychopaths," or "sexually dangerous persons" who need to be treated until they are unequivocally "cured." This challenges mainstream thinking that maintains that some human beings have difficulties with certain behaviors (e.g., deviant and/or violent sexual behaviors). They can be taught ways to control those behaviors but will have to utilize what they have learned on a daily basis. If they forsake the tools of their recovery, they may lose the ability to control their behaviors.

Despite the outmoded philosophy under which the system functions, the men at the MTC are struggling to address their issues through a multifaceted treatment program. They also have had to deal with a very frightening transfer process that has taken them from the jurisdiction of mental health and placed them under the jurisdiction of corrections. Currently, the Department of Corrections has approved components of treatment that were not permissible under mental health, and in general it has been supportive of the therapeutic process. However, the eventual form that the center takes will be the result of fluctuating pressures between treatment, security, the courts, the legislature, the media, and the public.

REFERENCES

American Bar Association. (1984). *Criminal justice mental health standards.* Washington, DC: American Bar Association.

American Psychiatry Association. (1977). *Report of the group for the advancement of psychiatry: Psychiatry and sex psychopath legislation: The 30's to the 80's,* Vol. IX, No. 98. Washington, DC: Author.

American Psychiatric Association. (1994). *Diagnostic and statistical manual of mental disorders* (4th ed.). Washington, DC: Author.

Bernard, G., Fuller, K., Robbins, L., & Shaw, T. (1989). *The child molester: An integrated approach to evaluation and treatment.* New York: Brunner/Mazel.

Boucher, R. (1979). *Treatment of the sexually aggressive and dangerous person: A comprehensive plan.* Bridgewater, MA: The Massachusetts Treatment Center for Sexually Dangerous Persons.

Cohen, F. (1995). Introduction to legal issues: How the legal foundation is developed. In B. K. Schwartz & H. R. Cellini (Eds.), *The sex offender: Corrections, treatment and legal practice* (pp. 22.1–22.9). Kingston, NJ: Civic Research Institute.

Cohen, M. L., & Boucher, R. (1979). Special programs in treating sexual aggressive in residential settings. Presented at the First National Conference on Sexual Aggressive, Memphis, TN.

Jesness, C. F. (1984). *Jesness Behavioral Checklist.* Toronto: Multi-Health Systems.

Kivel, P. (1993). *Men's work: How to stop the violence that tears our lives apart.* Center City, MN: Hazelden.

Knopp, F. H. (1994, November). Keynote address. Presented at the Thirteenth Annual Conference of the Association for the Treatment of Sexual Abusers, San Francisco.

Lombroso, C. (1911). *Crime: Its cause and remedies*: London: Hernemann.

Marques, J. (1995, October). Future directions for sex offender treatment. Presented at the Fourteenth Annual Conference of the Association·for the Treatment of Sexual Abusers, New Orleans.

Petrella, R. C., Richardson, M. H., & Burney, J. S. (1989). *Final report: Commonwealth of Massachusetts Governor's Special Advisory Panel on Forensic Mental Health.* Boston, MA.

Pithers, W. D. (1993). Treatment of rapists: Reinterpretation of early outcome data and exploratory constructs to enhance therapeutic efficacy. In G. Nagayama-Hall, R. Hirschman, J. R. Graham, & M. S. Zaragoee (Eds.), *Sexual aggression: Issues in etiology, assessment and treatment* (pp. 165–203). Bristol, PA: Taylor & Francis.

Prentsky, R. A., & Burgess, A. W. (1991). Hypothetical biological substrates of a fantasy-based drive mechanism for repetitive sexual aggression. In A. W. Burgess (Ed.), *Rape and sexual assault III* (pp. 235–256). New York: Garland.

Schwartz, B. K., & Cellini, H. R. (1995). The sex offender: Corrections, treatment and legal practice. Kingston, NJ: Civic Research Institute.

Schwartz, M. (1995). "In my opinion: Victim to victimizer." *Sexual Addition and Compulsivity*, 2(2), 81–88.

Van der Kalk, B. A. (1995). Trauma, mercury and the integration of experience. Paper presented at the Fourth Annual Conference on Advances in Treating Survivors of Abuse and Trauma: Multiple Dimensions in Healing, Philadelphia.

Williams, H. G., v. Lesiak, M. USDC CA no. 72-571-8 ADM.

Yochelson, S., & Samenow, S. E. (1976). *The criminal personality, Vol. I.* New York: Aronson.

Young, 857 P.2d 989 (Wash. 1993).

17

C. Psychiatric Settings

Treatment of Adult Male Sexual Offenders in a Psychiatric Setting
Sexual Behaviours Clinic, Royal Ottawa Hospital

John M.W. Bradford and David M. Greenberg

The Sexual Behaviours Clinic located in the Royal Ottawa Hospital is committed to providing specialized comprehensive assessments, consultations, management, and treatment to our community in general. Our service provides assistance not only to a population of sexual offenders but also to individuals with various sexual dysfunctions, paraphilias, and gender identity disorders. Over the past 16 years, the clinic has gained an international reputation as a center of academic excellence. Staff hold university appointments and provide education resources and opportunities to the two major university programs in the city. We also provide consultation to professional colleagues and as an information resource center to the community at large. The interface with the community has included consultation to other professionals and also the media via our public relations office. The research component of our Sexual Behaviours Clinic has produced ground-breaking scientific information to further delineate the boundaries of this area of expertise and dispel myths and misperceptions about sexual offenders. It also affords the clinic the opportunity to provide a vehicle for quality assurance and quality control. Although the clinic has opportunities for admission to psychiatric beds, its primary focus has been to manage offenders on a long-term basis in a community setting. This we feel provides a more effective long-term solution to these serious behaviors compared to merely gating penitentiary dispositions. Objective psychophysiological measures of sexual arousal and psychopharmacological interventions are often overlooked or underutilized by other programs, although there is an extensive body of research to substantiate the efficacy, reliability, and validity of these modalities. Effective treatment and management of individual sexual abusers may include psychopharmacological treatments while not excluding other treatment modalities. Our clinical practice of providing comprehensive, multidisciplinary, and multifocused interventions will be discussed in this chapter.

John M.W. Bradford and David M. Greenberg • Forensic Service and Sexual Behaviours Clinic, Royal Ottawa Hospital, Ottawa, Ontario, Canada K1Z 7K4.

Sourcebook of Treatment Programs for Sexual Offenders, edited by Marshall et al. Plenum Press, New York, 1998.

HISTORICAL PERSPECTIVE AND PROBLEMS ESTABLISHING THE CLINIC

The Sexual Behaviours Clinic was established in 1981. Prior to this period sex offenders were assessed and treated at the forensic service on an ad hoc basis, and there was no structured assessment and treatment process or formal research component. Early challenges centered around lack of funding. There was no funding forthcoming to establish such a clinic from the hospital, Ministry of Health, or any of the traditional funding sources. As a result, the clinic was set up under a research mandate. A research grant was obtained to cover the initial equipment for the sexual behaviors laboratory. In 1981, this was a considerable expense, as sexual arousal testing was measured by a multichannel polygraph that costs approximately $15,000. The other equipment, such as slide projectors, tape recorders, and so forth, probably amounted to another $3,000–$5,000 in total. Furthermore, the laboratory accommodation needed renovation. Therefore, this initial start-up cost of approximately $20,000 was a difficult problem to overcome. There also was no money to pay for the technician to run the laboratory, and this had to come from other research grants. For the clinic to be viable, the technician's salary initially had to be funded on a yearly basis. One of the issues in attempting to overcome this was to look at whether there was any way of funding the clinic on a fee-for-service basis. The Ministry of Health was approached to see whether there was anything in the Ontario Health Insurance Plan fee schedule that would support penile tumescence testing. Although there was an item in relation to penile tumescence testing, the amount of money this would generate would in no way cover the costs of running the laboratory. There was a second problem in that the laboratory had to be approved by the Ministry of Health and had to be supported by the hospital for that approval. At that time, problems arose with the hospital not being supportive of the laboratory other than as a research laboratory. Fortunately, the clinic and laboratory survived on research money for a period of 5 or 6 years, which was critical as it covered the early period of this clinic while its reputation as an important clinical service was established.

As a research clinic, all subjects coming into the clinic were regarded as participants in a research project. Signing informed consent for their participation ensured that the database could be established along these parameters. When the hospital would not fund the clinic, attempts were made to seek out other sources of funding, such as billing third parties for the assessments completed in the clinic. Again, this proved to be either difficult or impossible, as at that time any direct billing would be seen as a health care service and was frowned upon, even if it was not covered by the Ontario Health Insurance Plan. In this particular case, there was a question as to whether it would partially be covered, which made the whole situation ambiguous and therefore third party funding simply never materialized.

After about 5 years in operation, the hospital was persuaded to contact the Ministry of Health to see whether the laboratory could receive the necessary approval. Even though the funds could possibly have been obtained, this would not have maintained the running costs of the laboratory. It was hoped they would at least contribute something, as the laboratory was becoming a considerable drain on research funds. There were considerable problems with laboratory referrals in general. The rules maintained that the person running the laboratory could not refer patients to the laboratory themselves. As in this case the principal person who established the clinic (author JB) was also the person who would at that time make the bulk of the referrals. This then prevented the laboratory from being considered by the Ministry of Health, as it breached the referral protocol. Fortunately at this point, the hospital through its board became more convinced of the value of the Sexual Behaviours Clinic. The hospital initially partially funded the laboratory technician, initially at 25% of the salary, and then after a further 4-year period, assumed 100% of the technician's salary. At some point the Ministry of Health was approached for funding and partial funding was eventually allocated to the clinic. This was assigned to staff positions in psychology and social work, without any physician remuneration in the form of sessional money. There also was no money to cover administrative costs. As this money was included in the global budget of the hospital, over the years a struggle to maintain a small amount of this money proved to be the next battleground. Fortunately, with program management and the decentralization of budgets in relation to programs away from a central budgeting process, this has been possible. Upgrading the equipment in the laboratory (in terms of computers and software) has required a combination of research grant money, although more recently the hospital has funded the same as a capital cost.

The assessments completed in the Sexual Behaviours Clinic have never been billed directly, since the mechanisms for this have been problematic and have not been established. The exceptions to this would be clients from the United States or from other provinces in Canada and occasionally private clients where there may be a legal issue involved. To summarize, were it not for research grants and other than relatively small amounts of money from the Ministry of Health, this clinic would not exist today. The research status has been a benefit to the clinic rather than a handicap. However, the present round of health care cuts once again threatens the survival of the clinic and the laboratory in particular. Its complete reliance on research grants is likely to be necessary for its future survival. Currently, attempts are being made to see whether the assessment in the clinic can be billed directly to third parties. One of the problems, however, is that because this has never been done previously, those who have made referrals to the clinic in the past and essentially received this service free are now reluctant to pay for this service. Also, most people have their own financial difficulties, given the present financial environment, and this is proving to be a considerable struggle. Although research grants could contribute to the clinic, even these sources of funding are now more difficult to obtain, and the ongoing existence of the clinic is going to depend very much on its financial stability.

The timely emergence of the clinic coincided with heightened public awareness of the media attention to the topic of sexual abuse. The clinic rapidly gained a local, national, and international reputation for professionalism in the treatment and management of this group of offenders. The need for a specialized clinic of this nature is of paramount importance because of the chronicity of these disorders and to decrease the high recidivism of these offenders.

THE PROGRAM

Referrals, Legal Status, and Consent Issues

The clinic's referrals come from a wide array of sources including judges, the courts, crown attorneys, lawyers, physicians, other mental health professionals, and various agencies that deal with young offenders and developmentally challenged persons. Although the bulk of referrals initially came from the courts and lawyers, this mix has gradually changed since the inception of the clinic. Almost one third of the clinic's referrals are now made primarily by physicians. These patients are often persons with serious sexual disorders who have never been criminally charged with a sexual offense. Most referrals are local, although a number are referred from other provinces. Almost all of our patients are voluntary. Prior to commencing any assessment, all patients must consent to an evaluation process. Informed consent from the patient to undergo assessment and enter treatment and management at the clinic is pivotal to the ethical running of the program. Consent issues are carefully explored prior to any intervention being undertaken. Some offenders are on probation or parole or are transferred on a temporary absence pass from a detention center. A very small percentage of institutionalized patients in various secure facilities are referred on 30- or 60-day orders for specialized sexual assessment or initiation of a treatment program. Those offenders who have committed very serious violent offenses are admitted to the medium-secure facility located in the hospital. The Sexual Behaviours Clinic also has access to less secure hospital beds. Admission needs of a patient are dependent on the mental health legislation and their potential for relapse and assessment of their dangerousness at the time of the interview.

Assessment

Interview

Prior to initiating any treatment program, it is essential that a detailed comprehensive psychiatric assessment be completed. Each patient referred to the clinic must undergo a full psychiatric assessment including a detailed sexual history, family history, personal history, and past medical and psychiatric history. The reason for referral is explored in detail at the onset of the interview. Individuals may be pretrial, presentence, prerelease from custody, on probation, or other position in the criminal justice process. Patients also undergo a full mental status examination to exclude other psychiatric syndromes as well as a physical assessment where indicated. The importance of this critical step cannot be overlooked, and exclusion of other pathologies that are often associated with sexual offenders is pivotal to the success of any assessment–treatment program. It is not uncommon for the clinic to uncover psychopathology that often has been previously overlooked (e.g., Klinefelter's syndrome, cerebral arteriovenous malformations, temporal lobe epilepsy, and psychotic illnesses).

Investigations

Patients undergo comprehensive investigations including blood and urine analysis. Requests for a full sex hormone profile including free testosterone, total testosterone, sex hormone binding globulin, follicular stimulating hormone, luteinizing hormone, progesterone, estradiol, and prolactin are routine. The clinic also may request a complete blood count and urea, electrolytes, liver function and renal tests in patients where there is likelihood of the patient having psychopharmacological interventions at a later stage in the treatment process. Where other pathologies are suspected, the appropriate biochemical and serum tests are also requested. Urine drug screen as well as urinalysis may also be indicated in certain patients to exclude other psychopathology. For research purposes the clinic also has access to sophisticated serotonin markers such as H3 imipramine, lysergic acid diethylamide, and paroxetine binding platelet uptake markers.

Subjects complete a variety of sexual history questionnaires. The clinic uses various structured self-report questionnaires including the Bradford Sexual History Questionnaire, the Forensic Assessment Form, Abel and Becker's Cognition Scale, Michigan Alcohol Screening Test, Drug Abuse Screening Test, the Greenberg Sexual Preference Analogue Scale, the Sexual Fantasy Checklist, and other questionnaires designed to elicit adversarial and coercive perceptions, among others. Each client also completes a computer-generated. Decision Base self-generated diagnosis (Long, 1992). Research has shown the extensive comorbidity between the various paraphilias and other psychiatric syndromes. The clinic has found this to be an invaluable tool in the assessment of these offenders.

Penile plethysmography remains the most objective measure of male sexual arousal (Zuckerman, 1971). Travin, Cullen, and Melella (1988) reported that nearly 94% of convicted sexual offenders tested positively for pedophilic arousal with penile phallometry. This investigation is a valid and reliable objective measure of erotic sexual preference (Murphy & Barbaree, 1988). The potential abuse or misuse of this instrument lies primarily in the use of this testing as the sole basis for deciding issues at the preconviction stages of legal proceedings. Standardization of the test equipment with normal controls has been completed at our clinic and is considered essential to the functioning of this procedure. Denial and clandestine modus operandi of these offenders make this tool invaluable in the assessment of sexual offenders.

Where indicated, patients are also seen by a social worker who obtains collateral information from family and friends. Police records and other relevant court documents are requested by the psychiatrist. Neuropsychological or general psychometric testing are also requested when indicated for intelligence scores, cognitive deficits, and personality inventories. The clinic also utilizes various neuropsychiatric investigations such as computerized tomographic head scans, single-spectrum emission tomography, magnetic resonance imaging, and electroencephalography where indicated. One of the unique features of the clinic is the access to consultations from a wide variety of psychiatric experts where there is comorbid psychopathology. Neuropsychiatry, alcohol and drug addictions, schizophrenia, mood disorders, and geriatrics are some of the psychiatric subspecialties from which additional assessments may be requested.

The clinic also has been assigned as a beta test site for the Abel Assessment screen for interest in paraphilias (Abel, 1995). This is a computerized physiological test in which subjects are shown 160 slides of clothed adults, teenagers, and children over a 30-minute period. Results are reported using z scores for objective interest in 22 paraphilias.

Interpretation and Debriefing

Once all of the data and information have been elicited and collected, patients are always debriefed on their results. Full comprehensive disclosure of all the results and investigations as well as the psychiatrist's diagnostic opinions are discussed during the debriefing session. This is a valuable part of any treatment program, since it provides an opportunity for patients to ask any questions, to dispel any myths, and to assess their motivation and insight. Motivation of subjects should be seen on a continuum ranging from highly unmotivated clients who may deny the offenses to persons who are so-called "admitters" with good insight and motivation for seeking treatment for their problematic sexual behaviors. As patients proceed through the assessment process and debriefing, they will often gain valuable insight into their psychopathology. Debriefing also provides an opportunity to provide information about the treatment and management program in the short and long term. Difficulties raised at this stage can then be identified and dealt with by the therapist and patient. Often one of the most fundamental problems in working with this population group is poor insight and denial of the offense or other unconventional sexual behaviors. It has been reported that in a group of sexual offenders, almost half admit to their sexual offense. However, following penile tumescent studies and debriefing, half of the nonadmitters will then subsequently admit to the offense. This therefore means that almost 75% of patients referred to the clinic admit to the offense. The remaining 25% are either returned to their probation or parole officers or to the courts or lawyers. It is not uncommon for some of these offenders to present at a later date with new charges or a reconviction for a similar offense and finally be willing to acknowledge their sexual difficulties and need for treatment.

Although patients are diagnosed using the *Diagnostic and Statistical Manual of Mental Disorders*, 4th edition (DSM) criteria (American Psychiatric Association, 1994), some behaviors do not fit into any diagnostic category. Examples of this include rape, some incest offenders, inappropriate sexual behavior in developmentally challenged persons, and hypersexuality. Diagnostic categories such as Paraphilia Disorder Not Otherwise Specified or Sexual Disorder Not Otherwise Specified are therefore utilized with these behaviors.

Treatment and Management

Principles

The essential principal in any treatment and management program is the least restrictive and least intrusive intervention needed to adequately control the offender's problematic behavior. This may change over the course of their involvement with the clinic. The primary focus of any treatment program is to empower the individual to take responsibility for his behavior. Initially this may involve external controls, but gradually during development of a program the offender is encouraged to take responsibility for his own symptoms and behavior. The offender must recognize early precipitating trigger or perpetuating factors that exacerbate lapse symptoms. The clinic interventions are initially short term but nevertheless are integrated with a long-term commitment to psychiatric follow-up and relapse prevention techniques. Adaptive consensual and "conventional" sexual behaviors are encouraged to provide a meaningful sexual outlet for these offenders' sexual drives.

Psychopharmacological Treatments

Psychopharmacological agents are frequently overlooked by the therapeutic community because of ethical concerns, clinical misperceptions, and lack of expertise with these agents or lack of clinical resources. There is a wide and extensive body of literature on the efficacy and effectiveness of these agents in treating these disorders (Bradford, 1985; Green, 1992). Psychopharmacological treatment of sexual offenders is based on the assumption that depression of the sexual drive will result in a decrease in paraphilic behavior. The fundamental elements of sexual drive are sexual fantasies, sexual urges, and sexual behaviors. If there is a global reduction of sexual drive, then the paraphilic fantasies, urges, and behavior will also be reduced. Testosterone is the principal androgen produced by the testes in most of the animal species. In animal studies, the higher the level of evolution of the species, the less direct the influence of hormones on sexual behavior. The effects of plasma testosterone are mediated through action on intracellular androgen receptors on target organs. Testosterone is metabolized to dihydrotestosterone, which binds to the androgen receptors. Testosterone is also converted to estrogens in the brain and then may act through estrogen receptors. The binding of the hormone to the receptor sites can be inhibited by competitive and noncompetitive mechanisms. Androgen receptors are found in the various androgen-sensitive organs such as the prostate and various parts of the brain including the limbic system and anterior hypothalamus. The behavioral effects of testosterone are the result of its action on the brain, although the principal site of action is a matter of some debate.

Cyproterone acetate (CPA) has antiandrogen, antigonatropic, and progestational effects. Its principal mode of action is on the androgen receptors where it blocks the intracellular testosterone uptake and the intracellular metabolism of the androgen. Spermatogenesis, erections, and ejaculation are all decreased. Sexual fantasies are suppressed or at times completely eliminated. CPA also has a strong progestational action. The specific mode of action of CPA is competitive inhibition of testosterone and dihydroxytestosterone at specific androgen receptor sites. Liver dysfunctional adrenal suppression and feminization are unlikely but are possible risks to the patient who is prescribed this medication. Other unwanted side effects observed during the first two months of therapy include fatigue, hypersomnia, depression, negative nitrogen balance, and weight gain. Various studies have shown a substantial reduction of sexual arousal patterns of various sex offenders with CPA. CPA can reduce deviant sexual arousal while having less of an impact on nondeviant arousal responses (Bradford & Pawlak, 1993). It has been well documented that CPA can substantially reduce the recidivism rates of sexual offenders, and these beneficial effects may continue even when treatment is terminated.

Medroxyprogesterone (MPA) is a hormonal agent that has been used to treat sexual deviancy since the mid-1950s. The principal mechanism of action of MPA is through the induction of testosterone-A-reductase in the liver. It enhances metabolic clearance of testosterone. Plasma levels of testosterone are reduced. It also has an antigonotropic effect. Potential side effects of MPA treatment have included weight gain, decreased sperm production, hyperinsulinemic response to glucose load, and gallbladder and gastrointestinal dysfunction. However, desirable effects on sexual functioning were observed including reduction of sexual drive, erotic fantasy, sexual activity, and possible aggressiveness. There have been numerous reports that MPA appears to be effective in the treatment of sexual offenders provided there is compliance with treatment. Compliance with treatment has been reported to be a difficulty with this type of therapy.

Unfortunately, these agents were initially used in high doses with the intent of obliterating all sexual behaviors. This attracted the label of "chemical castration," and therefore proved unpopular with patients. Our experience has been to prescribe these agents in low doses. Rather than obliterate all sexual behavior, the primary aim is to empower the patient to master control over his or her sexual urges and drives. Kafka (1991) reported that the paraphilias are associated with a high sex drive. Some subjects masturbate five or more times a day. Patients reduce their sexual activity (i.e., masturbation or coitus) with these agents while still maintaining adequate erections and ejaculatory ability. Patients are fully informed about the approved indications and potential adverse effects of these medications. However, in practice relatively few serious side effects are reported by patients, and patients are closely monitored clinically with periodic blood analysis.

More recently the selective serotonin reuptake inhibitors have been reported to have potential therapeutic benefits, although to date no double-blind placebo cross-over trials have been completed. Various studies have reported on the efficacy of these agents (Greenberg & Bradford, 1997; Bradford, Greenberg, Gojer, Martindale, & Goldberg, 1995; Greenberg, Bradford, Curry, & O'Rourke, 1996a,b). The underlying hypothesis is that the paraphilias are associated with the obsessive–compulsive disorders spectrum such that where patients have recurrent and persistent sexual fantasies, they should be responsive to these serotonergic agents.

Psychological Interventions

Various cognitive–behavioral techniques are used at the clinic including covert sensitization, masturbatory reconditioning, and restructuring of cognitive distortions. Aversion techniques are not used in this clinic due to ethical concerns with these interventions. Each patient receives relapse prevention training, supportive psychotherapy, and psychological counseling to provide a holistic approach to the individual and his needs in the community. Individual relapse prevention focuses on decreasing the occurrence of unconventional stimuli that often lead to the precipitation of a chain of events leading to relapse. Subjects are encouraged to avoid high-risk situations as well as to decrease visual scanning or visual staring at inappropriate sexual targets. Patients are also taught about thought-blocking techniques. They are counseled about the importance of abstaining from masturbation in association with unconventional sexual fantasies, visual material, or other stimuli. Individuals who report fantasizing about their unconventional sexual practices during coitus are strongly encouraged to discontinue such practices.

Social Interventions

The clinic has a wide variety of groups that are run concurrently with individual therapeutic interventions. These separate groups target deficits in patients, sex education, social skills, anger management, and family dynamics. Our relapse prevention group is based on the 12-step program adopted by Alcoholics Anonymous. The clinic also has access to a wide variety of groups that are available in a psychiatric facility, for example, anxiety management and various support groups for families with associated mental illness.

Consultation for Comorbid Psychiatric Disorders

Other professionals may be consulted to assist in the treatment program. For example, substance abuse cases may be referred to the alcohol and addiction program; patients with epilepsy referred to neuropsychiatric unit; and patients with various psychiatric disorders, including psychotic disorders, mood disorders, and anxiety disorders, to the appropriate clinics for concurrent interventions. This multiaxis intervention provides a holistic approach to our patients' problems.

Long-Term Follow-up and Relapse Prevention

Subjects are gradually empowered to manage their own sexual disorders. With improved insight, motivation, and understanding of relapse prevention techniques, subjects are encouraged to monitor their possible relapse symptoms. When individuals have lapse symptoms such as increased paraphilic sexual preoccupations, sexual fantasies, sexual images, sexual thoughts, sexual ideas, or use of coercive nonconsensual pornographic material, they can access the available relapse prevention resources. This provides for a long-term crisis intervention program. We provide a 24-hour psychiatric emergency service and the availability of the individual's treating psychiatrist during office hours. Eventually, patients may only see their psychiatrist once a year for booster sessions, but they are encouraged that should they have lapse signs or symptoms they can access their therapist or support resources in a timely manner. Self-directed relapse prevention interventions are encouraged as a way of life. These patients are given reassurance that the hospital will provide a safety net should their symptoms of sexual disorders again lapse.

EDUCATION AND RESEARCH

Education

The Sexual Behaviours Clinic provides education to a wide variety of individuals including medical students, nurses, criminology students, law students, psychiatric residents, psychology students, and others. The clinic has promoted a wide variety of educational initiatives including community-oriented education days as well as guest speaker opportunities, both locally, nationally, and internationally. The clinic also has a record for providing expertise to other programs both nationally and internationally to initiate similar sexual behaviors clinics. It is estimated that over 200 workshops, seminars, and academic presentations in the field of sexual disorders have been presented over the past 15 years.

Research

The research component of any sexual behaviors clinic is, we feel, fundamental and essential to the working of such a clinic. It provides a valuable opportunity to disseminate information to our peers and the public. Approximately 10 peer-reviewed papers are presented at both national and international congresses each year. The clinic has an impressive list of publications and continues to remain committed to this important area. All information obtained during the assessment and treatment of various offenders is collected into our database and maintained with complete confidentiality. Informed consent is obtained from all individuals. This has provided us with a very large database on this particular population. The clinic now has a database of almost 2500 subjects, collected over the past 15 years.

CONCLUSIONS

The assessment of sexual offenders requires good interviewing skills that will elicit detailed comprehensive information about the sexual offenders' pattern of behavior. Individuals with paraphilic disorders often have multiple paraphilias and comorbid diagnoses (Bradford, Boulet, & Pawlak, 1992). The problems of denial, minimization, and guarding need to be adequately dealt with during this process. A high index of suspicion is often warranted with certain sexual offenders. Prior to implementing any interventions, assessment of motivation, insight and commitment to treatment need to be addressed. The importance of aftercare and long-term follow-up has been addressed in this chapter. Some referrals are not suitable candidates for proposed interventions and may be best dealt with by the criminal justice system. In reality most candidates have a potential for rehabilitation, but community fears are often driven by highly publicized sensational cases.

REFERENCES

Abel, G. (1995). *Abel screening*. Atlanta, GA: Abel Screening, Inc.

American Psychiatric Association. (1994). *Diagnostic and Statistical Manual of Mental Disorders* (4th ed.). Washington, DC: Author.

Bradford, J. M. W. (1985). *Organic treatment for the male sexual offender*. Behavioral Sciences and the Law. New York: Wiley.

Bradford, J. M. W., Boulet, J., & Pawlak, A. (1992). The paraphilias: A multiplicity of deviant behaviors. *Canadian Journal of Psychiatry, 37*, 104–108.

Bradford, J. M. W., & Pawlak, A. (1993). The effects of cyproterone acetate on sexual arousal patterns of paedophiles. *Archives of Sexual Behaviour, 22*, 629–641.

Bradford, J. M. W., Greenberg, D., Gojer, J., Martindale, J. J., & Goldberg, M. (1995, May). Sertraline in the treatment of pedophilia: An open label study. Presented at the Annual American Psychiatric Association, Miami, FL.

Green, R. (1992). *Sexual science and the law*. Cambridge, MA: Harvard Press.

Greenberg, D. M., Bradford, J. M. W., Curry, S., & O'Rourke, A. (1996a). A comparison of treatment of paraphilias with three serotonin re-uptake inhibitors: A retrospective study. *Bulletin of the American Academy of Psychiatry and the Law, 24*, 525–532.

Greenberg, D. M., Bradford, J. M. W., Curry, S., & O'Rourke, A. (1996b, March). A controlled study of the treatment of the paraphilias with selective serotonin re-uptake inhibitors. Presented at the annual Canadian Academy of Psychiatry and the Law, Mt. Tremblant, Quebec, Canada.

Greenberg, D. M., & Bradford, J. M. (1997). Treatment of the paraphilic disorders: A review of the role of the selective serotonin reuptake inhibitors. *Sexual Abuse: A Journal of Research and Treatment, 9*, 349–360.

Kafka, M. (1991). Successful antidepressant treatment of nonparaphilic sexual addictions and paraphilias in men. *Journal Clinical Psychiatry, 52*, 60–65.

Long, P. W. (1992). Decision Base Version 2.5. Vancouver, BC: Decision Base.

Murphy, W. D., & Barbaree, H. E. (1988). *Assessments of sexual offenders by measures of erectile response: Psychometric properties and decision making*. Washington, DC: National Institute of Mental Health.

Travin, S., Cullen, K., & Melella, J. J. (1988). The use and abuse of erection measurements: A forensic prospective. *Bulletin of the American Academy of Psychiatry and the Law, 16*(3), 235–250.

Zuckerman, M. (1971). Physiological measures of sexual arousal in the human. *Psychological Bulletin, 75*, 297–329.

II

Diverse Populations

18

An 11-Year Perspective
of Working with Female
Sexual Offenders

Jane Kinder Matthews

I met my first female sexual offender in May 1985. Probation officers in Hennepin and Ramsey Counties, Minnesota, were looking for therapeutic resources for women coming out of prison or through the court system who had been convicted of sexual abuse. Based on my experience with adult male sexual offenders and Ruth Mathews' experience with adolescent male sexual offenders, we were asked to develop a treatment program for these women. Funding via a 2-year start-up grant from the General Mills Foundation had been secured.

We had no idea what elements of male treatment would transfer to the women. Neither did we have any idea how women would respond to treatment. We could only guess at the backgrounds of these women and hope that we could delineate the myriad contributing factors that led to their behavior and plan our therapeutic interventions accordingly. Being optimists, we met and worked backward, making our best guess about who these people were and what was going on with them, using our intuitions to devise an intake interview that we hoped would get the information we needed.

Late on a Friday afternoon, our speculations about these women would be tested, as I was about to interview the first woman candidate for treatment. I knew her name well in advance; hers was a highly publicized case. I expected a hostile, unrepentant monster as I armed myself with my notebook and our well-reasoned intake interview. What I found when I entered the interview room was a tiny woman curled in the corner of a large leather sofa. She looked almost childlike herself, with her knees tucked up close to her and her feet to her side. Ruth and I had decided that our first question must be about the sexual crime. We believed that we needed to get that out of the way as soon as possible. It would give us a barometer of the woman's willingness to be honest and also remove the tension and expectations as she waited for the inevitable, terrible question.

I introduced myself and sat down across from her. "Tell me about the sexual abuse," I said, and tell me she did. Without a flinch, without an excuse, and totally without rationaliz-

Jane Kinder Matthews • Transition Place, Minneapolis, Minnesota 55414.

Sourcebook of Treatment Programs for Sexual Offenders, edited by Marshall et al. Plenum Press, New York, 1998.

ation, she told me everything. She took total responsibility for what had happened and when I asked her how she believed her victims felt she replied, "It was horrible for them, and they didn't deserve it."

My concept of a hostile, resistant, denying monster faded fast, and my curiosity and fascination were piqued. As I went on with the interview she related a background of unbelievable pain and tragedy with the same matter-of-fact delivery with which she had described her crime. She asked for no pity and made no excuses. She made no attempt to blame the victim and made no attempt to blame society or a coercive husband. "I should have known better, and I should have done better" was her explanation. At the end of the interview when I asked her why she was so forthright, she explained that she had nothing to lose; she had lost it all already and that telling the truth was easier than lying. "The lies are really hard, and this is the only way I can get help."

I emerged from my first encounter with a female sexual offender emotionally drained and awed. She was not what I expected, and the subsequent 11 years have not been what I expected. There have been those who were resistant, who minimized their culpability in the crimes, who blamed the victim, who saw no reason to change or get help, and who undermined our efforts, but the majority of the female offenders won my respect and I have constantly been impressed by their dignity and strength.

I like them very much, but that is not to say that I like what they have done or that I excuse what they have done. They have hurt other people, and I fully acknowledge that they have caused a great deal of pain. They also have suffered a great deal of pain, and we acknowledge that as well.

Sexual abuse is a complicated subject and many factors are involved. Sexual abuse perpetrated by a woman is often seen as more complicated, more bizarre. However, this is not the view we have developed. We do not regard female sexual offenders as bizarre, because we have learned that their behavior is based on very human frailties. They are motivated by anger, fear, revenge, and by accepting as normal what the rest of society knows is abusive. They act out of their own experiences and out of the experiences of the men in their lives. They respond to adolescents as though they were adults and ascribe adult abilities and skills to them. They desperately seek contact and affiliation. Whatever the motivation, we believe it is important to try our best to help these women alter their abusive behavior and repair as much of the damage as possible.

Some of our clients participate in treatment for sexual abuse even though they do not have a criminal conviction. If it is abusive, we call it a crime. If it could have resulted in a criminal conviction, we refer to it as a crime. We delineate our women according to their behavior, not according to their status as a referral from criminal justice or child protection agencies. Referring to them all as criminals may not be technically correct, but I have chosen to do so. Dividing them according to their legal status could compromise their anonymity, and the behavior is the same, regardless of the consequences that a woman may suffer because of it.

TYPOLOGIES

We have developed a system for categorizing our clients into one of three types. These three types are: teacher–lover, predisposed, and male-coerced. While there are many commonalities in the lives of these women, the different types present different developmental backgrounds and different therapeutic requirements.

Our first group of six women was evenly divided between those who had been coerced into sexual abuse by a male and those who had initiated the sexual contact themselves and acted alone. Later, a woman was referred who had been charged with sexual abuse because of sexual contact with an adolescent male. In this case she seemed to play the dual roles of teacher and lover toward the youth.

Subsequently we have consistently seen female sexual offenders who appear to fall naturally into one of these three types. The women also seemed to divide along these same lines in terms of their backgrounds and their adjustment to life. These three basic typologies have held for 11 years. There certainly are areas of overlap and there are individual differences within a typology, but they provide separations that have been helpful in dealing with these women. We utilize them as a means of organizing our data and deciding on our therapeutic approach. As we gather more data and meet more female offenders, these typologies and subsets are likely to change. The literature also cites a severely disturbed type of female sexual offender whose motivation is based on psychosis and a failure in her ability to differentiate between herself and her child(ren). We have not worked with any women in this category, and therefore will have no discussion of that type of sexual abuse perpetration.

Table 18.1 describes the characteristics of our three types.

TABLE 18.1
Characteristics of Female Sexual Offenders

	Teacher—lover	Predisposed	Male-coerced
Chaotic childhood	X	X	X
Tenuous relationship with family members	X	X	X
Emotionally/physically abused as a child	X	X	X
Low status member of childhood peer groups	X	X	X
Victim of childhood sexual abuse within family		X	
Victim of childhood sexual abuse by stranger			X
Poor school performance	X	X	X
Desperate need for affiliation		X	X
Marginal adjustment as an adult	X		
Poor adjustment as an adult		X	X
Sees herself powerless in adult relationships	X	X	X
Tenuous and difficult adult relationships	X	X	X
Physically and sexually abused by partners as an adults	X	X	X
Isolates as a way of protecting self		X	
Severe emotional problems		X	
Many self defeating and self-punishing behaviors		X	X
Self-hatred		X	X
Chemical problems as an adult			X
Low self-esteem	X	X	X
Male dependent			X
Feels unlovable		X	X
Easily threatened		X	X
Stays in abusive relationships because she feels no one else will have her			X
Bothered by deviant sexual fantasies when angry hurt or lonely		X	
Sexually abuses her own child		X	
Coerced into sexual abuse of others			X
Elevates an adolescent to adult status in her mind	X		
Falls in love with her victim and sees abuse as an expression of love	X		

DIFFERENCES BETWEEN MALE AND FEMALE OFFENDERS

I have previously listed (Matthews, 1993) the apparent differences between male and female sexual offenders based on my work with both. None of the women we have worked with has coerced others into being accomplices. Women use force or violence in committing their crimes far less often than men. When they do use physical force, it is of a lesser degree than males. Women tend to use fewer threats in an attempt to keep their victims silent. Fewer women initially deny the abuse and they are more willing to take responsibility for their behavior. Men tend to start sexually abusing at an earlier age (i.e., in adolescence). Only 2 of our 36 clients acted out as teenagers. Women tend to act out on themselves through self-punitive and self-destructive behavior, such as starving and cutting themselves, prostitution, and placing themselves in very dangerous situations before they act out on others.

In responding to therapy, men tend to forgive themselves more quickly than the women, and they tend to move more rapidly from shame to guilt, giving themselves permission to heal sooner. Men tend to develop empathy for the victim later in the course of their therapy; but even after women have developed empathy, they tend to continue to feel ashamed for their abusive behavior. Women's anger toward themselves tends to be more deeply entrenched and more difficult to alter.

Victims of both male and female sexual offenders sometimes include adolescents. In the case of females, this victimization pattern indicates the abuser with the least pathology. In the case of males, it indicates a great deal of pathology. The women in this category take the least time in therapy, but the men take as long as other perpetrators.

In addition to these differences and similarities it should be noted that, in our experience, women self-report abuse perpetration more often than men, and women who self-report are more likely to successfully complete treatment.

EVALUATING TREATMENT

Therapeutic Strategies

A major therapeutic decision revolves around the question of whether, with female sexual offenders, we are dealing with perpetrators or victims. The answer, of course, is that they are both. Given the often devastating backgrounds of these women, they could present themselves at any mental health clinic and ask for help in resolving those issues. We suggest that focusing only on the perpetration issues will deny the basic humanity of these women. Focusing only on their status as victims will absolve them of responsibility for their own crimes and make it attractive to remain in the victim role. We also believe they are probably unable to develop genuine empathy for their victims and truly to understand the impact of their behavior until they have received empathic support for their own pain. They have practiced suppressing their feelings for so long that being numb is natural for them. They learned first not to feel for themselves, and this generalized to others. They need to experience the developmental support that they missed in order to rebuild themselves first. The natural progression is that they voice their own pain, restore some of the damage that was done to them, and then begin to be strong enough and sound enough to develop empathy for their victims. We say that they must cry for themselves before they can cry for others, and when those tears do come they are likely to be genuine. When focusing on their own pain we do not negate the pain they have caused. Addressing it is merely deferred. To force them into mechanical statements of remorse is to teach them that they must once again comply with empty commands and compromise their own reality. Our therapeutic approach is supportive without being coddling, confrontive without attacking. We do not yell, demean, use sarcasm, or pit the women against each other. We believe that they must learn to trust and they cannot trust if they fear us. They also cannot respect us if we are so flexible and easy that we do not require them to face their issues. We try to model honesty and require that in our clients.

All clients must meet the following therapeutic goals: They must acknowledge the abuse; take responsibility for it; define, with the help of therapy group and therapist, individual emotional–behavioral issues; address issues specific to their typology and self; complete victim empathy work; devise exit criteria with the help of the therapists; and devise a prevention plan and aftercare plan.

THERAPY GOALS FOR EACH TYPOLOGY

Teacher–Lover

In most instances this type of offender is quite easy therapeutically. The main goal is to get these women to understand that what they did caused harm. These women often present with the statement, "I'm really angry. I've got a criminal charge and he got off scott free." They believe that, if the sexual contact was wrong, then the adolescent who was also involved was equally to blame. Once the offender understands that there was a power differential and that she, as the adult, was responsible for keeping the boundaries, she can move on quite quickly. Having these women understand that adolescents may experience confusion and a sense of failure and inadequacy as a result of the sexual contact is a major goal. When they come to understand that they may have added to the stress and trauma of a youngster who was already stressed and feeling inadequate, they often make a statement such as, "What could I have been thinking." Recently we have encountered women in this category who did require a longer time in treatment in order to address deeper, more complex psychological problems. The primary goal is still for them to acknowledge and understand the abuse and the impact of the abuse on the victim. They have the additional challenge of rebuilding a more shattered self.

Predisposed

These clients have the most devastating backgrounds and the most damage to repair. They have very few coping skills and very few positive associations. Their families may be nonsupportive and may not want the offender to deal with her abuse issues, as, all too often, it is a family member who abused her. The primary goal is to build the self-confidence of these women. Their self-esteem must be elevated and they must start believing that people can care for them. Their affiliation needs must be met by someone other than their children.

The most important therapeutic goal is for these women to voice their own childhood pain and sort out all the conflicting emotions of their chaotic experiences. They may both love and hate their parents, hate the parents for their abuse or nonsupport, and at the same time desperately hope that their family has changed and can finally offer love and support to them. These offenders often want but fear an adult partner. They can be rejecting and clinging in regard to their own child, and they may vacillate between confidence and withdrawal.

Our goals with these women include the development of a social network, which is a very tall order. They typically fear rejection and find it difficult to trust. In addition, they must address their extremely self-abusive or suicidal behavior, and reduce their own self-hatred. They must also develop a method to deal with deviant sexual fantasies.

Male-Coerced

Women of this type may not have abused initially without the coercion of a male, so a primary goal is to decrease their male dependence. They must learn that they have worth even if there is no man in their lives. We also assist them to learn that their voice is important and that they have an obligation to speak up and practice assertive behavior. They need to recognize that they do not have to please everybody. Most importantly, these women need to develop job skills and the skills necessary so that they can be self-supporting.

REACTIONS TO FEMALE-PERPETRATED ABUSE

In speaking about his adolescent sexual contact with an older woman, an adult male sexual offender stated, "I knew if felt weird and yukky to be involved with her. I was scared to death of her boyfriend, and I just hated being around them both. It was just a real nervous, embarrassed feeling." What this young man is describing are some of the results of sexual abuse. The term *sexual abuse* is such an inflammatory term that we hear it and imagine sexual intercourse forced with gun or knife. We tend to think only of the physical consequences of sexual abuse, but the emotional consequences are also devastating. The crimes of the predisposed and male-coerced offenders conform with the traditional concept of sexual abuse. The victims are children, there is force, and the damage is apparent to all. With the teacher–lover offender we must confront mainly the psychological trauma.

Why is this kind of contact devastating? An adolescent certainly has sexual curiosity and sexual arousal. The adolescent may have done some sexual experimenting, but most adolescents view adults as old, over the hill, unexciting, and unattractive. The sexual contact often brings a sense of shame and failure. A boy who has not established sexual relations with a peer may be attracted to an adult female but may conclude that he has settled for sex with someone who is second best, and he may want to deny it. His willingness to accept what he considers to be an inferior relationship may cause him to think he also is inferior.

Sexual contacts of this kind may undermine an already shaky self-esteem. Adolescent boys who become companions of older women, befriend their children, and help with chores are very likely to be needy and to have feelings of inadequacy. The adolescent may be isolated from peers and rejected by family. He may also have been the victim of sexual abuse earlier and have sexualized behavior. He is likely schooled in the art of acting tough and talking big, projecting a competent facade that belies his vulnerability. To the teacher–lover female he is a younger, smaller, and therefore less threatening version of the men she has had in her life. She assumes that she can be involved with him, have the love and companionship that she desires without having the pain, abuse, and degradation that have accompanied many of her other relationships. He seems perfect and she falls in love.

For the female adolescent who gets involved with a female teacher–lover, she often comes from a chaotic background, has low self-esteem, and is in desperate need of affiliation, affection, and acceptance. She, too, may have been the victim of sexual abuse and may have learned that sexual contact will keep people around and keep them involved. Her sexualized behavior may be seen by the offender as seductive and purposeful.

The sexual response for these adolescents is overshadowed by what they lose. What the teacher–lover takes from them is the time to explore sexuality and relationships with their peers. They do not get to experience falling in and out of love, negotiating and renegotiating associations. They do not get to decide when and how they will develop their sexuality. The older person may be demanding and coercive if the younger person wants to leave; therefore, the adolescent is asked to give up his or her desires and wishes in order to accommodate the adult. Male adolescents usually react in two ways: they resent the restrictions or they become desperately clingy and demanding. If the woman sees the sexual contact as merely a transient affair, the needy boy may be devastated and feel abandoned all over again. He may also make unrealistic demands of his future sexual partners, expecting the experience and focus that the older woman was willing to give him. Because of his discomfort he may try to get out of the relationship by creating crises and forcing her to push him away. If that does not work, he may become physically abusive. So, in many cases, the peaceful, loving relationship that a woman had hoped for becomes as violent as her relationships with older men. His resentment may be fueled in other ways. She can be ready to settle down and he does not even know who he is.

There are certainly times when the adolescent believes he or she is in love with the older woman. If the offender merely views their sexual contact as an affair of no significance, the young person can be devastated. The adult may want to move on, forget about the event, and get on with her life. The vulnerable adolescent will be deeply hurt, often feeling convinced that she or he is worthless and unlovable. The teacher–lover's attempts to find a nonabusive love match often backfires. She often can feel rejected or suffer physical abuse and the young person inherits a heavy load of emotional baggage that may be carried for a long time.

REUNIFICATION

Perhaps no other aspect of working with this population offers as much frustration as trying to determine if they should be reunited with their children. There are assumptions that once a woman has acted out sexually, every person she meets is a potential victim. Nothing could be further from the truth, but it is the argument that we lose the most often.

One client had sexual contact with her teenaged son. She replicated the abuse that was rampant in her own family for generations. She lived for 35 years without abusing any other child in any other manner. If past behavior is the best indicator of future behavior, it would be safe to say that the critical aspects of her case would indicate that her danger situations would be contact with her own son or with someone in a surrogate son position. Family therapy with her son was begun and went well. The foundations for a positive, healthy relationship were established. Her victim showed no fear and expressed gratitude that this once-abusive relationship was being repaired. She could have contact, in a therapeutic setting or planned structure, with her victim, but the restrictions placed on other aspects of her life by corrections officials were quite stringent. She was to have no contact with any child. She was to have no contact with any vulnerable adult. She was to have no contact with any adolescent. Her probation could have been violated for merely riding a bus or walking down a street. Try as we might, the probation officer and I could not get those restrictions altered. I wrote letter after letter to potential employers stating that she was not a threat to customers or co-workers. None were willing to take a chance until a very courageous probation officer gave her permission to work in an occupation that was technically off-limits to her. We set up very strict parameters under which she would interact with those around her and determined ways that she could protect herself from false allegations. It worked, and her very long struggle to become a positive member of society was rewarded.

There is also an assumption that once a woman has sexually abused someone, that her own children are vulnerable. For the teacher–lover offender, who has not harmed her own children, this poses a particularly difficult situation. Her children certainly do suffer because of the sexual abuse, and we classify them as secondary victims. As her victims are often the friends of her children, they lose a friend and are acutely embarrassed by the behavior of their mother. However, the mother–child bond between these women and their children is sometimes extremely strong and we work very hard to reunify. Resistance often comes from well-meaning foster families and guardians who believe that we are advocating placing these children back into dangerous situations. We have no desire to do so and believe that decisions about the mother's ability to meet her children's needs must be made on a case-by-case basis. Where the bond is strong, every effort should be made to reunify. In chaotic situations, the mother may have offered love, support, and guidance under extremely trying circumstances and this primal bond is a part of the child's memory. We certainly believe that, whatever the issues, family therapy should be a part of any reunification plan, for sexual abuse is seldom the only problem in these families. Healthy family relationships mean that the children need to be able to discuss their problems, fears, and difficulties in a supportive, accepting atmosphere.

When the woman's own children are her victims, the decision to reunify is more difficult. The age of the children at the time of the offense and at the time of possible reunification is important. The severity and duration of the abuse is also important. Of paramount consideration are the attitudes and skills of the mother and the feelings of the victim(s).

Some children of our clients have threatened to commit suicide and to run away if they were kept in foster care any longer. They want to be with their mother even if their lives will not be easy. They hate the idea of being regarded as "foster home freaks" at school. Children have been known to play foster parents and biological parents against each other, stating to their mother that they want to come home and stating to foster parents that they want to remain with them. Teenaged victims report more ambiguity when it comes to reunification. They may be enjoying the material comforts of a more affluent home and may be loathe to relinquish them. They may want to bring their mother into their sphere while continuing to live with foster parents. They may also dread the embarrassment of reunification if they are to return to the community where their mother's crime is known. They sometimes want to avoid family therapy, which is mandatory in any reunification plan. They want to avoid the pain of revisiting the abuse and confronting their mother with their feelings and reactions to the abuse. In most cases the desires of the children will become known, and while there are many difficult issues in reunification, we try to achieve it if the mother can meet the children's needs and protect them from further abuse. Getting all involved to agree on when this should happen is a challenge.

ADAPTING THE PROGRAM TO PRISON

In April 1995, I was asked to provide treatment and to develop a program for the prison population of female sexual offenders at the Minnesota Correctional Facility in Shakopee. I initially saw these women individually. Most of them had been in the institution for at least 6 months and had had time to learn that sexual offenders were on the lowest rung of the ladder in the eyes of their fellow inmates. Only a few were comfortable with other people in the institution knowing what they had done. Those tended to be the ones whose cases had received wide publicity before they came to prison. The other inmates knew details of their crime before they appeared in the population, so they only had to match the name to the newspaper article.

All of the women responded very well to individual treatment. They expressed gratitude at the nonjudgmental attitude and were generally relieved that they could finally talk about themselves. They could identify many deficiencies and problems that plagued them, and they were clear that they wanted help. When financial constraints dictated that we change to a group format, the women reacted negatively. A few were very resistant, stating again and again that they did not need treatment, that they had put their own abuse and the crimes they had committed behind them. Others expressed fear and anger that the work they had been doing individually must now be done in group and they were more timid in bringing up their issues. Confidentiality was of utmost importance to them, and we spent many sessions struggling with this issue. They were absolutely terrified that word of their sexual crimes would get out and that other inmates would know about them.

When these women were questioned closely, very few of them had ever been directly threatened. Their fear seemed to be more that people would know about them and demean them verbally or behind their backs. In the discussions, it occurred to me that this situation was rather like a very mean junior high school. Being talked about seemed horrible to some of these women, and status was basically the only thing that they had left. This situation defined one of our goals that outpatient women do not need to confront: that of maintaining one's dignity in spite of what people may say or do. We worked very hard to help them hold their heads up regardless of what anyone said or regardless of what they thought someone was saying about them. We did role-plays and brainstorming about replies that they might give if another inmate made a derogatory remark about their crime. One important concession that I made to the prison population was to alter the requirement that the women state their crimes to the entire group. It was understood that they would have to share their crime, but they could do so with a small number of group members, usually three or four, that they trusted. My hope is that eventually the prison women can discuss their crimes in a supportive group atmosphere just as the outpatient women do.

The types of sexual crimes that the women in prison committed were not very different from those of our outpatient clients. One can only speculate about why prison was a part of their sentences and the other women were placed on probation. Prison seems an appropriate response to those women whose sexual crime involved violence. It also seems appropriate if the level of violence in other areas of their lives is so great that they cannot function in society and participate in therapy on an outpatient basis. Women whose drug addiction is very severe probably need the confines of prison-based drug treatment and prison-based sexual offender treatment because of their inability to achieve stability.

When I transferred the Shakopee treatment program to prison psychology personnel, I made the recommendations that the women be introduced to treatment very early and that the bulk of their initial treatment be individual. Sharing their sexual crimes with the psychologist early in their incarceration can get them accustomed to talking about their crimes before they become acquainted with the unofficial prison mandate of silence, especially about sexual crimes. Our hope is that the women will be strong enough to then enter a group that is already in existence and feel comfortable in sharing their crimes with fellow group members. We firmly believe that acknowledging the sexual crime is of paramount importance in treatment, and this strategy should make that possible even in a prison setting. I found the women in prison just as touching, hurt, sad, strong, and intriguing as I have their outpatient sisters. One of the exciting results of working to develop the prison program is that we have many consistent responses to the same population in two different settings. My hope is that we can coordinate our efforts and learn more about these women.

FUNDING

The first 2 years of our community treatment for female sexual offenders was underwritten by the General Mills Foundation. This was a start-up grant and was designated to last for only 2 years. When the grant expired, funding was a nightmare, and these women became our (Ruth Mathews and myself) *pro bono* work. Some of the women were eligible for medical assistance, but many were not, as a requirement for medical assistance was that the woman have her children with her and many of our clients did not. Medical assistance programs have undergone drastic changes over the past 10 years, but it is still very much a hit-or-miss proposition for our women. Therapy was often court-ordered for these women, but the court made no provision for payment. When we were affiliated with a community-based organization, funding was often provided for the basic treatment program, with the assumption that the agency would then pay for any specialized therapeutic needs that their population might have. In time we learned that if we could be consulted early enough in the dispositional process, we could have payment for sexual abuse treatment written into the court order. In these cases we got paid, but we were often referred clients who had no ability to pay and there were no provisions in family or criminal court documents for payment.

In 1990, we wrote a joint proposal with Hennepin County, Minnesota, in response to a legislative mandate that the state Department of Corrections fund pilot projects for the treatment of sexual offenders. We were awarded that grant, and payment for women in Hennepin County was provided. In 1995, we wrote another proposal that would make women from all counties in the state of Minnesota eligible for payment under the grant. We were funded under that proposal and women from all over the state can now attend. The Department of Corrections grant is stipulated as the payer of last resort, so medical assistance, insurance, and health maintenance organization resources must be exhausted before we can bill the remainder of the costs to the Department of Corrections.

While this is the best we have ever had, there are still challenges. No money can be spent for transportation and the amount of money is very specific. Corrections money is also available only for women who have a criminal conviction, and yet we have had several women who were referred and entered the treatment program voluntarily. They are not eligible for funding, so, unless they have medical assistance or insurance funding, we are faced with taking their cases for free or at a reduced amount. We cannot exceed the amount of the grant; so, as we project the amount of money left, we must make decisions that are sometimes painful. In fiscal 1995, we had to limit adjunct therapy for a client's children, limit the number of individual sessions for our women, and limit the amount of psychological testing that was done. We know that, with each new legislative session, the budget could be cut and money for our program could end.

RESPONSES TO TREATMENT

Most of the women have responded very well to treatment. They often report that it is the first time in their lives that they have had someone to listen to them and the first time that they have been accepted for who they are. During the past 11 years, we have only had to terminate services to four women. The specifics of the terminations will be discussed later.

For the most part the women have been very supportive and helpful to each other. For some it is a tremendous relief to know that there is someone else who has done something horrible. The group helps tremendously because it is a safe place. Often they have become the pariahs of their communities. Family members are often divided in their hatred of, or support of, these women. Sometimes family members or friends support these women based on their belief that the abuse did not happen. So, if she is to continue to enjoy family acceptance, the subject of the abuse allegations is off limits. The group, on the other hand, offers support based on accepting the woman who has acknowledged the abuse.

The male-coerced and predisposed offenders never question the need for therapy. The teacher–lover women often wonder why they are being placed in a treatment group with "those real child molesters." They often state that they do not belong here, and the thought of sexual contact with a young child is really "perverted" to them. In time, they usually accept the fact that their behavior hurt the adolescent with whom they were involved and, as a consequence, they feel very comfortable with the group. We have, when the number of referrals allowed, divided the women and facilitated a separate teacher–lover group. This was based on the fact that some of these women were fairly high functioning when they came into treatment, and therefore could do their therapeutic work at a much faster pace. These groups lasted from 12 to 14 weeks, with the main therapeutic objective being an increase in awareness of the effects on her victim of the sexual contact. We learned from this approach that it was very effective for many of the teacher–lover women. However, there seemed to be a subset of these women who had more psychopathology and were not ready to be discharged after the time-limited group. This subset of women had backgrounds almost as devastating as the other categories of offenders and their adjustments were no better. This subset of teacher–lover women were transferred to the longer-term group and utilized the extra time to more thoroughly address their issues.

Of the six women who have left treatment, four were expelled and two self-terminated. Two of the expelled women were very self-centered and tried to sabotage the group process and use the group in the expression of their own egocentric purposes. Their goal seemed to be to strengthen their psychopathology instead of diminish it. They sometimes contrived to ask for most of the group time, with the idea that, even if they had to reduce the amount of time that they had, they would still get more than their share. They were both noncriminal justice referrals; therefore, there were no consequences if they failed treatment. They both initially presented with statements of exaggerated gratitude for having a place to get help. They both told of being misunderstood in other treatment venues and feeling accepted and nurtured by us. Eventually, however, we could not meet their need for constant attention and constant assurance, and they expressed anger toward us and the group. Two other women who were under criminal sanctions have been terminated for noncompliance. One failed to follow her case plan at the community agency where she was a client, and the other failed to follow the case plan devised by us. Two other women decided to stop participating in treatment. One believed that she had addressed her issues and the other did not see any point in continuing after her husband went to prison and she saw no hope of reunification. Both were non-criminal justice referrals.

In spite of the fact that four of the six noncompletions have been clients who had no involvement in the criminal justice systems, we still believe that it is important to try to treat them. Many of the women who do come to therapy through self-referral or a child protection referral do stay and complete treatment.

THERAPEUTIC OUTCOMES

Taking into consideration the limitations imposed by privacy statutes on recidivism statistics, therapy outcomes have been positive. We have learned from informal feedback from probation officers and child protection personnel that only 1 of the 40 women treated has committed a new sexual crime. This woman was actively involved in treatment when she reoffended. She was removed from treatment and sent to prison. After serving her sentence she returned and successfully completed treatment. One woman has reoffended by committing a nonsexual crime.

At the end of treatment the women report higher self-esteem, more confidence, less anxiety, more assertive behavior, increase in empathy, and less dependence on alcohol, food, and men. Many of them are able to hold a job for the first time in their lives. Most importantly, they are more able to respond to the needs of their children. Posttesting also indicates a marked decrease in psychopathology and an increase in positive coping skills.

SUGGESTIONS FOR CRIMINAL JUSTICE
AND CHILD PROTECTION

We have dealt with cases that were handled well by professionals involved in both the criminal justice and child protection systems and we have also been involved in cases that were absolute nightmares. In most instances the problems came from mistaken assumptions about female sexual offenders such as: once a sexual offender, always a sexual offender; you cannot trust what these women are saying; they have no interest in giving up their abusive behavior; and they will always be at risk to abuse.

Some difficulties have also arisen because of agendas of punishment and anger. Others assume that the offenders' victim issues are irrelevant to the dialogue and that the only thing we are to deal with is their perpetration issues. When we were referred our first cases the messages we got from other professionals were that these women were so beyond the pale and such a problem that we needed to find a way to get them out of society and keep them out. Their children were taken swiftly, with no discussion of reunification, and the press vilified them. In 11 years of listening to female sexual offenders, their victims, and their children, we hope that we have learned something about all sides of this complicated issue. We hope that society can learn to seek what is best for the offender as well as what is best for the victims of their crimes. From our experiences with female sexual offenders and case management in which the outcomes were positive and negative, we have several suggestions for effective intervention.

First get the facts. Listen to the victims. When allegations are made, investigate as objectively and thoroughly as possible. Nothing takes the place of good, objective fact finding. Children can be easily led or misinterpreted, and interviewing a child is a specific skill that not every police officer or social worker possesses. It is imperative that the job be done right and done right in the very beginning. It is also important to listen to the victims when they express their desires to be back with their family. If reunification cannot be achieved, it should be clearly because the mother or family cannot meet the needs of the child, not because people involved in the case have staked out a position that they do not wish to vacate.

It is also important to charge the woman with a crime if a case can be made. A criminal charge is a clear, cogent message that what she has done is not acceptable behavior. With this recommendation we want to make it clear that we support prosecution, not persecution. Criminal sanction forces the woman to address her abusive behavior, but professionals in the criminal justice system need to refrain from abusive, derogatory statements and treatment that is demeaning. The comment made to one of our clients by the arresting officer—that he did not want to transport her to the police station in his squad car but had to since the dog catcher's van was tied up—was totally unnecessary and added nothing of value to the disposition of the case. A judge's exclamation at sentencing that he could not believe that our client was a mother also set the tone for others in the system to deride her and dismiss the authentic progress that she made. It was easy for them to assume she had violated the terms of her probation when she had not and that she was lying when she was not.

A brief jail sentence also seems to have a positive effect. Unnecessarily long sentences, however, may validate in the minds of these women their worthlessness and allow them to hate themselves more than they already do. If we want them to change, we must give them the message that we believe they can change and we expect them to change. Holding the women accountable with the shortest possible jail sentence will give them the message that we want them back in society but we want them back as changed people. Many of the women have told us that serving some time in jail gave them time to think, to reflect, and, since they were "paying" for their crimes, it gave them permission to forgive themselves and move on. They could then pay attention to their issues and focus on making the necessary changes.

We believe it is best to pair legal sanctions with treatment. A criminal sentence gives the clear message that they must change, but it is likely that these women do not know how to change. They have tried to change before, but they do not have the emotional and/or financial resources to put their lives on a different path. A criminal conviction helps with the therapy process. Therapy is hard work, and the legal leverage helps them face what they probably would not otherwise be willing to face. Knowing that they could spend more time in jail provides the motivation to get the work done. A lot of good therapeutic work can be done when a person's back is to the wall and they know they must address issues of extensive pain.

If the woman is involved with an abusive male, we believe it is best to separate them and not allow reunification until both partners have made progress in treatment. If the woman has children, whether they are her victims or not, a foster placement is probably required. She needs to focus on rebuilding her life. However, we do not assume that these children must stay in foster care forever. Female sexual offenders may not be able to adhere to arbitrarily defined permanent limits. They may be extremely damaged people who take a long time to heal and improve their functioning.

CONCLUSIONS

Working with female sexual offenders for the past 11 years has been a very rewarding experience. They are generally very grateful for the chance to get help in altering their abusive patterns. For some of them, being listened to is a first in their lives, and they have difficulty in believing they deserve it. They love the attention, fear it will be withdrawn, demand that it not be, and eventually ask for what they need. Initially, they tend to avoid therapeutic assignments, but gradually they are able to face horrible backgrounds, support each other, learn to trust, learn to be honest, work hard, face reality, panic, cry, become strong, face the world with dignity, and give us a good run for our money. I would not have missed it for the world.

REFERENCES

Matthews, J. (1993). Working with female sexual abusers, in Elliott, Michele *Female sexual abuse of children: The ultimate taboo*. Harlow, Essex, UK: Longman Group.

19

Adult Intellectually Disabled Sexual Offenders
Program Considerations

Emily Coleman and James Haaven

To begin, an explanation of the language and focus of this chapter is in order. The term *intellectually disabled sexual offender* can be a daunting one. It is used here in the interests of both accuracy and efficiency. To write, "individuals who are intellectually disabled and who have sexual offending problems" each time is prohibitive. Yet concern about labeling is real and can be legitimate. Use of the term *intellectually disabled sexual offender* is not meant to imply that the individual has no other characteristics or importance. The authors' intent is to see each person in a respectful, holistic perspective, though the language may be lacking.

This chapter focuses on adult male sexual offenders who are in the mild to borderline ranges of mental retardation. The treatment approach utilized involves cognitive–behavioral group therapy and relapse prevention. In contrast, persons with more severe cognitive deficits may be more likely to benefit from an approach utilizing environmental contingencies and operant-based techniques such as response cost, time out, and differential reinforcement of other competing behaviors. It is important to acknowledge, however, that IQ can be overemphasized as an indicator of appropriate treatment strategies. Certainly, IQ alone does not adequately describe a person's abilities. Also, there usually is overlap between use of self-control and external control systems.

In working with the intellectually disabled sexual offender, it is important first to understand the experience of being intellectually disabled in today's society. Society values achievement, wealth, knowledge, and power on a scale that eludes many intellectually disabled persons. In order to survive intact in this often unappreciative environment, the intellectually disabled person develops and hones particular adaptive skills. For example, learning to anticipate the wishes of others is handy when you have been taught dependency. If your well-being is often dependent on pleasing others, knowing and delivering what they want is crucial. In addition, learning to fake understanding, much as a hearing-impaired person might extrapolate from every other word, becomes necessary in certain situations in

Emily Coleman • Clinical and Support Options, Greenfield, Massachusetts 01302.   **James Haaven** • Oregon State Hospital, Salem, Oregon 97310.

Sourcebook of Treatment Programs for Sexual Offenders, edited by Marshall et al. Plenum Press, New York, 1998.

order to manage. It is also important to understand that the intellectually disabled person is more likely to use categorical thinking rather than logical, inductive, or deductive thinking. Therefore, labeling becomes an important teaching method. Because the intellectually disabled person has fewer adaptive skills, he may overemphasize them, and because generalization to new situations is so difficult, changes can be particularly threatening. All of the above have implications for assessment and treatment approaches. An understanding of the world of the intellectually disabled person provides a needed frame for the therapist working with this population.

In comparing intellectually disabled sexual offenders and nondisabled sexual offenders, there are more similarities than differences. For example, intellectually disabled sexual offenders are as adept as nondisabled offenders at creating cognitive distortions in an attempt to justify offending behavior. Although there is as yet no plethysmographic database on an intellectually disabled normal control group, clinical experience indicates that the intellectually disabled sexual offender also develops a deviant sexual arousal pattern. Certainly, the intellectually disabled sexual offender frequently has deficit interpersonal skills as does his nondisabled counterpart. This includes a lack of social skills as well as skills involving assertiveness, empathy, stress management, anger control, and impulse control. The intellectually disabled sexual offender also shares problems of inadequate knowledge about sexuality and low self-esteem with the nondisabled offender.

However, significant differences do exist. These differences can affect accurate diagnosis and effective intervention strategies. Certain differences derive from societal response to the intellectually disabled person rather than directly from the intellectually disabled person himself. The sexual offender therapist is more likely to encounter both false-negative and false-positive diagnoses of paraphilia in the intellectually disabled population. Because society is frequently uncomfortable with the sexuality of the intellectually disabled person, "normal" behaviors may be regarded as deviant ones. Residential rules may levy equally negative consequences to consenting peer age sexual intimacy and to forced sexual abuse. A person may be referred for engaging in public masturbation when his problem is actually a lack of privacy in the institution. On the other hand, an intellectually disabled person may repeatedly sexually abuse children and suffer no negative consequences because his caretakers perceive the child as the emotional peer of the intellectually disabled person or because they believe he is not capable of controlling his behavior. Therefore, the therapist must be alert to the influence of the attitudes of the referral agent.

The intellectually disabled sexual offender presents with certain internal differences as well that are independent of societal attitudes. Compared to the nondisabled offender, the intellectually disabled sexual offender may use denial as a general defense mechanism to avoid painful differences rather than as a discrete self-protective maneuver in response to committing a sexual offense. For example, the intellectually disabled sexual offender may deny he is intellectually disabled, let alone that he has offended. To confront denial in an intellectually disabled sexual offender is to potentially challenge an entire adaptive style. In addition, the intellectually disabled sexual offender may have an even lower sense of self-esteem than the nondisabled offender. Repeated experiences of failure and derision contribute to this low self-esteem.

Certain diagnostic errors occur commonly among the intellectually disabled. Several diagnoses tend to be unrecognized and other conditions overdiagnosed. The confusion regarding diagnosing paraphilias in the intellectually disabled person has already been noted. In addition, character disorders, substance abuse, depression, organicity, and post-traumatic stress disorder are frequently missed. Conversely, schizophrenia appears to be overdiagnosed. The intellectually disabled person may be inaccurately judged as hallucinating because he is more prone to illusions and sensory misperception.

Because of the differences in working with the intellectually disabled sexual offender, certain intervention strategies have been found to be particularly effective with this population (Coleman & Haaven, in press). One of the most crucial strategies is teaching effectively. Sexual offender treatment is more closely aligned to education than to traditional therapy. Unfortunately, intellectually disabled sexual offenders are often more hampered in treatment progress due to ineffective teaching methods rather than by their cognitive deficits per se. Teaching that involves lengthy didactic presentations and abstract discussion is usually boring and beyond the attention span and concentration ability of the intellectually disabled sexual offender. Teaching effectively involves linking emotion with learning and includes elements of entertainment, fun, and even the bizarre. Treatment should involve doing rather than simply talking whenever possible. Use of art therapy, drama therapy, music therapy, and therapy animals is beneficial. Making projects related to therapeutic goals facilitates learning. For example, making posters describing "Old Me" and "New Me" concepts engages the client more than a discussion of his typical cognitive distortions. One of the pleasures of working with this population is the pull for the therapist to be creative in order to effectively intervene.

In developing programming for the intellectually disabled sexual offender, however, one should not assume that strategies used with nondisabled offenders are not appropriate. In fact, the intellectually disabled sexual offender should be provided access to any treatment strategies that are available to the nondisabled offenders. In addition to "positive" programming, cognitive–behavioral approaches that may be seen as aversive should also be utilized. This includes covert sensitization, minimal arousal conditioning, behavioral rehearsal, odor aversion, biofeedback, and use of the penile plethysmographic assessment. Both hormonal drug therapy (medroxyprogesterone acetate) and selective serotonin reuptake inhibitors (Prozac, Zoloft, Paxil, and Lurox) can be considered as well.

The following categories have been rather arbitrarily selected into one of three time frames: start-up, implementation, and maintenance. In reality, there is considerable overlap. Certain issues, such as funding and staffing, require attention throughout the life of a program. Others, such as choosing clients and surviving relapse, are somewhat more discrete and lend themselves more easily into categories. Therefore, the outline provides an organizational format to ease presentation but should not be interpreted strictly. The outline is relevant to both outpatient and inpatient settings.

Assessment and treatment may be provided in various settings depending on the level of risk that the client poses. The intellectually disabled sexual offender may receive individual or day treatment in outpatient clinics, within residential living situations (i.e., group homes or foster care), or in inpatient mental retardation–developmental disability (MRDD) institutional settings. It is important to note that significant numbers of intellectually disabled sexual offenders are in correctional and psychiatric facilities without the benefit of the traditional MRDD service continuum. Although there are only limited data available, Brown and Courtless (1967) found that up to 9% of inmate populations are intellectually disabled. Another study by Steelman (1987) indicated 3% of the New York prison population was intellectually disabled.

START-UP

The beginning of a program is probably the most crucial as it largely determines the structure, process, and tenor of what follows. It is an exciting and challenging time in the life of a program. A culture composed of motivated clients, competent dedicated staff, and supportive administration is being created. This culture will evolve and later guide and support the program through its inevitable trials. The beginning is the time to lay the groundwork for a sustaining culture.

Finding Funding

One of the most commonly voiced objections to sexual offender treatment is that it is too costly. Close supervision group homes can cost as much as $125 to $300 per day and inpatient settings as much as $450 per day. In contrast, outpatient sexual offender services may include assessments ($250 to $1000) and ongoing treatment ($200 to $400 per month). This cost is put into perspective when one considers the cost of incarceration: an annual $20,000 per inmate. The inmate's subsequent lost productivity needs to be considered as well as the financial cost to the victim in terms of medical, mental health, and legal fees. Finally, it is impossible to fix a financial cost to the emotional trauma that the victim has undergone. Effective treatment reduces the financial and emotional costs of future victims. If provided treatment, the intellectually disabled sexual offender can be housed in settings that are less restrictive and costly.

However, treatment programs do require money that may be increasingly hard to acquire. A recent survey by the Public Policy Committee of the Association for the Treatment of Sex Abusers (ATSA) found that 75% of ATSA member respondents felt that lack of funding for treatment is currently a serious problem or becoming one (F. Henry, personal communication, April 1996). Eighty-five percent felt that lack of funding for research is a serious concern, and more than half were concerned about financial constraints on clients. In the United States, the medical and mental health picture is under considerable flux with the advent of managed care. Increasing privatization of mental health services looms ahead and is drastically changing expectations. For example, Massachusetts has privatized the provision of mental health services and reimbursement amounts depend on the diagnosis. Currently, clients diagnosed with a paraphilia are given a total of six outpatient visits annually. Given that most sexual offender treatment programs are minimally 1 to 3 years in length, treatment in this area is clearly drastically underfunded. However, clients who are diagnosed with mental retardation and come under the auspices of the Department of Developmental Disabilities usually have more resources allotted.

In some state systems, there has been disenchantment due to the continued recidivism in spite of costly state-of-the-art services. Therefore, restrictive settings become the "treatment" of choice. Unfortunately, what is overlooked is the greater likelihood of reducing the high recidivism rate with this high-risk group in treatment and the subsequent cost savings. In contrast, creating close supervision settings without treatment is very costly.

In order to cope with dwindling financial resources, it is helpful to develop multiple funding sources so that the elimination of one does not necessitate the demise of the program. Private grants, state and federal monies, insurance companies, and fund-raising efforts by the board should all be tapped. Often, unfortunately, self-pay is overlooked. Although the intellectually disabled sexual offender is not usually in the higher socioeconomic level, it is important clinically as well as financially for the client to pay for services. Accepting responsibility for sexual offending includes paying for sexual offender services.

Overcoming Societal Attitudes

Societal attitudes toward the intellectually disabled in general and toward the sexuality of intellectually disabled persons in particular often present a serious obstacle to effective intervention. Often persons who are intellectually disabled are seen as either sex-crazed or asexual. On one extreme, the client is perceived as ridden with strong sexual impulses that are impossible for him to control. On the other hand, he is regarded as a holy innocent, forever a child and completely devoid of sexual stirrings. In fact, most intellectually disabled persons, as most nondisabled persons, fall somewhere in the middle of this curve. However, this unrealistic categorization can have disastrous consequences and is reflected in administrative, community, and legal arenas.

Convincing Administration

Administrations exist in part as a self-protective barrier against perceived threats to existence. Administrators in both outpatient and inpatient settings can be quite reserved about new programs addressing a group seen as having high liability and low payoff, both financially and politically. As noted above, administrators are not immune to stereotypical attitudes toward intellectually disabled sexual offenders. Yet administrative support is critical when starting a program. Administrators must be able and willing to address concerns expressed by advocates and the community who are not familiar with sexual offender treatment. Fortunately, administrators can be responsive to logical information based on sound clinical experience and research. Administrators need to be provided with data indicating the effectiveness of both sexual offender treatment in general (Marshall, 1993) and sexual offender treatment for the intellectually disabled in particular (Haaven, Little, & Petre-Miller, 1990). Bringing in outside leaders in the field as consultants who come armed with facts and credibility can also be helpful. In many cases, clients who are intellectually disabled sexual offenders are already being treated or are otherwise under the care of the agency but have not been acknowledged. Often, it is not a matter of taking on a new population, but treating an existing one with state-of-the-art care. In fact, administrators may be at far greater liability if a specialized program is not instituted. There has been increased attention leading to class-action suits to provide intellectually disabled sexual offender treatment services in correctional and psychiatric settings.

Another understandable administrative concern is that the numbers of clients in need of such specialized services are too low for financial viability. However, resources are so scarce in this field that insufficient referrals would be unlikely. Usually, when information about the program is disseminated, clients appear and are referred so that there is soon a waiting list. Making the program eligible to out-of-state clients further encourages this. In large rural areas, transportation may be an issue and services may require centralization.

A concern of state-funded inpatient programs may be increased costs due to greater community pressure to have offenders committed to those facilities if programs are available. However, providing institutional programs also increases the attention, demand, and acceptance for outpatient services. A continuum of treatment services from secure, locked facilities to community-based group homes promotes flexibility and support among programs.

Organizing Community Support

Although the establishment of residential treatment facilities for the intellectually disabled sexual offender is often a lightening rod for controversy, lower-profile outpatient programs can also receive a share of unwelcome limelight. Interestingly, programs can be seen and criticized for either mollycoddling or violating this group. Some people in society feel offenders are not "deserving" of help, while others see treatment coupled with consequences as unnecessarily restrictive. In either case, education regarding this population and treatment effectiveness is again essential.

Often organizations exist within the local area that support services to intellectually disabled persons, such as the Association for Retarded Citizens. If such organizations are not available, mobilizing the family members of prospective clients to support programmatic efforts can be invaluable.

Addressing Legal Obstacles

In outpatient settings, the percentage of intellectually disabled offenders having no legal involvement is usually much grater than the percentage of nondisabled offenders having no legal involvement. The majority of nondisabled sexual offenders are court-mandated for treatment. Treatment noncompliance can then result in violation of probation or parole and reincarceration. This provides a powerful incentive to work and change in treatment. Unfortunately, intellectually disabled sexual offenders are often denied this form of external support because of attitudes toward the intellectually disabled. The legal system feels ill-equipped to deal with this population and often refuses to take them under their auspices. This speaks to the need of administrators to educate the legal system and to find safeguards from commitments of intellectually disabled sexual offenders to settings lacking adequate basic care and protection.

Understanding the differences between the adversarial nature of the legal system and the multidisciplinary nature of the mental health system is a first step toward comprehensive care (Finn, 1993). Mental health practitioners need to educate themselves regarding the legal process from arrest through arraignment, pretrial, trial, and sentencing. Understanding the nuances and clinical impact of the altered plea, continuance without a finding, and other dispositional alternatives to trial is important for the mental health practitioner. Similarly, judges, defense and prosecuting attorneys, and probation and parole officers need information regarding specialized mental health services for intellectually disabled sexual offenders to guide their decisions. Networking and mutual education is essential to provide the clinical and legal support clients need to change. Forming a joint task force of respected community legal and mental health professionals can be very helpful in this regard.

Finding and Training Staff

It is rare to find a mental health professional who is familiar with both sexual offender and mental retardation issues. Yet knowledge and proficiency in both arenas is needed to work effectively with this population. In searching for staff, we may look at professionals experienced in either one of these field who are also open to learning about the other field. When hiring staff for MRDD programs, the staff seeking the position generally have experience with this population but not sexual offender experience. It is important that these staff receive a broad experience in sexual offender strategies. This should include nondisabled sexual offender treatment and juvenile sexual offender treatment. In this manner, traditional MRDD paradigms, which can be barriers to effective treatment, can be reevaluated.

Look for someone with the appropriate attitude and aptitude rather than a particular degree. In working with sexual offenders, a person should be comfortable with sexuality, able to combine confrontation and support as indicated, and be compassionate yet have a strong sense of boundaries. In working with the intellectually disabled, many of these qualities also apply. In addition, a person must be comfortable using nontraditional therapeutic methods. For example, rather than talking through an issue, the staff person should be willing to use art or drama therapy. Working effectively with the intellectually disabled person requires someone who does not feel sorry for their client, but feels respect, is aware of limitations, and is able to follow through on consequences.

In some ways, choosing to work with intellectually disabled sexual offenders is a response to a calling rather than making a career decision. What is needed in staff is an attitude, an openness, and a commitment rather than particular academic credentials.

Arranging Service Continuum

When designing a service continuum, there are a number of organizational components to be developed. A data collection system is needed for ongoing program evaluation purposes and policies need to be established for admission, continued-stay, and discharge criteria. Policies also should be established to guide the exchange of information, services, and responsibilities with all service providers. Agreement between service providers, especially those with different jurisdictional boundaries, is needed to implement the delivery system of services. In addition, policies should be established to address crisis intervention, medical emergencies, unapproved absences, inappropriate emotional outbursts, incidents involving law enforcement personnel, and reoffense (Ward & McElwee, 1995).

Protocols need to be developed for "invasive" treatment techniques: covert sensitization, masturbatory conditioning, physiological assessment, aversive conditioning, and so forth. In inpatient settings, a human rights board is usually required by accreditation standards to review individual programming and techniques. When this is not required, an advisory board might be formed to address these issues. This is especially relevant in correctional and psychiatric settings not designed specifically for MRDD clients.

Oftentimes when starting a program, attention is first focused on developing treatment techniques. A more effective approach is articulating the guiding treatment philosophy and model. This model should be understandable and user-friendly for other providers, advocates, and clients. Having first developed the treatment model, it is important to then design an organizational system to provide an efficient and effective delivery of services and supervision. This is especially relevant in inpatient programs where the organizational system is often already in place and the delivery system must therefore adapt to existing structure. In inpatient settings, the organizational system is often a much greater barrier to an effective program than lack of expertise.

The treatment model can be adapted from existing models of nondisabled sexual offender programs. Two such models are the four preconditions model (Finkelhor, 1984) and relapse prevention (Pithers, Marques, Gibat, & Marlatt, 1983), which can be incorporated into one approach. Relapse prevention focuses treatment on arranging supports around high-risk situations that may lead to relapse. The client learns self-management skills. These self-management skills then focus on conditions leading to reoffense: affective states (anger, depression, etc.), deviant sexual arousal, inappropriate relationship skills, cognitive distortions, disinhibitors (alcohol/drugs), and access to potential victims. The central tenet is that the offender is accountable for his behavior.

It is important in developing the program that the treatment focus on sexual problem behavior not be eroded or minimized. Too often programs without clarity of purpose evolve into habilitative skill building that may increase self-sufficiency but have little or no effect on control of problem sexual behavior.

IMPLEMENTATION

Program implementation requires a steady hand. It is a time of action, of both unexpected obstacles and of gathering momentum. The program director needs to be able to improvise and prioritize among a seemingly endless array of decisions. Guiding and witnessing the actual birth of the program is a powerful experience.

Designing Motivational Systems

Often, the intellectually disabled sexual offender does not have sufficient reason to change his offending behavior. Perhaps it is the only sexual outlet open to him. Perhaps he no longer believes admonitions of dire consequences that have never come to pass. Perhaps he is unaware of how to meet his needs in appropriate ways. As noted above, the legal system does not consistently provide the consequences needed for motivation. Therefore, the treatment agents in coordination with case managers must create their own motivational systems.

In supervised residential or inpatient settings, the management of the environment offers an important motivating factor. The role of the milieu is often overlooked in program design. The milieu should be a warm, respectful, humane, and consistent environment and should include the development of a communal feeling between clients and staff. It should be a safe environment where the client can take the risk of changing his behavior. The living environment should reinforce the change process. The setting should be thematic with visual representations of treatment accomplishments and reminders present. Focusing on the client's "New Me" identity can motivate the client to meet his own new perceptions of self. Treatment attention to the client's sense of identity should not be neglected.

Another motivating strategy is to foster a sense of "groupness" and culture among clients. To facilitate this, we utilize the buddy system so clients learn to work together and help each other in and out of the facility. Reciprocity should be a theme of the environment.

Motivational systems can be based on access to freedom or privileges. For example, a person may remain on one-to-one supervision until significant progress is made in treatment. However, smaller, more immediate rewards are needed sooner. Often, level systems are used in which the client must meet specific criteria for each level with a corresponding individual menu of reinforcers. This can be an effective motivating system, but it has disadvantages as well. It can become another external control and become a "goal" in itself rather than an internalized change. This is even more problematic if the client is character disordered. Level systems can be misleading in that the individual meaning of the experience to the client is overlooked. One suggestion is to use a level system for a client at the onset of treatment to initiate motivation, and then fade to a more generalized and internal reinforcement—the client's positive sense of identity.

Also, motivating is the process of ritualizing or recognizing "breakthroughs" or insights in treatment that may not necessarily be part of a specific plan. Such breakthroughs may include the client's sharing personal unsolicited information, deferring immediate gratification to help others, or taking responsibility for his mistakes not observed by others. Staff should facilitate the client in evaluating and judging his own behavior through, for example, self-charting. Most importantly, a culture in which status is gained by participation in the program needs to be nurtured and a sense of responsible self-identity encouraged.

Choosing Clients

Administrators are keenly aware that "controlling the doors" of a program is critical. To have control of client selection and discharge allows a program to focus its resources efficiently on specific types of client issues as well as reducing risk. Outpatient programs generally have this latitude, but political and financial pressures can compromise this control. Similarly in inpatient settings, the pressure of overcrowding and internal territorial politics can be problematic.

When developing a program, administration must decide what level of risk it is capable and willing to accept. This determines what program components are necessary to provide comprehensive treatment. In this regard, an initial and ongoing risk assessment is essential. Although there are many components in a risk assessment, possibly the most important in outpatient treatment is the client's willingness and ability to comply with direction and authority.

Treatment Coordination

In an outpatient setting, the intellectually disabled person usually is involved with a multitude of service providers and systems. This may include vocational, educational, legal, and residential care systems. Responsibilities often overlap different departments, such as the Department of Mental Health, the Department of Mental Retardation, and the Department of Social Services. There may be family members, guardians, or work supervisors involved as well. The outpatient therapist may best consider this a vast therapeutic network that requires coordination. To be effective in providing ongoing consistency of programming and public safety, a collaborative and cooperative approach is required. Comprehensive and consistent care is needed with the intellectually disabled sexual offender. All too often the therapist must confront the cognitive distortions of the client's lawyer, parent, and/or case manager who may inadvertently sabotage treatment through minimizing the client's problem. Ongoing and regular network meetings are required to identify problems, clarify positions, unify responses, and problem-solve issues. Finally, it is important to set aside collateral time for this networking. This collateral time usually exceeds the direct care time and should be planned in advance.

Safety Concerns

The essence of outpatient programs is that they are located within the community. The opportunities to relapse are myriad. Even for clients who are under the close supervision of alert and trained staff, offenses can occur quickly and seemingly without warning. Incidents may occur in the waiting room before an appointment or while traveling with staff to work. Initial and ongoing sexual-offender-specific evaluations help to determine the nature and level of risk so that effective interventions can be made.

The issue of safety in inpatient settings is less problematic since the settings are usually secure with little client movement to the community. In outpatient settings such as group homes and foster care, safety and security must be provided by structural controls and monitoring systems to continually evaluate the client's potential risk and the system's ability to make timely interventions. The structural controls lie primarily in providing mechanisms like door alarms, electronic monitoring, and location of the facility so that access to potential victims is limited.

When assessing the safety issue, it is necessary to evaluate how attentively the staff can and do monitor client activity. Programming also includes assessing the work site, day treatment facility, and other client activities. Transportation routes to these activities need to be evaluated. As these issues are incorporated into the program design, system controls of supervision and monitoring of clients must be developed. These monitoring systems might include behavioral tracking to monitor loosening of internal controls of clients. Signs of relapse may be mood changes, cognitive distortions, or structural stressors. Other behavioral indicators may include particular television viewing, collecting children's pictures, or staring at children. Having data collection systems to assist staff in continuous risk evaluation is an important component of program design. Relying solely on unguided staff awareness is risky. Not to be neglected is fostering client involvement through their understanding of high-risk situations; clients may sometimes identify risk situations that staff miss. Public safety must be paramount in any program design.

Ongoing Training and Support of Staff

Competent and dedicated staff are a treasure to be carefully protected and nurtured. Sexual offender treatment takes a toll on its practitioners (Coleman, 1992). Sexual offender therapists may experience vicarious traumatization through repeated exposure to harrowing accounts of sexual abuse recounted coldly by perpetrators. Personal experiences of being sexually victimized can be resurrected in therapists during their work. Paralleling the isolation the sexual offender client often experiences, the sexual offender therapist may feel isolated from colleagues. Therefore, it is crucial that support include not only practical training but also an understanding of the potential deleterious effects of sexual offender work and an avenue in which to address those concerns. Supervision may involve helping the therapist determine the particular self-control technique needed for a client as well as exploring, for example, the therapist's nightmares of being raped.

It is also important to care for every member of the sexual offender team. This includes the administrative assistants and laboratory technicians. The secretary who types the sexual offender reports and the technician who listens to audiotaped cues in the lab may also experience vicarious traumatization through their work. In addition, there is a different kind of stress related to having an important but auxiliary position to the sexual offender client. The adjunctive staff is repeatedly reminded of the presence of sexual abuse but does not have the same direct opportunity as therapy staff to observe positive changes in clients.

In addition to individual supervision, regular team meetings and retreats provide significant support. Team meetings are helpful not only in following an individual client's progress and problem-solving program issues, but also in providing a forum for processing team concerns. Time to ventilate frustration, celebrate successes, joke, and commiserate is important. No one can understand quite as well the joys and pain of sexual offender work as a fellow team member. In addition, crucial decisions about recommendations regarding family reunification, job site, and decreased supervision should not be made independently. Sharing perspectives and ideas makes for the most thoughtful decision as well as for sharing of responsibility. Finally, regular review of the new literature in the field and attending outside trainings and conferences allows for the necessary continual updating of knowledge in a field that is still evolving. Regional and national conferences also give the opportunity to network and validate experiences on a broader scale.

Staff training should include attention to monitoring client progress and regression. Complacency can be the greatest program failure. When staff think that things are "going smoothly," opportunities for complacency abound. Therefore, indicators of clients' increased use of disinhibitors, elementary controls not used, and increased chances to offend may take place without notice.

MAINTENANCE

Although the maintenance sections fits chronologically at the end of the chapter, attention to maintenance issues should occur at the program's inception. Development of follow-up care, protocols after relapse, and program evaluation systems are needed early to provide consistency. Researchers know that the choice of independent and dependent variables and data evaluation systems occur well before the actual intervention in a study. Similarly, planning for program maintenance should not be an after-the-fact affair.

Follow-up Care

Intellectually disabled sexual offenders are more in need of transitional services than nondisabled offenders. Easily overwhelmed by change in structure, the intellectually disabled sexual offender is more likely to regress to previous patterns of dysfunctional and inappropriate behavior. Any change can be threatening, and generalization is more difficult. Without adequate transitional planning, the intellectually disabled sexual offender is particularly vulnerable to relapse during this time. Also, there usually are fewer resources for the intellectually disabled person in the community. It is difficult to find social, political, and vocational niches where the intellectually disabled person is welcomed. The practitioner may need to take a more proactive approach and to help generate such opportunities. For example, developing a computer dating service or a newsletter with a personal advertisement section for the intellectually disabled might be helpful.

Three requirements in providing follow-up care programming are: (1) adequate external monitoring, controls, and support systems; (2) continuity and consistency of treatment processes; and (3) the ability to make timely interventions. To facilitate this, "user-friendly" monitoring systems need to be developed across providers and agencies. In addition, relapse prevention approaches must be utilized in order to make necessary interventions and maintain treatment consistency. Relapse prevention plans offer the client a self-management process and provide a means to monitor and intervene for the providers.

Resources to provide follow-up care often seem woefully inadequate. It is helpful in this regard to change our thinking paradigm of existing resources. Anyone who can be brought into the delivery of treatment should be considered as potential "staff." Practitioners often limit themselves by only looking at resources they formally control. The entire community is a potential staff pool: church, family, friends, volunteers, landlords, and other advocates. Practitioners may not have chosen them for staff. However, it is important to overcome the potential bias of, "If they are not under our supervisory umbrella, they are unable to help." The more support systems involved and coordinated, the more effective care can be.

Surviving Relapse

The ultimate goal of every sexual offender program is to prevent future sexual abuse. When that goal is not reached and a client relapses, the consequences affect the victim, the offender, their families, the treatment staff, the other clients, and the program as a whole. In spite of the most diligent treatment program, relapses will occur and a process for surviving relapse needs to be planned.

A relapse should be critiqued with the benefit of feedback from other providers and support people. A healthy program is able to put itself under the microscope. It is important to recognize the need to learn from mistakes and to realize that relapse can happen even when there has been no mistake on the providers' part. Free will, the ability to choose, does exist within the intellectual disabled sexual offender. Relapse, as well as success, is not in and of itself a measure of the therapist's ability or professionalism. The therapist's performance needs to be evaluated by the quality of the skills he or she demonstrated.

Working in advance with the media can help place a relapse in perspective. Every administrator fears the headline alerting the public to the failure of their program. Drastic responses, including closing down a program, can result from one client's reoffense in spite of an overall high success rate. If the community has been informed previously of the program's existence and its success rates through newspaper, radio, and television, the tendency of the public to leap to unwarranted conclusions can be stemmed. It is also important for the therapist and/or program director to warn their supervising administrator of a client's relapse before he or she gets the information from another source. While being careful not to violate client confidentiality, processing the impact of a client's relapse with other group members in the program is crucial as well. It can be a reminder to other group members not to become complacent about the recovery process. The wish to preserve their treatment program can contribute to the motivation to avoid relapse.

Program Evaluation

With fewer financial resources available, treatment programs are facing greater scrutiny. Additionally, public attention has been shifting from rehabilitation to punishment for all offenders. It is increasingly important that a program have an ongoing evaluation component to demonstrate therapeutic effectiveness and cost efficiency.

Program evaluation should answer two basic questions: (1) are we providing the services we say we are; and (2) are those services making a difference? Data collection systems need to be implemented that indicate what services are being provided, to whom, how often, and by whom. It is crucial to collect information regarding the impact of the program, including utilization of less costly settings and recidivism rates. Documentation of continuous quality assurance measures and procedures is necessary. Effectiveness of individual treatment strategies and consumer satisfaction (both of the client and the referral source) need to be addressed. Reduction of the need for expensive close supervision and incarceration and reduction of the community pain of reoffense are both critical. Review of individual treatment components allows for prioritizations, redesign, or elimination of components. This information also provides a means to identify what diagnostic and demographic types of clients benefit from the program. For example, Haaven et al. (1990) reviewed recidivism, skill strengths of clients, and diagnosis. One conclusion drawn from the data was that increased skills of the intellectually disabled sexual offender (the ability to develop and maintain relationships) was associated with recidivism reduction. This finding was then utilized to increase the needed skill building in the treatment program.

Program evaluation is no longer optional. It is essential in today's changing times.

CONCLUSION

Flexibility is essential throughout all three program phases: start-up, implementation, and maintenance. No one has definitive answers in this field. Assumptions should be regularly questioned. Because the field is so young and still evolving, researchers and clinicians must remain open and flexible, constantly incorporating promising new ideas and empirically testing their effectiveness. The therapist's assumptions can be greater obstacles than the actual problems faced. Especially when working with the intellectually disabled sexual offender, the practitioner must be able to adapt to the clients' needs and the shifting resources available.

An example of a paradigm shift in this regard is to give more program attention to managing the formal and informal treatment monitoring network and less to direct-care treatment. It has been said that, "It takes a village to raise a child." It also takes a village to protect a child.

REFERENCES

Brown, B., & Courtless, T. (1967). *The mentally retarded offender.* Washington, DC: National Institute of Mental Health, Center for Studies of Crime and Delinquency.

Coleman, E. (1992). Working with sex offenders: A therapist's survival guide. *SIECCAN Newsletter, 27,* 11–12.

Coleman, E. M., & Haaven, J. (in press). Assessment and treatment of the intellectually disabled sex offender. In M. S. Carich & S. Mussack (Eds.), *Handbook on sex offender treatment,* Brandon, VT: Safer Society Press.

Finkelhor, D. (1984). *Child sexual abuse: New theory and research.* New York: Free Press.

Finn, J. (1993). Perspectives on the judicial, mental retardation, law enforcement and correctional systems. In R. W. Conley, R. Luckasson, & G. Bouthilet (Eds.), *The criminal justice system and mental retardation* (pp. 8–16). Baltimore: Paul H. Brooks.

Haaven, J., Little, R., & Petre-Miller, D. (1990). *Treating intellectually disabled sex offenders.* Orwell, VT: Safer Society Press.

Marshall, W.L. (1993). The treatment of sex offenders: What does the outcome data tell us? A reply to Quinsey, Harris, Rice and Lalumiere. *Journal of Interpersonal Violence, 8,* 524–530.

Pithers, W. D., Marques, J. K., Gibat, C. C., & Marlatt, G. A. (1983). Relapse prevention with sexual aggressives: A self-control model of treatment and maintenance of change. In J. G. Greer & I. R. Stuart (Eds.), *The sexual aggressor: Current perspectives on treatment* (pp. 214–239). New York: Van Nostrand Reinhold.

Steelman, D. (1987). *The mentally impaired in New York's prisons—Problems and solutions.* New York: The Correctional Association of New York.

Ward, K., & McElwee, D. (1995, May). *Supporting individuals with inappropriate sexual behaviors in community based settings.* Training workshop at the ANCOR Conference on Intellectually Disabled Sex Offenders, New York, NY.

20

Evaluation and Treatment of Deaf Sexual Offenders
A Multicultural Perspective

Mario J.P. Dennis and Kathryn A. Baker

Imagine that you, a skilled clinician, are asked to evaluate a man who has committed a sexual offense and who cannot speak or comprehend your spoken language, and who reads and writes your written language poorly or perhaps not at all. He makes gestures with his hands and body that clearly have meaning to him. He appears to be upset, anxious, and angry. Both of you are aware that you cannot communicate easily. You are expected to conduct a forensic evaluation and perhaps treat this individual. As you contemplate your task, it occurs to you that you have many questions that you would like to ask your patient, such as how long he has been deaf, his level of education, if he experiences major psychiatric symptoms—all the questions we typically ask of a new patient. You wonder how you will establish rapport with someone who makes you feel anxious and perhaps inadequate. You may even feel a little frightened by the intensity of the man's attempts to communicate with you.

You are being confronted with what Wright (1969) has described as the dialogue between the deaf experience and the hearing experience: "It is the non-deaf who absorb a large part of the impact of the disability. The limitations imposed by deafness are often less noticed by its victims than by those with whom they have to do" (p. 5). The deaf patient with whom you are confronted has many years of experience dealing with the hearing world, while you may have encountered deafness for the first time. He does not recognize his inability to hear as a disability, although most likely you do.

We are hearing therapists who specialize in the treatment of hearing sexual offenders, but who over the past few years have been called on to evaluate deaf sexual offenders from all over our state of Virginia. The second author is also an experienced American Sign Language interpreter who treats deaf sexual offenders. She interprets for the first author when he conducts a forensic evaluation of a deaf sexual offender. Throughout the remainder of this chapter, the personal pronoun "he" will be used when discussing the deaf sexual offender, although there are female deaf sexual offenders as well. Additionally, a distinc-

Mario J.P. Dennis and Kathryn A. Baker • Shenandoah Valley Sex Offender Treatment Program, Harrison-burg, Virginia 22801.

Sourcebook of Treatment Programs for Sexual Offenders, edited by Marshall et al. Plenum Press, New York, 1998.

tion will be made between "deaf" and "Deaf" individuals. As will be discussed in greater detail later, members of each group have differing perceptions of themselves and their deafness.

Although the average citizen perceives deafness as a disability, there is an alternative perspective, held by many Deaf people, that deafness is a cultural issue. We believe that only by understanding this culture can a therapist effectively evaluate and treat the Deaf sexual offender. The inability to hear affects psychological and social development, family interaction, and community involvement. The deaf person's difficulties in developing communication result in problems in psychological, social, and educational development.

Steinberg (1991) points out that it is essential for mental health providers to understand Deaf culture. This chapter offers an introduction to deafness and it's impact on the development of deviant sexual interests and practices that result in arrest and incarceration. The second focus will be on resources and considerations for the evaluation and treatment of the deaf sexual offender. We will also attempt to provide an understanding of the role of Deaf culture and the influence of the Deaf community on the incidence, reporting, and treatment of deviant sexuality and sexual offenses.

DEAFNESS AND THE DEAF CULTURE

Scholars have long debated the anthropological and sociological factors that define a "culture" and the relative importance of those factors. We will not recapitulate those arguments here. Most importantly, there are a number of aspects of being deaf that Deaf people themselves cite as defining their culture. These include a shared language, values, and educational experiences that help create a sense of identity. Historically, Deaf adults have maintained this sense of cultural identity through involvement in the "deaf club." The deaf club is a social organization that introduces new members to the deaf culture, and helps to explain what members themselves call "the Deaf way." The role of the deaf club is changing, as Deaf people begin to move away from a Deaf-only culture and are increasingly assimilated into the hearing world. Likewise, enrollment in residential schools for the deaf is decreasing. Historically, these schools have served not only as educational institutions, but also as familial substitutes. These changes may have an impact on the reporting of sexual offenses, which in the past, due to the influence of residential schools and deaf clubs, may have gone unreported in an attempt to maintain the Deaf community's integrity.

Deaf Americans are witnessing many controversial changes in the ways they are perceived and how they perceive themselves. A cultural dichotomy has emerged, with members of the deaf and the Deaf groups having very different beliefs about their deafness, particularly as it relates to their identity as members of either the Deaf culture or the hearing world. For those who identify themselves as Deaf, the capital "D" reflects pride of membership in a culture that provides its members with a sense of personal power that they do not experience in the hearing world. Members of the Deaf community generally have Deaf parents, have attended residential schools for the deaf, and use American Sign Language (ASL) as their native language. They distinguish between themselves and those they describe as "deaf." The lower "d" is typically used to identify those who have lost their hearing after acquiring some degree of spoken language, most likely had hearing parents, and who often were educated in an oral or public school environment. Depending on their degree of proficiency with spoken language and the extent of their interactions with Deaf persons, those with acquired deafness may or may not know ASL. Finally, Deaf persons identify a third group–the hard-of-hearing—who function as hearing persons with a significant hearing loss that may be partially remedied with hearing aids. We have evaluated and treated Deaf, deaf, and hard-of-hearing sexual offenders, with most of our experience being with the first group. While we believe that it is important to understand the different background experiences members of these three groups have had, we believe that mental health professionals are likely to see men from all three groups. Understanding how these groups differ can help the therapist tailor treatment for the individual sexual offender.

A striking example of the cultural changes faced by Deaf persons occurred in 1988, when Deaf students at Gallaudet University in Washington, DC, asserted themselves in unprecedented fashion to demand that the only university for deaf persons in the United States name a deaf president. This event, now known as the "Deaf President Now" movement, was probably the first time that Deaf people united and spoke for themselves, insisting that the university be led by someone who shared their experience of deafness. Another perceptual change is the traditional view of hearing people that deaf people are suffering from a medical disability. An acrimonious debate continues between hearing parents of deaf children and Deaf adults concerning the medical procedure of cochlear implants. Dolnick (1993) cites a survey that found that 86% of Deaf adults would refuse a cochlear implant, even if it were free, because Deaf people do not see themselves as having a disability that requires remediation and treatment. In contrast, hearing parents of deaf children often seek ways of remediating and treating the deafness. They may consult with audiologists, physicians, and other professionals, hoping to fit their child into the hearing world. They may consider medical procedures, such as cochlear implants, as facilitating the development and understanding of spoken language. Such parents may enroll their child in a mainstream public school, determined to normalize the child's life as much as possible. They may demand that the child use aural amplification (hearing aid) even when it is of limited value. They may be reluctant to learn or have their child learn ASL, fearing that it will interfere with the child's attempts to learn English.

Language and Deafness

One of the significant determinants of a culture is its language, and it is no different in the Deaf culture where several methods have been developed to facilitate communication. The most widely used method by Deaf persons is ASL, a visual language incorporating handshapes, positioning, and body language to express ideas. In spite of its widespread use, for many years ASL was seen as a collection of isolated gestures with no connection to formalized language. On the other hand, ASL can be seen as a rich language in its own right. ASL has its own syntax, idioms, grammar, and rules just as other languages. However, ASL is different from English. There is no written form of the language, and any attempt to achieve a literal interpretation of an ASL sentence into written or spoken English would be confusing. For example, imagine that you are interviewing a deaf man who has admitted to fondling his young daughter.

Interviewer:
English Version: "What happened when you touched your daughter's vagina?"
ASL Interpretation: "Daughter's vagina touch you happened?"

Offender:
ASL Version: "Smile daughter smile, turn on me."
English Interpretation: "She smiled, and I felt turned on."

It can readily be seen that there is the potential for misunderstanding when native English speakers and native ASL speakers attempt to communicate without the assistance of an interpreter who is fluent in both languages. While this may not be of great concern during normal conversation, in the context of a clinical evaluation or treatment, the potential consequences of any miscommunication are tremendous. As will be discussed later, it is of the utmost importance that non-ASL speaking clinicians be aware of these difficulties and seek assistance from a certified interpreter.

With any spoken language, understanding the paralanguage is vital for an accurate interpretation of the speaker's message. The role of paralanguage may be even more important in ASL. The hearing speaker uses such things as tone of voice to convey emotional state; however, the ASL speaker must make greater use of facial expressions and body language and other nonverbal techniques. Two paralinguistic differences that distinguish English from ASL are the reliance on touch and the necessity of sustained eye contact. Deaf people often initiate communication using touch, which may include hugging as a greeting or leave-taking gesture, even with persons with whom they have limited familiarity. Likewise, the sustained eye contact that deaf persons depend on for understanding ASL can be uncomfortable for hearing people, who may experience such gazes as rude or intrusive. Deaf people may sometimes feel bewildered when their hearing counterparts respond negatively to these behaviors. For the Deaf person, touch is a natural and acceptable form of communication within their culture. It binds members of the Deaf culture, who have used touch in this way throughout their lifetimes. They may not recognize that uninvited touch may mean something quite different to the hearing person who is unfamiliar with Deaf culture.

Although ASL is the predominant form of communication for the Deaf person, other deaf persons may rely on lip reading, more properly referred to as *speechreading*, to understand what hearing persons are trying to communicate to them. Hearing persons often believe that speechreading eliminates the barriers for miscommunication, when in fact, it is heavily dependent on the skill of the speechreader, which can vary tremendously. Speechreading is of no value when the speaker is out of visual range, and the presence of a beard or mustache on the speaker's face can substantially interfere with even a skilled speechreader's ability to comprehend. The speechreader's job is made even more difficult by the fact that perhaps two thirds of spoken English is not visible on the speaker's lips.

Education of the Deaf

Just as ASL has assisted in maintaining the cultural identity of Deaf persons, so have the residential schools for the deaf. Thomas Hopkins Gallaudet is credited with establishing the first public school for instruction of deaf children in 1817 in Hartford, Connecticut. Then named the Connecticut Asylum for the Education and Instruction of Deaf and Dumb Persons, the school was later renamed the American School for the Deaf. Gallaudet studied with Laurent Clerc, a Frenchman, learned French Sign language, and then adapted it for use by deaf students in America. According to Pollard (1992), by 1892, 51 of the existing 61 public schools for the deaf used sign language, either in combination with oral communication or as the only form of communication. Since then residential schools for the deaf have played a prominent and invaluable role in the education of the deaf. However, that influence may be waning, as more and more deaf persons are attending public schools. The number of deaf students in residential schools has been steadily falling since 1970, and the pace appears to be accelerating. Schildroth and Hotto (1994) indicate that of the 47,014 deaf and hard-of-hearing children in the United States, only 20% are in residential schools.

Often, it is only in the residential school that deaf students learn language and have an opportunity to interact with other deaf peers. It may be the first time the deaf person has contact with a deaf adult who can serve as a role model, as it is estimated that 90% of deaf children are born to hearing parents (Schein & Delk, 1974). These parents cannot provide the gateway to the deaf culture that the residential school can. Although the school may appear to function as a surrogate for the family, nevertheless it cannot realistically provide the same degree of nurturing and socialization that hearing children receive within the family. Until recently, residential students often went for weeks or months without visiting their families.

Another disadvantage to growing up in a residential school is that some attitudes within the school may conflict with those of the hearing world. For example, many deaf sexual offenders who attended residential schools have reported to us that they were involved in sexual activity and were sexually abused in the school. Although most students who have been involved in such activity will not become offenders, those who do engage in deviant sexual activities as adults often have had very few nondeviant sexual experiences. They may assume that their sexual history is normal, when it is not.

Deafness, Sexual Abuse, and Sexual Offending

It should be noted that merely being deaf places children at a greater risk of being sexually abused. The deaf child's limited ability to communicate with hearing parents, teachers, or other adults often means that abuse may go unreported or undetected. Sullivan, Vernon, and Scanlon (1987) reported that while an estimated 10% of hearing boys were sexually abused, 54% of deaf boys had been molested. Comparable rates for hearing and deaf girls were reported, with 25% of hearing girls reporting that they had been sexually abused, compared to 50% of deaf girls. They pointed out that more deaf boys are abused than deaf girls, which is the opposite of the ratio in the hearing population. Sullivan and Knutson (1995) also examined the connection between disability and child abuse and neglect. They reviewed the records of 39,352 children in Nebraska who received services from the Boys Town National Research Hospital between 1982 and 1992. The records include cross-referenced databases from two social service and five law enforcement agencies. They determined that placement in a residential school substantially increases the risk for sexual abuse.

Klopping (1985) has noted that several residential schools for the deaf have had employees arrested and charged with sexual abuse, while superintendents of other schools have been charged with failure to report sexual abuse within the school. Klopping speculated that there may be several reasons for lack of reporting, including ignorance of the need to report, a lack of understanding of the harm done to the child victim if the problem is handled internally rather than by legal authorities, and the fear of negative publicity for the school.

It seems apparent that the prevalence of deviant sexual activity and sexual abuse among the deaf is probably more widespread than is reflected in the statistics. Many deaf offenders have reported to us that while attending a residential school they became involved in precocious sexual activities that they did not identify as abuse. These included consenting sexual exploration between peers, involvement in voyeuristic and exhibitionistic activities, and even outright sexual abuse by other students or staff. Some offenders have reported being sexually aggressive with female staff, exposing to them or attempting to fondle them. They appear to have been acculturated to deviant sexual activity beginning at an early age, and having no external frame of reference, assumed that they were engaging in appropriate behavior. Most residential schools are coeducational and have students ranging in age from 6–21 years; thus, the adolescent sexual offender or offending staff member has a large potential victim pool. There may be relatively few barriers to contact, sexual or otherwise, between older and younger students, between staff and students, and between males and females. As noted earlier, the common use of touch by Deaf persons can also provide a ready opportunity for a sexual offender to initiate sexual contact with a potential victim.

One man candidly told us of being involved in homosexual activity with other male students beginning when he was about 8 years old. He reported that older male students often molested younger boys, orally and anally sodomizing them. This activity was so common, however, that he did not consider it to be abuse, but a normal part of life at school. When he transferred to a residential school in another state he encountered a similar situation and was again involved in sexual activity with other male students. Thus, during critical periods of his psychosocial development, he was involved in sexual activities, first as a victim, and later as a perpetrator. As an adult, he was arrested several times for molesting young boys and is currently in prison.

Although we believe that sexual abuse may be prevalent within residential schools, those deaf children who do not attend residential schools may also be at risk for being sexually abused within the home. Green (1985) noted that deaf children who live at home present very difficult challenges to their hearing parents, which may have implications for child abuse. Parents who feel ineffective raising their hearing children may become very frustrated when dealing with their deaf child. Communication difficulties and a parent's negative attitude toward their child's deafness, which they may view as a disability, compound the task of child rearing and may be a causative factor in child abuse. Another contributor may be high rates of substance abuse in deaf parents of deaf children (Vernon, 1995).

ASSESSMENT OF DEAF SEXUAL OFFENDERS

The forensic evaluation of the deaf sexual offender is, in many ways, quite different from the examination of his hearing counterparts, due to the unique cultural and psychological forces that shape his development. This section examines the specific procedural and clinical issues that the examiner must consider throughout the evaluation process.

Using an Interpreter

Relatively few forensic examiners are fluent in ASL or have had experience evaluating a Deaf person. The first task, therefore, is to identify the communication abilities of the offender (i.e., does he use ASL and how fluent is he, and how well can he read English)? Once it has been determined that the offender uses ASL, it is then necessary to engage the services of a certified interpreter. The National Registry of Interpreters for the Deaf in Silver Spring, Maryland, can provide information about interpreter resources on a statewide or local basis, as well as a copy of the Code of Ethics for Interpreters. A local mental health agency or hospital may have an interpreter on staff or under contract, or may be familiar with using interpreter services in the area. Most states have a central agency for deaf services for referral and information that includes interpreting information.

Once a potential interpreter has been identified, it is important to develop a good working relationship between interpreter and examiner. Most interpreters will be unfamiliar with the nature of a forensic evaluation and may assume that the purpose of the interview is to provide mental health assistance. They may be put off by the relatively impersonal nature of the forensic interview, where the focus is to obtain information for possible use in a criminal proceeding. It is important to explain that the purpose of the evaluation is to help the court or referring agency to determine the offender's treatment needs and potential risk to the community. Equally crucial will be explaining the necessarily explicit nature of the interview, focusing as it does on deviant sexual behavior. The examiner should describe the sexual behaviors that will be discussed before engaging the interpreter for the evaluation. At the same time, the examiner should be aware that the deaf offender may use colloquial terms for body parts. This type of language should not be considered crude or vulgar but simply a reflection of how some members of the deaf culture refer to anatomy. It is preferable that the examiner use the offender's terms for sexual anatomy, which may help the interpreter feel more comfortable voicing these terms. Using euphemisms, such as "private parts" is not advisable, as the examiner will want to be more exact when discussing sexual activity. Interpreters who have had few opportunities to sign sexually graphic information, may be unfamiliar with the signs used by deaf offenders. One useful resource the examiner can share with the interpreter is Woodward's (1979) compilation of detailed signs of sex-related vocabulary.

Even skilled interpreters may find themselves being sympathetic to the deaf offender's plight, and may have difficulty maintaining their usual professional objectivity. Given the relatively small size of the Deaf community, the interpreter may know the offender, his victim, or his family from previous contacts with him or other Deaf people. Likewise, the offender may have information about the interpreter that will influence his perception and his openness in the evaluation. If the interpreter feels that professional standards cannot be maintained, the examiner should gracefully accept the interpreter's withdrawal from the process, and appreciate the honesty being expressed. Once an evaluation interview has been completed, it can be very helpful to offer to debrief the interpreter concerning any emotional responses to a very challenging interpretive task.

Just as the interpreter must accept the forensic clinician's definition of the task at hand, likewise the clinician must understand that the interpreter's role is defined by a professional code of ethics. The interpreter's role as communication facilitator dictates that the interpreter must only sign that which is voiced by the examiner, and voice only that which is signed by the offender. Thus, interpreters are not permitted to offer opinions about the deaf person or the veracity of the information obtained during the interview. The examiner should refrain from asking the interpreter for any additional information about the offender. The interpreter must maintain confidentiality and may not disclose the identity of the offender or the nature of the interview to others. Neither can the interpreter disclose to the examiner the content of any professional or personal contacts with other Deaf persons who may be connected to the case.

Deaf people have limited opportunities to communicate with hearing people using an interpreter. The examiner may find that the deaf offender sees the evaluation as an opportunity to communicate with the hearing world, and this may dominate the interview. Whereas the hearing sexual offender may be unwilling to communicate at all, the deaf offender may be only too willing to discuss everything in such detail that the examiner may feel overwhelmed. It is important, therefore, that the examiner take immediate control of the flow of the interview. Although it could be considered rude to repeatedly interrupt a hearing examinee, the interviewer should not hesitate to interrupt the deaf offender when he is providing too much or irrelevant information. The offender is unlikely to perceive this as hostile or inappropriate. The examiner may experience the unsettling feeling of being an outsider, unable to share in the direct communication with the client, and having to rely on the interpreter. It may be helpful for the examiner to keep in mind that he or she is the expert and can rely on his or her skills as a forensic evaluator, even though unable to communicate in the offender's language.

Assessment Issues

The evaluation of the deaf sexual offender presents additional challenges for the examiner when compared to the evaluation of the hearing offender. Hearing offenders who cannot read can usually complete standardized assessment inventories with the assistance of audiotape. This option is obviously not available for the deaf offender. Even determining the deaf offender's reading ability or level of intellectual functioning can be difficult. It cannot be assumed that a deaf person who has completed high school, for example, comprehends English sufficiently to complete standardized psychological assessment inventories. Golan (1996) points out that surveys conducted by Gallaudet University found that 60% of deaf 16- and 17-year-olds in the United States read at the third grade level. Undergraduate students at Gallaudet fared little better. Golan cited an internal study conducted at the university that found that 70% of the undergraduates could not read a college level textbook. If the offender's reading comprehension has been determined to be adequate to complete the inventories, the result of a standardized inventory still must be considered very carefully. The reader is encouraged to review Zieziula's (1982) guide to assessment instruments that are widely used with hearing patients and their appropriateness for deaf people. He found that few instruments have been normed for deaf persons, and the fact that many of them rely heavily on verbal skills may make them inappropriate for deaf people with poor reading skills. Unfortunately, the situation is unlikely to improve in the near future. Because it is extremely expensive to develop and norm psychological assessment instruments, test developers and publishers have been reluctant to take on the task for such a small population as the deaf. While videotaped versions of the Minnesota Multiphasic Personality Inventory and Multiphasic Sex Inventory are being developed; much more research is needed to determine the psychometric properties of these instruments when used in this medium.

Phallometric testing is typically a crucial part of the assessment of the sexual offender. Unfortunately, the use of the plethysmograph with deaf offenders is extremely difficult. The Association for the Treatment of Sexual Abusers Ethical Guidelines (Isaac, 1994) believes that the use of sexually explicit pictures of children is inadvisable, as they may violate child pornography laws. Many programs now use only audiotaped scenarios during phallometric assessment. The deaf offender is prevented by his deafness from participating in this form of assessment. Examiners may wish to consider the use of card sort techniques, although these lack the relative objectivity and precision of physiological evaluations. Again, however, limited reading ability may not permit even this approach.

Conducting the Interview

As with the hearing offender, the examiner should first collect offense information, the offender's educational, psychiatric, and legal history and any available clinical data from third parties. Deaf offenders often communicate at a very concrete level and may not understand more abstract concepts. The examiner should frame questions in simple, straightforward, concrete terms. Asking, "Were you involved in extracurricular activities?" may need to be rephrased to, "Did you go to any clubs at school or after school?" Similarly, questions about interpersonal relationships should also be worded in very simple terms. Rather than ask, "How did your mother treat you?" it may be necessary to use close-ended questions, such as, "Was your mother nice to you? Did she punish you?" Although wording questions in this way can be helpful, the deaf offender may not respond or may appear to sidestep the examiner's inquiry. It may be necessary to reword the question several times before obtaining the requested information or deciding that the offender is unable or unwilling to reply. It may be difficult to determine whether this reflects a lack of understanding or resistance. It can be helpful to compare the deaf offender's apparent comprehension of relatively benign questions (e.g., about his family background) and his sexual offenses. We have observed that some offenders appear to understand the examiner's questions quite well until the interview turns to a discussion of the offenses. The offender then may become vague or report that he is unable to understand the questions. Some deaf people may use their deafness and language deficits defensively when involved in treatment. With the deaf sexual offender, this tactic may be used to prevent him from experiencing painful feelings when confronted with his sexually deviant behavior.

We have found that the following questions can provide the examiner with a greater understanding of how the offender's deafness affected his psychological and psychosexual development:

- Did you have hearing parents or deaf parents?
- Are you the only deaf member of your family?
- If your parents were hearing, what did they think about your deafness?
- If your parents were hearing, how did you communicate? Did they know ASL?

If the offender attended a public school:

- How many other deaf children attended your school?
- Did the hearing children tease you? Were they nice to you?
- How did you communicate in school with teachers and other students? Speechreading, ASL, or writing?
- If you had an interpreter at school, did you like your interpreter?
- Did you play organized sports? Did you join scouts? Did you join clubs in school?
- Did you play with children who lived nearby your home?

If the offender attended a residential school:

- Did you always go to the residential school?
- Did you like the school? Did you have friends there?
- How long did you go to the residential school? Did you graduate? How old were you when you graduated? What grades did you get?
- Did you ever get into trouble at school? If so, what happened?
- Did you visit home? Did your family visit you at school?

These questions should help the examiner understand how well the offender adjusted to the public or residential school. This in turn can provide insight into the offender's self-esteem, degree of social isolation, and development of interpersonal skills, all of which are relevant to his potential response to treatment. The deaf offender who enjoyed a supportive family while attending a public school likely experienced very different social and developmental influences than the offender who attended a residential school. The former is likely to be more familiar with the values of the hearing culture, while the latter may have only been exposed to the hearing culture after living in the relatively insular world of deafness. With this understanding of cultural differences, the examiner should then explore the deaf offender's sexual history.

As noted above, deaf children in general are more at risk to be sexually abused than their hearing counterparts, and those who attended residential school may have been at even greater risk. However, rather than asking the deaf offender whether he was sexually abused, it is preferable to engage him in a detailed discussion of all of his early sexual experiences, many of which he may not have experienced as abuse. The examples below represent only a few of the questions we ask of deaf and hearing offenders. The chief differences in how we frame these questions for deaf offenders are the terms often used by deaf persons, which are in parentheses:

- Did anyone ever try to touch your penis (dick)?
- Did anyone ever put their mouth on your penis (dick)?
- Did anyone ever try to touch you with their penis (dick) or put their penis (dick) in your mouth or anus (asshole)?

For offenders who attended residential schools:

- Did you ever see anyone at school touch another student's penis (dick), vagina (pussy), or breasts (tits)?
- Did you ever try to see the girls naked in the shower or in the dorm?
- Did you or your friends at school every play grabass?
- Did any staff at your school get into trouble for touching students?
- Did any students at your school get into trouble for touching staff or showing their penis (dick) to staff?

In addition to asking about deviant sexual experiences, it is of course important to ask about normal sexual activities, such as dating, masturbation, consenting sexual activity with girlfriends, use of erotic materials, and sexual intercourse. It can be helpful to contrast the offender's involvement in deviant sexual activity with his participation in age-appropriate, consenting sexual activity.

Discussing the Circumstances of the Offense

It cannot be overemphasized that a victim statement and other investigation records must be available to the examiner prior to the interview. These materials provide the most accurate account of the offender's sexual offenses, but more importantly for the deaf offender they can help the examiner reconstruct the sequence of events leading up to and following the offense. Like hearing offenders, deaf offenders are eager to defend themselves or proclaim their innocence and may be difficult to follow as they present information in a haphazard, rather than an orderly fashion. It is at this point in the interview that the examiner will probably want to take clear control over the pace and direction of the discussion. Again, simple directive questions are more likely to elicit information than more abstract inquiries. For example, rather than ask, "Tell me about what you did to (victim's name)?" it is preferable to say, "(Victim's name) says that you put your hand on her vagina (pussy). Did you do that?"

Particularly when the offense involves a child victim, the authors generally begin the discussion of the offense by asking the offender about his relationship with the victim. With hearing offenders, the question can be relatively general and open-ended, such as, "Tell me about your victim." Many deaf offenders may not be familiar with the concept of a "victim," so it is preferable to use the victim's name, rather than refer to him or her as "the victim." Again, with the deaf offender questions should be specific and concrete: "Did you know (victim's name)? Where did you meet (victim's name)? Where did (victim's name) live? Did you like (victim's name)? Did (victim's name) like you? Did (victim's name) ever make you mad? Did you ever play with (victim's name)?"

Like hearing offenders, deaf sexual offenders rationalize and justify their offenses, using cognitive distortions to minimize their responsibility for their behavior. Both groups often maintain that their victims initiated the sexual abuse, that the abuse was really a form of play, and that the victim enjoyed the encounter. However, deaf offenders may offer additional rationalizations. Deaf offenders we have evaluated claim more often than hearing offenders that they were not molesting their victim but were merely "curious," although they are unable to explain this curiosity. One deaf man we evaluated molested four preadolescent females over a 10-year period, sexually abusing them countless times. When asked about his motives for fondling them, he insisted that he was only "curious." While curiosity may be a legitimate explanation for some sexual behaviors in a naive adolescent, for an adult this explanation is implausible and serves only to minimize the sexual intent of the perpetrator.

Deaf offenders often claim that their offenses, if they admit to them, are a result of their deafness and that they were never taught proper sexual behavior. They may have learned that in the past, in other contexts such as in their job or with their family, this explanation enabled them to avoid responsibility for their behavior. The general public is understandably sympathetic to the deaf person and may be reluctant to hold him accountable for his behavior. Judges, probation officers, and mental health professionals are equally likely to adopt this patronizing attitude with the deaf offender. The forensic examiner who is unfamiliar with deaf defendants may have to struggle with this as well. Certainly, deafness does have an impact on social competence, self-esteem, and interpersonal relationships, all of which may be implicated in the development of deviant sexual behavior, but it must be borne in mind that deafness is not a *cause* of sexual offending. The examiner's report can educate judges, probation officers, and child protective service workers about the lack of a causal relationship between deafness and offending.

The deaf offender's denial and minimization may have been reinforced by other members of the deaf community. They may believe that the offender has been wrongly accused and harshly treated by a judicial system insensitive to deafness. In contrast to the hearing offender, who is often shunned within the community and who may lose the support of friends and family, the deaf community may continue to support the offender. One offender we evaluated had molested several girls over a span of years and had been convicted of a previous sexual offense. Nevertheless, he maintained his status within the Deaf community and held a responsible position within the Deaf club. To the hearing world, this support of a convicted child molester may appear to be misplaced loyalty and trust. However, for the deaf community, the issue may not be the offense but maintaining the cultural integrity of the deaf community. Unfortunately, this may have the undesirable effect of placing the offender in proximity to potential victims, thus increasing the risk of future offenses.

Risk Assessment

The primary focus of the forensic evaluation of the deaf offender is his likelihood for future offending. The examiner is strongly encouraged to use the same risk assessment protocol that is used with the hearing offender. While all factors of a risk assessment should be considered, certain of these factors may be especially relevant for the deaf offender.

The offender's denial, especially when it is supported by family or the Deaf community, may place him at a higher risk for reoffending, not only because he may fail to recognize the seriousness of his acts, but also because members of the Deaf community may not recognize situations that place potential victims at risk. We have observed that many deaf offenders, especially adolescents, have not been prosecuted for deviant sexual acts, especially noncontact offenses such as voyeurism and exhibitionism. The deaf sexual offender therefore may believe that his offending carries few consequences, and he may repeat his offenses many times before being held accountable. He may be genuinely bewildered when he is finally arrested and convicted. He may ask himself why the police are charging him this time. It is often the legal system that first conveys to the deaf offender that he will not be held responsible for his offenses because of his deafness. Ironically, when he is finally arrested and the law attempts to hold him culpable, the offender then uses his deafness as a defense. To reiterate: Deafness should not be considered a cause of sexual offending; however, the offender may interpret others' tolerance of his behavior as tacit permission to continue the behavior. Allowing the offender to engage in deviant sexual behavior and not holding him accountable may encourage the offender to become involved in multiple paraphilias, which may raise his overall reoffense risk.

Similarly, we have observed that deaf persons may not be held accountable for other, relatively minor criminal behavior, and yet a history of nonsexual offenses appears to be a good predictor of future sexual offending. The examiner should not assume that lack of a formal criminal record means that the offender has not engaged in prior criminal activity. Again, it may be that authorities elected to overlook some criminal behavior because the perpetrator was deaf. It is important to question the deaf sexual offender about any contact with law enforcement and to ask if he has engaged in criminal activity, such as stealing or breaking and entering, that went undetected. One deaf sexual offender with a history of exposing also revealed to us a number of property crimes that were never prosecuted, even though the police were aware of the offenses. It was only after he broke into a business and stole panties and brassieres that they decided to arrest him.

Many deaf persons display emotional immaturity, impulsivity, lack of empathy, egocentricity, and a tendency not to be introspective. The reader is strongly cautioned not to conclude that these traits are universal among the deaf population. Still, the presence of these traits in a sexual offender will clearly have an impact on treatment response and recidivism. The examiner should question the deaf offender about behaviors that may reflect poor impulse control, such as unstable interpersonal relationships and frequent changes of employment or living situation. The offender's offense pattern may also reflect compromised impulse control, such as engaging in poorly planned offenses in situations where identification and apprehension are likely. One deaf offender molested a girl in her home while here father was in the next room. He reported lying on her bed with her for over an hour, while fondling her vagina. Years later, he fondled a young girl in clear view of two of her playmates in the front yard of his apartment complex in the middle of the day. Like many sexual offenders, this man claimed that because his offense was unplanned, he was unlikely to reoffend. However, a more accurate interpretation might be that each time he had an opportunity or urge to offend, he took advantage of the situation. This level of impulsivity led the examiner to speculate that there may be many other offenses that had never been reported.

Finally, recidivism risk should be considered in light of the presence of community supports, including probation and parole, and the availability of treatment. Just as law enforcement agents may be reluctant to make the deaf offender responsible for his criminal behavior, probation and parole officers may have similar problems supervising deaf probationers and parolees. The officer likely has had little or no experience with this population, and he or she may need to hire an interpreter or rely on notewriting to convey expectations of the offender's behavior while on probation. These additional difficulties may cause the officer to relax the rules ordinarily enforced for the hearing offender. If sexual offender treatment is ordered, the officer is unlikely to find a treatment program for deaf offenders or a mental health professional with expertise in both deafness and sexual offender treatment.

TREATMENT OF DEAF SEXUAL OFFENDERS

Treatment Issues

The mental health practitioner who is considering offering treatment to deaf sexual offenders will face many challenges. Because there are few practitioners experienced in sexual offender treatment and fewer still with skills in deafness, it follows that professionals with skills in both areas are extremely rare. Professionals treating deaf persons may be unwilling to treat deaf sexual offenders. At the same time, sexual offender treatment providers may have no experience with deaf people, including deaf sexual offenders. Thus, the practitioner will likely experience isolation, navigating very unfamiliar waters with little or no support or supervision. Whenever possible, the therapist should arrange for supervision and consultation with both a sexual offender expert and a clinician knowledgeable in working with deaf clients. This will help the therapist cope with feelings of isolation and the stress associated with treating this challenging population.

Generally, the therapist will have to rely on an interpreter to facilitate communication in therapy. As noted above, this can raise a number of issues. First, the pace of therapy with a deaf client is generally much slower, given the nature of the communication process. The pace slows even more with the introduction of an interpreter. Additionally, introducing an interpreter into the therapeutic setting transforms a dyad into a triadic relationship, which can cause confusion. The University of California Center on Deafness (1987) guidelines for using interpreters in mental health settings emphasize that the presence of a third person, plus the use of two languages and two channels of communication, will undoubtedly have an impact on the therapeutic process. The therapist must be sensitive to transference and countertransference that emerges between the three parties. It may be necessary for the therapist to explain these dynamics to the interpreter, who may be unfamiliar with these therapeutic issues.

It will be necessary for the clinician to modify treatment techniques and materials designed for hearing sexual offenders for use with deaf offenders. This may have to be done on a case-by-case basis, as it is likely that the clinician will be working with one deaf offender at a time. Even in urban areas, at any one time there may be too few deaf offenders to form a treatment group. Establishing regional treatment programs for deaf sexual offenders may ultimately be the only way that group treatment can be provided.

Integrating deaf sexual offenders into a group of hearing offenders presents other therapeutic difficulties. Unless the group leaders and deaf offender are fluent in ASL, it will be necessary to provide an interpreter, which raises potential problems. The hearing offenders may not accept the interpreter as a member of the group or may be reluctant to openly discuss personal issues in the interpreter's presence. Group dynamics will likely be affected by the interpreter's personal qualities, such as physical appearance, gender, and affect. In a similar way, the interaction between the deaf offender and his interpreter may influence the group. The hearing offenders may not understand that the interpreter is a professional who has been hired by the clinician and who must follow a strict ethical code. They may experience discomfort watching the communication occurring between the deaf offender and the interpreter and may feel a sense a resentment at being excluded from this communication. Hearing group members may be experiencing communication with a deaf person for the first time and may be unwilling to confront the deaf offender as they would another group member. This can have the unwelcome effect of supporting the deaf offender's denial and minimization.

There are other potential obstacles to effective deaf sexual offender treatment. The deaf population in general has a high rate of substance abuse, but there are very few substance abuse treatment programs for deaf people. The deaf sexual offender who also has a substance abuse problem, which should be addressed before sexual offender treatment commences, may be unable to find inpatient or outpatient drug and alcohol treatment.

The deaf offenders' communication skills and limitations will have a substantial influence on which treatment modalities can be used. Poor English skills will make it difficult for the offender and therapist to use such techniques as keeping a journal, writing an autobiography, reading assigned materials, and describing his offense cycle. The process of helping the offender understand the intent of these exercises may be one of successive approximations, and the therapist will have to patiently help the offender understand the concepts being presented. For example, the therapist will want the deaf offender to describe his offense cycle in detail, so that the therapist can understand what the offender was thinking and feeling before, during, and after his offenses. The offender may continue to reiterate that he was "curious" and may have great difficulty identifying specific feelings and thoughts he had before, during, and after his offenses. This reflects a lack of introspection, as described above. Thus, the therapist may have to teach the offender that thoughts, feelings, and core beliefs precede behavior.

Other standard treatment approaches that rely on oral communication and feedback may also be unsuitable. One example would be masturbatory satiation tapes. These are especially valuable for hearing offenders, enabling the therapist and offender to gain insight into the offender's fantasy world. Additionally, the technique is used to teach the offender the difference between appropriate and inappropriate fantasy, while diminishing his arousal to inappropriate stimuli. We are unaware of any substitute for this technique that may be suitable for deaf offenders. Another common component of sexual offender treatment is involvement in a support group. It is extremely unlikely that there will be a support group such as Sexaholics Anonymous for deaf offenders in the area. Thus, even while in treatment, the deaf sexual offender will remain isolated from other sexual offenders who could provide support while confronting him about his deviant thinking and behavior.

Guidelines for Treatment

Whenever possible, the therapist should also work with the offender's spouse and family. The wife of a deaf sexual offender lives in a minority culture and potentially faces a greater degree of social isolation and loss if her marriage fails, compared to hearing spouses of sexual offenders. Deaf women are more likely to be underemployed than hearing women or deaf men. They are often in the lowest income bracket and may have few incentives to seek employment. This makes the prospect of being alone even more daunting. On the other hand, she will feel loyalty to her children, who are likely to be hearing, while at the same time she will want to support her husband, a member of the deaf community, which may be the only source of social support for husband and wife. She may be understandably reluctant to accept her husband's guilt, fearing that not only could she lose her marriage if she does not support him, but her standing in the deaf community as well. In child molestation cases, this reluctance could affect her ability to protect her children. It will be necessary to educate her about the seriousness of her husband's offending and potential for reoffense and what she should do if she suspects that her husband is reoffending.

Much of the initial stages of treatment should utilize a didactic approach. The therapist should explore the deaf offender's fund of knowledge about such things as empathy, victimization, and basic sexual information. The deaf offender's experience and understanding may be different than the hearing offender's and may require education about role-taking and what it means and how it feels to be a victim. The very meaning of the word "victim" may be unfamiliar to the deaf offender, as there is no specific ASL sign for the term. Heller (1987) refers to a number of psychologists in the field of deafness who have described a number of distinctive personality characteristics of deaf mental health clients. These qualities include egocentricity, a lack of empathy, emotional immaturity, dependency, poor impulse control, and poor emotional adaptability. We have consistently observed these traits in deaf sexual offenders, and these traits should be the subject of intense clinical focus.

A major treatment goal with sexual offenders is the development of victim empathy. As noted above, deaf sexual offenders often attribute their offending to "curiosity" or ignorance and adhere tenaciously to these beliefs. Deaf offenders in turn often attribute this curiosity and ignorance to their deafness. The therapist will be required to not only challenge these beliefs, but also to educate the offender about the impact of his behavior on his victims and on society as a whole. The deaf offender who has been involved in deviant sexual activity from an early age and who did not perceive the activity as harmful may not understand why society places such negative sanctions on those who participate in this behavior. For example, they may not understand how old a person should be before giving consent to engage in sexual behavior with another. They may have difficulty distinguishing between aggressive sexual behavior and consenting sexual interaction. Deaf persons often hold more conservative, traditional sex role attitudes than their hearing peers. These attitudes can contribute to the offender's belief in male dominance and a sense of entitlement in meeting his sexual and relational needs. Similarly, the acceptance by the deaf offender's spouse of these same values can help maintain his distorted thinking, allowing him to continue with his behavior and rationalizations unchallenged. The deaf community's attitudes can influence the offender in a similar fashion, supporting his denial and minimization. The hearing therapist may encounter resistance from the offender as attempts are made to challenge these traditional values.

For deaf offenders whose English skills are sufficient, many of the same treatment techniques used with hearing offenders can be employed. Typically, these include writing an autobiography, keeping a journal, and reading assigned materials. Other treatment techniques are virtually identical to those used with hearing offenders. It is crucial to help the offender identify high-risk situations that could lead to a reoffense and to develop concrete plans for dealing with those situations should they arise. The deaf offender's therapist may be his only support during these times, and the therapist should develop a crisis plan with the offender that details how to contact the therapist at any time. As treatment nears termination, the therapist should encourage the client to return to counseling in the future if he feels that he is at risk to reoffend or if he faces other problems.

By now, the reader may be completely discouraged about the prospect of treating deaf sexual offenders. The therapist who takes on the challenge of working with deaf sexual offenders and who demonstrates an understanding of the deaf experience will be rewarded by earning the respect of the deaf community and the appreciation of the offender and his family. The deaf client may have experienced for the first time a hearing person's willingness to devote time and energy to his welfare. The opportunity to communicate his experience in a shared language to a hearing therapist who understands the Deaf way without being patronizing may have far-reaching benefits, enhancing the deaf client's self-esteem, while protecting the community and potential victims.

REFERENCES

Dolnick, E. (1993, September). Deafness as culture. *The Atlantic Monthly*, 37–53.

Golan, L. (1996, March 10), Dialogue of the deaf: What Gallaudet won't teach. *The Washington Post*, pp. C1–C2.

Green, B. (1985). Child abuse among the deaf and their families: Etiological considerations. In G. Anderson & D. Watson (Eds.), *Counseling deaf people: Research and practice* (pp. 55–82). Little Rock: University of Arkansas. Arkansas Rehabilitation Research and Training Center on Deafness and Hearing Impairment.

Heller, B. (1987). Mental health assessment of deaf persons: A brief history. In H. Elliott, L. Glass, & J. W. Evans (Eds.), *Mental health assessment of deaf clients. A practical manual* (pp. 9–20). Boston: Little, Brown.

Isaac, C. (1994). *Letter to members.* (Available from The Association for the Treatment of Sexual Abusers, P. O. Box 866, Lake Oswego, OR 97034-0140.)

Klopping, H. (1985). The deaf adolescent: Abuse and abusers. In G. B. Anderson & D. Waton (Eds.), *Proceedings of the National Conference on the Habilitation and Rehabilitation of Deaf Adolescents* (pp. 187–196). Washington, DC: National Academy of Gallaudet University.

Pollard, R. (1992). 100 years in psychology and deafness: A centennial retrospective. *Journal of Rehabilitation of the Deaf, 26,* 32–46.

Schein, J. D., & Delk, M. T. (1974). *The deaf population of the United States.* Silver Spring, MD: National Association for the Deaf.

Schildroth, A. N., & Hotto, S. A. (1994). Inclusion or exclusion? Deaf students and the inclusion movement. *American Annals of the Deaf, 139,* 239–240.

Steinberg, A. (1991). Issues in providing mental health services to hearing-impaired persons. *Hospital and Community Psychiatry, 42,* 380–389.

Sullivan, P. M., & Knutson, J. D. (1995). *The relationship between child abuse and neglect and disabilities: Implications for research and practice.* Omaha, NE: Boys Town National Research Hospital.

Sullivan, P. M., Vernon, M., & Scanlon, J. (1987). Sexual abuse of deaf youth. *American Annals of the Deaf, 132,* 256–262.

University of California Center on Deafness. (1987). *Guidelines for mental health professionals: Use of interpreters for the deaf.* San Francisco, CA: Author.

Vernon, M. (1995). An historical perspective on psychology and deafness. *Journal of the American Deafness and Rehabilitation Association, 29,* 8–13.

Woodward, J. (1979). *Signs of sexual behavior.* Silver Spring, MD: T.J. Publishers.

Wright, D. (1969). *Deafness.* New York: Stein & Day.

Zieziula, F.R. (Ed.). (1982). *Assessment of hearing-impaired people: A guide for selecting psychological, educational, and vocational tests.* Washington, DC: Gallaudet College Press.

21

Clergy Offenders

Andrew F. Kelly

This chapter is concerned with the particular aspects of treating clergy sexual offenders. Procedures that are rather "standard fare" for the treatment of sexual offenders are not delineated, although passing mention may be made of certain treatment techniques.

SOCIETAL ROLE OF THE CLERGY

Sexual misconduct among clergy is one of the most sensitive and emotionally charged topics facing society today. This fact is not missed by the media, who spare no opportunity to publicize another story about a priest or minister purportedly engaged in sexual misconduct. This is as true when there is only an unsubstantiated allegation made as it is in the unfortunate cases in which misconduct has indeed occurred. There is no mystery why public scrutiny in this matter is so great; the trust placed in religious professionals is truly sacred. Adults and children alike rely on clerics as members of society who are incorruptible by the concerns of everyday life. It is these individuals with whom people can share their darkest secrets and transgressions, without fear of retribution or shame. It is the clergy to whom many turn in their most difficult times. It is natural, therefore, for society at large to feel betrayed when the sacred trust we place in the clergy is violated. This represents an abuse of the power we accord religious professionals. Many in society are quite unsympathetic to the individuals who have violated this trust and feel they should banish them from the church and not be concerned with treatment or rehabilitation for the offenders. It is understandable they feel this way. Many of the clergy feel this way, and this issue, perhaps more than any other, is a source of disunity within the clerical body itself.

STEREOTYPE OF PAST CHURCH RESPONSE

Institutional Denial and Misunderstanding of the Nature of Sexual Abuse

The public trust in clergy and in the church hierarchy has not been helped by the manner in which clerics accused of sexual abuse have been handled by their ecclesiastical

Andrew F. Kelly • Clergy Consultation and Treatment Services, Outpatient Mental Health Services, St. Vincent's Westchester, Harrison, New York 10528.

Sourcebook of Treatment Programs for Sexual Offenders, edited by Marshall et al. Plenum Press, New York, 1998.

superiors in the past. The news media publicizes the cases in which accused clerics have denied the allegations to their superiors and were then reassigned to other locations. Worse still is the public perception of reported cases in which the men have admitted their abusive action, explained it in some manner, and were then reassigned after promising never to do this again.

Such behavior on the part of the authorities appears quite unsympathetic to the victims of abuse and to the people whom the clerics serve. It is hard to understand the naiveté of the church authorities at the time these abuses were taking place. In attempting to relate the naive stance of the church, an official once commented, "You know, 5 years ago I thought a pedophile was some kind of bicycle." It is only in the recent past that the public perception of sexual abuse in society has begun to change, as it has for the church hierarchy. The good news is that things have changed dramatically in the church.

Reform

General Policy and Procedure for Dealing with Allegations

Reform concerning the manner in which to deal with allegations of sexual abuse was led by Catholic institutions. This was clearly in response to the need for such reform when "priest pedophiles" became a buzzword in the press and public consciousness as Catholic institutions garnered most of the media attention. The reform began on an individual, diocese-by-diocese basis as dictated by local incidents of abuse. The most far-reaching reform began in the Chicago archdiocese in September 1992, with a formal policy of removal of any clergy against whom an allegation of sexual abuse had been lodged. A review board, with a lay majority not employed by the church, was established to consider all complaints of abuse, thus addressing the issue of the church attempting to police itself. The board is composed of three professionals (a psychiatrist, a psychologist, and an attorney), three priests, and three lay nonprofessionals. Chicago also set up a Victim Assistance Ministry designed to refer victims of abuse to professional help paid for by the archdiocese.

Review boards similar to Chicago's have been established in the larger dioceses throughout the United States. In smaller dioceses or religious orders (which may be composed of only 60 members), standardized policies and procedures are being established to deal with abuse allegations.

In June 1992, the Canadian bishops' Ad Hoc Committee on Child Sexual Abuse released a 90-page report to the Catholic Church of Canada (Canadian Conference of Catholic Bishops, 1992). The report contained 50 recommendations for responding to the problem of sexual abuse of children. Among the recommendations was the establishment of a review board process similar to that instituted by the Chicago archdiocese. The report recommended that Canadian Catholics become educated about sexual abuse and it provided principles and action plans to bishops concerning the handling of abuse cases, as well as making suggestions concerning the formation of clergy. In particular, the report recommended the involvement of women in training priests. The report also addressed the issue of abuse prevention, loneliness among diocesan priests, and the need to strengthen the support available to diocesan clergy.

In February 1993, a group of 31 psychiatrists, psychologists, priests, social workers, and victim representatives met to develop recommendations to the National Conference of Catholic Bishops (NCCB) regarding policy for responding to the "problem of child sexual abuse." They developed recommendations in three general areas: (1) care of victims, including offers of direct assistance, openness, and community education; (2) prevention, including upgrading priest candidate screening procedures, wellness promotion among clergy, treatment for abusers, and training in abuse recognition and research; and (3) principles for relapse prevention and reassignment.

Abuse of Power and the Denial Process

Shifts in perspective concerning clergy abuse of power are clear in the document as noted in the following passage (Canadian Conference of Catholic Bishops, 1992, Section E, point 46): "... a model of church life in which priests live their ministry as if it were an undebatable power provides a more favorable environment for committing and continuing acts of child sexual abuse." This passage makes clear the recognition that abuse is made possible by the cleric's role in society, and as such the institutional church is involved. It is therefore true that clergy offenders are abusing the power inherent in their position; sexual misconduct by a cleric is not just a matter of an individual who loses control temporarily and who can be trusted to "never do it again." Recognizing that the dynamics of the problem extend beyond the particular individuals involved is a paradigmatic shift.

The recognition of the power of denial and the need for treatment is illustrated in another section of the report (Canadian Conference of Catholic Bishops, 1992, Section B, point 17):

> There is one prerequisite before a priest implicated in child sexual abuse can begin specialized treatment: He must have begun to reexamine his own emotional, spiritual and sexual life. He should be capable of recognizing that this admission of his own limitations and failings is a sine qua non and that it is vital for him to cooperate with competent people in the field of psychiatry, counseling and spirituality who are ready to help him. It is of paramount importance that he seek to overcome denial and resistance to truth if he wishes to be as free as completely possible for the rest of his life.

In a sense, this passage may be seen as directed to the psychological process of denial, which may have been practiced by some church authorities as well. The offenders are troubled men who desperately need professional treatment to overcome their psychiatric disorder. The question now becomes where to send them for treatment.

PROBLEMS IN THE ESTABLISHMENT OF TREATMENT CENTERS

Social Stigma

The treatment of those guilty of sexual abuse is itself an emotionally charged issue. In American society a debate currently rages concerning the public registering and identification of adjudicated sex offenders in local communities to "warn" the public of the whereabouts of such individuals (Megan's Law). As is well known, among the prison population those guilty of child sexual abuse are often segregated from the general prison population for their own protection. Clearly, society looks down on this population. It is not hard to imagine, then, how this stigma becomes magnified even further among the clergy.

In establishing a treatment center for this population, it is necessary to contend not only with the societal stigma, but with the added negative attitudes of the public toward clergy who have "sinned" in this manner. In a hospital setting, the attitude of the hospital administrative staff may be expressed by marked ambivalence concerning the marketing of the program. Two competing agendas often exist within hospital communities regarding this specialty service: to have "those who need to know" be aware of the program, but not to let the general public or perhaps even the hospital staff know too much about it. This is not necessarily an openly expressed attitude, but rather an unstated, implied posture. This "feeling" has been expressed by members of small community-based hospital programs, and larger, more general hospital-based programs. There is also good reason for this beyond simple prejudice: clergy sexual abusers are a titillating story, and most hospital administrators do not desire to draw the attention of the press to such a program. The press have been known to go to great lengths to interview offending clergy, including obtaining visitor passes as a "relative," with elaborate stories of the need for an emergency visit, just to work their way into the treatment facility to get a "scoop," disregarding the confidentiality of the patient.

There is also the issue of the surrounding community. Recently a treatment center that treats clergy encountered some community protest regarding their moving to that community. The local community were afraid that their children would be at risk by being close to a facility that may treat some pedophile offenders. In the case of another clergy treatment facility, offending clergy tended to stay in the state where they received treatment. Some of these clergy were hired by the treatment facility itself as recovering counselors. Community protest grew at having such a population located in the state, especially when further allegations surfaced about some of the clergy who had settled there.

Attitude of the Clergy

Bias against the Offender and the Treatment Center

There is also the attitude of fellow clergy to consider. While they generally feel quite badly for their brothers who have committed these acts of abuse and have difficulty understanding how they could have done it, many are quite unsympathetic. They will not stand in the same room with them, feeling that these men have damaged the reputation of the church and, by extension, their own reputation. They not only want nothing to do with them, but nothing to do with any treatment facility that treats them. This can extend as well to religious retreat centers that often house the offending cleric, at least temporarily. Fellow clergy fear that if someone sees them at the treatment facility, they are automatically presumed to "have a problem" (i.e., a paraphilia of some kind). Given the reality of the closeness of the clergy community, rumors can travel fast. Very few want to take the chance of their reputation being needlessly tarnished, when all they came to talk about was a recent anxiety attack. Thus, treatment providers must deal with the resistance of the clergy population to attend the facility voluntarily.

Confidentiality

The closeness within the clergy community can be both a help and a hindrance to the treatment program goals. As noted above, fears of a damaged reputation can prevent those contemplating the need for help to seek it, thus reducing the available treatment population and leaving unmet the needs of the clergy. The closeness can help in that those who are supportive of the individual may be more readily available than friends in the lay community. This does, however, raise to an extreme level the need for confidentiality. Among the clergy, everyone knows everyone. The slightest description of an individual, piece of history, circumstance, or event can identify a cleric to other clergy in ways one might never suspect. Thus, the care mental health professionals practice in maintaining patient confidentiality must be accomplished with particular vigilance with this population.

Referral for Treatment: Mandated versus Voluntary

Adding to the social stigma of attending a treatment center is the fact that individuals are often mandated to receive an evaluation at the facility. The obligatory nature of such attendance raises even higher the suspicion that an individual may be "guilty" of something, or at least is accused of some kind of impropriety.

Therapeutic Alliance

While not unique to clergy, the attitude of the evaluee is likely to be much less compliant in those situations in which attendance has been mandated by a superior. As would be the case in the general public if an employer mandated an evaluation after an allegation had been lodged, the cleric may be resentful and protest that "the whole thing is political." The tendency for an accused to feel that this may be political is particularly intense for the clergy population, since this is a much more tightly integrated subculture than is the general public. Thus, the evaluee may claim that there are ulterior motives behind the referral and be resistant to cooperate or reveal much of himself. The "political" argument may be seized upon as a process of denial by the accused, either consciously or unconsciously.

The ability to maintain an open, cooperative attitude is probably easier with the clergy than among the general population, as there is already a built-in alliance and sense of caring and community. After all, if the cleric is innocent, then he should be able to get through this and return to his good work of ministry. If he is guilty, he is clearly in need of help, and everyone wants to prevent further harm to victims, the cleric, and the church community. Thus, the community nature of the life of clergy can be a very positive force if used in a curative manner.

ASSESSMENT

The assessment of sexually offending clergy should consist of at least a series of clinical interviews addressing general psychopathology for the assessment of comorbid diagnoses outside of the paraphilias (including addictions), a complete sexual history, personality assessment via self-report and examiner-administered testing, cognitive and neuropsychological testing, and a physical examination. General parameters of assessment will not be covered here, as we are limiting our discussion to issues that are unique to the assessment of clergy.

Initiating the Assessment

The treatment center must be careful to develop and maintain a neutral position with respect to the cleric and church authorities while conducting the assessment. As there may be mistrust between these authorities, the center must avoid being perceived as allied with either party. This may be accomplished by having the allegation clearly spelled out by a church official, usually the director of personnel, with the evaluation team (or one team member) and the accused cleric present. This fosters clarification, reduces the ambiguity that can breed suspicion, and sets a tone of openness and cooperation. Such an outright delineation of the allegation also serves as a first step in reducing the shame inherent in the evaluation process. With everything out in the open, the pressure to keep things hidden or unmentioned is greatly reduced. The message to the offender is, "Yes, we know all of this, and we still care about you and want to help you." To optimally set the stage for this process, before the church official describes the allegation, the offender should be instructed that he is not expected to say anything in response. It is better in fact if he saves any response for later in talking to the treatment team, after the official has left. Small-group studies in social psychology have clearly established how much more difficult it is to retract a falsehood after it is uttered before a group, and this should be prevented during this initial "setup phase" of the therapeutic alliance. The internal pressure is for the offender to publicly deny the allegation when first hearing it systematically presented to him and the treatment team by an "authority" figure, especially as the cleric is likely to be in great denial at this initial phase of treatment.

Special Assessment Considerations

Spiritual Assessment

The cleric's perceived relationship to God and the things of God must be improved for his full recovery. One of the first things clergy will often admit is that during the time they committed the offense(s), their prayer life was very seriously neglected or nonexistent. A personal spiritual history that addresses when they first heard the calling to serve God, their formation toward ordination, and where they served and how they faired at their various assignments are crucial pieces of information. An assignment history organizes the cleric's story in a way that often reveals where things began to go wrong in their spiritual life. How did they get along with the people with whom and to whom they ministered? What were the frustrations they experienced? What helped and hindered their own intimacy with respect to God? Do they view God as harsh and retributive or can they believe God to be compassionate and forgiving, especially with respect to themselves?

False Accusations

The clergy population is in the somewhat unique situation of having to deal with false allegations. While false accusations of sexual abuse do exist among the laity, especially in business settings, this is a particular problem among clergy. Often, the church is viewed as a "deep pocket" that may settle out of court rather than risk bad publicity, especially in the current climate. Clergy who are accused must be assessed, since this is good practice and is part of what appears to be an emerging standard policy of ecclesiastical communities around the world. Apart from the protection of potential victims and the clarity that an assessment will hopefully bring, the church is almost obligated in the current litigious environment to undertake an evaluation if the allegation can be considered in any way to be credible. The church is also interested in clearing the good name of clerics falsely accused and needs to stand behind them in such cases. While the treatment center cannot and should not attempt to determine the guilt or innocence of the accused, the evaluation is an important element in responding to an allegation, and some degree of cleric credibility assessment is involved.

Vague Criteria

Complicating any evaluation is the rather vague criteria concerning the characteristics of an effective cleric. What are we measuring when determining effectiveness? There are certainly "rule-outs" such as psychosis, antisocial character traits, and paraphilias, but what exactly are the positive criteria we are looking for and how do we measure them? It is quite difficult to write a concise job description for the clergy.

Plethysmography

There is considerable resistance among clergy organizations to the use of penile plethysmography. In the past, the stimulus materials were often of a pornographic nature, thus placing the cleric in the "occasion of sin." As the stimulus materials become less pornographic in nature, this objection may lessen; but compared to the general population, this assessment technique is not often used with clergy.

TREATMENT

Incidence/Prevalence

While there have been many statistics reporting the incidence of sexual abuse by clergy, so far no systematic, well-controlled studies have been completed to clarify this issue. In total, there appears to be more than 400 documented cases of child sexual abuse by Catholic clergy in the United States. Catholic clergy have drawn the most media attention, but there are allegations against Episcopal, Methodist, Lutheran, Presbyterian, and Greek Orthodox clergy as well (Jenkins, 1996).

The most systematic study to this point is the Chicago study conducted by a commission appointed by Joseph Cardinal Bernardin (Dempsey, Gorman, Madden, & Spilly, 1992). This study examined the priest personnel files of the archdiocese of Chicago between 1963 and 1991 ($N = 2252$). They found allegations of sexual abuse against 57 incardinated priests and 2 priests from other dioceses (visiting priests). Using the less stringent standards of civil law in which allegations do not have to be proven beyond a reasonable doubt, they found allegations against 39 priests and 2 visiting priests to be credible. This averages to 2.6% of the Chicago archdiocesan clergy having allegations against them, with 1.7% credible. In general, it is thought that between 2 and 3% of all Catholic clergy may have acted out sexually against minors (children and teenagers), with by far the greater incidence of abuse being against teenage males.

Stereotype of Clergy as Pedophiles

Perhaps one of the most distorted public perceptions of clergy sexual offenders is that they overwhelmingly abuse children. The public tends to view clergy offenders as "predator pedophiles," actively seeking out available children. This perception is likely the result of the extensive publicity that cases of pedophilia receive in the media. Father Canice Connors, former Director of St. Luke's Institute (he stepped down in December 1996), a residential treatment center for clergy, estimates that about 0.3% of American Catholic clergy might be active pedophiles. He reports that of the more than 500 priests and brothers who have been evaluated at Saint Luke's during a 10-ycarperiod, 44 received a diagnosis of pedophilia, 185 ephebophilia, 142 as compulsives, and 165 with "unintegrated sexuality" (Connors, 1994, p. 15). The fact that true pedophilia is in fact rather rare among clergy certainly runs counter to the current public perceptions.

Parish Trauma: The Removal of Clergy from Their Assignments

For parishioners, the removal of a cleric from their parish is devastating. This is the individual who ministers to them every week. They feel comforted and secure in his presence. When a cleric is removed from his assignment, the removal is usually swift and sudden, without warning. An announcement may be made by the cleric that he will be going on retreat for spiritual renewal or he may simply disappear, depending on circumstances. It is optimal for there to be some explanation, but if an allegation is made publicly and is blasted across the front page of the local paper, "the "optimal" situation may not be possible. If the allegation is credible and there is no doubt the cleric has abused a minor sexually, it is not helpful to either the cleric or the community to have him stand before the congregation at this time of emotional crisis. At that point, everyone feels confused, hurt, shamed, angry, and betrayed. Threats against the cleric's life in such situations have been made and should be taken quite seriously. At this time of spiritual crisis, the collective intellect and judgment of the parishioners is overwhelmed by raw emotion.

Intervention Team

In such a situation, the treatment center must have an intervention team ready to give information about the nature and effects of sexual abuse, to listen to the concerns of the parishioners, and to answer questions. A meeting with the parish staff should occur first, as the staff itself will usually be quite devastated. The meeting should include an official from the clergy personnel office, the treatment intervention team, and staff from the school, if one is affiliated with the parish. Next, the same group should meet with the parishioners. A brief presentation on the nature of sexual abuse should be made to provide information to supplant the fantasy and misinformation that may be present. This provides a grounding experience to help stabilize the crisis atmosphere and fosters a focus for the ensuing questions and discussion. Next, the team should be available for individual screening sessions to determine if parishioners need individual treatment. A referral network should be available to facilitate immediate treatment. Meetings of the team should be organized with the school staff to provide information they can share with the children. Small-group meetings led by the teachers with the students should be held in which the children's fears and worries can be addressed openly and forthrightly. The tendency for staff to feel they need to protect the children by not openly talking about the crisis, particularly in cases of child abuse, is misguided. Treatment referrals for children should be available.

If the case has been in the papers, the town will be crawling with reporters asking all kinds of questions. After the reporters leave, the people feel exploited, angry, and embarrassed. Children have expressed feelings of being rejected by neighboring communities. In the case of pedophilia and ephebophilia, children and adolescents who were seen as particularly close to the offending clergy may be suspected by their peers of also having been abused and subsequently may be shunned. Parish staff will often remark they "missed signals" and "should have known," feeling guilty that they did not intervene. In cases of child abuse, parents often feel responsible for "letting" this happen to their children. Crises of faith occur; people wonder if they truly believe anymore, and they question the validity of the services performed by the offending cleric. There is much to be done by the treatment center in responding to these crises.

The Relation of the Treatment Center to the Religious Organization

For the most part, the relationship between officials of the eccelsiatical community and the treatment center are quite cordial. As noted above, the treatment center must be careful to maintain a position of neutrality in the relationship between religious superior and cleric. If any bias is present, it should be as advocate for the cleric, since he is often unable or unwilling to advocate for himself, especially early in treatment. Limits must be set by the treatment team for successful treatment to occur. The limits to set with the cleric are part of standard practice. The limits with the religious organization are unique.

Limits concerning the parameters of communication between the treatment center and church officials should be clearly delineated in the first meeting in which the allegation is presented. As distrust of self and others is often present in the troubled cleric, a good policy is to have the cleric read every written communication and sign it before it is shared with anyone. Usually this will be treatment progress reports. In this initial session it should be quite clear to both cleric and superior what the process and content of communication will be.

In cases of milder boundary violations such as inappropriate hugging, kissing, or touching, there may be pressure to have the cleric "back to work" sooner than he is ready. When an acute episode of depression or anxiety has passed and the cleric looks and sounds better, it may be difficult for the non-mental health professional to appreciate the more subtle issues of shame, grandiosity, low self-esteem, alexythymia, and the like that set up the acute episode and/or boundary violation. The cleric, not wanting to disappoint his superior (whom he already feels he has disappointed), may also be eager to acquiesce to the superior. Issues of shame and poor assertion may be operating here, so this becomes "grist for the mill" in the treatment itself. Thus, it is essential that communication be clear to the superior why further treatment is needed. There can be pressure on the treatment center to acquiesce, since this is a future source of referrals, but this pressure cannot be a factor in the successful completion of treatment. At these times, the center acts more as an advocate for the cleric and educator of the superior.

Characteristics of Clergy Offenders

Just as there is no one type of alcohol abuser, offending clergy are individuals with diverse backgrounds and motivations for their actions. The characteristics that do tend to recur likely have more to do with their grouping as offenders than as clergy.

Subjugation of the Self

One of the most difficult issues in beginning treatment with this population is that often clergy who get into trouble have a very poorly defined sense of self. Among other things, this implies they may have limited awareness of their own emotional life, poor use of their leisure time, poor physical health, and undeveloped social relations. They may view their role in life as being concerned with the needs of others to the exclusion of themselves. In treatment, one of the first axioms for them to accept is that they cannot effectively minister to others if they cannot minister to themselves. Living one's life without regard for the development of self leads to a fragmented personal identity, especially with regard to needs for nurturance, intimacy, and sexuality.

Intimacy Failure

Intimacy has many connotations; in common parlance this term has been "sexualized" in that it often refers to some sexual interchange between individuals. Here, the term is more strictly applied, meaning the ability to feel, understand, and freely exchange aspects of the person's emotional life with others. Intimacy requires a feeling of interpersonal safety, a sense that sharing deeply felt thoughts and feelings with others will not produce negative reactions. Intimacy allows for spontaneity; action without appeal to an advanced censor. Within a spirit of intimacy, there is no need for external validation of emotions since there is an understood acceptance and ready expression of feelings.

Let us consider a case to illustrate:

> William is a Catholic priest in his late 30s who was stationed alone in a busy parish usually staffed by several priests. He was arrested for masturbating in public. William engaged in this activity knowing that he would be seen by children as they passed by. Following his arrest, William presented himself for treatment in accordance with the terms of his probationary sentence. When he entered treatment, William was a soft-spoken introvert who was mildly depressed, guilt-ridden, and notable for his complete inability to process or discuss his emotional life with anyone.
>
> William, a man consistently beaten as a child by his father and protected by no one, had an extremely negative self-image. He viewed others, especially those in authority, as threatening and not to be trusted. And yet, he found a home in the church and was extremely well-liked by those he served. A hard worker, he was devoted to those to whom he ministered. William's sense of internal self-worth was largely based on the accolades he received from others. However, when faced with a continuing conflict with his superiors, from which no relief was forthcoming, William felt powerless, hurt, and shamed. He was convinced that the reason his problem was not addressed was because he was worthless. Rejected, William's negative sense of self was activated, and all of the accolades from others were a dim shadow. When he exposed himself, William said he thought little about the children, but instead wanted to revel in his own shame. He sought to demean himself, and after committing this act, William isolated himself completely from friends and family. He had an extremely negative sense of self and felt others were good: that people in general were much better than he. There could be no better way to reinforce his own worthlessness (a familiar and in that sense comfortable view of himself) than to have others vilify and criticize him. William could not get the approval of others, and in this ineffective and self-destructive way, he expressed his anger and frustration. His action also expressed the anger and resentment he felt toward children who had a better life than he had as a child and that he felt he had now.
>
> We have been working with William to enhance his sense of self and to explore with him his own emotional life, which heretofore was unknown to William or mattered little. All that he cared about was getting the approval of others. When such approval by his superiors was not forthcoming, William self-destructed. Only as his sense of self became developed did he care to learn about his emotional life. William began to understand that the image he formed of himself, from his father through beatings and continual shaming comments, was not deserved. When asked during therapy what

William did to deserve this treatment by his father, he searched his mind. That this was a question based on an invalid premise was unknown to him. It served as a revelation when he was informed, "William, there is nothing you could have done to deserve the treatment you received." With this thought in mind, he began to cry, shedding decades of tears.

In this particular case, the children were pawns in a game of shame and self-loathing that William was lost in. He did not seek to terrorize them or establish any kind of relationship with them, but was passively exposing himself in the shameful, solipsistic world in which his image of self resided. While this certainly does not serve in any way as an excuse for William exposing himself (this is still a reprehensible act toward the children), it does cause us to target our treatment to the self-image of the offender, and to teach him healthy strategies to deal with anger and frustration. It also allows us to view the offender as a human being, rather than a monster to be permanently branded. We can perhaps appreciate his good qualities too, and see that, yes, it is possible he may have been a good priest as well.

Shame

It is important to support the good work the cleric has done in the past, as the impact of shame on clergy is particularly powerful, more so than in the general population. The reasons for this are rather apparent, as the role the cleric fulfills in society is as spiritual guide and leader. This point is made by a survey conducted of 1810 active Catholics in the United States and Canada (Rossetti, 1994). Among other questions, they were asked if they agreed with the statement: "I expect a priest's moral conduct to be better than other people's conduct." Of the 1013 lay Catholics who replied, 80.9% agreed. Of the priests who responded, 87.5% agreed. Rossetti makes the point that

> ... a large majority of active Catholics in North America still expect their priests to act better than the laity. The presbyterate shares their belief. Priests expect their own conduct to be better than the laity's conduct. In fact, priests are even more likely to set a higher standard for themselves.

For clergy to "fall from grace" is to lose a part of their sense of self or identity. For clergy like those described above who have a poorly developed sense of self apart from their vocation, it may represent a complete annihilation of the self. Thus, they may be unable to reflect on any of the positive aspects of self once they acknowledge their offense, and the offenders' choices become either denial or annihilation of the self. This process of shame is to be differentiated from guilt, as shame represents a rejection or negative evaluation of the *self*, whereas guilt is an evaluation of one's action or *behavior*. Thus, shame serves to perpetuate the initial stage of denial and must be addressed early to make progress in treatment. The offender must use guilt in a healthy manner to help reject and prevent the behavior from taking place again, whereas shame can only perpetuate actions of abuse.

Grandiosity

Grandiosity is another difficult barrier to treatment. While most clergy may praise the benefit of humility among those whom they counsel, the cleric whose sense of self is rather fragile may need to identify with a process of idolization of self and his distorted view of his role as a cleric. An inflated sense of self can greatly contribute to a resistance to acknowledge abusive acts. If such abuse is acknowledged, the abuse may be minimized and the victim blamed. While this dynamic can operate across all sexual offenders, clergy are in the unique circumstance of being able to "hide behind the church" and limit their awareness to the percentage of the parish who may back them no matter what they have done. They may be preoccupied with demonstrating to the treatment team how loved they are, dwelling on past accomplishments and parading incoming correspondence of praise from parishioners wondering when they will return to their ministry.

Blurring of Boundaries

Troubled clergy often cover over their own pain by their concern for others, thereby neglecting themselves. This defensive operation is similar to nonclergy who "throw themselves into their work." Those in the helping professions, however, run the risk of becoming dependent on their patients or parishioners for the nurturance and support they did not receive as children or perhaps are not presently receiving. Idolization by parishioners can become a danger as the boundaries between parishioner and the cleric can become blurred by the past deprivation of nurturance and current intimacy deficits in the cleric. Among healthy clergy, such idolization is recognized as reflecting an unmet need within the parishioner and is ministered to in an appropriate manner. For the wounded clergy, it can be mistaken as an opportunity to meet a need within the cleric, resulting in a violation of boundaries.

Psychosexual Immaturity

The need for nurturance may become sexualized, as intimacy becomes confused with sexual gratification. In clergy who have had little to no experience with exploring their sexuality at a young age, their psychosexual development may be arrested and therefore immature. Their sexual object of choice may therefore be an adolescent (ephebophile) or a child under the age of puberty (pedophile). In such cases, denial is often quite extreme; the cleric continues to view himself as displaying affection for the child. The dynamics of denial and psychosexual immaturity are similar to nonclergy populations, but often compounding the problem is an entrenched grandiose image of the self exacerbated by the cleric's own distortion of the affirmation received from his parishioners and the attendant abuse of the power accorded to the cleric's position in society.

Flight into Health

Another complicating factor is that clergy guilty of abusing their position of power are usually quite motivated to do no more harm, once they admit what it is they have done. Once through this initial denial stage, they can appear to truly understand what they have done and vow to never commit such an act again. In decades past when little was known about the characterological dynamics of the paraphilias, superiors were often taken in by such flights into health, believing what the cleric may have believed themselves: that they would never do it again. Clergy tend to be rather intellectualized, and their lack of awareness of their own internal emotional state only compounds the problem. They may have made up their minds, but not their hearts. In treatment, they must first be given the tool of an awareness of their own emotions.

Alexithymia

As noted, clergy are often quite intellectualized, having little awareness of their internal emotional life. As they lack this awareness and find it difficult to commune with themselves along an emotional dimension, they may not have developed a language to communicate these feelings to others. Thus, they need to develop this awareness so they may first understand how they feel themselves. Once this is accomplished, they have a tool necessary for their own recovery.

Empathy Deficit

Troubled clergy who have crossed boundaries have a poor appreciation of the effect of their action on the object of their violation. Once they are able to recognize their own emotional life, they can begin to develop empathy for their "victim(s)," along the model proposed by Marshall, Hudson, Jones, and Fernandez (1995). The stages of empathy they propose include: (1) emotional recognition, which is the ability to accurately discriminate the emotional state of another; (2) perspective taking, which is the ability to put oneself in the observed person's place and see the world as they do; (3) emotional replication, which involves the vicarious emotional response that replicates (or nearly replicates) the emotional experience of the target person; and (4) response decision, which concerns the observer's decision to act or not on the basis of their feelings.

The healthy cleric has no difficulty with empathy, and this ability is likely, in fact, part of what makes an effective cleric. The unhealthy cleric, as has been described above, is in a desperate struggle to meet his own needs and has lost touch with the needs of those to whom he ministers. It can be seen, therefore, that the development of internal emotional awareness is an important aspect of treatment.

Rebellion against Authority

Adding to the dynamics may be struggles with authority. As in the case noted above, the cleric's own issues with authority may be played out in his behavior toward those less powerful than himself. This is a clear abuse of the power of his position, and as such represents a displacement of his struggle with his religious superior to an arena in which he can feel potent.

Effects on Therapists

What is the effect on therapists who deal with clergy offenders? In comparison to the general offender population, these are ideal patients. They are generally bright, overtly cooperative, and do not have a history of violence or overt coercion. Working with any sexual offender is still a stressful experience, however, and an important question for this population is what is the effect on the faith of the therapist? This question was studied directly as part of a carefully designed structured interview of the staff of treatment centers working with Catholic clergy (Holmes & Meehan, 1995). The interviewers asked if treating priests with such scandalous histories shook the therapists' faith in church and God. In interview after interview they were surprised to hear how working with these men had reawakened the spirituality and fortified the faith of the treatment staff:

> One psychologist spoke of the "theology of tragedy" and how he had come to understand grace and suffering in a new way. Catholic therapists, and those with no identified religion, consistently replied that they had never worked in an environment that gave them more satisfaction, fulfillment and even wonder at God's love and mercy. (Holmes & Meehan, 1995, p. 23).

This finding is consistent with conversations the author has had with the staff of clergy treatment centers across the country. It may be that in seeing these men fiercely struggling to recapture the spirituality they have lost, the value of spirituality is enhanced in the observer.

AFTER TREATMENT

Continued Psychotherapy

Follow-up treatment is essential for the clergy offender to maintain gains and for implementing relapse prevention. Certainly individual therapy should be continued for a minimum of 6 months to a year, first weekly or twice weekly, then eased to biweekly when appropriate.

Support Team

An aftercare support team should also be constructed by the treatment team along with the patient prior to discharge from the treatment program. The support team should include a member of the church hierarchy, usually an individual from the office of personnel or the equivalent who has some degree of authority. This keeps the lines of communication between cleric and superior open. Friends whom the cleric trusts should also be part of the team. These people should be a mixture of friends from the clergy and laity. The team should be small enough to convene reliably, as continuity from meeting to meeting is essential; five or six members is appropriate.

The purpose of the team is to support the cleric, by giving him the opportunity to talk about his life, struggles, and feelings and by knowing that any one of them is available to be called on at any time, should the need arise. It is less formal than treatment and allows the cleric to talk about what is on his mind no matter how trivial it may seem. The support team helps prevent the cleric from falling back into old patterns such as working compulsively or isolating himself and becoming lonely. Suggestions can be made in an atmosphere that is "lighter" than the treatment setting allows, especially as the meeting will take place in the parish, at someone's home, or some other location of the cleric's choice.

12-Step Meetings

Attendance at 12-step meetings such as Sexaholics Anonymous (SA), or Sex and Love Addicts Anonymous (SLAA) is also helpful, especially for the compulsively driven paraphilias. The cleric may not share with this group his vocation if he does not wish to do so, but he must share himself in all other ways and be part of the group. These 12-step groups, however, should be viewed as treatment adjuncts and not as replacements for treatment. These meetings also vary considerably in their level of sophistication and in the messages they deliver. The primary individual therapist should ask about the meetings to ensure that the cleric is receiving appropriate information and interpreting what is being said in a helpful manner.

Reassignment and Its Legal Implications

There is a full range of opinions on what the church should do concerning the reassignment of a cleric following treatment. Some feel that clergy guilty of sexual misconduct should never be returned to ministry in any form (Fortune, 1989). This view represents one extreme end of the continuum of options. There is good evidence from empirical research conducted at the Saint Luke Institute (Connors, 1994) that such a dire approach is unwarranted. Connors' 10-year follow-up research on priests treated in St. Luke's residential program who had achieved sexual sobriety showed no incidence of reoffending. Connors points to a number of risk factors, however:

> Favorable indications include these factors: At the height of the disease, the priest involved sought older victims, showed little overt aggression, had a small number of victims, and now has better neuropsychological function; is conflicted about his behavior, shows remorse and victim empathy during treatment, enjoys improved peer relationships, and is active in constructing support for his ongoing recovery. (p. 15)

Certainly the less compulsive the behavior, the more confident one can be of a positive treatment outcome. Implicit in improved peer relations is an ability to tolerate a healthy intimacy and to let others in to share feelings, thoughts, and values. The better the cleric's peer relations and social support network, the less the drive to assuage the ache of loneliness through sexually offending.

While the religious authority may, in a particular case, feel rather confident in reassigning that individual, they are also faced with the reality of being sued in civil court for punitive damages of negligence should that individual reoffend. If the cleric offends and the superior had no reason to suspect such an event, the church will be unlikely to be held liable for damages. Once it can be shown in a court of law that there was reason to be suspicious of that individual (such as past offending), then the organization is liable for punitive damages. The manner in which different superiors deal with this is up to them, but the trend is to increasingly assign clerics with any history of offending to administrative office jobs or to decide they are technically "unassignable." The superior is placed in the extremely difficult position of having to choose between legal liability and the devastating financial effect such liability can have on the entire religious organization and the vocation of the cleric. To be a cleric is not a job, it is a way of life. It is calling that the individual feels from deep within. For the superior to deny the cleric the opportunity to resume his ministry is to literally to take away the meaning of his life. It is a very difficult decision to make. In the case of the pedophile, there is no question that the cleric can no longer have any ministry to children. For the cleric who is guilty of sexual misconduct with adolescents or adults and who in the opinion of the treatment center has been successfully treated, the decision is much more difficult.

CONCLUSION

The stereotype of clergy as "predator pedophiles" is quite strong. The zeal of the media in publicizing a relatively few number of cases and the readily identifiable nature of the clergy contributes to the genesis and maintenance of this stereotype. Many clerics will never touch a child at any time because of the overwhelming fear that they will be accused of sexual misconduct. Elder clergy are genuinely aghast at the extent to which fear has created a culture in which they must keep children at a distance, preventing them from carrying out a part of their ministry that in the past has been so vital to themselves and to families of the parish. But what of the clerics who have sexually offended?

While there are no formal studies, cases of true "predator pedophiles" seem relatively rare among the clergy population. This is likely due to the extensive ecclesiastical training and screening process that will tend to "weed out" frank antisocial character pathology among candidates. These are individuals who tend to live in some kind of community at some point during their training, thus permitting more extensive observation of their behavior than would be the case with other "employers."

In terms of treatment, while clergy tend to be rather intellectualized, thus presenting their own set of treatment difficulties, clergy offenders are likely an easier population to treat than the offender population in general. Once through the denial stage, they are ready to evaluate, introspect, and deal with the moral and interpersonal aspects of their action. This reflective posture is, after all, a part of their training. While there are certainly treatment failures among this population, there is good reason to be optimistic about successful treatment. These are individuals who have chosen to lead a life devoted to the care and ministry to others; now they must learn how to minister to themselves. With the proper amount of time, their issues of shame, intimacy failure, and grandiosity can be successfully explored and resolved.

REFERENCES

Canadian Conference of Catholic Bishops. (1992). *From pain to hope*. Publications Service, Canadian Conference of Catholic Bishops, 90 Parent Avenue, Ottawa, Ontario K1N 7B1, Canada.

Connors, C. (1994, October 21). The moment after suffering. Lessons from the pedophilia scandal. *Commonweal*, pp. 14–17.

Dempsey, J. Q., Gorman, J. R., Madden, J. P., & Spilly, A. P. (1992). *The Cardinal's Commission on Clerical Sexual Misconduct with Minors: Report to Joseph Cardinal Bernardin, Archbishop of Chicago*. Chicago: The Commission.

Fortune, M. (1989). *Is nothing sacred?* New York: Harper & Row.

Holmes, P. A., & Meehan, M. J. (1995, September, 9). Broken glass. *America*, pp. 22–23.

Jenkins, P. (1996). *Pedophiles and priests: Anatomy of a contemporary crisis*. New York: Oxford University Press.

Marshall, W. L., Hudson, S. M., Jones, R., & Fernandez, Y. M. (1995). Empathy in sex offenders. *Clinical Psychology Review, 15*, 99–113.

Rossetti, S.J. (1994, October, 29). Priest suicides and the crisis of faith. *America*, pp. 8–12.

22

Professionals

Gene G. Abel, Candice A. Osborn, and Brent W. Warberg

Protecting the public from sexual victimization should be the primary goal of treatment programs for sexual perpetrators. We should be particularly protective of those who are the most vulnerable, such as the very young (Abel, Lawry, Karlstrom, Osborn, & Gillespie, 1994) or old, those with physical or emotional impairments, and those who seek professional assistance. In the professional setting, clients are particularly vulnerable since they have virtually no knowledge of what constitutes appropriate professional conduct, they are in some degree of stress, and they are in need of assistance from the professional. The professional, after years of training and immersion in the professional role, can develop considerable professional arrogance and insensitivity to the vulnerability of clients. Some professionals also fail to appreciate that they are never on an equal power base with a client seeking their assistance. They may rationalize that their professional interaction simply involves two adults communicating with one another, when in actuality the professional relationship requires a level of trust and personal intimacy not present in other stranger-to-stranger relationships. Thus, the very nature of the professional relationship places professionals in a position in which they can exploit their client's trust. In some cases, this leads to inappropriate sexual behavior perpetrated by the professional against a very vulnerable client. This chapter attempts to clarify how such victimization can be prevented.

According to the Ad Hoc Committee on Physician Impairment Report on Sexual Boundary Issues (Schneidman, 1995), professional sexual misconduct (PSM) "exploits the physician–patient relationship, is a violation of the public's trust, and causes immeasurable harm, both mentally and physically, to the patient" (p. 208). This committee identified two levels of sexual misconduct: sexual violation and sexual impropriety. Sexual violation includes physician–patient sex, whether or not initiated by the patient, and engaging in any conduct with a patient that is sexual or may be reasonably interpreted as sexual. Sexual impropriety includes behavior, gestures, or expressions that are seductive, sexually suggestive, or sexually demeaning to a patient. These definitions may be applicable to sexual behavior between professionals in any field and the clients they serve. Approximately 20% of these offending professionals carry out activities traditionally viewed as paraphilias (such as frottage, fetishism, pedophilia, and voyeurism), but the majority are involved in

Gene G. Abel, Candice A. Osborn, and Brent W. Warberg • Behavioral Medicine Institute of Atlanta, Atlanta, Georgia 30327.

Sourcebook of Treatment Programs for Sexual Offenders, edited by Marshall et al. Plenum Press, New York, 1998.

sexual activities with their adult clients that, if they occurred independent of the professional relationship and were by mutual consent, would not warrant further attention.

The professionals involved in PSM cover the broad spectrum of individuals given special access to clients, most of whom require a professional license, ordination to holy orders, or certification to practice. Examples include social workers or therapists providing counseling, lawyers providing legal services, clerics providing spiritual counseling, physicians or nurses providing diagnosis or treatment, psychologists providing psychological evaluation and/or treatment, and educators teaching students, to name but a few. Although all combinations of genders become involved in PSM, the majority of these cases involve a male professional perpetrating upon a female client (Gartrell, Herman, Olarte, Feldstein, & Localio, 1986). For this reason this discussion will refer to the perpetrator as he and the client–victim as she.

What makes treatment for such perpetrators challenging is that many of them have devoted the majority of their lives to the acquisition of various professional skills and, as such, are highly trained and competent in the practice of their profession, excluding their PSM. In many cases, the professional views his activities with his client not as sexual misconduct, but as mutual sexual activity between two consenting adults, one of whom happens to be a professional. In many cases, the professional ethics that govern such activity have been vague to nonexistent or not addressed during the professional's training. The professional often denies the inappropriateness of his sexual behavior with a plethora of cognitive distortions and professional arrogance. By the time the professional comes to the attention of others, he frequently has been sexually involved with more than one client, on a number of occasions.

We have extended our traditional sexual offender treatment to this population for a number of reasons. First, others had failed to see the similarities in the assessment and treatment of perpetrators of PSM and those diagnosed with paraphilias. In both groups, the perpetrators are primarily males; there is a compulsive quality to the perpetrators' behavior; the perpetrators operate from an unequal power base between them and their victim; attempts are made by the perpetrators to conceal their sexual activity from others; treatment is frequently not self-motivated, but results from others becoming aware of the sexual misconduct; stress, anxiety, depression, drug misuse, or skills deficits are common antecedents to the sexual behavior; paraphilic arousal patterns sometimes lead to the misconduct; victims are generally selected because of their helpless, vulnerable or suffering state; there is an organized, planned grooming or seduction of the victims; cognitive distortions are almost always used by the perpetrators to justify their behavior; the perpetrators demonstrate an inability to empathize with their victims' plight; the perpetrators are usually absent when the victims become symptomatic as they begin to appreciate the inappropriateness of the perpetrator's sexual behavior; and the perpetrators' initial presentation is that of a hostile, angry individual who denies the accusations against him/her.

A second factor was that the regulating agencies that inevitably became involved in such cases had minimal knowledge or understanding of the already-existing extensive professional literature regarding the evaluation and treatment of inappropriate sexual behaviors. Many such organizations have either minimized the misconduct by viewing it as a sin, a misunderstanding, or a simple issue of morals or have overreacted by discarding the professional out of hand. In some cases, the regulating agencies have seen no relationship between their handling of these cases and their own responsibilities as professionals. Most regulating agencies have failed to appreciate the reality that the very nature of the professional relationship brings the professional into frequent contact with vulnerable clients, a situation that is ripe for possible exploitation. The most common deficit of these organizations has been that, once the PSM behavior was exposed, there was no organized, systematic means of checks and balances to protect future potential victims or to provide treatment to the professional to prevent future occurrences of PSM. The professional involved was admonished by his profession, told not to do is again, and returned to the profession without an organized plan for preventing reoccurrences, or was automatically removed from the profession. This is not to say that all perpetrators can be safely returned to the practice of their profession; some, indeed, are so severely impaired that they should be restricted from ever practicing again. However, this decision should not be arbitrary, but based on a systematic assessment and an examination of treatment outcome.

RESPONSE TO PSM BY REGULATING AGENCIES

Each regulating agency appears to handle PSM within its own structure. In some respects, the regulating agencies have responded to PSM in a fashion consistent with the profession that they represent. In most cases it is impossible to discern the rules by which each of the professions deals with PSM within its ranks, since the discussion preceding the decisions often occur in closed hearing. This issue is highly politicized and strongly influenced by national attitudes regarding crime and punishment and society's view of the professional. Since the perpetrators of PSM often have no spokespersons, the disposition of such cases can be highly idiosyncratic and unpredictable.

The Health Professions

Physicians, psychologists, social workers, chiropractors, optometrists, and so forth require a license to practice their profession. These licenses are regulated by the respective licensing boards, under the auspices of the Secretary of State's office of the state in which the license is granted. Some state professional licensing boards also have professional wellness or recovery programs that advocate for the perpetrating professional. These organizations were originally developed to assist professionals impaired by substance abuse or dependency. Their traditional approach has been to require the professional (if allowed to return to the profession) to practice under a consent order, in which the individual is to limit their practice as defined in a written contract; failure to do so can lead to revocation, suspension, or other actions taken against the professional's license. Some of these recovery programs have embraced evaluation and treatment programs for PSM based on the model employed with chemically dependent professionals. However, the efficacy of the addiction model has not been documented in the scientific literature. Additionally, the Ad Hoc Committee on Physician Impairment (Schneidman, 1995) views sexual misconduct as a violation of the public trust rather than as an impairment. It was noted that although a mental disorder may be a basis for sexual misconduct, they concluded that sexual misconduct is not caused by physical or mental impairment and specifically stated that the frequently used term, "sexual addiction," is not recognized as a disease in the *Diagnostic and Statistical Manual of Mental Disorders*, 4th edition (American Psychiatric Association, 1994).

The professional who is required to complete a PSM evaluation by his regulating agency is placed in a double-bind. If he is forthcoming with his sexual misconduct, this previously unverified information becomes available to the licensing board since, in most states, when a professional's license is being investigated, there is no confidentiality. Thus, any acknowledgment can markedly increase the professional's risk for loss of his license. On the other hand, if the professional does not reveal his involvement in PSM, he may be labeled as being in denial and this label is frequently interpreted as evidence that the patient cannot be treated. To confound this issue ever further, the professional faces an additional dilemma: whether to reveal victims who are not already known or suspected by others. By revealing this information, he may place himself at even higher risk for loss of his license as well as for civil malpractice lawsuits.

The Religious Community

The religious community is in a tremendous period of flux regarding PSM. Professional sexual misconduct has been particularly problematic for the Roman Catholic Church in which a priest is attached to the church for life, unless specific action is taken by the Vatican to sever that attachment (laicization). Although media coverage suggests that the greatest sexual problem in the religious community is sexual molestation of adolescent boys, the majority of PSM involves sexual interactions between the clergy and adult parishioners.

Historically, religious communities have viewed PSM as a sin, a sin that could be forgiven, and perpetrators of PSM remained within the church but were relocated. However, as cases of PSM have become more public and the cost of litigating such cases has risen, most religious organizations are taking a very hard look at their disposition of cases of PSM. Many now ask their clerics to sign agreements indicating whether they have a history of inappropriate sexual behavior and, if so, to disclose this on their insurance forms, promise not to act upon these proclivities, or both. In this fashion the religious communities hope to exclude insurance coverage for PSM so that the religious organization will not be liable should misconduct occur.

Most churches are now reluctant to retain individuals who have been involved in child molestation or have had affairs with members of the congregation. However, some religious organizations are attempting to examine the issue of rehabilitation following PSM. This move appears to be less of a therapeutic issue, given the low recidivism rates posttreatment of professionals involved in PSM, and more a risk management issue for those providing insurance coverage to the religious organizations.

As noted previously, the disposition of perpetrators of PSM in the religious community has been either to accept and forgive them or to reject and remove them from religious life. These decisions have been handled within the church structure. Treatment of PSM by clerics traditionally has been provided within the religious community and primarily has consisted of spiritual counseling. However, there are no published data to support the effectiveness of this intervention. For the religious hierarchy to rely on another profession to implement psychotherapeutic treatment requires the development of trust outside the religious community. Working through this trust and relying upon other professions is not an easy task for the religious community and these relationships have yet to be worked out.

The Educational Profession and Volunteer Youth Organizations

Some perpetrators of PSM are sexually attracted to youth. Contrary to what is generally presented in the media, most cases of child molestation occur with a child or children that are well known to the perpetrator. In these cases, the molestation of the child requires the opportunity to interact with the child over time in a setting where the potential perpetrator is seen as nonthreatening to the child. During the course of such contact, the perpetrator grooms the child, moving the relationship from a nonsexual one to a relationship in which touching, then sexual touching, and in some cases intercourse occur. It should not be surprising that some individuals with a specific sexual attraction to children put themselves into settings where youth education occurs, such as school systems, and youth-oriented organizations such as Boy Scouts and Girl Scouts of America, Big Brothers and Big Sisters, and summer camps or after-school activity centers.

Youth-focused activities and the institutions that support them are quite varied and, not surprisingly, how accusations of professional sexual misconduct are handled is likewise quite variable. When accusations are made against a member of a voluntary youth group, there is usually an informal investigation and, in recent years, more formal reporting of such allegations to child protection agencies. Youth groups run by volunteers have come under greater scrutiny since some of these organizations have prided themselves on offering youth the opportunity to interact with a surrogate parent on a one-to-one basis. Another characteristic of such organizations is the designated power structure within the organization, sometimes reflected by the uniforms worn and designations on these uniforms indicating a chain of command. This appears to contribute to the perpetrator being able to gain compliance in sexual activity from a child, since the child is taught to obey those higher up in the chain of command of the organization.

When it is ascertained that the perpetrator has been sexually involved with a youth, he is frequently simply dismissed by the organization. Rehabilitation of the perpetrator generally is not attempted since the pool of replacements for the perpetrator is extensive, requires minimal training, and the perpetrator is not considered to actually be a member of the national volunteer organization but as operating at the local level of the organization.

Historically, at the primary, middle, and secondary school level, accusations of child molestation often were not believed, and thus, were not acted upon. More recently, while these accusations are frequently still considered suspect, the alleged perpetrator is usually suspended pending investigation. When the accusations are determined to be valid, the teacher is usually fired and his teaching certificate is rescinded. These perpetrators are seldom allowed ever to teach again. At the college level, there has been minimal attention to sexual misconduct in the past. Even today, most colleges have no specific restrictions against social or sexual interaction between faculty and students and social interaction is often encouraged. However, the enactment of laws related to sexual harassment has brought greater attention to sexual interactions between students and faculty members or administrators.

Certification to teach at the primary, middle, or secondary levels is rarely allowed after a teacher has been found guilty of sexual interaction with a student. Therefore, specific treatment for PSM is, for the most part, irrelevant and the individual is better served by more general sexual offender treatment. However, this is not necessarily the case for teachers at the college level who are more likely to be allowed to continue teaching. The biggest challenge in the treatment of college teachers is combating the traditional view held by college faculty and administrators that sexual interaction between faculty and students is acceptable.

The Legal Profession

The authors are not aware of any ethical restrictions against or systematic response to regulate PSM within its membership by the American Bar Association.

THE LEGAL RESPONSE TO PSM

Many states have recently criminalized professional sexual misconduct between adult clients and health care providers and, in some states, clerics. Perpetrators can now be charged with a felony or misdemeanor and fined, incarcerated, or both. In other cases, PSM is viewed as a variant of sexual harassment and civil lawsuits are brought against perpetrators. This has resulted in some exceedingly high awards being granted to victims, primarily as punitive damages, but the impact of such lawsuits in preventing PSM is unclear.

EVALUATION OF PSM

Allegations of PSM require careful and comprehensive evaluation. Like other sexual offenders, professionals are often reluctant to admit having engaged in inappropriate sexual behavior due to their fear of the consequences of such an admission. Not only do they risk losing the privilege of practicing their profession, as noted above, they may also risk criminal charges. Often, professionals are required by their regulating agency to waive their right to confidentiality of their psychiatric records. Therefore, it is ethically mandatory that professionals undergoing evaluation be informed of their potential loss of confidentiality and that a waiver of confidentiality be obtained before the evaluation begins.

In addition to the clinical and social history, possible paraphilic interest should be explored in detail. Review of the allegations and/or depositions by the victim(s) regarding the professional's inappropriate sexual behavior is of great assistance in identifying specific areas of inquiry for the clinician conducting the evaluation. Collateral information, obtained from family and co-workers, can provide valuable information regarding the professional's general level of functioning, emotional stability, possible history of prior boundary violations, practice procedures, and so forth. However, the collection of collateral information cannot be obtained without the professional's written permission. Even when great care is taken in the gathering of this information, there is a significant risk that others will become aware that the professional is under investigation.

Psychological testing should include assessment of the professional's sexual interests, cognitive distortions regarding sexual interactions with clients, personality and psychological disorders, and other variables of interest to the evaluator. A medical history and physical examination, as well as a blood chemistry evaluation, and a comprehensive drug screen are recommended. Neuropsychological screening should be conducted to rule out possible organic impairment.

Psychophysiological evaluation may be helpful in identifying pedophilic interest, but since most incidents of PSM involve sexual interaction with adult partners, it is of less assistance than in cases of paraphilia. As an alternative, a polygraph examination may be used to cut through the alleged perpetrator's denial.

TREATMENT FOR PSM

Some regulating agencies dealing with PSM have been supportive of cognitive–behavioral treatment of the professional provided that relapse prevention and long-term surveillance is included in the treatment program. Others, unfortunately, have been reticent to consider any form of treatment for perpetrators of PSM.

Perpetrators of PSM are generally better educated than the average paraphiliac, since the acquisition of a license necessitates extensive intellectual skills. Individuals involved in PSM are also generally more compliant with treatment and are willing to modify their professional practice guidelines to enable themselves to be considered for the possibility of returning to professional work. The relationship between the perpetrator of PSM and the therapist therefore is generally more amiable and less adversarial than usually exists between a paraphiliac and therapist. Unfortunately, the professionalism of the perpetrator of PSM is often accompanied by considerable arrogance. Professionals are accustomed to special treatment and to special privileges being given them because of their professional status. Perpetrators of PSM often initially find it difficult to assimilate the role of a client and instead attempt to join alliances with the therapist, as a fellow professional.

Some treatment components are similar for paraphiliacs and perpetrators of PSM. These components of treatment can be divided into:

1. Components to modify the perpetrator's sexual interests and behavior

- *Odor aversion*: The perpetrator is taught to identify and pair the antecedents of his inappropriate sexual behavior with an offensive odor.
- *Covert sensitization*: The perpetrator learns to pair the potential negative consequences of his inappropriate sexual behavior with the imagined antecedents to that behavior.
- *Satiation*: The perpetrator is taught to repeatedly verbalize specific components of his inappropriate sexual fantasies to the point that boredom replaces sexual excitement.
- *Medication*: Medications are sometimes employed to decrease sex drive and to afford the client more control over his sexual urges. Serotonin reuptake inhibitors are prescribed, not for their antidepressant action, but rather for the common effect of reducing sex drive and/or obsessive sexual thoughts. Hormonal agents such as medroxyprogesterone acetate (by mouth or injection) and leuprolid acetate injections are rarely used with perpetrators of PSM because their inappropriate sexual behavior is rarely so out of control or so dangerous that hormonal treatment is necessitated. A professional whose sexual behavior is so out of control would probably be prohibited from returning to practice.

2. Components that target social adjustment

- *Cognitive restructuring*: The perpetrator confronts the incorrect beliefs and rationalizations that have supported his involvement in inappropriate sexual behavior.
- *Victim awareness*: The perpetrator learns the full impact and negative consequences of his inappropriate sexual behavior for his victims and others.
- *Assertiveness training*: The perpetrator learns and rehearses to communicatie more effectively with others without aggression or passivity.
- *Anger management*: The perpetrator learns to identify the triggers for his anger, appropriate responses for coping with his anger, and strategies to avoid becoming excessively angry.
- *Sex education*: The perpetrator is taught what constitutes appropriate sexual behavior in our culture, the ethical guidelines regarding sexual interaction between professionals and clients within his specific profession, and improved relationship skills.

3. Components that target maintenance

- *Relapse prevention*: The perpetrator learns to identify situations that place him at risk for reoffending and strategies to appropriately cope with these situations.
- *Surveillance*: Individuals from the perpetrator's family and social life are taught to recognize cues that indicate the perpetrator has started the chain of events that may lead him to commit inappropriate sexual behavior and are asked to report their impressions by completing a short questionnaire, which they send to the therapist twice per month.

The details of these components of treatment will not be elucidated since they are available in the published literature (Abel, Barrett, & Gardos, 1992; Abel & Osborn, in press; Warberg, Abel, & Osborn, 1996).

ENSURING SAFE PRACTICE

The guiding principle of PSM treatment is protection of future clients. Thus, in addition to treatment of the professional, specific methodologies are implemented to help ensure that the professional is not able to reoffend. These methodologies are employed as necessary.

Expansion of the Knowledge Base Regarding PSM and Prevention Measures

Evaluation and treatment of PSM is a fairly new area of specialization with relatively little published literature on the subject. A guiding principle of treatment of perpetrators of PSM is that they in some way help correct the problems that they have caused. To further the professional's knowledge of the literature and to expand our understanding of specific issues related to individual cases, the perpetrating professional is asked to do a literature search and develop a referenced article on a component of PSM specific to his case. This article is reviewed and critiqued by the treatment staff and is added to the treatment program's literature so that other perpetrators of PSM can read and review these topics. Typical topics have included screening seminary applicants for pedophilia, how to develop a sexual-harassment-free office, professional arrogance and its relationship to PSM, and the role of denial in the treatment of PSM. To expand the perpetrator's knowledge of the impact of PSM on victims, each professional is also required to complete 4 hours of continuing education in the content area of PSM.

Finally, those completing treatment are asked to broaden their profession's knowledge of PSM by suggesting curriculum changes in their professional school's training program and by participating in lectures on PSM (such as Grand Rounds). The goal of such endeavors is to heighten the awareness of professionals in training regarding the consequences of boundary violations in the practice of their profession.

Some regulating agencies, upon receiving copies of the perpetrator's literature review, have falsely assumed that the perpetrator is so arrogant that he has written an article to teach others (who have not been involved in PSM) how to avoid it. It is the perpetrator's responsibility, as well as that of the therapist, to clarify that such articles are not intended to reflect a vast knowledge of the entire area, but have been developed only to ensure that the perpetrator grasps, in detail, an area specific to his particular PSM behavior. Since boards frequently change membership, this clarification needs to be reiterated frequently.

Warning the Future Client

When individuals seek professional care, they generally have limited information regarding standards of care, ethical guidelines, or the nature of the professional relationship. Because of this naiveté, clients may not recognize that the early grooming behaviors of the professional are inappropriate or that they are leading to more explicit sexual interaction. However, disclosure of the professional's past PSM could be expected to frighten off potential clients and result in the destruction of the professional's career. A viable solution involves providing clients with descriptions of standards of care and ethical practice in the form of printed principles of practice. This document is given to clients by the professional or his staff. Imbedded in the principles of practice are details regarding the professional's duty to protect clients from sexual harassment, his request that any suspected professional sexual misconduct be reported to office staff immediately, and informing them that social relationships and sexual activities between professionals and clients are unethical and prohibited. In this way, the client is made aware of appropriate professional–client interaction.

The decision to return the professional to practice frequently rests not only with the regulating agency but also with the administrative board of the institution for which he works. Should the perpetrator reoffend posttreatment, it is generally the regulating agency or the institution, or both, not the perpetrator himself, which suffer the greater barrage of the media and the risk of legal liability. Under these circumstances, members of both groups often, no doubt, opt for the seemingly safer decision to remove the perpetrator from practice or decline employing him.

Surveillance by Clients

The effectiveness of a practice plan for PSM necessitates feedback from the consumer— the client. The problem of obtaining such feedback from clients again is the risk of destroying the professional's practice. For this reason, feedback from the client is cloaked under a client satisfaction survey. Similar surveys are common professional practice today. The questions relevant to inappropriate behavior by the professional are included among other general questions about the quality of service received (see Abel et al., 1992; Warberg et al., 1996).

To gather these responses from a representative sample of clients, all clients seen in a 1-week period are asked, by the professional's office staff, to fill out the survey. This procedure is completed at least once within each quarter, but the professional is not informed when the surveys are being distributed. Results of the surveys are advanced directly to the professional's supervising therapist. Clients identify themselves only by their initials (for confidentiality purposes) and problematic replies are investigated by the supervising therapist through questioning of the professional's staff and the professional himself. The source of the questionable response is not identified to the professional.

In this way feedback from the consumer can be integrated with other methods of assessing the professional's ongoing practice to assist the supervising therapist in therapeutic intervention. Obviously, breaches of safe practice are immediately reported to the regulating agency so as to ensure the safety of the public.

While this procedure has high acceptance in other professions, it is often problematic within the religious community. Since members of the clergy are supposed to epitomize moral, religious, and ethical behavior, churches frequently believe that the members of the congregation, in addition to the lay administrative staff, must be notified regarding the details of the cleric's past history of professional sexual misconduct. This poses a significant problem because confidentiality of such information is unprotected. Since PSM is seen as a sin or moral deficit, such disclosure may poison the congregation for the return of the cleric or necessitate his placement with another congregation. In some cases, church members accept the cleric back into their congregation. However, problems can occur when new members join the congregation since, by principle, they also need to be informed regarding the cleric's past PSM. This subsequently leads to the reopening of this old wound, with increased anxiety for all involved, and results in the placement of the cleric being continuously tenuous.

Surveillance by the Professional's Staff

For adequate surveillance of the professional, the details of his prior PSM must be disclosed. Full disclosure of this information must be made to those individuals working closely with the perpetrator, including information revealing ways in which his behavior might have been detected. Professionals usually work closely with an office staff, office managers, or professionals who cross-cover for them. This affords the supervising therapist a rich opportunity for gathering information regarding the perpetrator from individuals educated regarding the perpetrator's past PSM behaviors. The staff and cross-covering professionals are admonished not to be "little detectives" and are not asked to go out of their way to watch the perpetrator. However, they are asked to provide feedback to the supervising therapist regarding their knowledge of the professional's interactions with clients.

The perpetrator identifies the individuals with whom he works, acquaints them with the details of his past PSM behavior, and develops, with the supervising therapist, a staff surveillance form that is completed by the staff and cross-covering professionals once per month and is sent to the supervising therapist. The questions on this form can be made very specific to the perpetrator's antecedent behavior that has led to PSM (see Abel et al., 1992; Warberg et al., 1996). The perpetrator signs the form before it is distributed, indicating his awareness and approval of the surveillance, and gives his permission for the form to be sent to his supervising therapist, irrespective of the consequences for him. The responses are reviewed by the supervising therapist and summarized on a quarterly basis, and the summary is sent to the perpetrator's regulating agency. As with the client feedback forms, problematic areas are discussed with the staff and any apparent gross misconduct is reported immediately to the professional's regulating agency.

Monitoring of the professional by his own professional staff is potentially problematic. Since the staff's employment often depends on the functioning of the professional, they may be reluctant to report his inappropriate sexual behavior. Although there is a potential confound of supervision provided by the professional's staff, it appears to be less an issue than expected. Experience indicates that, since most staff members are females and most victims are females, female staff feel a strong dedication to protecting female clients from a perpetrator, even when he is their employer.

Small churches or offices may have only part-time support staff. In such cases, the professional will need to restrict the times he meets with clients or members of his congregation to those times when support staff are present. Supervision by staff is more difficult, if not impossible, when the professional's practice extends outside of office confines. Professionals who work in hospitals or nursing homes, visit members of their congregation in the members' homes, serve their clientele in the community, and so forth, are more difficult to adequately monitor. Clerics, for example, may need to be restricted to only visiting with or counseling members of their congregation in their office or may need to be accompanied on home or hospital visits by a colleague or lay member of the congregation. Other professionals may need to be prohibited from working outside of an office environment.

Occasionally, cases of PSM are treated in which no one is aware of the perpetrator's prior PSM behavior, such as when a perpetrator voluntarily enters treatment and no complaints have been lodged against him. Under these circumstances, it is impossible to inform staff about the perpetrator's prior behavior. In these cases, the surveillance forms completed by the staff and cross-covering professionals give feedback regarding sexual harassment, under the guise that the professional is a strong believer in prevention of sexual misconduct and the avoidance of any behavior that could be construed as such. Since prevention of sexual harassment is a major issue in most businesses, this serves as an excellent vehicle for providing feedback regarding the professional's (and his staff's) behavior. A sexual harassment free office helps protect clients from PSM.

Alterations of the Office Layout

Grooming and/or seduction of clients typically begins in the office setting. Under the guise of being very personally concerned about the client, the perpetrator disregards the usual physical or emotional distance between himself and the client and begins to breach the professional boundary by moving closer to the patient, touching the patient first in nonsexual ways, then eventually touching the patient in sexual ways and discussing personal, nonprofessional issues with the client. Since the professional's office staff members are aware of the inappropriateness of such physical closeness with clients, the professional conceals such activity behind closed doors.

The grooming sequence of increasing emotional and physical proximity to the client can be deterred by changes in the office layout that allow staff members to see and possibly hear what is occurring in the professional's office. For example, the professional's desk and chair are placed so that he is readily visible through a window or an open door. The client's chair is placed at a point from the door where it is not visible to passersby, thereby maintaining the client's confidentiality. The office staff is educated regarding the professional's past history of PSM and, within the normal course of office practice, is able to monitor the professional's behavior with clients. Staff members are admonished not to be detectives or go out of their way to monitor the professional, but instead are asked to ongoingly assess the professional–client interaction and provide feedback to the supervising therapist. Generally, this office arrangement is utilized for all clients. Again, such supervision has high acceptance by professional regulating agencies and, surprisingly, by most clients. Those clients who are not comfortable with this arrangement are referred to another professional.

Institutions may be reluctant or unable to make changes in the physical layout of their facilities due to the expense or bureaucratic procedures involved. In these cases, the perpetrator may need to pay for the alteration himself, if allowed by the institution. A viable alternative is the open-door policy mentioned above. Some institutions, however, may not be amenable to this alternative and the perpetrator will have to seek employment with another institution.

Chaperoning Physical Examinations

Some procedures require physical examinations of patients, including patients of the gender that the perpetrator has offended upon in the past. Indeed, physical examination in many cases serves as a catalyst for the perpetrator initiating greater intimacy between himself and the client. The use of chaperones during all physical examinations is becoming an increasingly common standard of care for clinicians whose professional activity demands physical examinations of clients. Perpetrators of PSM generally obviated the system by either not having a chaperone or by diverting the chaperone with other activities during the physical examinations, while they carried out their inappropriate sexual behavior. Adequate chaperoning demands that the chaperone be aware of the perpetrator's past history of PSM and also be acutely knowledgeable about what constitutes an appropriate physical examination protocol.

Once the chaperone is adequately knowledgeable of these two issues, he or she supervises all physical examinations. The chaperone signs the professional's note in the patient's chart with the word "chaperone" following his or her signature. When chaperones are used, the patient is protected from improper actions by the professional and the professional is protected from spurious accusations of improper examinations by clients. Chaperones increase the professional's overhead costs, but they are a necessary expense when the professional has been involved in PSM.

Proper chaperoning demands a complete appreciation of the professional's past PSM. Some perpetrators are reluctant for the individual(s) chaperoning him to have this knowledge because it may contaminate the professional–staff relationship. One of the professional's fears is that this knowledge will place the chaperone in a one-up position and make it difficult for the professional to be in charge. However, once the professional has been involved in PSM, in order to return to practice, the supervision is necessary and it does change the relationship. If the chaperone cannot supervise the professional during physical examinations while still taking orders from him, then the professional will need to hire someone who can or refer physical examinations to other professionals.

Protocols for Physical Examinations

When professional sexual misconduct has occurred within the context of physical examinations done by professionals (such as physicians, chiropractors, nurses, optometrists, and so forth), descriptions of appropriate examination procedures should be detailed in written protocols. During the course of medical training, for example, physicians learn in great detail the sequence of examinations and the specific procedures for conducting various types of examinations. Indeed, hours are spent in medical training repeatedly practicing these protocols so that physicians follow these specific steps in order not to miss evidence of organic disease. The presence of a chaperone, the use of examination gowns, the use of latex gloves, the protection of privacy while the patient disrobes and puts on the examination gown, chaperoning of the entire examination, and the step-by-step protocol of the examination are all part of this detailed training process.

Clients are provided with a written, step-by-step description of the examination protocol to educate them regarding what constitutes an appropriate examination. The protocol also advises the patients of the necessity of immediately reporting any variances from the protocol, under the guise that the professional prides himself on his abilities to always conduct such examinations in a systematic manner. Therefore, these protocols are given to all patients undergoing physical examinations and are also posted in the examination rooms.

The professional cannot guarantee that his clients will read and remember these protocols. Therefore, these protocols are not only given to all patients undergoing physical examination, but are also posted in the examination room. However, some patients are not able to read and the protocol must be explained in detail by the chaperone. With patients for whom English is not their first language, this may not be possible and the professional will need to refer them to others.

Restriction of Clientele

In some cases, perpetrators of PSM have such a chronic history of PSM, such intense attraction to certain client ages or genders, or such poor impulse control regarding their sexual behavior with a specific subgroup of clients, that they must be restricted from working with certain types of clients altogether. This also may be necessary due to the nature of the perpetrator's practice or to the difficulty in establishing adequate surveillance of the professional. For example, professionals with pedophilic arousal usually need to be restricted from working with children, those with a breast fetish restricted from conducting physical examinations of females, and so forth.

Such restrictions have received considerable acceptance by perpetrators and the licensing boards or supervisory organizations, since these steps significantly reduce the risk of subsequent PSM. It is possible, for example, for a professional who is at high risk with female clients to work in a prison setting that houses only males or for him to refer physical examinations of females to other physicians. Limiting access to clients of a specific gender or age group is feasible when the professional operates entirely within the confines of an office setting where his contact can be monitored. However, this approach is problematic when the professional's practice extends outside of such office confines. Previously, regulating agencies have failed to recognize the effectiveness of these restrictions and have simply prohibited these professionals from practicing.

Some professionals' training is so narrow that restriction of their clientele allows them no alternative populations. For example, the obstetrician–gynecologist with poor control of his impulsivity with females may have insufficient training to treat male patients. In these cases, the professional may have to drop out of clinical service and function in an administrative or other nonpatient contact role only, retrain, or else leave the profession.

Polygraphs as Adjuncts to Surveillance

Ideally, supervision of perpetrators of PSM would include an objective instrument to assess whether the perpetrator has relapsed, but no such instrument exists. Those involved in supervising the professional who has returned to practice rely on a variety of feedback mechanisms regarding his ongoing performance, including those described above. Since PSM generally involves sexual behaviors that, if occurring outside his professional realm, would not be considered inappropriate, deviant, or paraphilic, indicators generally used to monitor paraphiliacs are not applicable. Even when paraphilic interest is the motivator for the PSM, measuring such interest cannot determine whether the perpetrator has acted on this interest.

One potential means of gathering information regarding whether a perpetrator has relapsed is through the use of polygraph examination. There is considerable debate regarding the sensitivity and specificity of polygraph assessment and whether it can be used to assess relapse behavior. In the majority of cases, however, polygraphs have been found to be of assistance in providing additional feedback to the supervising therapist. Polygraphs generally cover the 6-month period since the prior polygraph and investigate not only whether the individual has been involved in touching patients for sexual gratification, but also whether the perpetrator has attempted to groom clients for subsequent PSM.

When listed as one element of the perpetrator's practice plan, it is clarified that polygraphs should not be viewed as lie detectors, but only as adjuncts to gathering further information to be integrated by the supervising therapist in evaluating the professional's continued fitness to practice. There is a danger that some regulating agencies will view polygraphs as perfect indicators of the truth or validity of the perpetrator's self-statements. However, this is not supported by the scientific literature. The limitations of polygraph examinations, therefore, need to be clarified in the practice plan.

OTHER PROBLEMATIC ISSUES

Treatment of the Ultrareligious

Some religious groups have beliefs or practices that place severe limitations on standard evaluation and treatment. Hasidic jews, for example, are forbidden to undergo psychophysiological assessment that would require them to see slides of nudes. Other beliefs preclude their participating in some components of treatment such as satiation or sex education.

Treatment of members of ultrareligious groups requires working closely with the client's religious leader, since the religious laws of the perpetrator are frequently unknown to the therapist. Detailed discussions with the perpetrator's religious leader allow the therapist to possibly obtain approval for various aspects of the perpetrator's treatment and to differentiate client resistance from religious prohibitions. Such religious clearance prolongs the treatment process but is a necessary step.

Disability

Most professionals carry disability insurance policies. Some of these policies provide substantial payments to the professional if he is no longer able to practice his profession in the manner he has always practiced it. If a perpetrating professional's practice normally involved a specific clientele, and as a result of his PSM the professional can no longer treat that clientele, he may seek disability payment. Opinions of course differ as to whether a treated PSM perpetrator can safely return to practice. The treating therapist may become embroiled in such determinations, since the insurance specialists may attempt to negate disability coverage on the grounds that sexual misconduct is a choice rather than an impairment and that not returning to practice, or returning to a limited rather than full practice is a choice, even when this action is supported by the treating therapist or regulating agency. Insurance specialists may also suggest that the professional is malingering in order to receive disability coverage. The professional's disability status is periodically reevaluated by the insurer across the course of treatment, often requiring the treating therapist to spend substantial amounts of time completing the associated paper work.

The Personality-Disordered Professional

Professional training is frequently a long, arduous task requiring a considerable commitment from a strong-willed, hard-working student. The meeker student falls by the wayside under the rigors of professional training. The very personality characteristics that allow the student to complete professional training may also contribute to his professional sexual misconduct.

Individuals involved in PSM are frequently confrontive, with a high likelihood of having significant personality disorders and considerable professional arrogance. These personality characteristics may interfere with treatment and reduce compliance, and therefore must be treated along with other contributors to PSM. The therapist has a number of treatment options. First, supplementary individual therapy during the course of cognitive–behavioral treatment can focus on personality disorder and noncompliance components as major issues needing to be resolved before treatment can be successful. Second, the perpetrator's literature review can address his specific personality characteristics as a way to focus a significant portion of treatment on this issue. Finally, perpetrating professionals can be referred to local psychotherapy resources for longer-term therapy to deal with their chronic personality issues for whatever duration needed.

THE EFFECTIVENESS OF TREATMENT AND ITS RELATIONSHIP TO THE RETURN TO PROFESSIONAL PRACTICE

When a professional is temporarily barred from the practice of his profession, when he is identified in the media as a perpetrator of PSM, when he is arrested and charged with a felony or misdemeanor, when he loses the support of his professional colleagues and/or regulating agency, or when he undergoes an integrated cognitive–behavioral treatment with strong relapse prevention and surveillance components, his professional practice changes forever. Recidivism studies comparing treated versus untreated cases of PSM are unlikely to be completed, since allowing an untreated professional involved in PSM to return to professional practice is unethical. As a result, evaluation of the effectiveness of treatment must rely on uncontrolled outcome studies of treated PSM cases without a control group comparison.

When the professional's inappropriate behavior has come to the attention of regulating agencies, these individuals are generally scrutinized very closely by the agency's investigative arm. Recurrences are exceedingly unlikely to go undetected, since the regulating agency is already aware of the prior conduct, as are his staff, colleagues, and family. PSM treatment outcome from the Behavioral Medicine Institute of Atlanta reveals that 52.3% of referred professionals were removed from professional practice. This 52.3% was composed of 32.3% who were excluded by their regulating agency, prior to treatment; 10.8% were unable to practice due to arrest and/or convictions; 4.6% were removed by the treatment program because of their poor response to treatment: they were too impulsive, they had irreparable central nervous system disease, or the intensity of their proclivities remained high posttreatment; 3.1% due to both the regulating agency and arrest and/or conviction;

and 1.5% voluntarily elected to remove themselves from professional practice. Of the 47.7% of treated cases who returned to practice, identified recidivism in the last 7 years has been less than 1%.

Treatment appears to be successful for a number of reasons. First, the most outrageous perpetrators usually are removed from further professional practice by their regulating agencies before they are even assessed or treated. These cases may have been those most likely to relapse; however, since they are out of practice, it is impossible to determine what their recidivism rate would have been. Second, the treatment model (cognitive–behavioral treatment with a strong emphasis on relapse prevention and surveillance) used to treat these cases has demonstrated itself to be effective with individuals with even more severe sexual problems than most perpetrators of PSM.

Finally, since the vast majority of PSM cases are known to their regulatory agencies, compliance with treatment protocols is exceedingly high. Involvement of these regulatory agencies no doubt significantly reduces recidivism.

CONCLUSIONS

The most problematic area of working with perpetrators of PSM is the disparity between the exceedingly low recidivism rate and the professional's ability to return to practice. It is impressive that individuals with extensive histories of PSM, individuals who have been involved with multiple victims or at a high frequency, and individuals whose PSM behavior is strongly influenced by paraphilic interests have done exceedingly well in returning to practice. This suggests that factors traditionally considered to be predictive of high risk are actually rather poor predictors with this population.

Decisions regarding whether professionals are allowed to return to professional practice posttreatment are generally made behind closed doors. These decisions frequently are not based on the evaluation of the level of risk of relapse but instead on the societal climate regarding inappropriate sexual behavior, the misperception that PSM cannot be corrected, fear of costly lawsuits should recidivism occur, and the availability of other professionals to take over the responsibilities of those who are removed from the profession.

Various studies of the prevalence of PSM among physicians and psychologists indicate a rate of approximately 6% (Gartrell et al., 1986), while the percentage of recidivism among treated professionals is less than 1%. These data suggest that returning treated PSM perpetrators actually lowers the overall rate of PSM. It would appear that returning treated perpetrators of PSM to practice serves the dual purpose of reducing the overall likelihood of PSM and rehabilitates those same professionals to productive careers.

REFERENCES

Abel, G. G., Barrett, D. H., & Gardos, P. S. (1992). Sexual misconduct by physicians. *Medical Association of Georgia, 81*, 237–246.

Abel, G. G., Lawry, S.S., Karlstrom, E. M., Osborn, C.A., & Gillespie, C. F. (1994). Screening tests for pedophilia. *Criminal Justice and Behavior, 21*(1), 115–131.

Abel, G. G., & Osborn, C. (in press). Cognitive–behavioral treatment of professional sexual misconduct. In J. Bloom, C. Nadelson, & M. Notman (Eds.), *Current dilemmas in the approach to sexual misconduct among physicians*. Washington, DC: American Psychiatric Press.

American Psychiatric Association. (1994). *Diagnostic and statistical manual of mental disorders* (4th ed.). Washington, DC: Author.

Gartrell, N., Herman, J., Olarte, S., Feldstein, M., & Localio, J. B. (1986). Psychiatrist–patient sexual contact: Results of a national survey. I: Prevalence. *American Journal of Psychiatry, 143,* 126–131.

Schneidman, B. S. (1995). Ad hoc committee on physician impairment: Report on sexual boundary issues. *Federation Bulletin: The Journal of Medical Licensure and Discipline, 82*(4), 208–216.

Warberg, B. W., Abel, G. G., & Osborn, C. (1996). Cognitive–behavioral treatment for professional sexual misconduct among the clergy. *Pastoral Psychology, 45,* 49–63.

23

Children Who Molest

Toni Cavanagh Johnson

This chapter will discuss treatment programs for children under 12 years of age who sexually molest. Many important issues arise and will be discussed, such as the need for a thorough assessment, the overidentification of children as offenders, the need for a mandate to treat the child and the parents, funding, age-appropriate treatment, and the availability of suitable out-of-home treatment facilities.

The identification of a young group of children with significant sexual behavior problems was only sparsely alluded to in the literature until the late 1980s, when several articles appeared in close succession. The articles written by Johnson (1988, 1989) and Friedrich and Luecke (1988) described children who molest. Johnson called them "child perpetrators" and "children who molest"; Friedrich called them "sexually aggressive." Johnson and Friedrich's work was independent of one another. Johnson was in Los Angeles and Friedrich in Washington State and then Minnesota. Both authors had seen these children in outpatient mental health clinics. The children presented with serious sexual problems along with very disturbed and aggressive behaviors in all aspects of their lives. Criteria for inclusion of the subjects in the three studies was almost identical. There was a pattern of overt problematic sexual behavior in the child's history, an age difference of at least 2 years between the children involved, and force or coercion was used in order to obtain the participation of the other child in the sexual behavior (see Johnson, 1993a, for review).

CHARACTERISTICS OF CHILDREN WHO MOLEST

A brief summary of some of the characteristics of children who molest as described in the studies by Johnson (1998) will provide a backdrop for understanding their treatment needs. In addition to the features outlined in Table 23.1, the following features are valuable to note.

School Performance

Overall, the children in the studies had average to low average IQs. None were mentally retarded, yet a large percentage had severe learning problems. Many were in special education classes.

Toni Cavanagh Johnson • 1101 Fremont Avenue, Suite 101, South Pasadena, California 91030.
Sourcebook of Treatment Programs for Sexual Offenders, edited by Marshall et al. Plenum Press, New York, 1998.

TABLE 23.1
Descriptive Features from Studies of Children Who Molest[a]

	Johnson study 1	Friedrich study	Johnson study 2
Subjects	47 boys	14 boys, 4 girls	13 girls
Ages	4–12	4–11	4–12
Race	44% Caucasian	Not specified	62% Caucasian
	28% Black		31% Black
	28% Hispanic		75 Hispanic
Average age at intake	9.7 years old	7.3 years old	7.5 years old
IQ	Average to low average	Range 70–139	Average to low average
	No MR	Mean IQ 98	No MR
Victimization history	50% sexually abused; pervasive, harsh physical punishment and emotional abuse; parental violence	75% of boys, 100% of girls sexually abused	100% sexually abused; pervasive harsh physical punishment and emotional abuse; parental violence
Average age at first perpetration	8.7 year old; range 4–12	Not specified	6 years old; range 4–9
Average number of victims	2.1; range 1–7	2 for boys; 2 for girls	3.3; range 1–15
Average age of victims	6.7 years old	Not specified	5 years old
Average age difference between perpetrator and victim	Boys and female siblings, 4.5 years; boys and male siblings, 3 years	Not specified	Girls and siblings, 4.2 years
Relationship to victimized child	46% Siblings, 18% cousins, 16% schoolmates, 6% foster siblings	Not specified	First victims: 54% siblings; 23% cousins; 23% friends

[a]Adapted from Johnson (1993a).

Peer Relations and Skills

Aggression apart from the sexual problems, was also characteristic of most of these children. They had very poor peer relations and very few, if any, had a best friend. Their relationship to other children was generally characterized by antagonism, fear, uncertainty, and continual disagreements. Social skills were few and these children had very limited ability to control their impulsiveness. Frustration tolerance was very poor. Problem-solving and positive coping skills were virtually nonexistent.

Sexual Preoccupation

Children in all three studies showed a high degree of sexual preoccupation. On projective tests, these children saw more sexual content than expected. On the Projective Storytelling Cards (Caruso, 1987), which pull strongly for sexual themes, sex and aggression arose regularly in their stories. The majority of these children did not report elaborate fantasies about sex. A few had frequent thoughts about consensual sexual behavior with same-aged peers or adults. A few fantasized about forced nonconsensual violent sex or physical aggression. There were other children who had no conscious access to any sexual undercurrent in their thoughts, but were aware of physical aggressive fantasies.

Diagnoses

Children in all three studies could be given a *Diagnostic and Statistical Manual of Mental Disorders*, 4th ed. (DSM-IV) (American Psychiatric Association, 1994) diagnosis. By far the most prevalent diagnosis were conduct disorder and oppositional defiant disorder. Adjustment disorder was less prevalent. In the Friedrich and Luecke study, one girl was given a diagnosis of dysthymic disorder. Although many of the children were depressed, few reached the level of major depressive disorder. Only one child had a thought disorder. Some children had suicidal thoughts, but this was not a persistent issue. Most of the aggressive feelings and destructive behaviors were directed outside the children.

Relationship to Adults

Most of these children had no satisfying relationships with persons of any age. In virtually all cases, a history of long-standing parent–child problems existed even before the child molested. The children's relationships to adults in the family and outside the family were generally stressed and fraught with conflict. Nurturance was clearly lacking in the relationship between the parents and children. Since most of the children lived in single-parent families headed by their mothers, this was the primary relationship from which to derive nurturance. Unfortunately, this was frequently not the case, because the mother–child relationships were mainly characterized by highly ambivalent and strained feelings.

Victimization Experiences of the Children

Although there was little documentation of reported physical abuse, descriptions by children and their caretakers showed clear signs of severe and erratic physical punishment for the majority of the children. Most of the children, both boys and girls, were molested by family members, their fathers being the most prevalent offenders, yet few fathers were living in the homes when the children began their molesting behavior. Of the 60 children in the Johnson studies, only one of the children was still living in the home with the offender when the sexually aggressive behavior was discovered and treatment began.

Sexual Behaviors

The sexual behaviors in which these children engaged included the full range of adult sexual behaviors. The sexually abusive behaviors noted in the Johnson studies were vaginal penetration with fingers, penis, and other objects; oral copulation; fondling; genital contact without penetration; exposing genitals; intercourse; and French kissing. The sexual behaviors of these children are comparable to those of adolescent and adult offenders.

Victim Selection

All of the children knew their victims, who were readily available to them.

Age of Aggression and Overt Victimization

An interesting aspect of the Johnson (1988) study of 47 boys was the relationship between sexual abuse of the children and sexually aggressive behavior. The children were divided into those who began to molest between ages 4 and 6, those who began between ages 7 and 10, and those who began between ages 11 and 12. The data indicate that the children who began molesting at the younger ages were more likely to have been victims of sexual abuse. Seventy-two percent of the children who began molesting between 4 and 6 had documented histories of sexual abuse, whereas 42% of children 7 to 10 and 35% of children 11 and 12 years old had similar documented histories. The figures may underestimate the number of children who had been overtly sexually abused. The molestation behavior by the children did not begin immediately after their victimization. In most children, a several-year period occurred between the termination of the victimization and the onset of perpetration. Sexually reactive behaviors (Johnson, 1993a) are more frequently noted in children currently being abused or soon after the abuse has ended. The intense anger and its pairing with aggressiveness and anxiety that is seen in children who molest appears to take many years to develop and is generally not concurrent with the abuse.

Characteristics of the Parents of Children Who Molest

There was a preponderance of single-parent mothers in all three samples. Descriptions of the mothers indicates a propensity toward personality disorders and depression, with minimal evidence of psychotic processes. Many of the mothers suffered from dependent personality disorder, narcissistic personality disorder, or borderline personality disorder. Many had a combination of these personality disorders, with varying intensity of each type. A substantial number of the parents were dysthymic at the time of the child's treatment. Some of the mothers had major depressive episodes. Virtually all of the mothers had some history of emotional and sexual abuse and had grown up in highly confused and disrupted environments. The fathers of these children were mainly absent. Many of the fathers had been emotionally, sexually, and physically abused as children. Many had been involved in the criminal justice system. In some cases, the fathers were unknown because the mothers had multiple sexual contacts at the time of conception. Virtually no children had memories of a positive relationship with their father, and few children had any positive male role models. A history of substance abuse was noted in the majority of the families.

Family and Home Environment

Most children who molest have massive confusion about all facets of life and additionally have paired sex with aggression, jealousy, vindictiveness, cruelty, pain, and sometimes pleasure. Their confusion has occurred mainly from living in environments that have fostered these associations while providing no stability from which an organized and balanced view of life, relationships, and sexuality could develop. Unable to make sense of their chaotic environment, these children act out the cognitive and emotional confusion about everything, including sexuality, onto others.

The families and homes of these children were generally very unstable. The emotional life of the family was chaotic. Relationships between family members were highly stressed and distrustful. Adults could not depend on the children to tell the truth, and the children could not depend on the parents to be consistently truthful. Child rearing was very rudimentary and generally based on an authoritarian model. Parents attempted to exert total control in an environment in which the parent was always correct and no questions were to be asked. Some families had transient people living in their home.

There was a pervasive quality in the families of very sexualized relationships. A covert sexualized atmosphere was found in virtually all the homes. The subtle and not so subtle sexualized relationship between adults and children was frequently the most salient force that educated children toward sexualized and aggressive behavior or sustained it. It was often difficult to determine whether the sexualized behaviors by many of the mothers was abuse. If done by males, it would have been considered abusive.

DIFFERENTIATING CHILDREN WITH
SEXUAL BEHAVIOR PROBLEMS

Before the mid to late 1980s, children with sexually aggressive behaviors were not labeled and given a specific diagnosis that focused on their sexual behavior. After it became accepted and recognized that this group of children existed, there has been a tendency to overdiagnose children with less severe sexual behavior problems as children who molest. Some professionals have tended to describe any child who displays problematic sexual behaviors with other children as a child who is molesting. Not only does this hurt the children, it misdirects their treatment needs, causes their parents enormous distress, and has in some cases caused the children to be stigmatized and isolated from other children needlessly and for long periods of time.

This tendency to overdiagnose appears to stem from a misperception that there only two groups of children: those whose sexual behaviors are normal and those who are molesting. Johnson (1993b) describes children on a continuum from natural and healthy sexual behavior to children who molest; consequently, it is possible to divide children who have sexual behavior problems into three groups: "sexually reactive," "children who engage in extensive, mutual sexual behaviors," and "children who molest other children."

Sexually reactive children engage in self-stimulating behaviors, in sexual behaviors with other children and sometimes may touch adults in sexually suggestive ways. Generally, this type of sexual behavior is in response to stimuli in the environment or feelings that reawaken memories that are traumatic, painful, or overly stimulating or that they cannot comprehend. The child may respond by masturbating or engaging in sexual behaviors alone or with children or adults. The sexual behavior is a coping strategy against the feelings and/or thoughts. This type of sexual behavior is often not within the full conscious control of the child. The sexual behaviors may represent a partial form of reenactment of sexual abuse the child has sustained or witnessed and may be the child's way of trying to understand, master, or work it through. Shame, guilt, anxiety, and fear may be related to the upsurge and aftermath of the sexual behaviors. Confusion about sex, driven by the child's history, is fundamental to this type of sexual behavior. There are no threats and there is no attempt to hurt the other person involved in the sexual behavior. These children do not coerce others into sexual behaviors but act out their confusion on them. While there is no intent to hurt others, being the object of such sexual behaviors can be confusing and the other person may feel abused, misused, or confused. Many of these children do not understand their own or others' rights to privacy.

Often distrustful, chronically hurt and abandoned by adults, children who engage in extensive mutual sexual behaviors (group 2) do so to relieve their pain. The extensive sexual behaviors become a way of connecting to others, usually children but sometimes adults. They use sex as a way to cope with their feelings of abandonment, loss, hurt, sadness, anxiety, and often despair. These children do not coerce other children into sexual behaviors but find other similarly lonely children who will engage with them. Almost all of these children have been sexually and emotionally abused and look to other children to help save them emotionally. When connecting sexually with other children they feel less vulnerable and lonely.

The sexual behaviors of children who molest (group 3) are frequent and pervasive. A growing pattern of sexual behavior problems is evident in their histories. Intense sexual confusion is a hallmark of their thinking and behavior. Sexuality and aggression are closely linked in the thoughts and actions of these children. Unless the other child is too young to understand, children who molest use some type of coercion to gain the victim's participation in the sexual behaviors. Bribery, trickery, manipulation, or emotional or physical coercion are used. Physical force is not commonplace nor necessary because the children's victims are selected owing to special vulnerabilities, including developmental delays, social isolation, and emotional neediness. The victims may be older, younger, or the same age. There is an impulsive, compulsive, and aggressive quality to many of the behaviors of these children, including the sexual behaviors. These children generally have problems in all areas of their lives.

ASSESSMENT INSTRUMENTS

Because the diagnosis of children with problematic sexual behaviors is quite new and complex, it is helpful to use instruments specifically developed for this purpose. The Child Sexual Behavior Checklist (CSBCL)—Second Revision (Johnson, 1995a) was specifically developed for children 12 years of age and younger referred for assessment of sexual behavior problems. It offers a descriptive history or summary record of a child's sexual behaviors from the perspective of the parent–caregiver. When treatment related to sexual behavior problems is implemented, it provides the baseline data from which to develop a treatment plan. Target sexual behaviors can be chosen from the data provided by the CSBCL and progress can be measured by repeated assessment with the measure. The CSBCL provides a framework for discussion about sex and sexuality with the parents–caregivers and alerts them to behaviors that should be brought to the attention of the therapists during the course of treatment.

Part I of the CSBCL contains over 150 behaviors of children related to sex and sexuality ranging from natural and healthy childhood sexual exploration to behaviors of children experiencing difficulties in the area of sexuality. The behaviors are grouped by type for ease of evaluation. Part II asks about aspects of the child's life that might increase the frequency of sexual behaviors (e.g., access to pornography, nudity, abuse history, sleeping arrangements, and whether the child has seen violence between people he or she knows). Part III provides a more detailed description of sexual behaviors engaged in with other children. Part IV is completed by the therapist–evaluator with the parent–caregiver if, after reviewing section I and III, it appears the child may have a sexual behavior problem. Section IV is composed of 26 characteristics of children's sexual behaviors that raise concern (Johnson, 1995a, 1996a). The greater the number of these characteristics that describe the child's sexual behavior, the greater the likelihood that the child has a sexual behavior problem. After completing and analyzing the CSBCL, assessment interviews (Johnson, 1993c) and other assessment instruments (Johnson 1996a), a working hypothesis of which of the four groups a child falls can be made. Computer scoring of the CSBCL is available through the author.

Other assessment instruments, especially developed for assessing children who molest and their families, include: Family Roles, Relationships, Behaviors, and Practices I and II;

Family Practices Questionnaire; Children's Sexual Behaviors: A Survey; Adults' Sexual Behaviors as Children; and the Children's Temperament Scale (Johnson, 1996a). These instruments evaluate the home environment, focusing on boundary violations; the age at which the parents think that bathing, showering, sleeping, and being nude with other children is acceptable; parents' attitudes toward sexual behaviors in children in general; the parents' own early sexual histories; and the temperamental characteristics of the children. Each of the instruments is filled out by both the parents or other caregivers for the child separately. This allows the evaluator a separate view of the child from each parent–caregiver's perspective. A shortened questionnaire on the emotional, physical, and sexual boundaries entitled Family Roles, Relationships, and Practices III is available for children (Johnson, 1995b, 1996a).

The instruments described are specific to the sexual behavior issues. Assessment of other areas of the child's functioning will also be useful and should be done as needed.

DEVELOPMENT OF TREATMENT PROGRAMS
FOR CHILDREN WHO MOLEST

Referral Sources

Treatment programs, both outpatient and inpatient, have experienced significant problems with appropriate referrals. Prior to opening their doors, the lore in the community was that there are "hundreds of children who molest without adequate treatment." After the program opened its doors, referrals were few. This has been a consistent theme around the United States and in England, Canada, New Zealand, and Australia. The "droves" of children who molest does not materialize. Many of the children who are referred do not meet the criteria for molesting other children, but do have problematic sexual behaviors. It appears that there has been an exaggeration of the size of the problem. While the number of children who molest is not large, each one of the children is a risk to others and requires very careful, thorough, and extensive support to stop the behavior.

Referral sources are child protective services, schools, parents, pediatricians, day-care centers, churches, and, in some jurisdictions, police and probation. School systems are excellent referral sources as they are often struggling to maintain the children in school with little success. Most children who molest require special education services.

An additional issue is the variable response of the "system." In almost any locale in the world, it is difficult to predict what will occur when a report is made of a young child molesting. A particular problem is a young child who molests children outside his or her home. Because child protective services generally has a mandate to protect children in their homes, they may simply refer the child to counseling. Because of the young age of the child, most police departments do not arrest or provide probation service to the child. Hence, no system will assist the family to get help for the child. This variable response also makes it difficult for treatment providers to "find" the children who require treatment. Although referred for treatment, they are unlikely to call and make an appointment.

Funding

Funding for inpatient and outpatient programs has come from a wide variety of sources: Department of Children and Family Services, Department of Mental Health,

United Way, probation, Department of Corrections, Department of Health Services, specialized grants from county and state governments, and grants from private foundations. Funding problems have been extensive. In addition to the difficulty in finding the children and keeping them and their parents in treatment, it is difficult to track these children to look at long-term success and failure because of the highly transient nature of their families; thus, it is difficult to provide evidence of the value of treatment to referral sources.

Because of the volatile and dangerous nature of the children's problems, the staff–child ratio is low. This provides additional funding problems. As managed care takes over mental health funding and requires short-term solutions, this population will require special funding methods, because there are no short-term solutions to their problems.

Some dramatic funding crises have occurred. In Broward County, Florida, a residential treatment program for children who molest was established in January 1996, by a nurse whose young adopted son was molesting other children. Told that there were hundreds of young molesting children in need of treatment and in despair of finding abuse-specific treatment for her son, the nurse used her own money to fund the project and hired a program director, only to find out that the county had cut several million dollars from the children's services budget and that referrals were scarce. Five months after it opened, it had only two of its five beds filled, one by her son.

Location

Most outpatient treatment programs are housed within mental health agencies. Some take great care not to have children who molest mix with the general child client population. If this may occur, it is stressed to the parents not to leave their children unattended or to allow them to go alone to the bathroom. Group homes are frequently in single-home neighborhoods and have to fight to be allowed to remain there. Residential neighborhoods characteristically do not want this population of children.

While some residences look like regular homes, other programs are in more institutional settings. Some residential programs stress the importance of having the clinical staff available in the residence, not stationed in another building or off campus. This decreases the splitting between line staff and clinicians and provides more containment and clinical development of the milieu.

Treatment Providers

Critical to the success of treatment programs are the clinicians and care providers. Because there are not many clinicians who have a history of working with children who molest, many programs look for people with good clinical skills and some or all of the following: experience with adolescent offenders, experience working with young children, familiarity with the relevant systems, experience with all types of victims, expertise in working with parents, knowledge of child development, and an ability to teach effective parenting. One of the more salient requisites is a balanced view about sex and comfort with their own sexuality. This assists the individual to tolerate the pervasive and intrusive sexual material of the children and to talk about sex without embarrassment. If a person has a history of abuse of any kind, this must be resolved prior to working with these children. Working with children who molest is very difficult. Transference is powerful and frequently disquieting both from the child to the therapist and from the therapist to the child. Persons who believe that all the children need are love and hugs to surmount their problems fare poorly in this work. Working with abused and abusive children is not a way for people to work out their own histories of abuse.

Mandate to Treatment

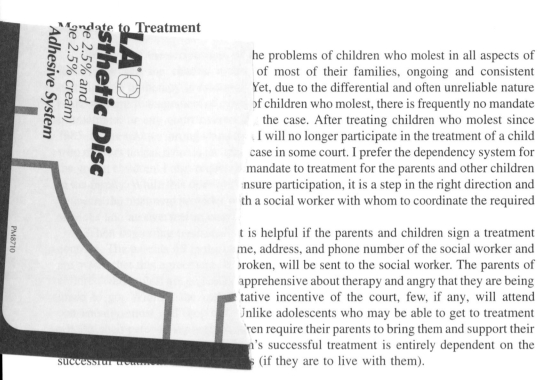

he problems of children who molest in all aspects of of most of their families, ongoing and consistent Yet, due to the differential and often unreliable nature of children who molest, there is frequently no mandate the case. After treating children who molest since I will no longer participate in the treatment of a child case in some court. I prefer the dependency system for mandate to treatment for the parents and other children nsure participation, it is a step in the right direction and th a social worker with whom to coordinate the required

t is helpful if the parents and children sign a treatment me, address, and phone number of the social worker and roken, will be sent to the social worker. The parents of apprehensive about therapy and angry that they are being tative incentive of the court, few, if any, will attend Unlike adolescents who may be able to get to treatment ren require their parents to bring them and support their n's successful treatment is entirely dependent on the successful treatment s (if they are to live with them).

Format of the Treatment Program

In the majority of cases of children who molest in the United States, treatment is provided by therapists in mental health centers, in group homes, and in residential facilities. Most of these therapists do not have specialized training and do not work in specially designed treatment programs. A national survey (Freeman-Longo, Bird, Stevens, & Fiske, 1994) indicated that there were 390 treatment programs for children who molest in the United States. A more accurate statement would be that 390 agencies and individual treatment providers responded in the affirmative when asked if they provided treatment to children who molest.

Outpatient treatment programs specifically developed for children who molest number far fewer and vary widely in what they include (Araji, 1997). Program elements that are helpful include: group, individual, family therapy, and multifamily therapy; groups with children who molest and their parents; and outreach to the various systems involved and to the child's school and any day-care program the child attends. Resources to provide in-home treatment and parent-aides are very beneficial. Group therapy is provided for the parents, the children who molest, and sibling victims. Individual therapy may be essential for the parents to provide them with an understanding of themselves and to support them as they help their child. Children who molest and sibling victims may also profit from individual therapy on an as-needed basis. Family therapy occurs throughout the treatment process. This initially may be with only the child who molests and the parents. Family therapy with the sibling victim will occur when the sibling victim is ready. Other children may join the family at the same time as the victim or afterward. Multifamily groups and groups with children who molest and their parents are used throughout the treatment process to meet specific treatment goals.

Because the boundaries in these families are very diffuse, it is helpful to define the parameters of information exchange between therapists and parents at the outset of treatment. Some children who molest have not been allowed any physical or emotional privacy, and sexual boundaries are almost nonexistent in their homes. Development of good boundaries is essential. Whereas parents are the holder of the privilege for children, therapists need not disclose to them everything that occurs in treatment. The children need to understand the limits of confidentiality (in jurisdictions with mandatory abuse reporting) while also knowing that not everything they say in therapy will be disclosed to their parents. Children can tell their parents what they choose, although it is best if they only relate what they and the therapists said, not specific items discussed by the other children. Confidentiality is an important concept to teach without having the children think there are any secrets about therapy material that they cannot tell their parents.

Generally, the outpatient treatment of children who molest is quite long. Many programs require 18 months of once or twice weekly meetings. This will depend on the seriousness of the child's and family's problems, the amount of adjunctive treatment, consistency of attendance, desire of the family to address the problems, and experience of their therapeutic team.

Treatment Modalities and Goals

Some programs have as an underlying assumption that victims become perpetrators. While it is true that most children who molest have been victimized, it is not true that most children who are victims of sexual abuse become perpetrators. In fact, very few child sexual abuse victims become perpetrators. Using this mistaken assumption will confuse the children who are molesting and who have not been abused and will provide a prophecy for children who have been. Understanding each child and the factors that contributed to the child's sexual offending behavior is a far more helpful means of assisting the child and family.

There appears to be little argument that the treatment of children who molest must directly discuss the sexual offending behavior, as well as many other issues. Nonspecific play therapy is not recommended as the primary treatment modality. While play therapy can elucidate and ameliorate the intrapsychic struggles and the worldview of the child, children need a great deal of information in order to stop the sexual offending behavior and need to acquire skill development to allow them to be liked and trusted by their peers, parents, and other adults. Play therapy can be a helpful adjunct.

An essential element of the treatment of all children who molest is working with their parents (if the children are to return home). Treatment for children in out-of-home placements, which has not been able to include their parents, is almost certainly doomed. Children who molest are not born this way. The home in which he or she grows up provides the fertile soil for the child to develop the sexually aggressive behavior patterns. When a child's parents live a long distance away, residential programs can coordinate the treatment and consult regularly with the parents' therapist.

Most providers agree that the mainstay of a treatment program for children who molest is group therapy. These children have often been made to feel very bad about themselves. It is helpful for them to see other children with similar problems. The group also provides an opportunity for the children to make friends, learn to communicate, see others' problems, and develop appropriate ways of interacting. Since young children learn best by doing, the group provides an interactive environment in which to learn the skills and meet the treatment goals (Johnson, 1995a).

It is important that the groups be fun. These children are often hyperactive, learning handicapped, angry, and impulse disordered. The group needs to have momentum and energy; the children need to interact with one another to learn. It is useful for the children to learn to ask one another pertinent questions about precipitants and sustainers of problematic sexual behavior and other problematic interactions. In this way, they know the questions to ask themselves. Much of what the children need to learn is how to think and problem solve. Asking each other the pertinent questions forces them to be active and not passive recipients of the therapist's knowledge. Beware of the child who knows all the right answers but none of the right questions. They know what to say, but have not integrated it into their behavior or thinking. The therapist acts as a facilitator of the direction of the content and a modulator of the process, but essentially the work is done by the children interacting with one another, observing each others' behaviors, and catching the problem thinking and actions of other group members. While some therapists provide individual therapy in a group, this does not appear to be a useful tactic, because the children not receiving the attention get bored and disruptive and little learning takes place.

Parallel group therapy for the parents is very important (Griggs & Boldi, 1995). When the children are in group treatment, the parents will meet. Because the children are young, the majority of their values, attitudes, and feelings regarding sex and sexuality are derived from their parents. This, as well as a host of other issues, are important to address in parents' group therapy.

Many programs struggle with referrals and do not have an adequate number of children for group treatment; hence, they do individual work. Two children form a group for purposes of treatment. Two children are superior to one, because the interaction between them stimulates discussing, exchanging ideas, socializing, playing games, sharing the time, listening, empathizing with each other's struggles, and more.

Individual therapy is useful for intrapsychic conflicts, interpersonal struggles, attachment issues, family problems, the discussion of embarrassing or shameful material, and other troubles or worries the child feels uncomfortable bringing up in group. In general, it is most helpful to deal with the sexual issues in a group setting. Because many of the family interactions are very sexualized and many of the children have been sexually abused, the children sometimes become apprehensive being in a closed room with one person talking about sex.

Family therapy is essential because most of the precipitants of the sexually aggressive feelings and behaviors emanate from the family environment. The elements that sustain the aggressive behaviors are often found in the interpersonal relationships between nuclear and/or extended family members. Family therapy provides an excellent opportunity to assess issues important to the health of the family and an environment in which the child can heal and grow.

It is essential that all material used with children who molest be age and stage appropriate. They are not "little" or "short" adult or adolescent offenders. Prepubertal children frequently do not have the reinforcing sexual pleasure which accompanies the offending of older persons. The hormones that drive sexual behaviors are not yet prominent in these children. The fantasy life of children is generally far less prominent. Their sexual response patterns to sexual material are not yet developed. Their seeking sexual contact with others is generally due to modeling rather than a developmental desire. Children have not reached the stage in which dating and the development of romantic attachment are developmental tasks.

Concepts, format, and treatment styles from adult and adolescent sexual offender treatment have frequently been used with the children without being adequately modified. While many of the issues are similar, at least at face value, there are major developmental differences that require modification of treatment approaches. Cognitively, children cannot grasp abstract concepts as older people can. Affectively, children are far less sophisticated and more labile. Whereas older offenders can move away from the family's disturbed behaviors, children cannot. Their values, attitudes, and feelings are mainly shaped by the family in which they live and it is virtually impossible for them to see the family as separate from themselves. Influences outside the family are less strong.

Interfacing with the community is an essential feature of the treatment of children who molest. If a child is molesting, he or she is not safe in a school environment without supervision. It is important to go to the school with the parents and develop a safety plan with the principal, teacher, and other staff (as needed) similar to that used at home. A feedback loop between teacher and parents and therapist can be devised. Most molestation occurs in the bathrooms at school. Hence, these children are generally restricted from bathroom use with other children. Close supervision on the playground is necessary.

Children who molest should be assessed for special education needs. Many of these children have attention deficits, hyperactivity, learning handicaps, and a general inability to be contained in a large group.

SPECIAL ISSUES IN RESIDENTIAL PROGRAMS

Most residential programs for children who molest with which I have consulted have not carefully assessed the children and have mixed children with all levels of sexual problems together. This may exacerbate the sexual confusion of sexually reactive children or children engaging in extensive but mutual sexual behaviors. It also decreases the use of the milieu as a laboratory of change, because the treatment needs of the less disturbed children are quite different. In some cases, the pressure for 100% occupancy/utilization has forced programs to have child victims housed with children who molest. Both situations present a very high risk of molestation and are a supervision nightmare.

This problem is even more serious in residential facilities that do not have the expertise to work with children who molest. Worldwide, most residential facilities and group and foster homes that house children who molest have no specialized supervision or plans in place to help remediate the sexual problems. Placing children who molest in out-of-home care with abuse victims can cause extremely serious problems. Some providers do not tell the other children in the residence they are living with a child who molests, which exacerbates the problem and increases the risk. This is done erroneously in the name of confidentiality.

After hours of discussion with judges and other professionals in many countries, I am convinced that the best interest of the nonoffending children is served by giving them information about the molesting children with whom they live who may hurt them. This information can be given in a sensitive manner with all children in the living unit present, and a plan of protection for everyone can be set up during the discussion. This provides protection (deterrent) for the child who molests and the other children. This can be done without denying the rights of the child who molests.

There are residential programs with between 4 and 16 beds on the same unit. The smaller units are better suited since there are not large numbers of these children, and thus nonmolesting children will not be placed with them. Individual attention is also more available in a smaller unit; because attachment is a fundamental problem with these children, this is important. It is preferable to keep children who molest of similar ages together. If other children need to be added to make up the census, perhaps same-aged children with aggressive behavior problems would be best suited.

Finding, training, emotionally supporting, and supervising line staff (care providers) for residential care is arguably the most difficult aspect of providing good residential treatment for children who molest. Caring for these children on a daily and hourly basis is exceptionally challenging and requires large reserves of emotional health and physical stamina. Line staff are generally the least adequately compensated in residential settings; hence, highly qualified people may look for other positions. People who take the line staff positions as a way of learning about children while they are doing undergraduate studies or as a backdrop to entering degree programs are often good candidates for these positions.

Because the most effective treatment occurs in the milieu, the integration of the clinicians and line staff into an effective treatment team in the units is essential. The importance of the milieu cannot be downplayed, as this is where the learning occurs. Children learn best in the moment, as they have great difficulty understanding concepts in their abstract form. Many programs include the line staff in group therapy to assure the continuity between milieu and treatment.

Difficulties frequently arise between treatment team members owing to differences in their theoretical understanding of children who molest, their philosophy of treatment, their philosophy of child rearing, and their experience. Ongoing training and clinical supervision of the treatment team is essential to avoid team members from becoming harsh, punitive, and shame-based in their interactions with the children.

Some residential programs house children who molest with adolescent sexual offenders. In fact, many programs are designed for 8- to 14-year-olds. Adolescents are significantly more advanced physically, sexually, emotionally, and developmentally. Children under 10 years of age are significantly different from adolescents in terms of their cognitive functioning, skills, and interests and in terms of the tasks that are developmentally appropriate. Although they share the same problem of sexual offending, this is often expressed and felt very differently by pre- and postpubertal offenders. Children frequently cannot defend themselves from adolescents and may be vulnerable to molestation. The thought processes and content of discussions of adolescent sexual offenders is beyond what the young children know or should know. Milieu treatment is far less effective in these situations and can be highly detrimental.

Most residential centers are aware that single rooms are the best way to manage children who molest, but unfortunately only a few have them. Others try to compensate by using laser beams near the beds and doors that set off an alarm when crossed. Others have pressure sensitive alarms under the carpets near the beds and doors. Some use cameras to monitor; some use sound or light systems. Virtually all require awake staff who make rounds at irregular time intervals.

A significant problem for residential programs is the removal of children before they have completed treatment. It is not infrequent that a social worker, probation officer, or the court will place a child with parents or other family members prematurely. Frequently, this has to do with budget constraints. Because of the scarcity of facilities with specialized programs, some children are sent to treatment programs that are too far away for the parents to participate in treatment, and they do not complete treatment in their home town. Returning a child who molests to his or her untreated family of origin is risking immediate failure.

Some programs stress open spatial designs to minimize the occurrence of staff being alone with children, to reduce any fears the children may have of being abused or false allegations of abuse. Most programs do not allow any staff in bedrooms with the door closed. Some do not allow staff to sit on children's beds or to engage in any prolonged touching of the children.

Physical contact is essential for healthy emotional and psychological growth in children. Some programs for children who molest have made rules for physical contact that do not allow the children to learn healthy ways to touch both children and adults. Frequently, no physical contact between the children is allowed and any that occurs is suspect of a sexual connotation. Programs should define their rules for types of physical contact between staff and children and encourage the children to learn healthy ways to be in physical contact with others. This may require an individualized plan for some children that is constantly revised as they learn about healthy ways to be in physical contact with adults and peers. A goal of treatment is healthy physical, emotional, and sexual boundaries.

As virtually all children who molest have difficulty trusting adults and have varying degrees of attachment disorders, some programs focus on attachment. "Holding" is a technique developed in Colorado, which is very controversial. Children are restrained for long periods of time while being physically poked or while being forced to look in the eyes of the person holding his or her upper torso. The child is apparently supposed to give over control to the adults. The theory behind the technique is not well articulated and the success of the technique has never been empirically tested. This appears to be highly problematic and perhaps a dangerous approach with children who molest. It could easily be misinterpreted as a sexual or physical assault and may cause extreme fear, anger, or dissociative reactions. It is far more appropriate to structure a program in which there is respect for the children by the adults and a system in place to empower the children to control their own behavior.

EFFECTS ON THERAPISTS AND CAREGIVERS

While it is exciting to intervene early in the life of a child and prevent the child from developing an ongoing sexual problem and to observe the children's resilience, it is also worrisome to have no well-studied methods of intervening in the problem. Working with children who molest is complex, physically exhausting, emotionally draining, and can affect the adults' worldview. Some treatment providers begin to see sexual offenders everywhere, others doubt that healthy families exist, some treatment providers may begin to see men or sex in a negative light. Intrusive recollections of the children's traumas may invade the adult's waking and sleeping hours. Anger at the "system" and the children's parents can get in the way of good treatment. The inhumanity in the lives of these children becomes evident when observing the pervasiveness of the effects of all of the abuse and traumatic events that they have lived through. The goal of treatment with many of these children may not be a complete recovery but rather a diminution of the symptoms, which may take many months, often years, with frequent dramatic regressions throughout the treatment process. Therapist and line staff burnout is high in this field.

SUGGESTIONS FOR IMPLEMENTING PROGRAMS

The first principle in this field is that you must make sure you want to work with this population. It is both very difficult and very rewarding, but on any particular day, the difficulty may outweigh the rewards. High frustration tolerance and the ability to see the progress and supply hope to the children and parents are essential. Learn about the systems' response to these children in your area and develop contacts with all of them. Educate the systems about children who molest and develop protocols between these systems to coordinate a response, identify referrals, and provide services. Develop a clear mission statement for the treatment program, stay focused, and develop outcome measures and a good data collection system before you begin.

Extensive interviewing of potential treatment providers and providing them with clear information about the children and the problems attendant to their treatment is useful. Thorough background checks, intense training, and high levels of supervision are all necessary. In residential treatment, frequent treatment team meetings with clinicians and care providers, working together to develop the clinical and milieu plan for each child, will encourage cooperation and decrease splitting. Clinicians will profit by spending extensive time in the milieu to appreciate the struggles the children present and to provide supervision and suggestions to care providers. Punitive responses that can lead the children to negative feelings about sex and sexuality may surface when support for the line staff who are on the firing line is inadequate.

Power struggles are frequent with children who molest. Learn to disengage. Members of the treatment team cannot control the children's behavior; only they can. Give the children the skills and knowledge they need to control their own behavior. Look at what is behind the struggle; see the need that is being expressed by the conflict, and help the child meet the need in socially appropriate ways.

Believe in the children's ability to overcome their pain and struggles by having hope when they are hopeless, give them knowledge when they do not understand, and teach them skills by which they can overcome their problems. When at all possible, teach their parents how to love and emotionally support them.

ACKNOWLEDGMENTS. I would like to acknowledge the contribution of Dennis R. Pickering, MA, CPC, Mary M. Kowalski, BSN, RNC, Dori Martinale, MSW, ACSW, CISW, from Arizona Youth Associates; Janet Eder from the CAT-Team, New Zealand; Patrice Crawford, RN, from the Crawford Center, Inc., Florida; John Eckstein from Experiment with Travel, Massachusetts; Diane Johnson from Teams, Minnesota; Michael L. Barrow, MS, Hiram Rivera-Toro, MFCC, Karen Shipley, MFCC, from St. Anthony's Group Home, California; and Mary Seabloom from the Institute for Child and Adolescent Sexual Health "Storefront/Youth Action," Minnesota.

REFERENCES

American Psychiatric Association. (1994). *Diagnostic and statistical manual of mental disorders* (4th ed.). Washington, DC: Author.

Araji, S. (1997). *Sexually aggressive children*. Thousand Oaks, CA: Sage.

Caruso, K. (1987). *Projective storytelling cards*. Redding, CA: Northwest Psychological Publishers.

Cunningham, C., & MacFarlane, K. (1991). *When children molest children*. Orwell, VT: Safer Society Press.

Freeman-Longo, R., Bird, S., Stevenson, W., & Fiske, J. (1994). *Nationwide survey of treatment programs and models serving abuse-reactive children and adolescent and adult sex offenders*. Orwell, VT: Safer Society Program and Press.

Friedrich, W., & Luecke, W. (1988). Young school-age sexually aggressive children. *Professional Psychology Research and Practice, 19*, 155–164.

Griggs, D.R., & Boldi, A. (1995). Parallel treatment of parents of abuse reactive children. In M. Hunter (Ed.), *Child survivors and perpetrators of sexual abuse: Treatment innovations* (pp. 147–165). Thousand Oaks, CA: Sage.

Johnson, T.C. (1988). Child perpetrators—children who molest other children: Preliminary findings. *Child Abuse and Neglect, 12*, 219–229.

Johnson, T.C. (1989). Female child perpetrators: Children who molest other children. *Child Abuse and Neglect, 13*, 571–585.

Johnson, T.C. (1993a). Preliminary findings. In E. Gil & T.C. Johnson (Eds.), *Sexualized children: Assessment and treatment of sexualized children and children who molest* (p. 68). Rockville, MD: Launch Press.

Johnson, T.C. (1993b). Sexual behaviors: A continuum. In E. Gil & T.C. Johnson (Eds.), *Sexualized children: Assessment and treatment of sexualized children and children who molest* (pp. 44–45). Rockville, MD: Launch Press.

Johnson, T.C. (1993c). Clinical evaluation. In E. Gil & T.C. Johnson (Eds.), *Sexualized children: Assessment and treatment of sexualized children and children who molest* (pp. 137–178). Rockville, MD: Launch Press.

Johnson, T.C. (1995a). *Treatment exercises for abuse victims and children with sexual behavior problems*. South Pasadena, CA: Author.

Johnson, T.C. (1995b). *Child sexuality curriculum for abused children and their parents*. South Pasadena, CA: Author.

Johnson, T.C. (1996a). *Assessment packet for children with sexual behavior problems*. South Pasadena, CA: Author.

Johnson, T.C. (1996b). *Understanding children's sexual behaviors—What's natural and healthy and what's not?* South Pasadena, CA: Author.

Johnson, T.C., & Berry, C. (1989). Children who molest other children: A treatment program. *Journal of Interpersonal Violence, 4*, 185–203.

24

Adolescent Sexual Offender Treatment at the SAFE-T Program

James R. Worling

Adolescent sexual offenders are responsible for approximately 20% of sexual assaults against teens and adults and between 30 and 50% of sexual assaults against children (Barbaree, Hudson, & Seto, 1993). Most adolescent sexual offenders referred for an initial assessment have a history of previously undetected sexual offenses, suggesting that isolated incidents of sexual aggression are relatively uncommon. Although it is not known what proportion of adolescents continue to commit offenses as adults, it was found recently that 37% of a small sample of untreated, violent adolescent sexual offenders reoffended sexually as adults (Rubinstein, Yeager, Goodstein, & Lewis, 1993). Furthermore, it is a widely held belief that many adult sexual offenders began offending during their teenage years (e.g., Prentky & Knight, 1993).

THE SAFE-T PROGRAM

In response to the obvious need for the treatment of adolescent sexual offenders, treatment programs proliferated in North America during the mid-1980s, and this is also when the Sexual Abuse: Family Education and Treatment (SAFE-T) Program was created. In brief, in 1982, a handful of interested staff from the Adolescent Services Program at Thistletown Regional Centre volunteered their time to work with adolescent victims of intrafamilial sexual abuse as a pilot project. During the next 2 years, they were inundated with referrals and saw the need to establish a specialized program to provide sexual-abuse-specific assessment and treatment resources. Despite the opposition of some senior clinicians who believed that adolescent sexual abuse victims and offenders did not require specialized services, the SAFE-T Program was formally established in 1985 through the tenacity of its founding director (R. Berry) and the dedication and interest of a small group of clinical staff.

James R. Worling • SAFE-T Program, Thistletown Regional Centre for Children and Adolescents, Toronto, Ontario, Canada M9V 4L8.

Sourcebook of Treatment Programs for Sexual Offenders, edited by Marshall et al. Plenum Press, New York, 1998.

The SAFE-T Program is a community-based, outpatient clinic that is one of several specialized programs at the Thistletown Regional Centre for Children and Adolescents in Toronto, Ontario, Canada. Thistletown Regional Centre is directly funded and operated by the Provincial Government of Ontario. SAFE-T has a staff of 12 clinical positions (child care, social work, psychology, and art therapy), 1.5 support staff, and a part-time consulting psychiatrist. SAFE-T is a sexual-abuse-specific program that provides assessment, treatment, interagency resourcing, and long-term support to two client groups: (1) children and families in which incest has occurred (including adult incest offenders), and (2) adolescent sexual offenders (both intrafamilial and extrafamilial) and their families. During the average year, 75 cases receive direct clinical services. This represents approximately 220 individuals, as SAFE-T strongly encourages inclusion of family members, where appropriate, in offender and victim treatment. The average length of treatment is approximately 2 years, and clients are able to return at times of crisis following their discharge. Currently, half of the cases in the program are adolescent sexual offenders and their families, and half represent child victims of incest and their families. Given the long-term nature of treatment, 30 of the 75 cases serviced each year are new admissions. SAFE-T provides consultation and training to other professionals, and offers sexual-abuse-specific internships to students in social work, psychology, child care, and medicine. SAFE-T also conducts research in the area of sexual assault and victimization.

Several philosophical ideals guide our assessment and treatment procedures. In particular, we believe that the need to prevent further sexual offenses is the prime consideration in the provision of services and forms the basis for decisions regarding clinical interventions; sexual victimization/offending has a profound and long-term impact on individuals and families; in families where sexual abuse/victimization has occurred, treatment is best addressed through an integrated, holistic, and comprehensive model that has a sexual-abuse-specific focus; treatment interventions reflect the unique strengths and needs of families and individuals and include appropriate aspects of cognitive–behavioral, family-systems, group, insight-oriented, play, and art therapies; all individuals and families have strengths that will foster positive changes with the appropriate direction, support, and encouragement.

Client Group

To date, adolescent sexual offender referrals to the SAFE-T Program have come from Probation and Community Services (51%), other treatment agencies or group homes (33%), child protection agencies (12%), or parents (4%). Given our special relationship with Probation Services (described below), we continually hold 24 places in our program for probation referrals. Offenders are accepted for assessment if they are not actively psychotic and are at least of borderline intellectual functioning. Although we have accepted developmentally delayed offenders in the past, we found that we were unable to provide adequate services to this specialized population within the structure of our program. For example, we found that weekly outpatient therapy was insufficient to maintain therapeutic gains and that much of our expertise and treatment methodology were not appropriate for this client group.

Of the adolescent sexual offenders accepted for assessment and/or treatment, approximately 93% are male, and the modal age at the time of assessment is 15 years (range: 12–19 years). The offenders reflect the cultural diversity of metropolitan Toronto and, given that SAFE-T is a publicly funded program, the majority (75%) of our offenders are from lower socioeconomic groups. Approximately 80% of the offenders receive criminal charges for their sexual offenses, and almost half have previous nonsexual criminal offenses. To date the offenders were, at the time of initial assessment, living either at home (50%), in secure-custody facilities (26%), group homes (15%), foster care (5%), with family friends (3%), or on their own (1%). With respect to family composition, the offenders were living with the following parental figures prior to the detection of their offenses: mother and father (biological, adoptive, or long-term foster care) (42%), single mother (24%), mother and stepfather (23%), father and stepmother (9%), or grandparents (2%).

Despite the prevalence of noncontact offenses such as exhibitionism, 98% of the offenders at SAFE-T are referred for "hands-on" offenses (although many have also committed noncontact offenses for which they were never charged). This figure likely reflects our society's propensity to view noncontact offenses as nuisances rather than as sexual assaults. It is important to note, however, that Longo and Groth (1983) found that 33% of adult sexual offenders began with exhibitionism and voyeurism in adolescence and progressed to more intrusive contact offenses. The victims of our adolescent offenders are intrafamilial (34%), extrafamilial (51%), or both (15%); female (62%), male (17%), or both (21%); children (53%), peers (27%), adults (4%), or from two or more age groups (16%).

Assessment

SAFE-T's offender assessment takes approximately 2 months. Included in this process is the collection of reports from other treatment agencies, schools, Probation Services, child welfare, and police (when available). Several clinical interviews are conducted with the adolescent offender and, wherever possible, interviews are also conducted with the adolescent offender's family and various family subsystems, depending on the nature of the case (e.g., parents, father and son, siblings). We also meet regularly with other significant individuals in the offender's life, such as the child protection worker, probation officer, and group home worker, to gain a more complete understanding of the adolescent. Offenders complete a number of psychological tests focusing on issues such as anger, depression, loneliness, sexual offending, sexual attitudes, family relationships, self-esteem, and personality. We also ask parents and siblings to complete questionnaires, as our focus is not solely on the adolescent offender. We view sexual offending as a behavior that is multidetermined; therefore, the goal of our assessment is to understand the cultural, biological, familial, individual, and situational factors that have contributed to the development and maintenance of the adolescent's sexual aggression and to devise treatment plans according to the needs and strengths of the offender and his or her family.

Although many programs in North America utilize phallometric assessments with adolescents, SAFE-T does not employ this procedure for several reasons. First, as a treatment program that also works with sexually abused children, we are particularly sensitive to the fact that the children depicted in the visual stimuli are being further exploited despite Canadian laws that permit the use of pornography for research purposes. Several programs have stopped using visual stimuli as a result of similar concerns and have substituted auditory stimuli in their place. Second, adolescence is a period of emerging sexual development, and teenagers are continuously developing and refining their sexual scripts, identities, and preferences. Exposing adolescents to visual or auditory images of deviant sexual activities could negatively affect their emerging sexual development. As Laws and Marshall (1990) noted, "any initial deviant contact, random deviant fantasy, or exposure to textual or visual representations of deviant behavior may supply sufficient material for later elaboration in masturbatory fantasy" (p. 221). Despite the proliferation of phallometric laboratories, there are no data in the literature regarding the adolescents' experience of the process or of the potential for negative residual effects. Several adolescents at SAFE-T have participated in these examinations at other centers, and many have described the experience as humiliating. Third, there is very little evidence regarding the reliability or validity of this procedure with adolescents (using visual or auditory stimuli), and there are no normative data from nonoffending adolescents. Indeed, results from phallometric assessments of adolescent offenders suggest that arousal data are significantly influenced by such variables as the offenders' age (Kaemingk, Koselka, Becker, & Kaplan, 1995) and history of physical and/or sexual abuse (Becker, Kaplan, & Tenke, 1992). Furthermore, variables traditionally correlated with deviant sexual arousal in adult sexual offenders such as the number of victims and degree of force are not reliably correlated with arousal in adolescent sexual offenders (Hunter, Goodwin, & Becker, 1994). Becker et al. (1992) also found that adolescents who denied their offenses tended to provide invalid deviant-arousal data. Finally, given our holistic view of sexual offenders, deviant sexual arousal is but one aspect of sexual offending—although perhaps critical in some cases—and focusing assessment and treatment efforts on the role of the genitalia erroneously takes the focus off other core issues such as self-esteem, intimacy deficits, and the thoughts and emotions that perpetuate sexual-offending behaviors (Marshall, 1995).

To gather information regarding sexual arousal (and other sensitive information), we rely on establishing a caring and supportive therapeutic relationship with the offender and then asking questions. File information regarding previous offenses and updates from the probation officer, group home staff, and parents also provide a rich array of data regarding the offender's sexual preferences and practices. Of course, there are some offenders who will only acknowledge deviant sexual fantasies after considerable involvement in therapy, and there are others who will deny any sexually deviant fantasies. Although some would label our humanistic philosophy as naive, we cannot justify exposing teenagers to an intrusive and potentially harmful procedure with no established reliability or validity that would, in any case, provide information regarding only one of many critical treatment goal areas.

Treatment

From the results of our assessment, treatment plans are individually tailored for each client, and treatment goals are reviewed every 4 months. On average, these goals are addressed through concurrent weekly group therapy for 18 months, weekly individual therapy for 24 months, and biweekly family therapy for 12 months. With respect to sexual-offender-specific treatment goals, we utilize the repertoire of cognitive–behavioral and relapse prevention strategies that are currently popular in adolescent sexual offender treatment and we address issues related to denial and accountability, sexual arousal, sexual attitudes, and victim empathy. Given that sexual deviance is only one aspect of the adolescent's life, related treatment goals often include the enhancement of social skills and friendships, self-esteem, family relationships, body image, appropriate anger expression, trust, and so on.

Funding

Given that SAFE-T is directly operated by the government of Ontario, we are subject to the changes in government and, therefore, the resulting changes in government philosophy and fiscal planning. This environment of uncertainty adds considerable stress to the already challenging work of providing services to children and families in which sexual abuse has occurred, and it often makes it difficult to begin long-term treatment with individuals and families. In hindsight, it would have been advantageous for our program to have moved at least "arms length" from government funding during the late 1980s by seeking divestment options that would have provided some autonomy.

On a more positive note, the SAFE-T Program has had tremendous success obtaining additional funds to provide services for adolescent sexual offenders. With an ever-increasing demand from probation officers in Toronto to provide services for adolescent sexual offenders, the SAFE-T Program proposed a 3-year pilot project with Probation and Community Services in the Toronto area. In particular, it was proposed that in exchange for funding three new staff positions at SAFE-T (one part-time researcher and two social workers), assessment and treatment services would be offered to adolescent offenders and their families.

Although originally intended to be time-limited, this joint venture with Probation Services is now in its ninth year. Furthermore, the money originally allocated for the project has gradually been increased and added into SAFE-T's base budget. For an average annual cost of approximately $130,000 (Canadian) from Probation Services added to SAFE-T's base budget, this project has provided the following each year: assessment and treatment for 24 adolescent sexual offenders and their families; local, national, and international training workshops for students and professionals; supervised student internships regarding sexual-abuse-specific treatment; psychological assessments for adolescent sexual offenders at other community agencies; psychological assessments of additional clients at SAFE-T (child, adolescent, and adult victims/survivors of sexual abuse, adult incest offenders, and family members); and research regarding the etiology, assessment, and treatment of adolescent sexual offenders. Note that the annual average cost of the above services is equivalent to the cost of housing one teenage sexual offender in a local custody facility for 1 year—without sexual-offender-specific treatment.

This project has also created a strong alliance between the SAFE-T Program and our biggest referral source: Probation and Community Services. Through our workshops, project meetings, and our joint clinical work we have gained an appreciation of the roles, skills, and needs of the probation officers. Many probation officers in the Toronto area have also gained a better understanding of the roles and limitations of a sexual-offender-specific treatment agency and have received sexual-offender-specific therapy instruction through the internship program and workshops. This enhanced communication and understanding has resulted in more coordinated treatment for adolescent offenders at SAFE-T and in our community. We believe that this joint project between the legal system and a community-based treatment program could serve as a model for other sexual offender treatment providers.

Intake Process

With respect to our intake process, we have experienced two significant difficulties in the past. First, SAFE-T used to keep a waiting list for services; however, we soon found that the list was growing too rapidly, given the long-term requirements of comprehensive therapy and the demand for sexual-abuse-specific services. During 1994, for example, SAFE-T had to turn away 20 referrals for every one taken into the program. Once clients (both self- and agency referrals) were placed on the waiting list, they stopped looking for alternative resources. When we could finally take the case into the program, so much time had passed since the original disclosure that many clients were resistant to "reopen the past." The solution adopted for this problem was twofold: First, the waiting list was discontinued, and cases are now taken only when there is an opening. Second, our intake position has evolved into a clinical role in that the intake coordinator (a social worker) provides those seeking services with names of alternative resources, ongoing clinical support, and reading materials when appropriate. Although far from ideal, this solution encourages clients to participate actively in locating (and advocating for) resources and helps to reduce the time from initial disclosure to treatment.

The second major difficulty regarding our intake procedures involved incest offenders: particularly, sibling incest offenders. During the early history of our program, we would agree to conduct an assessment without significant consideration of the offender's place of residence. In cases where the offender was still living with the victim(s) or potential victim(s), we often found ourselves completing our assessment and recommending that the offender be removed from the home because there was significant risk of reoffense. In several instances, our concerns were not shared by the child protection worker, probation officer, or family members, and this put us in the position of advocating for the removal of the offender: that is, we were often performing the role of child protection workers. Needless to say, this often fostered an adversarial relationship between the SAFE-T Program and the clients and made subsequent treatment efforts more challenging than necessary. After a client reoffended in the home, we decided to adopt the policy that we would not become involved in a case in which the offender currently resided with his or her victim(s) or a potential victim(s). With this arrangement, it is the responsibility of the child protection agency, Probation Services, and the family to seek appropriate placement in the interest of safety for both the offender and his or her victim(s). Although our intake policy has been more widely accepted within the community over the years, there are still several referral agents who have difficulties with our guidelines. We seek some comfort, however, in the knowledge that we are not alone in this policy and that the National Adolescent Perpetrator Network (1993) suggests that "in cases of sibling incest, the sexually abusive sibling should be removed from the home until both siblings' therapists approve reunification" (p. 33).

Involvement of Other Agencies

There are often many individuals and agencies involved in the lives of the adolescent sexual offenders at the SAFE-T Program, and we need to be cognizant of the frequently competing needs and objectives, given our belief in a comprehensive and holistic approach. It could be quite tempting for a treatment program to conduct its sexual-offender-specific treatment in isolation, and thereby avoid the potential headaches of collaboration by simply working with the offender. However, adolescent sexual offenders spend at most 5 hours per week at our clinic when they are involved in concurrent group, family, and individual treatment—they spend about 100 waking hours each week in other environments. Given that high-risk factors such as anger, depression, boredom, loneliness, and deviant sexual arousal occur in environments such as family, school, or residential settings, treatment that directly includes these systems will undoubtedly be more effective. In one of the only studies with random assignment to treatment conditions, Borduin, Henggeler, Blaske, and Stein (1990) found that after 3 years, 12.5% of those adolescent sexual offenders who completed multisystemic therapy reoffended sexually compared to 75% of those who completed individual therapy.

Many cases will involve the offender's parents, siblings, probation officer, child protection worker, and the group home staff. Whenever we have provided treatment without addressing the concerns of these individuals, we have experienced difficulties at the offender's expense. For example, parents, the probation officer, and the SAFE-T team may agree that an offender presents considerable risk to young children in the community, yet continually battle with a group home that is permitting many unsupervised hours in the community. SAFE-T, the custody facility, and parents may agree that the adolescent is not ready to return home, yet the child protection worker may disagree and fail to provide an alternative residence. To minimize difficulties such as these, we now typically have a "business meeting" with all parties (including the family) before we begin an assessment, and this meeting serves several purposes simultaneously. First, all individuals and agencies are given the same information regarding our assessment and treatment procedures, limits of confidentiality, and expectations for a coordinated approach to reoffense prevention. Second, the meeting provides an opportunity for the important individuals in the offender's life to make known their mandates, biases, and long-term goals. Third, all participants have the opportunity to receive updated information concerning the offender, as there are often recent details not included in the file. Most important, this meeting begins a process of working collaboratively with the many individuals and agencies, and it underscores our belief in the importance of working together on these cases as a multisystemic team.

Following the business meeting, we ask key individuals such as the referral source and the group home worker to attend the initial assessment meeting. After introduction to the clients—and only with the clients' permission—these individuals sit behind a one-way mirror with our clinical team and, in many cases, continue to participate in the assessment in this manner until treatment commences. Having this expanded team during the assessment not only enriches our assessment with the added clinical input, but it further enhances our efforts to work together with other agencies as a collaborative team. Furthermore, the offenders and their families often find it supportive to have a familiar face present when they are beginning at a new agency.

Working collaboratively extends well beyond the assessment, as we typically review treatment goals every 4 months in a meeting that includes all agency and family stakeholders. We also encourage open communication throughout the team wherever possible, and we frequently speak with staff from residential settings and parents throughout the course of treatment. For instance, we contact the group home when an offender requires extra support or monitoring as the result of a particularly difficult session, and parents or other agencies will contact us with concerns they feel are relevant to the risk of sexual reoffense.

Our multisystemic meetings, assessments, goal reviews, and ongoing discussions are certainly not a panacea for interagency conflict; however, we find that they go a long way toward setting the stage for a coordinated approach to adolescent sexual offender treatment. Some level of disagreement is certainly welcome, as this encourages all parties to continually reassess their goals and objectives. When we have had significant difficulties reaching agreement with an agency (often regarding such issues as the need for sexual abuse specific treatment), one solution that has helped is to offer workshops and consultations to the agency regarding the relevant issues.

Even when all of the external agencies and individuals are working collaboratively, orchestrating the sexual-offender-specific group, family, and individual therapy for adolescent sexual offenders can be a challenging task. This is made somewhat easier at our program, however, as SAFE-T offers all of these services under one roof. Furthermore, each case is supported by a multidisciplinary team with therapists from all components of the family's involvement in treatment. For example, a sibling incest offender's team may consist of the family therapist, the offender's individual therapist, a co-leader from the adolescent offender group, the victim's individual therapist, and a co-leader from the parents' group. In this way, communication regarding sexual-offender-specific issues is enhanced and specific interventions are more easily timed and coordinated. We also work in this collaborative and multisystemic fashion with the adult incest offenders at our program; however, there are certainly unique aspects of our work with adolescents given their stage of development.

Role of the Family

One of the most significant differences between adolescent and adult sexual offenders is the relationship to the family of origin. As noted earlier, approximately half of the offenders seen at SAFE-T are living with their families, and many of those in residential settings will return home following probation. Even though some offenders will never return home, family issues (past, present, and future) are salient for every adolescent at SAFE-T.

Adolescents are at the developmental stage of separating from the family and establishing an independent identity through closer attachments to peers. This is often a source of conflict for all adolescents (whether offenders or not) and their families, and the struggle for independence is often exacerbated with the addition of sexual assault issues such as the need for parents to monitor high-risk factors. Another essential reason to involve families in the treatment of adolescent sexual offenders is that family difficulties that may have contributed to the development of the adolescent's sexual aggression need to be altered if risk is to be reduced. The family environments of many adolescent sexual offenders are often unstable and involve physical and emotional violence. For the adolescent, these interaction patterns foster low self-esteem, loneliness, depression, anger, and the inability to form intimate relationships with others: factors that are said to contribute significantly to the development and maintenance of sexual aggression (Marshall, Hudson, & Hodkinson, 1993). As such, family therapy is often focused on assisting families to change interaction patterns, roles, expectations, and boundaries in an effort to enhance family relationships and reduce the risk of further offending. It is crucial to note, however, that we do not hold parents accountable for their child's sexual offending; rather, we view family dysfunction as contributing to the development of factors that increase the likelihood an adolescent will choose to offend sexually. Furthermore, we view family therapy as an important adjunct to sexual-offender-specific treatment, not as a replacement.

The need for interventions that include the family is particularly evident in the case of adolescent sibling incest offenders. Families of sibling incest offenders are characterized by excessive levels of marital discord, parental rejection of the offender, physical discipline, and verbal aggression (Worling, 1995a). In addition to the obvious need for treatment for the sexually abused sibling(s) and the adolescent offender, parents of sibling incest offenders are often struggling in their ability to support simultaneously their offending and victimized children. Nonvictimized siblings are also grappling with issues of loyalty, and many have witnessed the sexual abuse within the family. Finally, all family members are attempting to cope with the removal of the offender from the home and with the possibility and timing of the offender's return.

Whether assaults are intrafamilial or extrafamilial, parents need to be included in any relapse prevention plans if interventions are going to be successful for the adolescent intending to maintain family relationships. Although these sessions are typically very challenging, we have found it particularly helpful for the adolescents to explain to their parents their offense chains, their high-risk situations, and their development of coping mechanisms. They also need to enlist parental support in the prevention of further offenses. This intervention should be timed appropriately in that the offender should have successfully mastered much of the sexual-offender-specific work and be sufficiently prepared to present this information to his or her parents. Furthermore, parents need to be adequately prepared to hear information about their child that could be highly disturbing. For example, we often find that parents react negatively upon learning the degree of planning their child engaged in before each offense, as they had previously assumed that the offenses were spontaneous and, therefore, "less serious." We have also found that the adolescents' descriptions of their offenses contain more detail than the parents were aware of. It is also essential that family communication patterns be altered in family therapy, if necessary, before this work is attempted, as it is important that parents listen to their child's thoughts, feelings, and explanations.

Although we strive to include the offenders' families whenever possible, this can prove to be a challenging task in some cases. Many parents coming to our program have already experienced adversarial relationships with a child protection agency, police, courts, schools, and other community treatment programs, and thus are wary of an additional involvement. To facilitate their participation, we offer flexible meeting times (and, sometimes, locations), provide honest assessment feedback, and emphasize the importance of their participation in the assessment and treatment of their children. We have also engaged some parents in therapy by offering them access to our groups for parents of adolescent sexual offenders, adult survivors of childhood sexual abuse, or parenting workshops. Most important, however, we work hard to establish a caring and nonjudgmental relationship, as most parents come to our program feeling ashamed, guilty, and embarrassed regarding their child's sexual offenses. Of course, some parents will not engage in any therapeutic process, and we must struggle to provide therapy, which includes family issues, in their absence. In the case of adolescent offenders who have been abandoned by their families, we often need to assist them in dealing with this reality and help them to learn to avoid further sexual offenses in the absence of family relationships.

One of the most powerful indicators of the salience of family involvement is that almost all offenders at SAFE-T mention the loss of family relationships when devising aversive scripts for covert sensitization exercises. The following is a typical scenario developed by an adolescent sexual offender:

> If I ever reoffended the worst possible thing that could happen to me is my mother would have me thrown in jail. I wouldn't have a family left. The door which marks my position in my family would be shut and locked. I would be left out in the cold of penattentary [sic] life … I would become alone and I expect that I would die a painful death of being lonely.

Developmental Factors

Adolescence is a developmental period marked by significant biological, social, and cognitive changes. With respect to biological changes, the adolescent male, for example, must contend with rapid changes in height, weight, enlargement of penis and testes, onset of ejaculatory capacity, growth of pubic hair, and possibly feelings of appearing unattractive. Within the space of several months, there is a 20-fold increase in serum testosterone levels for males in early adolescence (Vaughan & Litt, 1990). Socially, young adolescents are beginning to form heterosocial friendships and intimate relationships and they are moving from close family attachments to closer bonds with peers. In terms of cognitive changes, adolescents are developing the capacity for abstract thought, a more mature sense of time, enhanced metacognition, greater information-processing and memory capacity, higher-order moral reasoning and mutual role taking, as well as increased self-control. Adolescence is also a time of heightened interest in sexual matters, and this produces a need to incorporate sexuality into both personal identity and social relationships. With this multitude of change, it is not surprising that adolescence is also a time of increased risk for the development of such problems as depression, substance abuse, eating disorders, and norm-breaking behaviors.

One area that requires an awareness of the developmental limitations of adolescents is victim empathy training. The enhancement of victim empathy is a component of virtually all sexual offender programs, as it is assumed that victim empathy will inhibit further offending. Although very young children can demonstrate empathic behaviors in response to distress in others, the cognitive and emotional capacities to empathize continue to mature during adolescence in conjunction with developmental changes in moral reasoning, abstract thought, and role-taking abilities (Davis & Franzoi, 1991). Furthermore, many adolescent sexual offenders have been abused physically, emotionally, and/or sexually, and these harmful experiences appear to impede the development of empathy. Given these factors, the development of empathy will be a challenging task for many adolescent sexual offenders. Of course, we still spend considerable time during therapy on the enhancement of victim empathy, and we have noticed significant shifts when an adult survivor has come to speak with the offender group. However, we find that offense prevention is heightened when we capitalize on their natural adolescent egocentrism and self-preoccupation by assisting them to highlight the negative personal consequences for continued offending (e.g., loss of family, loss of freedom, loss of friends, etc.).

While developmental factors need to be taken into account in treating adolescent sexual offenders, there are many techniques developed for adult sexual offenders that can be easily modified to suit these clients. For example, although the offense cycle exercises developed for relapse prevention with adult sexual offenders are often too complex and abstract for many adolescents, we use an adaptation of a simplified offense chain: situation–strong feelings–sexual thoughts–thinking errors–planning–high-risk situation–sexual assault–strong feelings. Many adolescent sexual offenders agree that their offenses follow this progression, and they are able to discern identifiable patterns and develop appropriate alternative coping strategies for each stage in this chain. Similarly, many of the relapse prevention, cognitive-restructuring, and deviant arousal reduction exercises have been successfully adapted for use with adolescents by using more simplified language, more concrete tasks, repetition, briefer time frames, and the use of games (e.g., Becker & Kaplan, 1993).

Sexual Victimization among the Offenders

Another factor that appears to be important in adolescent sexual offenders is the current impact of childhood sexual victimization. As in the case of adult sexual offenders, many more adolescent sexual offenders have a history of childhood sexual victimization than do comparable nonoffending adolescents. In a recent investigation (Worling, 1995b), it was found that 43% of the adolescent sexual offenders at our clinic reported childhood sexual victimization. When examined according to the gender of their victims, 75% of those adolescents who had assaulted a male child reported sexual abuse compared to 25% of those who offended against females. This result suggests that sexual victimization may be an important contributing variable to adolescent sexual aggression against males. In their review of the literature, Hanson and Slater (1988) also found that sexual victimization was more common in the backgrounds of adult offenders against male children than among offenders against female children. It is important to note, however, that many sexual offenders do not report a history of sexual victimization and furthermore that most male victims of sexual abuse do not become sexual offenders.

Despite the similarities between adult and adolescent sexual offenders regarding the prevalence of childhood sexual victimization, there is necessarily a closer temporal contiguity between victimization and offending for the adolescents. This means that for the victimized adolescent offenders, the trauma symptoms typically associated with childhood sexual abuse may be far more pronounced than among adult offenders who may have attempted to "normalize" their past abuse (Briggs & Hawkins, 1996). As such, it is important to incorporate these issues into any intervention and to carefully balance the need for victim and offender treatment.

Minimization of Adolescent Offending

The most difficult issue in working with adolescent sexual offenders is the pervasive and systemic minimization of the importance of working with this population. Police are often reticent to charge the adolescent sexual offender; perhaps because they, as do many others, view sexual violence by an adolescent as a slight variation in the process of normal sexual development. This is particularly true for adolescents who are primarily exposing or peeping. Indeed, one of the cases at the SAFE-T Program was a 16-year-old rapist with a well-documented (yet untreated) history of exhibitionism (age 12), voyeurism (age 13), and many family difficulties related to violence and abandonment. This boy's offenses had been considered by other agencies as "experimentation" rather than as instances of abuse. Even when adolescents are charged, probation orders are often too brief to accommodate long-term therapy, and orders for treatment are often absent. Although some adolescents leave our program when their probation orders expire, most continue to participate fully in treatment. This is likely attributable to the fact that we strive to establish a caring and nonjudgmental therapeutic relationship, our treatment is comprehensive and holistic, and we are often successful in engaging the most crucial system in the adolescent's life: the family.

The minimization of adolescent sexual aggression is also evident in the relative dearth of information in the literature regarding adolescent sexual offenders in comparison to the knowledge amassed on adult sexual offenders. Furthermore, in contrast to the multitude of data regarding the sexual attitudes, fantasies, and behaviors of nonoffending adults and college students, we are often operating in a scientific vacuum when it comes to information regarding normal adolescent sexual development.

CONCLUSIONS

Despite the difficulties involved in working with adolescent sexual offenders, their developmental characteristics are often a positive force for therapy. Their need to form close associations with peers, for example, lends itself naturally to group therapy, and adolescent peer pressure is a powerful vehicle for confronting denial and minimization.

Similarly, the need to be independent and somewhat rebellious toward adults permits many opportunities in group therapy for the adult co-leaders to allow the offenders to take ownership of the group activities. We have found that, with appropriate support and encouragement, adolescent sexual offenders develop and follow excellent group therapy rules and expectations and can assist one another in making positive changes. In fact, when the group is running well, the adult co-leaders often provide little input aside from the introduction of offense-specific exercises and the assignment of homework.

Although the familial, cultural, and personal factors underlying adult and adolescent sexual aggression may be similar, many adult sexual offenders have established entrenched deviant sexual arousal patterns through more extensive masturbatory conditioning and sexual offending. Given that adolescents are still refining their sexual identities, preferences, and practices, there is considerable hope that sexual-offender-specific therapy will be highly efficacious, particularly when treatment addresses the adolescent's sexual aggression within the context of peers, school, society, and the family. Recidivism data (criminal charges) were collected for adolescents who completed at least one year of treatment at the SAFE-T Program and a comparison group of sexual offenders who did not receive treatment at our program (i.e., youth referred for an assessment only or those who refused, or dropped out of, treatment). With a mean follow up of 6 years (range: 2–10 years), the sexual assault recidivism rate for the comparison group was more than three times higher (18%) than the recidivism rate for the treatment group (5%).

ACKNOWLEDGMENTS. The preparation of this chapter was supported by a grant from Probation and Community Services, Ontario Ministry of Community and Social Services. The views expressed herein are the author's and do not necessarily reflect those of the Thistletown Regional Centre for Children and Adolescents or the Ontario Ministry of Community and Social Services. My sincere thanks to Sabrina Ramdeholl and William Marshall for their valuable comments on a previous draft of this manuscript.

REFERENCES

Barbaree, H.E., Hudson, S.M., & Seto, M.C. (1993). Sexual assault in society: The role of the juvenile offender. In H.E. Barbaree, W.L. Marshall, & S.M. Hudson (Eds.), *The juvenile sex offender* (pp. 1–24). New York: Guilford Press.

Becker, J.V., & Kaplan, M.S. (1993). Cognitive behavioral treatment of the juvenile sex offender. In H.E. Barbaree, W.L. Marshall, & S.M. Hudson (Eds.), *The juvenile sex offender* (pp. 264–277). New York: Guilford Press.

Becker, J.V., Kaplan, M.S., & Tenke, C.E. (1992). The relationship of abuse history, denial and erectile response: Profiles of adolescent sexual perpetrators. *Behavior Therapy, 23*, 87–97.

Borduin, C.M., Henggeler, S.W., Blaske, D.M., & Stein, R.J. (1990). Multisystemic treatment of adolescent sex offenders. *International Journal of Offender Therapy and Comparative Criminology, 34*, 105–113.

Briggs, F., & Hawkins, R.M.F. (1996). A comparison of the childhood experiences of convicted male child molesters and men who were sexually abused in childhood and claim to be nonoffenders. *Child Abuse and Neglect, 20*, 221–233.

Davis, M.H., & Franzoi, S.L. (1991). Stability and change in adolescent self-consciousness and empathy. *Journal of Research in Personality, 25*, 70–87.

Hanson, R.K., & Slater, S. (1988). Sexual victimization in the history of child sexual abusers: A review. *Annals of Sex Research, 1*, 485–499.

Hunter, J.A., Goodwin, D.W., & Becker, J.V. (1994). The relationship between phallometrically measured deviant sexual arousal and clinical characteristics in juvenile sexual offenders. *Behavior Research and Therapy, 32*, 533–538.

Kaemingk, K.L., Koselka, M., Becker, J.V., & Kaplan, M.S. (1995). Age and adolescent sexual offender arousal. *Sexual Abuse: A Journal of Research and Treatment, 7,* 249–257.

Laws, D.R., & Marshal, W.L. (1990). A conditioning theory of the etiology and maintenance of deviant sexual preference and behavior. In W.L. Marshall, D.R. Laws, & H.E. Barbaree (Eds.), *Handbook of sexual assault: Issues, theories, and treatment of the offender* (pp. 209–229). New York: Plenum Press.

Longo, R.E., & Groth, A.N. (1983). Juvenile sexual offenses in the histories of adult rapists and child molesters. *International Journal of Offender Therapy and Comparative Criminology, 27,* 150–155.

Marshall, W.L. (1995, October). *The sex offender: Monster, victim, or everyman?* Keynote Address, 14th Annual Research and Treatment Conference of the Association for the Treatment of Sexual Abusers, New Orleans, LA.

Marshall, W.L., Hudson, S.M., & Hodkinson, S. (1993). The importance of attachment bonds in the development of juvenile sex offending. In H.E. Barbaree, W.L. Marshall, & S.M. Hudson (Eds.), *The juvenile sex offender* (pp. 164–181). New York: Guilford Press.

National Adolescent Perpetrator Network. (1993). The revised report from the National Task Force on Juvenile Sexual Offending. *Juvenile and Family Court Journal, 44,* 1–120.

Prentky, R.A., & Knight, R.A. (1993). Age of onset of sexual assault: Criminal and life history correlates. In G. C. Nagayama Hall, R., Hirschman, J.R. Graham, & M.S. Zaragoza (Eds.), *Sexual aggression: Issues in etiology, assessment, and treatment* (pp. 43–62). Washington, DC: Taylor & Francis.

Rubinstein, M., Yeager, C.A., Goodstein, C., & Lewis, D.O. (1993). Sexually assaultive male juveniles: A follow-up. *American Journal of Psychiatry, 150,* 262–265.

Vaughan, V.C., III, & Litt, I.F. (1990). *Child and adolescent development: Clinical implications.* Philadelphia, PA: Harcourt Brace Jovanovich, Inc.

Worling, J.R. (1995a). Adolescent sibling-incest offenders: Differences in family and individual functioning when compared to nonsibling sex offenders. *Child Abuse and Neglect, 19,* 633–643.

Worling, J.R. (1995b). Sexual abuse histories of adolescent male sex offenders: Differences based on the age and gender of their victims. *Journal of Abnormal Psychology, 104,* 610–613.

25

Development of a Service for Sexually Abusive Adolescents in the Northeast of England

Finlay Graham, Graeme Richardson, and Surya R. Bhate

INTRODUCTION

In this chapter we describe the development of an integrated service for sexually abusive adolescents in England from its inception in October 1993, to the present. The service is based within the National Health Service, is staffed on a multidisciplinary basis, adopts an eclectic approach (albeit with a cognitive–behavioral bias), and sets out to integrate its service delivery with other relevant agencies, particularly social services. This development is described, problems identified, and resolution strategies discussed within a specific adolescent focus.

SERVICE DEVELOPMENT

History of the Service

The Department of Adolescent Forensic Psychiatry at Newcastle City Health National Health Service Trust was established as a result of an increasing awareness that the mental health needs of adolescent offenders were not being addressed. It was fortuitous that at the time we were advocating for the needs of this group (including sexually abusive adolescents) to be identified more clearly, a national review of forensic psychiatry was being undertaken by the Department of Health under the chairmanship of Dr. John Reed. The Reed Committee's recommendations in 1992 were both timely and helpful: "adolescents should not be assessed by adult criteria ... adolescents should be treated in a way which encouraged successful transition to adulthood ... each Health Region should form an Adolescent Forensic Psychiatry team."

The unmet needs of this group, coupled with the case for early intervention, was being advocated at this time by staff within the hospital, by the Regional Health Authority, and by

---

Finlay Graham, Graeme Richardson, and Surya R. Bhate • Kolvin Unit, Newcastle General Hospital, Newcastle-upon-Tyne, England NE4 6BE.

Sourcebook of Treatment Programs for Sexual Offenders, edited by Marshall et al. Plenum Press, New York, 1998.

purchasers of health services (i.e., district health authorities). The eventual outcome was acceptance of the need for a small adolescent forensic psychiatry team to be established and function as a specialist group within a region comprising a population of approximately 3 million. The mandate for the service was to provide a multidisciplinary, eclectic mental health service for children and young persons aged between 10 and 20 years who were in serious conflict with the law for person-centered offending and who displayed significant psychological or psychiatric disturbance and presented with a profile of already high and increasing risk. Sexually abusive adolescents were regarded as a primary target within this service profile.

General Legislative Context

Within England and Wales, health, criminal justice, social services, and probation services are quite separate agencies, often with poorly established links. Responses to sexual offending as a result lack integration and arguably present as ad hoc in comparison with the more integrated services found in North America. In England and Wales there is no legislation that specifically addresses how these various agencies tackle the problem of adolescent abusers or meet their needs. Since the majority of adolescent sexual abusers referred for assessment and treatment had not been prosecuted through the criminal justice system, they were technically not sexual offenders and few were subject to court-mandated treatment. It is for this reason that we have chosen to use the term *sexually abusive adolescents*. Most were dealt with through the civil law as it pertains to the care and protection of children generally (The Children Act, 1989). Consequently, the law designed to protect victims is the primary vehicle used to attempt to manage the risk young abusers present. This legislation is relatively weak and is not able to stipulate that the young person undertake a program of treatment.

The prevailing orthodoxy within the juvenile justice agency in England and Wales tends to advocate a policy of minimal intervention with young offenders in general. This is based on the beliefs that adolescence has always been a time of rebellion that young people grow out of as they get older and establish stable relationships (usually in their late teens, early 20s), and that interventions by the state tend to lead to negative outcomes. Empirical evidence does support this policy for the general run of young property offenders who do seem to grow out of the behavior as they grow older. Critics of the interventionist option also point out that over one third of all children placed in care end up in prison subsequently, suggesting that the state is an equally inadequate parent. However, this policy does not fit with the known evidence on sexual abuse career development, which indicates that sexual abuse is something individuals are more likely to grow into rather than grow out of (Abel & Rouleau, 1990). Gradually this argument is being accepted more with young sexual abusers, who are seen as an exception to the accepted orthodoxy.

The weaknesses of the legislative framework for working with sexually abusive adolescents within England and Wales is regrettable. A more powerful framework would be preferred, but as we argue later we are skeptical as to the benefits of coercive treatment with adolescents. The fundamental problem with young abusers is that they tend to abuse children younger than themselves and that offenses of this type have a very low detection rate. Even when the offense has been detected, evidential problems with child witnesses often preclude prosecution. These difficulties will not be overcome easily and it would be unwise to lobby for different rules in respect of sexual offenders as compared to other offenders. The inescapable reality, in our judgment, is that adolescents will continue to perpetrate about one third of the sexual abuse inflicted on children, that the majority will escape prosecution because disclosure will be delayed and evidence inadequate, and that sexual abuse therapists will have to grapple with this reality as best they can.

Funding for the Service

No simple recipe for securing funding emerged, but the following represent some of the arguments that have proven influential in the development of our service. Arguments to purchasers for funding an adolescent forensic psychiatry service, in which sexually abusive adolescents are a focus of need, have included references to national policy (Reed, 1992) and reference to international (e.g., Knopp, Freeman-Longo, & Stevenson, 1992) practice. Victim and victimizer have been presented as points on a developmental continuum and not as entirely separate factors. Sexual abuser career development, in which multiple victims can be involved in patterns of behavior originating in adolescence and continuing into adulthood, was cited as an indication of a case for early intervention in order to prevent further victimization. Empirical evidence reported in the literature (Marshall & Barbaree, 1990a) regarding positive treatment outcome in terms of risk reduction were cited, but in addition the moral case for assisting youngsters in difficulty was stressed. Reconviction as an evaluative yardstick was criticized and a challenge thrown down to apply an analogous measure to managed illnesses such as schizophrenia, depression, acquired immunodeficiency syndrome (AIDS), cancer, diabetes, cardiac, and other health problems that are managed but not cured. The dangers of ignoring adolescents who present risks to vulnerable children were pointed out as a closing argument.

In the end, such arguments have been partially accepted in that funding, although never as much as we consider sufficient, has been secured for the time being. The arguments may seem sound to professional clinicians, but gaining acceptance from budget holders depends on pursuing the case with vigor and determination. This was assisted by identifying the committees within which decisions were likely to be made, arguing for representation, submitting proposals and knowing what support existed within our own National Health Service Trust. Lobbying for the needs of the patient group among decision makers, fellow professionals, and other relevant agencies was essential for progress to be achieved. High-profile conferences and opening ceremonies with targeted invitations have presented useful strategies for gaining support. Links with the media have also proven useful but require careful management. Further positive strategies have included developing an extensive network of links with other services and publishing work in the field in order to demonstrate the quality of our specialist service provision. Above all, the case needed to be argued with determination, lobbying made effective, and expectations within our team structured toward success requiring a commitment to hard work.

In the development of our service a profile of support has been established in which we are funded to work with young abusers in health clinics, prisons, social services children's homes, privately run children's homes, and for the courts.

DESCRIPTION OF THE SERVICE

Sources of Referrals

Sexually abusive adolescents are referred from a wide range of sources including social workers, general practitioners, probation officers, consultant psychiatrists and psychologists, courts, and prison personnel. They are variously referred for risk assessment and advice on management of risk, advice regarding appropriate placement options, assessment of suitability for treatment, and court reports.

Patient Groups

The adolescent forensic psychiatry service sees a broad range of patients of whom sexually abusive adolescents are one subgroup, although one that makes up a significant proportion of our total number of referrals. The sexually abusive adolescents seen have engaged in patterns of abusive behavior ranging from indecent exposure to sexual murder.

The typical English sexually abusive adolescent was a 15-year-old Caucasian male, from a dysfunctional family, who had a history of contact with health and social services and who had displayed chronic difficulties across a broad spectrum of behaviors (Richardson, Graham, Bhate, & Kelly, 1995). The English sexually abusive adolescent appears more likely (than his North American counterpart) to have come from a home where parents have separated, presented with greater difficulties at school, and exhibited more generalized antisocial behavior. Multiple victims on multiple occasions were typical, but in general abusive behaviors did not lead to prosecutions. Abuse typically took place in a home location on a female victim 6 years younger than the perpetrator.

Service Provision Model

Our preference was for a continuum of service provision within which different models of direct and indirect treatment coexist within an integrated service. We have established what appears to be an adequate continuum of care provision appropriate to the estimated degree of risk, the nature and extent of the associated difficulties, and family functioning, including the degree of support provided by the family.

Psychologists within our team have taken the lead in developing programs and in training staff to deliver these programs. Psychologists also lead in the assessment of sexually abusive clients and in more specialized aspects of treatment conducted on an individual basis. The basic model of service delivery begins with a brief risk assessment aimed at establishing suitability for a program. This is followed by a comprehensive assessment to identify individual abuse profiles, etiologic factors, and treatment needs. Both stages of this assessment are conducted on a joint basis by a psychologist and residential social worker or by a psychologist and psychiatric nurse. The client is then allocated to a group program that best fits their needs. Assessment continues throughout the group program, and needs that are considered to remain are taken up subsequently in individual work. Psychologists provide regular support sessions for the psychiatric nurses and residential social workers who are the primary deliverers of group programs.

Those clients deemed by us to be low risk are those perpetrating predominately low-frequency, minor severity, intrafamilial abuse or single incidents of extrafamilial abuse that were nonviolent and did not indicate any preoccupation with deviant sexuality. They are likely to have supportive family backgrounds and to have shown adequate social integration. Such young people are seen in outpatient clinics and are offered structured programs of group work, individual therapy, and family work that are run by our own staff (psychologists and psychiatric nurses) in conjunction with the youngster's social worker.

Moderate-risk clients are those perpetrating higher-frequency, intrafamilial abuse of a more invasive nature or extrafamilial abuse in which violence was a limited factor. They are unlikely to have had the support of their family and are likely to present with many difficulties including poor social competency and social alienation. Such young people are seen on an outreach basis in children's homes where they are enrolled in programs that we have developed and assist in running with other agencies. Comprehensively structured programs of intensive therapy are delivered by residential social workers, who we have trained, within a supportive context of overall care.

High-risk clients have committed serious sexual offenses usually involving violence. At the younger end of the age spectrum (i.e., below 15 years), these clients tend to be seen in social services secure care accommodation. At the older end of the age spectrum, they are likely to be seen in prison. High-risk clients with mental health difficulties (e.g., psychosis, psychopathic disorder) are seen in our secure hospital unit. Again, structured programs of treatment including individual psychotherapy and psychiatric treatment appropriate to the clients' needs and the constraints of their situation are offered. These programs are delivered by psychologists, psychiatric nurses, and psychiatrists.

Staffing the Service

This has ranked as one of the most difficult problems in setting up a service for sexually abusive adolescents. In our experience no profession can claim adequate training for its members for work in this field. Arguably, forensic or clinical psychology approximates most closely to the ideal, but in reality within Britain there is at present no accredited training for work with abusers. Unless staff have gained specific experience in working with sexually abusive adolescents in previous employment, then the reality is that services will be established with inexperienced staff. Luckily, we began with two psychologists and a psychiatrist (the authors), all with significant prior experience in the field.

In order to combat this problem we have found that staff training is essential. Roles and expectations must be structured carefully and maintained by using developed and documented programs of therapy. Recording, monitoring, and auditing of service delivery is critical to the establishment of a degree of clinical consistency across personnel and an assurance that program integrity is not jeopardized by staff working beyond their competency level. Assessment of individual needs should be undertaken only by genuinely experienced staff. Above all, the service must be actively managed, as the autonomous clinician model favored by many, in our view, is unacceptable in this field. Staff support in terms of reviews of group dynamics, reviews of individual cases, and discussion of personal coping responses are essential.

Staffing the service has been approached in a genuinely multidisciplinary manner, although psychologists within the team have led the development of programs. Psychiatric opinion is sought where indicated clinically. Our analytic psychotherapist leads our thinking on the problematic area of prior victimization [since 41 of 100 clients surveyed had a recorded history of prior sexual abuse (Richardson et al., 1995)]. Social workers lead on work with families and on relapse prevention work in the community after discharge. Psychiatrists and psychologists lead on pretrial court work. Psychiatric nurses and residential social workers are the principal deliverers of the structured, group work component of our treatment program. We seek to work as a multidisciplinary team in which we attempt to harmonize these differing roles. However, clearly defined responsibilities and duties and an identifiable clinical hierarchy were put in place so that the team could function effectively.

Practice Manual

To facilitate our own clinical practice and our consultancy service, we have prepared a practice manual. This documents our clinical approach and practice and provides the framework and content for our training program. It consists of 13 separate sections: (1) theoretical explanations of abusive behavior; (2) characteristics of sexually abusive adolescents; (3) working with parents; (4) motivating abusive adolescents and their parents; (5) assessment; (6) sex education and sexuality; (7) behavioral therapy; (8) social skills training; (9) victimization work; (10) cognitive therapy; (11) self-esteem training; (12) victim empathy education; and (13) relapse prevention.

The aims and objectives of each treatment module are explicitly stated and a framework is provided for the sequence of sessions that comprise the module. The session focus and critical content of the sessions are documented, and any treatment strategies or techniques used in the sessions are described. Written exercises, discussion points, and visual and televisual presentations to be used during sessions are listed and a central resource library is available.

Training Program

As part of our consultancy service to other agencies and in order to develop a profile of high-quality and professionally defensible clinical practice, we have developed and run our own staff training program. This is a modular program consisting of five modules: (1) theory, risk assessment, and risk management; (2) assessment, motivation, and treatment models; (3) treatment I—psychoeducation, skills training, and victim issues; (4) treatment II—abuse cycles, cognitive restructuring, fantasy modification, and working with families; and (5) relapse prevention. The training is divided into three semester terms over a 1-year period, with each module consisting of a number of weekly sessions that last for 2.5 hours. The format of training follows a workshop model, combining lectures, seminar presentations from participants, case presentations, role-play, video presentations, and small-group discussions around key clinical issues and practicalities. Two assignments are required for each module, one is practical and involves work with a patient, the other is academic requiring a written submission. A reading list is prepared for each module.

Sexually Abusive Adolescent Core Group

A sexually abusive adolescent core group was formed that consisted of the key members of our multidisciplinary team who are involved in service delivery for this patient group. The group is chaired by an experienced clinical psychologist, and all other disciplines are represented. This group meets weekly. The core group has three primary objectives: (1) to ensure prompt delivery of a quality clinical service; (2) to facilitate the clinical development of group members; and (3) to facilitate the overall development of our service for sexually abusive adolescents. In order to meet these objectives, the group reviews case administration, identifies key clinical issues, and provides continuing professional development and supervision for staff.

PROBLEMS AND SOLUTIONS REGARDING SERVICE DELIVERY

Dearth of Residential Placements

Our service delivery model and clinical practice have been restricted by the lack of service provision within social services and child psychiatry for children and adolescents generally. Residential child placements are particularly scarce. Most local authorities had rundown state-funded residential placements, with funding reallocated to fostering and adoption services in line with minimal intervention philosophy. It was not atypical, as a result, to find young abusers placed with other children, some of whom had been victims of sexual abuse. In response to this problem, we had to initiate contacts and negotiate contracts with appropriate agencies, develop outreach programs, and find additional funding for our own secure hospital beds, in order to establish a viable continuum of clinical provision.

Renegade Training and Maverick Assessment

Unhelpful practices we have encountered in attempting to develop an integrated service include what we have termed "renegade training" and "maverick assessment." Integration of services needs to be planned if a range of different service elements are to come together to meet the overall spectrum of identified need. By renegade training we mean training run by people who are not specialists in treating sexual offenders and who provide a single course, while ignoring the overall service development objectives in the local area. They offer no realistic framework for providing support posttraining and are consequently unhelpful. Integration can be diverted and developmental themes started at one time only to become out of date as inexperienced staff religiously follow one particular theme but are unable to modify this in light of evaluation or empirical development in the field more generally. In raising this issue we are not arguing for parochialism or a single-model approach, but rather for planned, integrated development designed to meet the identified profile of patient needs.

Maverick assessments present similar difficulties and arise in cases where an individual assessor, not part of the integrated service provision and perhaps not experienced with sexual offenders, undertakes an assessment of a sexually abusive adolescent. Recommendations are made without consulting local service providers and may suggest services that are not locally available (e.g., long-term psychotherapy within a therapeutic community or arousal modifications) and that the assessor has no intention of providing personally. What is achieved by these assessments is confusion for the patient and his family and frustration for local service providers when presented with such recommendations. Our policy is not to accept such assessments but to reassess the case ourselves.

Consultancy Model of Working

Personnel from other agencies have tended to become overreliant on the psychologists from our service who act as program consultants and have generated an expectation that the psychologists should deliver the treatment. Psychologists have been flooded with staff anxieties about undertaking clinical tasks and been referred all requests for information regarding programs and clients. Unrealistic expectations of what the psychologists can and should deliver have developed as a result of this lack of confidence and anxiety.

We have overcome these difficulties to a significant degree through several strategies. A basic strategy was to establish good working relationships with the personnel of agencies for whom our psychologists act as consultants. The need to clearly define contract boundaries in which respective responsibilities and accountabilities are pinpointed has been critical. A formal training program for the staff from other agencies who deliver components of the treatment program has provided a vehicle for developing good working relationships, agreeing upon boundaries, and establishing the credibility of the psychologists. This training program also has helped to build the consultant's confidence in the ability of staff from other agencies to deliver components of the treatment program. A framework for providing ongoing clinical supervision of staff from other agencies has been developed. Joint selection of program staff has proved highly beneficial. Continued development and refinement of clinical practice through empirical research is important to maintain a position as a specialist service capable of providing consultancy. This is more likely to be achieved in practice when psychologists acting as consultants are not totally responsible for the direct delivery of treatment and have time to evaluate practice and conduct research.

Staff Complaints

The following staff complaints, specific to this area of work, have been encountered: lack of confidence or feeling anxious; assessment work perceived as high status, treatment work as low status; feeling dumped on if asked to take a case on for treatment if the assessment was not conducted personally; and feeling undervalued if engaged in structured group therapeutic practice as opposed to more autonomous individualized practice. Such feelings are to be expected and have no guaranteed resolution strategies, but do require sensitive management and honest description of jobs at the recruitment stage.

Multidisciplinary Practice

Work with young sexual offenders should be multidisciplinary, because no single profession or theory can claim to provide an adequate approach to the broad spectrum of need presented by young sexual abusers. In practice the multidisciplinary approach has proven problematic to create and sustain. Cross-professional supervision is often necessary and in our experience simply has to be accepted. Teams need a hierarchy of some kind, but in this field the basis for that may be challenged. Our view increasingly is that this must be made explicit and established on the basis of knowledge, skill, and experience in the specific field. The creation of a subgroup of highly experienced staff who lead on assessment, perhaps conducted jointly with less experienced staff, has been found to be invaluable. Intraprofessional support networks have had to be established in addition to cross-professional supervision even when this has necessitated going outside the service. An open management system, including multidisciplinary allocation and review of cases, has been found to facilitate teamworking. An acceptance that multidisciplinary work is based on the richness that is derived by having different viewpoints represented has been cultivated. The danger can be that staff perceive multidisciplinary working as implying absolute equality and as each team member offering the same skills. The flaw in this argument must be confronted, although the underlying dynamic needs to be understood. We do not endorse a generic worker approach and have found that the practical difficulties in sustaining a multidisciplinary approach can never be overlooked.

Developing a Service while Running a Service

This has been a major problem, but it was probably unavoidable when setting up a new service. Staff expectations need to be structured toward a developing service having numerous advantages, but the price to secure these is a flexible approach and at times an "all hands to the pump" outlook. Staff selection bearing the above in mind was critical. Care needed to be taken to help staff manage their time and to prevent research becoming the repeated casualty. A developing specialist service will not, and should not, develop far unless underpinned by empirical research. Specialist services live on professional credibility that is developed and sustained by research.

CLINICAL PRACTICE

Theoretical Models

Our approach to providing sexual abuse therapy is based on both generic and specific models of patient problems and treatment. We maintain that the clinical enterprise is essentially informed by psychological theory and research and ought to reflect the basic principles of any psychotherapeutic practice. Generic models of clinical problems and therapy, such as behavior therapy and cognitive therapy, are considered relevant. Specific models of sexually abusive behavior and treatment include: (1) the sexual assault cycle (Ryan, Lane, Davis, & Isaac, 1987); (2) the model of deviant sexual behavior (Becker & Kaplan, 1988); (3) the model of etiology and maintenance of adolescent sexual offending (Bera, 1994); (4) the multifaceted theory of adolescent sex offending (Marshall & Eccles, 1993); and (5) the relapse prevention approach to treatment (Pithers, Martin, & Cumming, 1989).

In translating this chosen approach into clinical practice, the basic principles of any credible psychotherapy are considered relevant. Clients must be treated with respect as individuals and a therapeutic rapport should be established prior to addressing sensitive issues. The majority of young people referred presented a profile (as described previously) of multifactorial difficulties within which sexually abusive behavior was but one presenting problem. This multifactorial conceptualization of abusive behavior combined with the absence, in our opinion, of any single, comprehensive, integrating theory necessitated a careful consideration of the individual needs of patients. A preparedness to adopt an eclectic approach to treatment was indicated while accepting that a cognitive–behavioral orientation would feature most prominently. Rigid belief systems centering on one model of causation spawning a recipe/conveyor belt approach to treatment in which individuals are all put through the same treatment program were considered inappropriate for sexually abusive adolescents.

Developmental Perspective

When working with adolescent abusers, it is important to adopt a developmental perspective in terms of theories and research regarding childhood and adolescent developmental stages, tasks, and adjustments. The stage of adolescence and the onset of puberty typically involve major transitions and adjustments to biological, personal, and social changes occurring at this time. Sexual and social maturation are critical areas of development. Marshall and Barbaree (1990b) and Marshall and Eccles (1993) have emphasized that puberty and adolescence are critical periods in the development of sexually abusive behavior, as it is then that the young male must learn to control his sexual behavior.

In our clinical work we see young people with histories of highly problematic childhoods who have not successfully coped with the developmental demands of childhood and who might be described as unsocialized in many aspects of behavior. They are, therefore, less able to cope with the developmental demands of emerging adolescence and predictably may fail to make the necessary adjustments that characterize social and sexual maturation. As a consequence, they are vulnerable to sexual maladjustment. Treatment may be seen in terms of helping the young person readjust to the developmental task of adolescence and to better cope with social and sexual demands so that they may more functionally make the next transition into young adulthood.

Case Formulation

Multifactorial theories of etiology promote multidimensional assessments and conceptualizations of the client's presenting problem(s). The case conceptualization when informed by both generic psychological models and specific models of abuse helps achieve understanding of the young person's abusive behavior. It hypothesizes the interrelatedness of predisposing, precipitating, and maintaining factors. It seeks to identify links between the client's predisposed vulnerabilities, personality characteristics, cognitive functioning, social functioning, immediate situational precipitants, and maintaining factors regarding abusive behavior. It also places abusive behavior in the context of early, possibly traumatic life experiences and the evolving dynamic within the young person's family.

The case formulation is fed back directly to the young person. It is important that he does not reject the formulation as relevant to him and his behavior. In subsequent treatment he is socialized into the generic psychological models and specific abuse models using a psychoeducational approach. When this is achieved, the clinician and the client have a common perspective from which to engage in the therapeutic process in a meaningful and collaborative manner. In our view, a case formulation approach guards against oversimplistic interpretations of the young person's presentation. It also helps prevent rigid adherence to any one therapeutic model, approach, or technique.

Assessment

If it is correct to conceptualize a multifactorial model of causation in respect of sexually abusive behavior and to judge that an adequate, integrative theory currently eludes us, then it follows that assessment must be conducted on a fairly comprehensive basis. This belief system has major implications for the assessment process adopted and who should conduct it. Our opinion that therapeutic work with sexual offenders should reflect good practice in any psychotherapeutic intervention increases the complexity of the assessment task being contemplated. For these reasons the normal practice adopted was for an experienced psychologist or psychiatrist to lead the assessment.

Belief in multifactorial causation requires the administration of a broad-based assessment, but the factors described in Table 25.1 are considered essential to a routine assessment. This routine assessment is supported by the administration of appropriate psychometric measures and made more consistent by the use of documented semistructured interview procedures. It is followed, if necessary (based on experienced clinical judgment), by assessment of less-frequently occurring factors such as mental illness, neuropsychological difficulties, learning difficulties, and other problems.

Risk assessment and risk management are fundamental features of our assessment model and are conducted jointly with other agencies (e.g., social services, police, courts). A documented manual (Graham, 1995) has been produced on a multiagency basis and is being piloted currently to ascertain utility, reliability, and validity.

TABLE 25.1
Assessment Factors

Specific	Generic
Are sexually abusive behaviors contained	Family history
Sexual knowledge	Parenting style
Sexual victimization	Personal and social functioning
Sexual beliefs	Behavior in school
Offense analysis	Intellectual ability
Sexual fantasy (if appropriate)	Personality and temperament
Deviant arousal (if appropriate)	Coping responses
Motivation to engage in treatment	Profile of relationships
Cognitive distortions	Psychiatric assessment (if clinically indicated)
Victim awareness	Intimacy skills

The assessment task is aided by processing in discrete stages. Stage 1 involves the collection of relevant background information from police, social services, education, and probation. Stage 2 involves initial interviews with the young person and their family. The aim of this initial phase of interviewing is restricted to providing information regarding the assessment process, anxiety reduction, and listening. Stage 3 involves information gathering interviews with the young person and their family (separately) in order to obtain a clear developmental history and profile of current general functioning. The allegation of sexual abuse is not discussed at this stage. Stage 4 involves detailed interviews with the young person that focus on the alleged incident of sexual abuse. We have chosen to process our assessment in this way through learning from experience that sexual issues can only be discussed with an adolescent after rapport has been established.

Treatment Program

A guiding principle in our clinical practice is that models of disorder and associated treatment approaches derived from work with adults cannot be applied to children and adolescents. We maintain that there are significant differences between adult sexual offenders and sexually abusive adolescents that need to be considered. For example, the role of deviant sexual arousal, abusive sexual fantasies, and cognitive distortions in the onset and early development of abusive behavior is far from certain in many adolescent cases.

Our treatment program is informed by hypotheses about the nature of the young person's abusive behavior and related difficulties derived from both generic and specific models incorporated into an individual case formulation. It is therefore model-driven, cognitive–behavioral in orientation, modular in structure, and with a relapse prevention component (see Fig. 25.1). The modular structure allows greater flexibility in terms of which modules are deemed appropriate and in what order of priority they are delivered. We have found this flexibility critical in several community based cases where expectations regarding duration of treatment for essentially voluntary clients need to be realistic and parsimonious. With our community-based clients, we introduce the relapse prevention model early in treatment and help the young person and his caregivers generate an initial relapse prevention plan to facilitate management of risk in the community.

We also provide offense-related treatment in individual sessions and groups. In the initial development of our service, individual sessions predominated. We do not fully

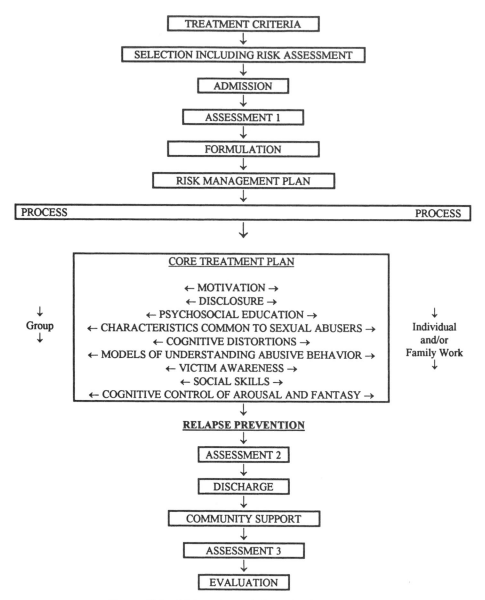

FIGURE 25.1. Adolescent sexual abusers treatment program.

accept that treatment of sexually abusive adolescents ought to be exclusively or predominantly group based. The empirical data supporting this position are not entirely convincing, although we appreciate it is more cost-effective in economic terms for the treatment provider service and that empirical data to support individual treatment models are lacking also.

Within this therapeutic structure, the therapeutic style is collaborative, with the therapist applying strategies and techniques in a directive style. The young person is required to adopt a focused, problem-oriented approach and is encouraged to take an active part in the therapeutic process. The ultimate aim is to help the young person develop his capacity for reasonable self-efficiency and self-help.

Working with the Youngster's Family

In principle, we are committed to working with the families of our sexually abusive adolescents. In practice this can be difficult to achieve, as families also become entrenched in denial, minimization, and rationalization. We aim to involve parents in our assessment, share our formulation and treatment plan with parents, provide educational handouts and facilitate discussion, possibly with other families in a similar situation if that is feasible, work through parental anxieties, review parental coping responses, and involve parents in relapse prevention planning.

Achievement of these aims depends on the level of motivation that can be developed in parents. Experience indicates fathers are more difficult to engage and that some parents are impossible to motivate. In most cases, however, success is achieved in engaging at least one parent in joint therapeutic work, although this falls short of systemic family therapy, for example. Formal motivational interviewing strategies have been found useful with parents, and empathizing with their difficult predicament further aids rapport.

PROBLEMS AND SOLUTIONS

Balancing Psychotherapy and Offense-Specific Treatment

During the development of our service we have attempted to integrate the provision of a client-specific psychotherapeutic service based on a case-formulation approach and on general principles of therapeutic practice, with an offense-specific service based on established structured programs of treatment. Our aim has been to formulate a forensic psychotherapy practice that integrates both generic and specific approaches.

We appreciate the importance of operationalizing therapy in a relatively structured and documented way, in order to facilitate clinical consistency and evaluative research. We also accept that the standardized, modular group treatment approach is more economical in terms of staff resources, when compared with the individualized psychotherapeutic approach. We believe both approaches need to be available in a broad spectrum of clinical options offered within a single service.

Absence of Incentives and Coercion

The rarity of court-mandated treatment because of the limited powers of current legislation is in marked contrast to the situation pertaining in many North American programs and has several implications for our clinical practice. We have placed an increased emphasis on motivating the client and his family. The pace of therapeutic intervention has been moderated to minimize anxiety or discomfort in the young person. Frequent explanation about the assessment and treatment process, coupled with feedback to facilitate more immediate indicators of progress, have been provided. Individual work in the early stages of therapy has been emphasized while a comfortable rapport is being established with the assessor/therapist.

In any case, we have a healthy skepticism regarding the ethics and merits of "coercive" treatment. We doubt its clinical utility and see it as in danger of encouraging young abusers to "go through the motions." Genuine positive motivation is preferred and can only be achieved after significant effort from both therapist and client. Passive resentment in clients, especially adolescent clients who developmentally are predisposed to resent adult authority and impositions, is a major risk in a coercive approach.

Unrealistic Expectations

Aims and objectives adopted by the team have tended to be set too highly. Individual needs in clients have been emphasized too strongly and group needs not sufficiently enough. A consequent drift toward more individualized programs of treatment occurred, leading to resourcing problems. The multifactorial etiology needs to be acknowledged, but an achievable balance between economically deliverable group-based treatment and highly costly (in staffing terms) individualized treatment must be acknowledged. A desire to achieve absolute standards of therapeutic practice has been evident, which again led to feelings of inadequacy and failure to meet objectives. Visits to other programs, conference attendances, and literature reviews have proven beneficial in identifying comparative standards of practice that are more achievable.

Clients of Differing Ability Levels

In our experience, young sexual abusers are heterogeneous in intelligence, attention, language, social skills, cognitive functioning, and personality. The emerging spectrum of functioning that we encounter in our clinical practice has been a problem that we believe must be reflected in our therapeutic provision. A specific program has been tailored toward the needs of learning disabled adolescent sexual abusers. For the majority, a core program of group therapy has been offered. An individually tailored program of therapy run on a one-to-one therapeutic basis has been overlaid onto the core program and is designed to address individuals need not covered sufficiently in the core program of group therapy.

Client Motivation

It has been stated previously that most of our clients attend on a voluntary basis and that we are skeptical of coercive treatment in principle. The inevitable consequence of this is that motivating clients assumes immense significance, and that without establishing a degree of positive motivation, both assessment and treatment are impossible. There are many techniques for trying to develop positive motivation, none of which guarantees success, but in our experience it is rare that we fail completely. In addition to our motivational work with the young abuser, we also collaborate with the youngster's parents, the court, the youngster's social worker, his defense solicitor, and finally through peer pressure in group therapy.

An acceptance that motivation in adolescents will be limited and that motivation at any level is likely to fluctuate over time, gradually declining as it does so, is essential. Treatment programs offered in particular community-based treatment with voluntary clients must acknowledge this fact. The strategy we prefer, based on our experience, is to offer intensive therapeutic programs delivered over weeks rather than months. Young abusers are offered half-day sessions in our day unit rather than weekly sessions, which might represent the norm in classic therapeutic approaches. Individual work to develop trust and a feeling of safety has been found to provide the most effective start and to provide an opportunity to prepare the youngster for entry into group work. The necessity of working with predominately voluntary clients, which is our usual practice [we very rarely use the Mental Health Act (1983) to compel treatment with adolescents] may be inconsistent with mainstream North American practice. Working with clients toward development of rapport and positive motivation is time-consuming but worth the effort, particularly with sexually abusive adolescents who we feel need to be treated more, not less, like adolescent clients with other difficulties.

Victimization

In our clinical practice with sexually abusive adolescents, it has been found that some of our adolescent abusers are so close to their own abusive experiences and so preoccupied with them that therapeutic progress is blocked unless the issues associated with their own victimization are addressed. A compromise is adopted on a case-by-case basis and, where judged clinically necessary, victimization is briefly psychotherapeutically addressed prior to focusing on offense-specific work. However, we take care to avoid allowing offenders to excuse themselves.

Opposing Views of Therapy

Opposing views frequently appear to be held by different practitioners, but they are seldom expressed openly, although a passive–aggressive stance has been apparent in our practice at times. These passive–aggressive responses have proven extremely disruptive and have impeded progress. We have found that an open management style has been helpful, but increasingly our view is that this needs to be combined with rigorous monitoring within explicitly stated boundaries of responsibility and accountability. Documented therapeutic procedures are a major aid, but these take time to develop.

CONCLUSIONS

Development of a service for sexually abusive adolescents as part of our comprehensive forensic service has been a positive experience, which after 2 years we cautiously judge to have been a success. Positive factors contributing to this perceived success have included an amicable relationship between the consulting psychiatrist and the consulting psychologist leading the team. The establishment of support networks and membership of the region's decisionmaking forum have been critical in gaining financial backing. Positive publicity from media, conferences, and research also have proven useful in securing financial backing. Tolerance and flexibility among our team in the development of an eclectic approach have proven a major advantage.

Negative factors impeding progress have included slowness in establishing a more rigorous management approach focusing on ownership of specific clinical duties and associated responsibility for elements of program delivery. A dearth of trained staff has been a difficulty, as have passive–aggressive strategies shown by staff when adjusting to a new style of working. Arguing for new funding within a cumbersome bureaucratic system, itself undergoing change, and within which the significance of sexual abusiveness in adolescents was underestimated required unbending commitment.

Overall, the case for early intervention at the beginning of sexually abusive careers is a powerful one. We have succeeded in gaining at least limited acceptance of this and have begun to develop a spectrum of service provision that we consider appropriate to the needs of sexually abusive adolescents.

REFERENCES

Abel, G.G., & Rouleau, J.L. (1990). The nature and extent of sexual assault. In W.L. Marshall, D.R. Laws, & H.E. Barbaree (Eds.), *Handbook of sexual assault: Issues, theories and treatment of the offender* (pp. 9–21). New York: Plenum Press.

An Introduction to The Children Act 1989. London: Her Majesty's Stationary Office.

Becker, J.V., & Kaplan, M.S. (1988). The assessment of adolescent sexual offenders. *Advances in Behavioral Assessment of Children and Families, 4*, 97–118.

Bera, W.H. (1994). Clinical review of adolescent male sex offenders. In J.C. Gonsiorek, W.H. Bera, & D. LeTourneau (Eds.), *Male sexual abuse: A trilogy of intervention strategies* (pp. 113–144). London: Sage.

Graham, F. (1995). *Assessing risk in sexually abusive young people*. Newcastle, England: The Derwent Initiative.

Knopp, F.H., Freeman-Longo, R., & Stevenson, W.F. (1992). *Nationwide survey of juvenile and adult sex offender treatment programs and models*. Orwell, VT: The Safer Society Program.

Marshall, W.L., & Barbaree, H.E. (1990a). Outcome of comprehensive cognitive–behavioral treatment programs. In W.L. Marshall, D.R. Laws, & H.E. Barbaree, (Eds) *Handbook of sexual assault: Issues, theories, and treatment of the offender* (pp. 363–385). New York: Plenum Press.

Marshall, W.L., & Barbaree, H.E. (1990b). An integrated theory of the etiology of sexual offending. In W.L. Marshall, D.R. Laws, & H.E. Barbaree (Eds.), *Handbook of sexual assault: Issues, theories and treatment of the offender* (pp. 257–275). New York: Plenum Press.

Marshall, W.L., & Eccles, A. (1993). Pavlovian conditioning processes in adolescent sex offenders. In H.E. Barbaree, W.L. Marshall, & S.M. Hudson (Eds.), *The juvenile sex offender* (pp. 118–142). London: Guilford Press.

Mental Health Act. (1983). London, Her Majesty's Stationary Office.

Pithers, W., Martin, G., & Cumming, G. (1989). Vermont treatment program for sexual aggressors. In D.R. Laws (Ed.), *Relapse prevention with sex offenders* (pp. 292–310). New York: Guilford Press.

Reed, J. (1992). *Review of health and social services for mentally disordered offenders and others requiring similar services*. Report of the official working group on services for young people with special needs. London: Department of Health, Home Office.

Richardson, G., Graham, F., Bhate, S.R., & Kelly, T.P. (1995). A British sample of sexually abusive adolescents: Abuser and abuse characteristics. *Criminal Behavior and Mental Health, 5*, 187–208.

Ryan, G., Lane, S., Davis, J., & Isaac, C. (1987). Juvenile sex offenders: Development and correction. *Child Abuse and Neglect, 11*, 385–395.

III

Ethnic Populations

26

Te Piriti
A Bicultural Model for Treating Child Molesters in Aotearoa/New Zealand

Jillian Larsen, Paul Robertson (Kai Tahu),
David Hillman (Tuhoe), and Stephen M. Hudson

There is now wide acceptance of what constitutes the core elements of an effective treatment program for sexual offenders against children. However, it has been recognized that there is a need to develop specific programs for special groups, for example, young offenders, offenders with intellectual disabilities, and offenders from non-Western cultural backgrounds, especially indigenous peoples. It is the provision of effective assessment and treatment for Maori, the indigenous people of New Zealand, that is the focus of this chapter.

The rationale for developing a bicultural treatment program for sexual offenders is presented, along with general concerns in cross-cultural and ethnic psychology. Issues relating to Maori and the process of colonization in New Zealand are reviewed, as well as efforts aimed at both increasing understanding and addressing difficulties facing Maori. We then outline a program for treating Maori men who have offended sexually against children. This program, which also caters for non-Maori clients, involves an adaptation of the standard form and consists of the widely accepted core components (e.g., relapse prevention, cognitive restructuring, sexual reconditioning, etc.). The program includes additional components and processes specifically focused on the needs of Maori. A cultural perspective policy has provided the blueprint for this development and is presented together with a review of progress to date.

CROSS-CULTURAL OR ETHNIC PSYCHOLOGY

Mental health professionals, both in New Zealand and overseas, are increasingly recognizing the need to consider cultural factors in their work. In addition, recent surveys

Jillian Larsen and David Hillman (Tuhoe) • Te Piriti Special Treatment Unit, Psychological Services, Department of Corrections, Albany, New Zealand. **Paul Robertson (Kai Tahu)** • Auckland Regional Office, Psychological Services, Department of Corrections, Auckland, New Zealand. **Stephen M. Hudson** • Department of Psychology, University of Canterbury, Christchurch, New Zealand.

Sourcebook of Treatment Programs for Sexual Offenders, edited by Marshall et al. Plenum Press, New York, 1998.

indicate that psychologists in New Zealand need to develop greater understanding of Maori in order to be able to work effectively with them.

However, while cross-cultural psychology has the potential to be a powerful vehicle for change, it can also be used to perpetuate structures and systems that have difficulty providing effective treatment for those outside of the dominant culture (e.g., Jackson, 1987). Traditionally, the positivist approach of cross-cultural psychology, with methods based in Western beliefs and values, emphasizing cultural dependent variables and deficits, has contributed to maintaining the status quo (e.g., Smith, 1991). Through ethnocentric processes, the dominant culture has been able to maintain its superiority and justify subjugation of "inferior" peoples by using their own standards to judge and draw conclusions about other cultures. Through use of such a framework, a hierarchy of knowledge has been established that places Western knowledge, values, and beliefs in superior position to that of indigenous peoples. These processes were not necessarily intentionally disempowering, but rather often the result of the difficulty researchers had in seeing the impact of their own values and beliefs on their work.

More recently, the development of indigenous or ethnic psychology has allowed the consideration of phenomena within parameters defined by the participants in the research, rather than by the researchers. This approach reduces stances of superiority, inaccurate assumptions about peoples, and the imposition of ill-fitting hypotheses. It also encourages the use of multiple methods and levels of analysis, as well as consideration of the role of socio-historic factors in the behavior of groups and individuals. Some of the results of this approach have provided the basis for developing the treatment program outlined in this chapter.

ISSUES FOR THE INDIGENOUS PEOPLE
OF AOTEAROA/NEW ZEALAND

Te Tiriti o Waitangi (The Treaty of Waitangi)

In New Zealand, the Treaty of Waitangi creates a unique focus on the partnerships between the *tangata whenua* (indigenous people, i.e., Maori) and the Crown, represented by the government. The use of the term *bicultural* rather than *multicultural* does not diminish the status of other cultures, but rather emphasizes the primacy of the relationship between Maori and the Crown. A bicultural approach to treatment reflects the desire to fulfil treaty obligations. Consideration of the role of the treaty in New Zealand's history and its place in present-day society is beyond the scope of this chapter (for a fuller coverage, see Yensen, Hague, & McCreanor, 1989); however, we present below a brief description of the core issues.

The Treaty of Waitangi (see Appendix 1) was signed in 1840 by representatives of many of the *hapu* (subtribes) of Aotearoa (New Zealand) and representatives of the Queen of England. Bringing whalers, seamen, escaped convicts, and other settlers under control and avoiding colonization by the French were significant motivating factors for Maori to sign the treaty. Preempting the French and facilitating peaceful settlement of a new colony provided significant motivation for the English.

Problems arose following the signing of the treaty and continue today as a result of different interpretations and relatedly the failure of governments to honor it. The different understandings have been in part due to differences in the Maori and the English translations, particularly related to the issue of sovereignty. The colonists considered that the Maori had ceded sovereignty, while the latter considered that they had agreed only to governance. Given their intimate relationship with the land, it is highly unlikely that Maori would have handed over sovereignty to the English. In relation to this, different perceptions of people's relationship with the land, including the concept of ownership, has also led to difficulties.

The debate over the provisions of the treaty and arguments over the failure to honor it continue today. It has been argued that the government and its agencies have manifested and reinforced monoculturalism, which has impeded the progress of biculturalism in Aotearoa (e.g., Ministerial Advisory Committee, 1988). While the treaty has gained a degree of acceptance, being seen as the founding document of New Zealand society by some, there are those who see it as irrelevant and wish to consign it to the history books.

The implementation of the treaty depends considerably on the attitude of those involved in its application. Sir Henare Ngata, a noted Maori scholar, has suggested that the treaty is capable of being successfully implemented and its obligations honored if it is approached with a positive attitude. Despite ongoing debate, the treaty is seen by many New Zealanders as providing the basis for a change to a bicultural society. It is therefore central to the development of a bicultural program for sexual offenders. A useful approach has been to consider the spirit and principles behind the words in the treaty, rather than their exact meaning. Partnership and *tino rangatiratanga* (power over resources, self-determination) have been identified as two fundamental principles that should guide bicultural development.

Development of Indigenous Psychology in Aotearoa/New Zealand

We believe that wider social and historic factors need to be considered if we are to fully understand the situation of Maori. This necessarily involves consideration of the impact of the dominant Western culture on the work of psychologists, both clinically and in research settings. It is easy for members of a dominant culture, subculture, or gender to forget the values and beliefs that guide their thoughts and behaviors. If the majority or the values of the most powerful group are accepted as the only valid context within which to investigate people and their behavior, there is no need to proceed beyond this point. However, we believe that there are many equally valid worldviews that need to guide investigation if the range of people populating the planet are to be adequately understood.

The position of Pakeha (i.e., non-Maori, but more specifically New Zealanders of European cultural background) and other Western psychologists, allows them to create knowledge by collecting and interpreting data in particular ways. Their dominance allows such people to define the parameters of a society or community, even if their understanding of it is incomplete. The resulting knowledge is often used to justify and continue the subjugation of a particular group (e.g., Smith, 1991). Therefore, it is essential to consider the power afforded those who develop and apply the dominant paradigm. Lack of consideration of such factors has meant that although Maori and other minority groups have been studied a great deal, their perceptions and worldview have not been adequately considered (Gilgen, 1994). Thus, the research has not necessarily led to better understanding of their needs or improvement of their situations. It frequently just retells the same old stories without seeking to answer the problems (e.g., high numbers of Maori with alcohol problems, high level of Maori imprisonment) (Gilgen, 1994). This is obviously inconsistent with the spirit of the Treaty of Waitangi and with any therapy system that emphasizes self-determination. It also neglects the impact of systems and sociohistorical factors, such as colonization and urbanization, that have resulted in alienation of Maori from traditional sources of wealth, power, and identity.

While there may be many factors motivating a search for better understanding of the impact of cultural factors in psychology, it is proposed that maintenance of professional and ethical standards should be of primary concern. Ethical codes of psychologists for example outline the need to maintain at least an adequate knowledge base to enable the delivery of effective treatment. It is clearly not possible to acquire or maintain such a knowledge base if cultural issues are not adequately understood. In short, how can adequate assessment and therefore treatment be undertaken if there is not sufficient understanding of the factors that predispose individuals to certain behaviors and subsequently precipitate and perpetuate these. Any comprehensive psychological theory necessarily accounts for cultural factors, and it has been suggested that such factors need to be considered, not just as categorical variables, but as part of a complex structure that is integral to a person's functioning.

CRIMINAL JUSTICE SYSTEM IN NEW ZEALAND

Maori in the Criminal Justice System

Currently, and historically, the number of Maori clients in the criminal justice system in New Zealand has been disproportionate to the number in the general population. The Psychological Services of New Zealand's Department of Corrections has been seeking to increase the understanding of this phenomena and improve the service delivered to Maori clients for a number of years. Initial steps have involved training to improve understanding of Maori in general and Maori in the criminal justice system in particular. More recently the process of developing models for working with Maori and programs for training Pakeha (non-Maori) psychologists in bicultural practice has begun.

As research is an essential basis for both model development and training, Psychological Services is closely considering the issues of undertaking research with Maori. This has led to the identification of a number of potential problem areas and subsequent development of principles and protocols for working in this field (Robertson, Larsen, Rush, & Doak, 1995). Developments in this area represent the beginnings of an effort to build a knowledge base that represents the realities of Maori rather than the biases of particular research methodologies. The aim is not to abandon scientific rigor, but rather to develop models that facilitate consideration of variables that have tended to be invisible in much past and current research and clinical work with Maori. The principles for doing research with Maori also provide guidance for the development of cultural policies and practices in treatment programs, such as the one described in the current chapter.

Developments in the cultural area have also been driven by practical motivations. In 1991, Maori made up less than 15% of the population; however, they made up nearly 50% of the prison population and were overrepresented in other areas of the criminal justice system. These rates reflect trends for indigenous peoples and minorities in other countries. Biased policies and practices within criminal justice systems may have contributed to this situation, but the factors contributing to the overrepresentation of indigenous peoples remain to be fully clarified. What is clear is that Psychological Services has a significant number of Maori clients, and it is essential to understand the factors that contribute to their high rates of contact with the criminal justice system if we are to work effectively with them.

Progress in Developing Bicultural Practices

There has been increasing effort to understand the overrepresentation of Maori in negative statistics. Additionally, as more Maori become involved in the research process, a greater understanding of the impact of cultural variables is emerging. Means are being developed to facilitate application of psychological and other health models in ways that are meaningful to Maori (e.g., McFarlane-Nathan, 1996; Peri, 1995). A cognitive–behavioral approach has been seen as being the most amenable to adaptation for working with indigenous people, as it promotes a collaborative approach aimed at eliciting meaning from clients.

In developing a model for working with Maori, McFarlane-Nathan (1996) draws on the experience of people working with Native Americans (e.g., Renfrey, 1992). He has suggested that similar issues have long been of concern to Maori, for example, the impact of colonization on the mental health of indigenous peoples and the need for them to be competent in both cultures in order to survive. Some Maori have suggested that Pakeha (non-Maori) get all the glory for being bicultural, while Maori, who are bicultural by necessity, not choice, get none (e.g., Stanley, 1993). McFarlane-Nathan considers the level of acculturation and deculturation into indigenous and mainstream societies as key issues that need to be addressed when working with indigenous and other ethnic peoples. He suggests that failure to acculturate into the mainstream and/or their own societies leaves individuals marginalized and susceptible to a range of difficulties, including poor health and imprisonment. He also suggests that failure to acculturate and deculturation contribute to chronic low self-esteem, difficulties with formal education, difficulty in communicating, and a generalized sense of resentment, frustration, and aggression.

McFarlane-Nathan has used these concepts as a basis for developing training for Pakeha psychologists in the Department of Corrections Psychological Service so that they are better able to understand issues contributing to Maori offending. In addition, the Bicultural Therapy Project (McFarlane-Nathan, 1996) aims to assist Pakeha psychologists and ultimately other health workers to develop relationships with "experts" in the Maori world to whom they can refer clients when issues are beyond the scope of their own expertise. The model proposed by McFarlane-Nathan requires an explicit acknowledgment of the ethnicity of the client. It validates Maori resources present in the community, as well as acknowledging the value of traditional and neotraditional healing processes. The model proposed requires that in assessing a client, consideration must be given to the factors associated with acculturation/deculturation. For many, Maori spiritual issues, a difficult area for Western psychology, are likely to be of significance in such an assessment.

Although there have been promising developments in research and clinical work with Maori, difficulties remain in working within an essentially ethnocentric framework and system. Significant changes to the research and clinical practices, as well as to underlying assumptions, are needed if we are to gain an accurate understanding of Maori and be successful in assisting them to deal with their difficulties. Smith (1991) points out that it is not enough to change the faces of the research and health workers. Herbert (1995) also warns against merely replacing scientific rigor with a cultural perspective. She suggests, rather, that the aim is that being Maori or taking a Maori perspective is a strength to be incorporated into existing skills, knowledge, and practices.

In an attempt to facilitate systemic changes, Psychological Services has introduced a bursar program to provide financial assistance for Maori to undertake training in clinical psychology. Introducing this system has been critical in ensuring ongoing bicultural development in the service via the input of the bursars and other Maori graduates. The development of a group for Maori psychologists within the service has also been important in providing a forum for addressing bicultural issues within Psychological Services, as well as providing mutual support to reduce feelings of isolation. Holding of regular *hui* (meetings) to discuss issues relevant to working with Maori, to increase understanding of Maori, and to contribute to the formulation of policy and practice has also been an important part of the efforts of Psychological Services to develop a partnership with Maori. Another key area of development has been in the formulation of principles and protocols for doing research with Maori (Robertson et al., 1995) that reflect Psychological Service's commitment to competent and ethical research and demonstrate accountability to Maori. These guidelines are not an original work, but rather an amalgamation of principles from various sources that have been formulated in a manner most appropriate to our service

TE PIRITI

Te Piriti is a psychological treatment program at Auckland Prison, New Zealand, designed to reduce the likelihood of reoffending among men who have been convicted of sexual offenses against children. The name Te Piriti means *the crossing*, which signifies the transition to a new and better life. The medium-security prison unit, which opened in May 1994, is a free-standing complex that includes a therapy unit within it. The program is staffed by psychologists, rehabilitation workers, and administrative staff employed by Psychological Services.

The Therapy Program

The assumption underpinning the program is that sexual aggression is multiply determined by a combination of social, cultural, developmental, biological, and conditioning processes. The treatment involves consideration of cognitive, behavioral, and social learning concepts and consists of two phases. In the first 3 to 4 months, the primary focus is on enabling the men to understand the facts that motivated their offending, challenging distorted beliefs concerning the offending, encouraging them to take responsibility for their offending, and developing empathy for their victims. The remainder of the program concentrates on sexual reconditioning, skills acquisition, and relapse prevention strategies.

Treatment is provided in a group format (ten men plus one or two therapists) over a 9-month period. The first and last weeks of the program are devoted to assessment. During the remaining weeks, the groups meet for 2.5 hours per day, 3 days a week. All participants in the program have voluntarily entered treatment for their offending and related issues. They remain at the unit for the duration of their treatment program, and on completion of their therapy are released or returned to another prison to await release.

The Te Piriti program was modeled on the Kia Marama sexual offender treatment program at Rolleston Prison, Christchurch (see Chapter 2, this volume). However, in developing the program at Te Piriti, a greater emphasis was placed on developing a program that would be seen as effective by Maori. The proportionally greater number of Maori in the Te Piriti catchment area needed to be considered in developing a program to service Auckland and the surrounding regions. There also was some early concern about the apparently high dropout rate initially of Maori men from the Kia Marama program. Therefore, a cultural consultant was appointed to work in conjunction with the psychologists and rehabilitation workers, both in terms of the details of their work as well as processes to increase the program's cultural appropriateness.

MISSION STATEMENT AND CULTURAL PERSPECTIVE POLICY

Mission Statement

The mission statement for Te Piriti makes explicit the bicultural emphasis of the program and the need to adhere to central principles of the treaty, especially partnership and *tino rangatiratanga* (self-determination). In this way, Maori values and beliefs are validated and the rights and responsibilities of both parties (i.e., Maori and the Crown) are acknowledged. In order to achieve these objectives, a cultural perspective policy with clear goals and aims in specifically defined areas has been developed. The first three goals relate to establishing a bicultural context, including an ethnically diverse and informed staff, and creating a culturally supportive environment and processes for consultation with local *iwi* (clans or tribes) and other Maori. The fourth goal relates more directly to bicultural service delivery.

The policy addresses important aspects of Maori culture, such as a holistic view of people including a spiritual dimension, and their intimate relationship with the land and nature in general. Kinship, extending to ancestors who have passed on, and collective responsibility are also of fundamental importance, as is *te reo* (language) and the following of appropriate protocols in various situations. Although these and other fundamental aspects of the Maori world (such as hierarchies of power and responsibility and the sacredness of women as the source of life) are enduring, their expression alters over time, especially with the influence of outside groups. In addition, while all *iwi* adhere to central beliefs and values, there is variation of expression and in detail between the different *iwi* of Aotearoa. This is by no means an exhaustive explication of the central aspects of Maori society, which is also beyond the scope of the current chapter, but this will give readers an idea of areas of importance. Incorporation of central aspects of Maori society in the program helps to reverse the negative impact of colonization by validating traditional beliefs and attitudes, thus facilitating acculturation into Maori society in parallel with increasing acculturation into Pakeha society. In addition, the program does not contribute to alienation for those who are secure in their identity as Maori.

Cultural Perspective Policy

Goal One: An Environment that Is Culturally Supportive of All Staff Is Created

This goal involves ensuring that: (1) appropriate methods of welcoming Maori and other cultures are developed; (2) all staff of Maori descent have the opportunity to attend network meetings; (3) all other ethnic groups have the opportunity to attend network meeting; and (4) all staff have the opportunity to attend bicultural and cross-cultural *hui* (meetings).

The team of ten staff at Te Piriti is increasingly achieving a balance in terms of its ethnic makeup. In addition to the cultural consultant, the two rehabilitation workers are Maori. In the planning stages for the unit a decision was made to include therapy staff from disciplines other than psychology, as there is still a grave shortage of Maori psychologists.

The rehabilitation workers typically have a social work background and a major focus of their work is to establish links with the clients' families and other supporters and to liaise with agencies that contribute to the external management phase of relapse prevention. The rehabilitation workers are also group co-facilitators, along with psychologists, in the first part of the program, which deals with the offense cycle and victim empathy. Every effort is made to achieve a gender and culture balance in the therapist dyads. The administrative support person is of Pacific Island origin and has an important frontline role in promoting positive cross-cultural attitudes.

In conjunction with local *iwi* elders and Psychological Services staff, including the Maori Roopu (Psychological Services staff of Maori descent), the cultural consultant has established protocols for *powhiri* (welcome). The positive outcomes of this practice include demonstration of respect for Tangata Whenua (indigenous people) and facilitating better understanding of the processes and practices of people of other cultures. It also conveys a warm welcome that facilitates dialogue and receptivity to the program. Artwork and posters depicting Maori and Pacific Island people and values, which are present throughout the unit, also create a more welcoming environment. The three group therapy rooms have been given names in both Maori and English, conveying positive values of Maori and Pakeha (non-Maori) cultures.

The last two annual bicultural *hui* (meetings) for Psychological Services staff had good representation from the Te Piriti team, all of whom were eligible to attend. The purpose of these meetings was to familiarize staff with traditional Maori procedures and protocols, to discuss the division's obligations under the treaty in order to improve service delivery to Maori, and to offer training in culturally appropriate research and therapy methods.

Goal Two: Bicultural Training to Be Undertaken by All Staff

This goal involves: (1) all staff to have an understanding of the Treaty of Waitangi; (2) all staff to complete the Maori and treaty awareness program (Te Iho, meaning *sapwood*) of the Department of Corrections; (3) all new appointees complete available Te Iho modules within 12 months of appointment; (4) each staff member performance plan has at least one career development goal directed to increasing his or her competence in cultural issues; (5) at least one staff training session each 2 months to be devoted to cultural issues; and (6) conduct a review and synthesis of available papers relating to Maori mental health issues and present at staff training sessions.

This goal has been achieved in various ways, including drawing on prior experience of staff, attending *hui* (meetings), and Te Iho training (see below). In addition, psychologists at the unit are currently participating in a bicultural therapy project, which includes examination of attitudes and beliefs about the impact of culture, promotes acceptance of differences, and addresses other relevant issues regarding assessment and treatment.

Te Iho is a three-stage program developed by the Department of Justice to help staff increase their awareness of Maori culture, traditional beliefs, and practices. The first component, Kete One (kete, meaning *basket*) looks at the influence the Treaty of Waitangi has had on the department and examines how the treaty affects the participants' work. The second stage, Kete Two, which examines the dynamic nature of culture, considers how, for Maori, the value of change is dependent on whether it is self-directed or imposed from outside and also on the rate at which it occurs. The third section, Kete Three, examines how the treaty defines the relationship between the Crown and Maori, as well as outlining the obligations that both must meet within this relationship. It is proposed that if staff are to meet obligations in the department, it is important that they look at themselves and their way of working in order that they can endeavor to provide better service to Maori. As this package is no longer readily available through the national office, the cultural consultant will play an important role in facilitating a regionally based program.

In addition to the above, staff have had fees paid for Maori language courses and seminars presented by Maori mental health practitioners. In 1995, the cultural consultant presented a series of lectures on the foundations of Maori psychology. The topics included important concepts such as: Maori cosmology, genealogy, kinship and social structures, *whanau hui* (family meetings), change and progress, sources of knowledge, and the different aspects of the person.

The cultural consultant also instructs staff regarding appropriate *powhiri* (welcoming) and *poroporoake* (farewell) processes for staff, visitors, and clients. This also involves teaching *waiata* (Maori songs) and *mihi* (formal introductions). Reviews on Maori mental health have been presented at annual meetings of Psychological Services and at bicultural *hui* (meetings). Examples are cited above. These were also discussed as part of the bicultural therapy project.

Goal Three: Process for Managing the Action Phase of Te Iho

This goal involves: (1) establishing a register of Maori/*Iwi* (tribe) resources; (2) in consultation with the cultural consultant, develop an action plan whereby all staff have the opportunity to establish ongoing contact with *iwi* resources; and (3) all staff work on establishing and fostering appropriate links with local *iwi* in conjunction with regional office, community corrections, and penal cultural consultants.

The action phase of Te Iho involves developing relationships with local *iwi* in order that they are consulted on an ongoing basis. This is still in the developmental stages. The unit has contacts with local *iwi*, namely Ngati Whatua and Tainui, and with Maori agencies that may be involved with the provision of a postrelease program, both cultural and therapeutic. *Iwi* representatives have been invited to Te Piriti to give feedback regarding the program and cultural initiatives. Also, contact has been made with other government agencies involved in working with Maori. Staff at Te Piriti also seek to maintain an ongoing relationship with local *iwi* (tribe) and the community through providing information about the program, attending *hui* (meetings), on *marae* (gathering place), and involvement in research projects.

In addition, action plans have been formulated for contact with the *whanau* (family), *hapu* (subtribe), and *iwi* (tribe) of program participants. Whenever possible *whanau hui* (family meetings) are arranged between the participant's family and the cultural consultant and other staff. Where necessary, staff assist inmates in contacting *whanau* member for support.

Goal Four: Revision of Policies and Processes to Improve Service Delivery to Maori

This goal involves the: (1) department cultural advisory officer, consultants and *kaumatua* (elders) being consulted on all matters pertaining to unit cultural policies; (2) consistent funding for cultural consultant being secured; (3) *powhiri* (welcome) and *poroporoake* (farewell) being conducted for each treatment group; (4) all Maori residents have opportunity to undergo assessment by the cultural consultant and receive ongoing input as required; (5) bicultural adaptation of treatment group process (e.g., *karakia*, or prayer) is encouraged; (6) bicultural adaptation of program content; (7) for each individual

Maori resident, contact is made with appropriate *whanau* (family), *hapu* (subtribe), and *iwi* (tribe) representatives to facilitate postrelease reintegration to tribal region; and (8) all Maori sexual offenders in Te Piriti catchment area are being encouraged to attend the program.

The cultural consultant at Te Piriti is now a permanent full-time position. It is clear that without such a position many aspects of the culture perspective policy could not be implemented. Tasks performed by the cultural consultant in addition to those already mentioned include providing training for prison staff, students, and probation officers who work with program graduates; developing protocols for liaison with the Children and Young Person's Service in relation to family reintegration; training staff of other government and community agencies; liaison with staff from Kia Marama; contributing to bicultural development of Psychological Services as a whole; and assisting with research including evaluation of the program at Te Piriti.

Powhiri to welcome new therapy groups take place in the therapy unit immediately prior to the commencement of the therapy program. Inmates from the Maori cultural group participate with staff in welcoming new program participants, as well as visitors to the unit. This is an opportunity for them to practice language and *powhiri* protocols.

Maori clients undergo a cultural assessment by the cultural consultant to determine the effects of colonization and the implications of this for the client. The assessment covers familiarity and comfort with aspects of both Maori and Pakeha (non-Maori) cultures and concludes with recommendations to address deficits [e.g., English or Maori language classes and instruction in *marae* (gathering place) protocols]. It is hypothesized that addressing symptoms of cultural alienation (e.g., poor communication skills likely to impede development of intimacy) will increase self-esteem and confidence and will contribute to the development of skills necessary to reduce the risk of reoffending. The recommendations from the cultural assessment are discussed with the client's therapist and incorporated into treatment goals. It is our practice to refer clients to Maori healers and teachers where appropriate.

When a Maori client is experiencing difficulties that cannot be resolved in the group setting, the cultural consultant may meet with him individually, with or without the therapists. He may recommend a consultation with a Maori person experienced in mental health phenomena. In addition, the cultural consultant convenes a weekly Maori caucus. In this 2-hour session, aspects of therapy are discussed and instruction is given in Maori beliefs and values. *Marae* (gathering place) protocol, *haka* (war dance) *waiata* (songs), and related issues are also focused on in order to reduce the individuals' sense of alienation from their own culture. This group is open to all residents regardless of ethnic background.

All groups decide on their own methods for opening and closing group sessions, which provides an opportunity to acknowledge the spiritual dimension. Some groups choose to have *karakia* (prayer), *waiata* (song), or *whakatauaki* (proverbs) relevant to the program. The proverb below, for example, stresses the importance of treating people with care and consideration:

Uia mai koe ki ahau	You ask of me
He aha te mea nui au te ao?	What is the most important thing in this world
Maku e ki ata,	My reply must be,
He tangata	It is people
He tangata	It is people
He tangata	It is people

In order to make the content of the program more accessible to Maori, it has been important that the cultural consultant achieve an understanding of the cognitive–behavioral and relapse prevention models. Therefore, group sessions have been observed by the cultural consultant and senior psychologist so that cultural concepts can be incorporated. For example, lifestyle balance in the relapse prevention model may be reconceptualized as the balance and interaction of Taha Hinengaro (mind) Taha Wairua (spirituality), Taha Tinana (body), Taha Whanau (social/family), Taha Whenua (environment), Taha Tikanga (rules), Taha Tangata (self), and Taha Pakeha (new world). The latter is included because it is a common factor genetically of many Maori.

In addition to the above, Maori myths and legends are referred to in order to increase understanding of Western concepts, for example, the story of Tane (God of the forest). Tane had an incestuous relationship with his daughter Hinetitama, whom he married. When she found out her husband was also her father, she fled with shame and became Hinenui Te Po (Goddess of Darkness). This and other stories can be used to demonstrate the impact of sexually inappropriate behaviors and to challenge assertions that incest was traditionally sanctioned by Maori. We intend to rewrite the treatment manual to include Maori translations, adaptations, and methods.

A comprehensive reintegration protocol has been developed for all participants in the program. For Maori clients it is particularly important to organize *hui* (meetings) with *whanau* (family) and *hapu* (subtribe)/*iwi* (tribe) representatives, as the concept of *whanaungatanga* (interconnectedness) permeates Maori society. The cultural consultant plays a role in organizing and facilitating these *hui* (meetings), and ensures that the visitors understand the goals and methods of the program and how they might best support the client on his release. To date, we have had two reintegration *hui* where we returned the client to his own *marae* and met with his *whanau* and representatives of support agencies. These *hui* were considered by all present to be worthwhile and signaled a positive development in the relationship between Maori and the Department of Corrections. We intend to conduct these whenever possible to increase Maori community awareness of and support for our program and its participants.

The cultural consultant has played an important role in motivating Maori offenders, who had previously been reluctant to volunteer for treatment. He has been part of the recruitment team that visits other prisons throughout the North Island. In presenting information about Te Piriti, he guides the team in following Maori processes, thus increasing the credibility of the program. In addition, he is able to clearly explain the bicultural aspects of the course.

CONCLUSION

While a considerable degree of knowledge and expertise has been developed in treating sexual offenders, specialist programs still need to be constructed for special groups such as indigenous and other ethnic peoples. Developments in indigenous psychology have contributed to redressing the skewed research and the resulting culturally inappropriate clinical practices of the past. However, there is clearly some way to go in constructing models to facilitate effective treatment for Maori and other indigenous peoples.

At Te Piriti, we believe we have made a good start in adapting a Western psychological program to meet the needs of Maori. Te Piriti has been successful in both increasing the number of Maori entering treatment (31% of intake) and retaining them in the program (30% of those completing the program). Initial assessment indicates that this success has been due to a number of factors, including having a bicultural staff, bicultural training, development of practices incorporating Maori beliefs and values, the bicultural adaptation of the program, and greater involvement of local *iwi* (tribes) and clients' family. The developments and successes described are consistent with North American models that have been further developed for the New Zealand context.

Developments within Psychological Services have also contributed to providing a climate amenable to applying the principles of the Treaty of Waitangi. Implementation of a Maori bursar scheme, development of principles for guiding research with Maori, and in-service training, along with other initiatives, have facilitated the process of developing a bicultural treatment program for sexual offenders at Te Piriti.

From the start of this process those involved have recognized that it was the beginning of a long journey. Predictably, developing a bicultural approach to treating sexual offenders has not always been easy and challenges, both personal and professional, have had to be met along the way. However, we believe that it is worth the effort and that we are making good progress in increasing the ability of Psychological Services to provide an effective and relevant service to Maori in Aotearoa.

Ko te pae taawhiti, Whaaia kia tata, Ko te pae tata, Whakamaua kia tina (Seek out the distant horizons and cherish those you attain) (*Metekingi*, cited in Durie, 1994).

ACKNOWLEDGMENT. The authors acknowledge the foresight of those who recognized the particular needs of Maori clients and proposed the position of cultural consultant at Te Piriti, particularly Robin Jones and Piero Gherardi.

APPENDIX 1

Te Tiriti o Waitangi/The Treaty of Waitangi

The Treaty of Waitangi is made up of four articles, the first three of which were presented in both the Maori and the English language. The fourth article is usually not cited when reference is made to the treaty, as it was included only in the Maori translation:

Article the First
(English translation)
The Chiefs of the Confederation of the United Tributes of New Zealand, and the separate and independent Chiefs who have not become members of the Confederation, cede to Her Majesty the Queen of England, absolutely and without reservation, all the rights and powers of sovereignty which the said Confederation of individual Chiefs respectively exercise or possess, or may be supposed to exercise or possess, over their respective territories as the sole Sovereigns thereof.
(Maori translation)
The Chiefs of the Confederation and all the Chiefs who have not joined the Confederation give absolutely to the Queen of England forever the complete government over their land.

Article the Second
(English translation)

Her Majesty the Queen of England confirms and guarantees to the Chiefs and Tributes of New Zealand, and to the respective families and individuals thereof, the full exclusive and undisturbed possession of their lands, estates, forests, fisheries, and other properties they may collectively or individually possess, so long as it is their wish and desire to retain the same in their possession; but the Chiefs of the United Tribes and the individual Chiefs yield to Her Majesty the exclusive right of preemption over such lands as the proprietors thereof may be disposed to alienate at such prices as may be agreed upon between the respective proprietors and persons appointed by Her Majesty to treat with them in that behalf.

(Maori translation)

The Queen of England agrees to protect the Chiefs, the subtribes and all the people of New Zealand in the unqualified exercise of their chieftainship over their lands, villages, and all their treasures; but on the other hand the Chiefs of the Confederation and all the Chiefs will sell land to the Queen at a price agreed to by the person owning it and by the person buying it (the latter being) appointed by the Queen as Her purchase agent.

Article the Third
(English translation)

In consideration thereof Her Majesty the Queen of England extends to the Natives of New Zealand Her royal protection and imparts to them all the rights and privileges of British subjects.

(Maori translation)

For this agreed arrangement therefore concerning the Government of the Queen, the Queen of England will protect all the ordinary people of New Zealand and will give them the same rights and duties of citizenship as the people of England.

Article the Fourth (Maori translation only)

The Governor says that the several faiths (beliefs) of England, of the Wesleyans, of Rome, and also Maori custom shall alike be protected by him.

English translation from the Treaty of Waitangi Act (1975)
Maori translation by Sir Hugh Kawharu

REFERENCES

Durie, M. (1994). *Whaiora: Maori health development.* Auckland, NZ: Oxford University Press.

Gilgen, M. (1994, August). *Ethnocentrism and its contribution to skewed research.* Paper presented to the Psychological Services Bicultural Research Hui, Auckland, New Zealand.

Herbert, A. (1995, October). *Psychology reality checks.* Paper presented at Hui 95, Maori and Psychology, Hamilton, New Zealand.

Jackson, M. (1987). *The Maori and the criminal justice system a new perspective: He Whaipanga Hou, Part 1.* Wellington, NZ: Department of Justice.

McFarlane-Nathan, G. (1996, May). *Developing a psychological model for working with Maori.* Paper presented at the Psychological Services Bicultural Training Programme, Auckland, New Zealand.

Ministerial Advisory Committee. (1988). *Puau Te AtaTu (Daybreak), the report of the Ministerial committee on a Maori perspective for the Department of Social Welfare.* Wellington, NA: Department of Social Welfare.

Peri, M. (1995, September). *Dynamics of whanaungatqnga.* Paper presented at the Psychological Services Bicultural Training Programme and Maori Psychologists Roopu, Auckland, New Zealand.

Renfrey, G. (1992). Cognitive behaviour therapy and the Native American client. *Behaviour Therapy, 23,* 321–340.

Robertson, P., Larsen, J., Rush, C., & Doak, J. (1995, March). *Research on or research?: Developing guidelines for doing "Maori research" in the Department of Justice.* Paper presented at the Annual Divisional Conference, Psychological Services, Rotorua, New Zealand.

Smith, L.T. (1991). Te Rapunga I Te Ao Marama (The search for the World of Light): Maori perspectives on research in education. In T. Linzey & J. Moiss (Eds.), *Growing up: The politics of human learning* (pp. 46–55). Auckland, NZ: Longman Paul.

Stanley, P. (1993, January). *The power and the glory and the great white hunter.* Paper presented at the Psychological Services Hui on Bicultural Issues in Psychology, Auckland, New Zealand.

Yensen, H., Hague, K., & McCreanor, T. (Eds.). (1989). *Honouring the treaty: An introduction for pakeha to the Treaty of Waitangi.* Auckland, NZ: Penguin.

27

Blending the Traditional with the Contemporary in the Treatment of Aboriginal Sexual Offenders

A Canadian Experience

Lawrence Ellerby and John Stonechild

While there has been a long-standing recognition of the overrepresentation of Native Canadians in conflict with the law, systems have been slow in attempting to identify, understand, and address this profound and alarming societal concern. Aboriginal people have the highest arrest, incarceration, and crime rates of any group in Canada, and native offenders are disproportionately represented in most provincial, territorial, and federal correctional institutions (LaPrairie, 1996). LaPrairie reports that, although the 1991 census revealed that only 3.7% of the Canadian population reported being of aboriginal ancestry, the averaged number of admissions of aboriginal offenders to federal and provincial correctional institutions between 1989 and 1994 was 11.8% and 20.2%, respectively (Canadian Centre for Justice Statistics, 1994). The level of disproportionality increases in certain regions of Canada, with the prairie provinces (Saskatchewan, Manitoba, Alberta) having the largest overrepresentation of aboriginal inmates. As of December 1995, 39% of the inmates incarcerated in federal institutions in the prairie region were aboriginal (Cowie, 1996). LaPrairie (1996) reports comparable and even higher percentages of aboriginal inmates as being found in provincial institutions within the prairies.

In Canada there has been increasing concern and attention toward aboriginal men who have committed sexual offenses. As of the end of 1995, 16.5% of the total number of sexual offenders incarcerated in federal correctional institutions and on parole were aboriginal, while 25.7% of all aboriginal offenders were identified as sexual offenders (Motiuk, 1996; Motiuk & Belcourt, 1996). Again, regional disparity is observed, with 64% of the aboriginal sexual offenders in federal corrections being located in the prairie provinces and with 40% of the aboriginal offenders in this region being identified as sexual offenders (Cowie, 1996; Motiuk, 1996). As a sexual offender program located in Winnipeg, Manitoba, part of

Lawrence Ellerby and John Stonechild • Forensic Behavioral Management Clinic, Native Clan Organization, Winnipeg, Manitoba, Canada R3C 0A1.

Sourcebook of Treatment Programs for Sexual Offenders, edited by Marshall et al. Plenum Press, New York, 1998.

the prairie region, it has been necessary to be mindful of the significant proportion of aboriginal sexual offenders and to strive to develop treatment approaches that will effectively respond to their needs while addressing criminogenic factors and risk.

PROGRAM EVOLUTION

In 1987, the Native Clan Organisation's Forensic Behavioral Management Clinic began providing community and institutional sexual offender assessment and treatment services for primarily moderate- to high-risk/need adult male aboriginal and nonaboriginal sexual offenders, most of whom had received federal sentences of over 2 years. While we recognized that at approximately 50% of the offenders who would be participating in our program would be aboriginal, at that time we were unclear as to what this would or should mean in terms of developing and delivering sexual offender treatment. Were aboriginal offenders different from nonaboriginal offenders? Did aboriginal offenders have unique needs and require specialized programming? These were questions we asked ourselves and continue to explore as our treatment program evolves.

The primary objective of our program has been and continues to be to reduce/prevent further sexual victimization. We attempt to realize this goal by assisting and supporting men to enhance their level of accountability and insight into their sexual offending behaviors and to assist them in developing and learning to implement a range of healthy coping strategies so that they are better prepared to avoid and/or manage their various risk factors. Components of treatment include: identifying and accepting responsibility for their history of inappropriate sexual behavior; identifying and developing insight into the emotional, cognitive, and behavioral factors that have contributed to offending and that are indicators of future potential risk; acknowledging and understanding the role of deviant sexual fantasy and arousal in offending and developing strategies to modify and manage inappropriate sexual fantasies and arousal patterns; identifying, challenging, and replacing denial, minimization, rationalizations, justifications, and cognitive distortions; developing an understanding of and emotional appreciation for the impact of sexual offending on victim/survivors; developing a host of functional coping skills (e.g., skills related to communication, problem solving, emotional awareness, anger management, assertiveness, managing cognitions, relationship and social skills, enhancing self-identity and self-esteem, and learning about healthy sexuality); addressing personal victimization/trauma, family of origin, and developmental issues; fostering healthy attitudes and respect for women, men, and children; and generating offense cycles and relapse prevention plans.

In the clinic's initial years we grappled with how effective a cognitive–behavioral sexual offender treatment program would be with aboriginal offenders. In considering the differences between native and nonnative offenders, we recognize that Native Canadians are not a homogeneous group. Canadian Aboriginals may be registered Indians, nonstatus Indians, Métis, and Inuit and may comprise a number of distinct tribal groups such as the Cree, Ojibway, Saulteaux, Mohawk, Algonoquin, and Micmac. As a result, the extent to which aboriginal offenders differ from nonaboriginal offenders, or in fact from each other, and the uniqueness of their treatment needs is largely determined by the individual's level of acculturation and racial identity.

Acculturation has been defined as "a multi-dimensional and psycho-social phenomenon that is reflected in psychological changes that occur in individuals as a result of their interaction with a new culture" (Marin, 1992, as cited in Casas & Casas, 1994, p. 25). In terms of Native Canadians, this would reflect the degree to which an aboriginal person accepts and adheres to Euro-Canadian and/or traditional tribal societal values, norms, and mores across cognitive, behavioral, affective/spiritual, and social/environmental domains. Waldram (1992) recognized the importance of defining cultural adherence and distinguished between three categories of aboriginal offenders in identifying how cultural issues are pertinent to treatment. He describes a "traditional" group as individuals who are born and raised in primarily aboriginal, typically reserve or remote communities, whose first and primary language is a native language, and whose identity is strongly linked to aboriginal culture. The "transitional" group consists of individuals who have a strong identification with their home communities, aboriginal culture, and language but who are also well-versed in Euro-Canadian ways. The "assimilated" group is characterized by individuals who are raised in a Euro-Canadian cultural milieu from an early age and have little knowledge of an aboriginal culture or language. All aboriginal people are seen as fitting along a continuum of cultural adherence from aboriginal traditional to Euro-Canadian assimilated. Other models of acculturation identify additional categories, such as a "marginal" group, which encompasses those individuals who do not adhere to the values of either culture (Choney, Berryhill-Paapke, & Robbins, 1995; Ryan & Ryan, 1989). Couture (1995) indicates that acculturation levels may affect how aboriginal offenders experience and present their difficulties as well as their responsiveness to interventions. Therefore, the type and style of intervention most appropriate for treating an aboriginal offender will largely be contingent on their acculturation level.

Although we initially considered separate treatment groups for aboriginal and non-aboriginal offenders, for pragmatic reasons we began by delivering a mixed group. Over the course of this group experience, we found that some of the native men were quite similar to the nonnative men and were comfortable with and responded well to a cognitive–behavioral approach. Others, however, demonstrated a need for an alternative process. These individuals tended to present as shy, quiet, and uncomfortable within the group setting. They rarely provided information spontaneously, had some difficulty with language, and when asked to contribute, did so awkwardly and reluctantly. The characteristics of the aboriginal men who had difficulty in group were associated with a traditional and to some extent transitional level of acculturation, while those who were comfortable with the process presented as assimilated and also to some extent transitional.

Having noted the differences in responsivity, it was decided that while treatment goals and targets would for the most part remain the same for all of the aboriginal and nonaboriginal men, the process of therapy (in both individual and group therapy) would be mindful of and attempt to adapt to meet the needs of the individual differences observed. For example, therapists needed to be aware of differences in the verbal and nonverbal communication styles of some aboriginal offenders. Long pauses or silences needed to be respected and answers waited for rather than giving into the urge to repeatedly ask questions, allowing other group members to answer or take over discussion, or assume that the silence was a sign of resistance. There needed to be a realization that a native group member sitting with his head leaning back as if he were asleep may be concentrating rather than daydreaming or sleeping, and that a lack or absence of eye contact did not mean the individual was being inattentive or deceitful. For group members with less developed language skills (aboriginal and nonaboriginal), treatment jargon and complicated terminology needed to be avoided.

The way in which some aboriginal offenders in the program best processed information differed from other aboriginal and nonaboriginal offenders. For example, some native men had difficulty with tasks such as written assignments and journaling but could do the exercises verbally. This is consistent with the oral tradition among traditional aboriginal people. Therefore, rather than inappropriately interpreting failure to complete written work as a lack of motivation and resistance, written assignments were replaced with oral assignments. Strategies that have assisted us in working with traditional and transitional aboriginal offenders have included being concrete and directive rather than nondirective or facilitative; using stories and metaphors to illustrate a concept or identify an issue relevant to the clients functioning; using circles to explain concepts such as offense cycles; being challenging in a supportive rather than confrontational manner; and working hard at attempting to develop a strong and sincere therapeutic alliance. These process techniques are also consistent with the literature related to multicultural counseling and counseling strategies for American Indians (Atkinson & Lowe, 1995; Merta, 1995).

In modifying the process of therapy as described, it is important to note that we have found these same therapeutic strategies to benefit assimilated aboriginal offenders and nonaboriginal offenders as well. In addition, shifting the process of therapy to adapt to the individual differences and needs of the client has assisted us in avoiding unwanted and unnecessary control issues that interfere with and disrupt the therapeutic process. Finally, when altering the process of therapy for both aboriginal and nonaboriginal offenders, we have found that clinicians must be cautious that the clients' style of presentation is, in fact, a reflection of cultural characteristics rather than manipulations in an effort to avoid addressing their offending behavior.

In addition to attending to the process of therapy, another way we have attempted to meet the needs of the native men in our program has been by introducing and addressing topics and issues of particular relevance to them. Over the course of treating aboriginal and nonaboriginal sexual offenders, some distinct differences between the two groups have emerged. The native men in our program have more frequently presented with issues related to abandonment, displacement, racism, and an absence of or confusion about their personal identity (Ellerby, 1994). They also tended to experience difficulties related to chronic exposure to and histories of maltreatment and abuse, substance abuse, poverty, and death (Ellerby, 1994; LeClair, 1996). These are all profound issues that must be addressed as part of the therapeutic process. They are also seen as relevant to our sexual offender program as, in our opinion, the impact of these experiences are linked to these men's offending cycles. As a result, attempting to diminish risk by focusing on a relapse prevention approach without taking into consideration and addressing these kinds of personal trauma is insufficient.

In addition to these pressing emotional issues, many of the aboriginal offenders in our program tended to be more disadvantaged in their education, employment skills and history, financial position, and social supports compared to our nonaboriginal clients (Ellerby, 1994). Given the significance of these deficits, addressing these very practical matters needed to become a target of treatment. As a result, therapy focuses on assisting men to develop skills to enhance their abilities to seek out educational, employment, or social opportunities, to address their anxiety related to these areas, and to problem solve difficulties they experience once involved in schooling, work, or social situations to enhance their ability to succeed in these situations. Clinicians also at times take on a case management role by initiating referrals to programs specifically designed to address upgrading, skills training, job searching, money management, and social skills. Again it must be noted that while these deficits have appeared more pervasive among the aboriginal men who have attended our program, many nonaboriginal offenders present with the same difficulties and are supported in the same manner.

After having run mixed groups of native and nonnative offenders, we no longer believe there to be a need to separate groups based on race. It was evident from our experience that all the men could learn from, care about, and support each other. The richness of diversity among the group members experiences, worldviews, styles, strengths, and areas of difficulty added to the group treatment experience and was seen as invaluable. Racially heterogeneous groups have been described as more productive, creative, and less superficial than homogeneous groups, as providing rich and diverse feedback, and as adept at challenging biases and stereotypes (Corey, 1990; Gelso & Fretz, 1992; Johnson & Johnson, 1994).

While we have not found it necessary or desirable to deliver homogeneous groups, either in our community or institutional programs, we do, however, attempt to ensure that the mix of each group is designed so that individual members will not feel alone or out of place. Factors such as offense type, acculturation, age, and level of intellectual functioning are taken into consideration in determining the group composition. To date, none of the offenders who have been in our treatment programs have expressed the need or desire to participate in an all aboriginal or all nonaboriginal group. This is consistent with a recent survey of aboriginal inmates in federal corrections in which native inmates reported that they did not feel excluded from or shy about attending nonaboriginal-specific programs, that any program that helped them was of value, and that aboriginal and nonaboriginal offenders could benefit from each other's programs (LaPrairie, 1996).

In addition to modifying the style and content of treatment to meet the needs of certain native offenders, we also attempted to support these individuals by encouraging, supporting, and assisting them to enhance their level of acceptance for, understanding of, and involvement in their culture. This has included addressing issues of shame about their native heritage with some men and assisting others to access native elders/healers and traditional ceremonies in the community. Although we viewed enhancing cultural/racial identity and involvement in traditional ways as important since the inception of our program, it was not until 1994 that we actually made a move to blend traditional healing into our approach, offering both contemporary cognitive–behavioral therapy as well as traditional native healing as part of our sexual offender treatment program.

A decision to look beyond what was considered to be "state of the art" sexual offender treatment programming and to approach native elders to see if there was a way to incorporate traditional healing into the program was made after reviewing our treatment outcome data. What we discovered was that while aboriginal and nonaboriginal offenders who had completed the treatment program appeared to have benefitted equally (in terms of recidivism rates), only half the number of aboriginal offenders completed the program compared to nonaboriginal offenders. Native offenders were more likely to be suspended during treatment for breaching conditions of their release (e.g., breaching abstain orders), more frequently dropped out of treatment at the completion of their sentence (after which there was no longer a legal mandate to attend), and were more likely to reoffend sexually while in treatment. We interpreted these data to be telling us that many of the aboriginal offenders in our program did not appear as invested or as engaged in the treatment process as did the nonaboriginal offenders, and that our emphasis on a cognitive–behavioral, relapse prevention approach did not appear as relevant or meaningful to them (Ellerby, 1994).

In order to respond to these findings, our program had to develop to a point where we were comfortable and able to look at various treatment alternatives. In beginning to provide sexual offender treatment services, we had to develop our skills and expertise in working with sexual offenders and, more specifically, with aboriginal sexual offenders. As the program grew and developed, we needed to adjust toward our changing client population, which included more difficult and higher-risk offenders who presented with chronic histories of both sexual offending and violent behavior and who exhibited a myriad of deficit areas. Histories of nonsexual violence and violent sexual offenses were particularly evident among the native offenders in our program, a finding that has also been identified in other samples of aboriginal sexual offenders (Ellerby, 1994; LeClair, 1996). We also began to provide services to high-risk juvenile offenders, developmentally delayed offenders, and female offenders, who other systems and programs were not prepared to accept. We experienced another adjustment as we expanded from providing primarily community-based treatment programming to also providing institutional sexual offender programming. As part of this expansion, further evolution of our skills was required in establishing a system in which there was a continuity of assessment and treatment services and a continuum of care from our programs in the medium- and minimum-security federal institutions to the community program.

Each of these changes and developments required the clinical team to enhance and broaden their skill base. At the point where we were comfortable, confident, and competent in providing treatment to a range of sexual offenders in various settings, we were also ready and able to explore alternative approaches to providing sexual offender treatment. The combination of our readiness to seek out new treatment strategies and our outcome data indicating a need to modify programming for aboriginal offenders resulted in the consideration, development, and implementation of traditional healing as part of the treatment program.

THE CLINICAL TREATMENT TEAM
AND THE ROLE OF THE ELDER

Our clinical team is multidisciplinary and consists of clinicians with backgrounds in social work, psychology, and psychiatry. In 1994, a native elder (second author) was added to the treatment team. The elder is an integral part of the clinician team and takes on a number of important roles including consulting with clinical staff regarding program development issues, offender assessments, and in case conferencing treatment clients. In addition, the elder provides direct service including individual counseling, traditional teachings, and traditional ceremonies. The elder's healing work is integrated with the individual counseling, group therapy (open and closed core and maintenance groups), couple and family counseling, and arousal modification sessions that are delivered by clinic therapists. The type of treatment modalities engaged in and frequency of session for each offender are determined on an ongoing basis according to their individual level of risk/need.

The working approach among the clinical team is a cooperative one, in which the mental health professionals are open to learning and seeking consultation from the elder, while the elder is open to learn and seek consultation from the clinicians. We feel that what this cooperative approach based on a mutual respect and recognition of the unique skills each treatment team member brings to the program is ideal, particularly when there has been a tendency for some mental health professionals to reject the utility of traditional healing and elder involvement in treatment and an equal rejection of contemporary treatment strategies and a disregard for the involvement of mental health professionals by some aboriginal people and communities.

While the roles of social workers, therapists, psychologists, and psychiatrists in the provision of mental health services and the treatment of sexual offenders is commonly known, the function of elders/healers in native communities and with aboriginal men who have engaged in inappropriate sexual behavior is less understood.

The role of the elder in any given community is to serve his or her people in a spiritual manner no less than a local minister. He or she must be a supporter, teacher, advisor, arbitrator, and healer for individuals, families, and communities. Elders perform various ceremonies and deliver the sacred teachings through the use of the sacred plants, the sacred talking stone, the eagle feather, the sacred pipe, and the sweat lodge. In their teaching, elders do not seek perfection, but rather strive to teach and to be an example.

Although we speak of native elders and their spiritual work, not all native elders are spiritual workers. Some individuals are referred to as elders out of respect for their age and wisdom, although they may not be spiritual workers. Among elders who are spiritual workers, there is diversity in the gifts they have been granted and the roles they perform (Ellerby, 1995). For example, elders/healers may be counselors, teachers, and medicine men/women who heal through the use of sacred medicines, sacred songs, and sacred ceremonies, or they may perform specific types of ceremonies. It has been said by the old and ancient people that spiritual elders are not made but rather they are granted divine gifts through visions and dreams. Some of these gifts are the ability to heal, to perform the Sundance, the shaking tent ceremony, the sweat lodge ceremony, to interpret dreams and visions, or to be a counselor. It should be noted, however, that a single elder would not perform all these ceremonies.

A person is not immediately granted spiritual eldership. Depending on their cultural heritage, he or she must go through a lengthy process that may include counseling with elders, learning the traditional teachings, fasting, attending sweat lodge ceremonies, and being asked to participate in specific rites (e.g., dance for 3 or 4 days at a Sundance and perform the chest-piercing ceremony). Even after this process, once the person is recognized as an elder or spiritual worker by the other elders, they will still apprentice under the guidance of an accomplished elder.

Elders do not work alone and will have one or two helpers, some of whom may be referred to as pipe carriers. The pipe carrier works for the elder for an unspecified amount of time anywhere from 1 to 8 years. Having gained experience and knowledge in the traditional ways, he or she will then seek permission to fast and plead for divine gifts through their visions or dreams. Few are chosen for this path and fewer yet are successful.

Through having the opportunity to work jointly with clinicians and elders we have come to see both significant similarities in our work with people as well as distinct differences. This combination of similarities and differences is seen as not only enhancing the quality of the treatment/healing we are able to provide in our sexual offender program, but has also enhanced and supplemented our own clinical skills and perspectives.

There are a number of important distinctions that appear to define the role and process of healing as practice by elders. One of the defining features of an elder's practice is a holistic approach to healing. Within this tradition elders make little or no distinction between physical, mental, emotional, and spiritual well-being. Human beings are seen as a whole rather than compartmentalized aspects of an individual. Any type of distress is an indication that an individual is out of harmony or balance with forces either internal or external to his or her total being (Torrey, 1986). In keeping with this holistic approach, we have attempted to minimize using the term "aboriginal sexual offender" and instead refer to men who have committed sexual offenses. While for some this may seem to be a semantic issue (or a failure to correctly describe, label, or diagnosis), within the native holistic tradition it is not seen as appropriate to identify an individual based on one aspect of their behavior. While sexual offending is clearly seen as inappropriate, the behavior is viewed in a larger context as one part of a whole human being.

Another characteristic of an elder's approach to counseling is their attempt to have a positive impact on each offender's self-esteem. Ross (1992) reported that elders view a negative and confrontational approach to working with offenders as counterproductive. Rather than constantly confronting the offender with how much damage he has done, how he has hurt others, and how his failure to control his harmful impulses is to blame for the damage caused, elders will focus on the individual's potential, their ability to heal and move forward, and the need to learn to respect oneself and to have respect for others around them.

Elders also emphasize in their practice of healing a very active role in the intervention process. Clients are rarely expected to independently identify, develop insights into, and resolve problems, but rather are often given specific solution-oriented advice by the elder that they are to follow in order to achieve the desired change and healing.

Another distinction, particularly in offender treatment, is that traditional healing cannot be mandated. The offender must request healing before they can be treated, by presenting the healer with tobacco. The elder uses this tobacco to communicate with the spirit world on the individual's behalf.

The elder's acceptance of a nonordinary reality and emphasis on the psychospiritual realm of personality are other defining features in their practice of healing. It is this spiritual orientation that provides the impetus for healing strategies. Elders possess a belief in different levels of human experience and conceptualize a reality that transcends the "normal" world while still influencing it (Harner, 1990). One of the functions of the elder is to enter this realm on behalf of other people and act as conduits of positive energy from this dimension. This energy is then translated into concrete insight or action leading to problem resolution or decision making (Lee & Armstrong, 1995). Traditional healers assume the spiritual aspects of life. Spirituality is highly valued and is seen as providing the basis for the relationship between mental and physical health and well-being. Elders are trained to intervene at a spiritual level to relieve the stress surrounding issues that affect body, mind, and spirit.

Thin Elk (1995) states that before healing takes place, a relationship of mutual respect must exist between the afflicted person, the healing process, and the healer. An important part of understanding the role of elders in healing is understanding the relationship between an elder and their clients. Elders are held in extremely high regard by those who seek their healing. Not only is there a great respect for the elder but also a high level of faith in the healing process and a confidence that the elder, through counseling, teachings, and ceremonies will be able to bring about the desired change. A good illustration of this is provided by Kottler (1993), who describes Don Jose, a healer in Peru. He identifies how, because of the confidence and authority Don Jose maintains with the people he heals, they come to him eager and ready to change and are confident in his powers to heal even before the ceremony begins. The healer conveys to them his certainty that they will see improvements and then engages in a series of rituals and chants as part of the healing process. Kottler (1993) points out that

> whether evil demons are really being exorcised or whether an active placebo response is being elicited by a sophisticated set of rituals, there is no doubt that Don Jose and his successful colleagues are powerful human beings. They have presence. They expect their clients to get better. Their clients have faith in their powers to cure. (p. 5)

In much the same way, the confidence, respect, and trust that many aboriginal people have in their elders sets the stage for change, facilitating both their motivation to change and their expectation for success. While part of this confidence in the power and expertise of the healer comes from the teachings, legends, symbols, rituals, and ceremonies that are part of the healing process, much of this respect and faith comes from the therapeutic relationship or alliance that is developed between the elder and the offender. The elder's approach, style of presentation, and, at times, familiarity with the offender's family or community, all work toward building a strong bond with their clients that enhances the offender's confidence and willingness to take the risks necessary to look at and change their lives.

The closure of healing by elders is also different from that of clinicians. The healing process that occurs is attributed to the creator and the elder reassures the client that treatment is effective and will continue to be effective, since the creator is always present. In our program, this is not done in a way that suggests a cure or that absolves the offenders from taking responsibility for managing their lives and their risk. The creator's presence is identified as being a constant source of motivation and a strength to draw from to assist them in managing their lives in a healthy manner.

While some aspects of the elder's philosophical orientation and approach toward healing are very different from the theoretical orientations and clinical practice of the clinical team, there are concepts we have learned from the traditional ways and incorporated into our contemporary treatment process and there are other traditional ways of practicing that are, in fact, very similar to how we as clinicians approach our work with offenders.

Throughout the years, we have come to learn and believe that we must broaden our treatment focus to address a host of issues that are beyond, yet undeniably linked to, sex-offender-specific issues. This position has come about from seeing the range of deficit areas that sexual offenders in our programs have presented with, our belief that there is a need to address these issues if change and risk management is to be maintained over time, and out of our affinity for the holistic approach practiced by elders and aboriginal communities.

The perspective of identifying the men we treat as more than the sum of their offending and the need to expand supports to include their community have also been adopted. In identifying what constitutes community, we have identified various levels. While family and home community (where the offender was born and/or raised) typically constitute community, often offenders are released to cities away from their home communities, and as a result must develop a sense of community outside of the original one. What is identified as community is expanded to include friends, support people, agencies, and other resources that are more immediately available to the offender. Part of attending to a holistic approach has involved attempting to assist offenders to develop or connect with various community supports to enhance their feeling of belonging. As a result, we attempt to engage external supports, both from their urban community and their home community, into the treatment process. This has involved securing the support of probation and parole officers, staff at other treatment facilities and in other community agencies, teachers, employers, friends, and family. In addition, the clinic regularly provides couple counseling and family sessions and has recently implemented a support group for partners, family members, and others who are part of an offender's community or support group.

If an offender intends to return to their home community, we attempt to recruit and include the community in the work we are doing. This involves providing the community with information about the offender's treatment/healing experiences (level of participation, treatment gains, areas of concern); providing them with information related to the offender's risk factors, cycle of offending, and relapse prevention plan; and attempting to determine the community's willingness and ability to support the offender upon his return and to assume some responsibility for monitoring and managing his risk. This process is consistent with the external supervision dimension of relapse prevention (Pithers, Cumming, Beal, Young, & Turner, 1989) and is employed both to enhance appropriate monitoring and support for the offender and to establish and enhance the offender's feeling of community acceptance and support.

Another common feature in the healing practices of elders and the treatment process of clinicians in our program is attention to the importance of the therapeutic alliance. While the significance of the therapeutic relationship in the process of psychotherapy is often noted, this important dynamic is rarely identified and discussed in working with forensic clients. This may be because of a blur between the role of punishment and treatment in some programs, or because of negative attitudes held toward sexual offenders by some clinicians and their resulting lack of desire to establish a therapeutic bond, or because of efforts on the part of the clinician to keep a distance between themselves and the offender to protect against being manipulated or from experiencing the stressors associated with working closely with sexual offenders (Gutkin, Ellerby, Smith, & Atkinson, 1993). In our work with offenders, we have found it crucial to nurture and develop a strong working alliance with our clients. The frequent absence of caring, supportive, and healthy role models in offenders' lives and the therapeutic need to develop a relationship in which there is a degree of trust, respect, and openness, all demand that attention be given to the therapeutic relationship.

A significant distinction between our clinicians' work and that of the elder in the sexual offender treatment program is the spiritual component of healing. While therapists do not tend to use spirituality as part of their treatment interventions, we have found that the perception of native offenders of the treatment program and their motivation for treatment and attitudes toward clinical staff have been positively affected since the inclusion of the traditional healing process. There appears to be an appreciation and respect for the fact that the program has recognized the importance and relevance of traditional healing, and there is gratitude for the opportunity to access culturally relevant programming.

As a final point in discussing clinical staff issues, there is a pressing need for more aboriginal people to become involved in training for and in the practice of counseling, social work, nursing, psychology, and psychiatry and to be providing assessment and treatment services to aboriginal offenders. All things being equal (e.g., therapists maintaining similar attitudes and values toward clients, clinician's level of education, age, and similar personalities), ethnic minority clients prefer ethnically similar counselors (Atkinson & Lowe, 1995). However, the current reality is that there are so few aboriginal clinicians that most native offenders are likely to be treated by nonnative therapists. While it is important for more aboriginal people to be involved in working with aboriginal offenders, it is also important to note that this does not mean that nonaboriginal clinicians cannot work effectively with native men who have committed sexual offenses.

Some native communities have asserted that only aboriginal therapists should be providing treatment to native sexual offenders because only they have the skills required to establish a relationship in which the offender will openly address their problems. In our experience we have not found this to be the case. What we have observed is that how successful a clinician is (native or nonnative), or even how successful an elder is in working with offenders is largely determined by their therapeutic style and approach, their ability to engage the client in a therapeutic relationship, and their experience in working with offense-specific issues. While native people must become more involved in the treatment of native offenders, the decision by some aboriginal people and communities to reject or dismiss the wealth of research knowledge related to sexual offenders and sexual offender assessment and treatment, as well as the expertise of nonnative practitioners, we believe, is unfortunate and counterproductive to providing healing for their people.

TRADITIONAL HEALING: PROCESS, TEACHINGS, AND CEREMONIES

In the traditional way, a person's life is considered a gift from the creator, and as a result each individual is expected to show respect for themselves and accept responsibility for their health. This entails learning to lead a healthy lifestyle through attaining an inner balance or achieving inner purification from imbalance in all aspects of the self (spiritual, mental, emotional, and physical) through traditional ways.

The clinic currently provides the opportunity for an offender to participate in traditional healing through smudging, use of the sacred talking stone and eagle feather, sacred circles, and sweat lodge ceremonies. Participation in traditional healing is voluntary and aboriginal men who are not interested in involving themselves in this aspect of the program are not required to do so. In addition, nonaboriginal men who are interested in participating in sacred teachings and ceremonies are welcome to attend.

Smudging is the burning of the four sacred plants (tobacco, cedar, sweet grass, and sage) for the purpose of purification and to drive out negative emotions prior to a ceremony or tribal meeting. It is believed that the aroma of the sacred plants puts one in conscious contact with positive spirits and results in the person becoming more receptive and open-minded. In the prairies, sweet grass or sage are often burned on their own for smudging during prayer. While smudging precedes all traditional ceremonies and teachings, aboriginal offenders have the option of also smudging prior to an individual or group session.

The sacred circle is a ceremony conducted by the elder that provides cultural understanding and spiritual growth through a process of individual and group counseling. Within our sacred circle ceremonies the elder teaches what is known as the medicine wheel or the circle of life. The circle of life describes the four directions: East, South, West, and North. Each sacred quadrant contains sacred elements of powers, spirits, and teachings that lead to personal balance. The circle of life shows and guides the many ways in which all things are connected and interrelated, both the outer and inner qualities of human beings. Although different tribes assign different qualities to different points on the circle or to different animals, they are similar in many ways (Correctional Service of Canada, 1993).

The circle of life, as taught in the prairies and within our program, may be described in the following manner. In the East quadrant we find the eagle who represents strength. The East offers the gifts of being able to focus on the here and now, to learn things at a different level of understanding, and to develop the ability to see through complex situations and over a long period of time. Its color is yellow, representing the dawning of a new life. Between the East and the South is the hill of infancy. In the South is where we find the mouse that represents fear. The South is the place of the heart and the place for testing our physical bodies. The South teaches us to discipline our feelings so they can be expressed in an open and honest manner that does not harm others. Its color is green, representing the path of the sun, which brings us the grass and green valleys. Between the South and the

West is the hill of youth and learning. In the West is the bear, who represents healing. This is the direction of dreams, prayer, and meditation. The lessons from the West are to take an inventory of oneself and move toward healing, both spiritually and physically. The color of the West is red, representing life. Between the West and the North is the hill of maturity. In the North is the buffalo, who represents teaching. The gift of the North is the wisdom of how all things fit together to create a balance. Its color is white, representing the purity of the spiritual path in life. Between the North and the East is where we find the hill of old age.

Within the sacred circle these lessons and much more are taught, discussed, and applied to the various problems and issues in the men's lives. During the sacred circle, the sacred talking stone and eagle feather, representing strength, are held to help give the individual courage to open up and talk about themselves, their lives, and their behavior. The stone and feather are also used for this purpose during sweat lodge ceremonies, and offenders can choose to use them during individual or group therapy sessions.

It has been said by the old ones that the sweat lodge is the oldest ceremony among North American traditional natives. The ceremony is a purification rite in which individuals can gain balance within themselves. The sweat lodge is a dome shaped construction framed with willow saplings and covered with hides or canvas. The dome may vary in height and circumference depending on a particular tribe or elder; however, most are sized to accommodate 10–12 individuals. A sacred fire is built in front of the lodge where the stones, representing the grandfather and grandmother spirits (very old and wise), are heated in the fire. The sacred fire represents the healing forces that cleanse the negative spirits that may dwell within a person. The number of doors a lodge has will depend on the region, the cultural heritage, as well as the type of ceremony being conducted in the lodge (e.g., a healing ceremony, thanksgiving ceremony, truth-telling ceremony, dream interpretation ceremony). Inside the lodge is a pit in the center where the stones, or grandfathers and grandmothers from the fire are placed. This hole has been said to be the door to mother earth from whence she sends her blessings. The grandfathers and grandmothers bring healing, wisdom, and knowledge and take onto themselves our trials and tribulations.

Before attending a sweat lodge ceremony many will fast, sacrifice, and/or pray. Prior to entering the lodge the elder must be presented with tobacco and in some regions prayer flags, so they are able to communicate to the spirit world on behalf of the individual. As each person enters the sweat lodge, they are said to be reentering the womb of the mother earth. The participants sit around the pit, and the red-hot stones are brought in and placed in the center hole. As each grandfather and grandmother enters, they are welcomed and a mixture of the four sacred plants are placed on them, creating a red sparkling glow as they burn and produce a calming odor. The door to the lodge is then covered over and closed leaving the participants in darkness, with the exception of the glowing grandfathers and grandmothers which slowly fade, leaving blackness.

The heat of the stones heats the inside of the lodge and causes the participants to sweat. The elder beings with a prayer and smokes the sacred pipe with its spiritual power and connections. Having honored creation, the elder then douses the red-hot rocks with water to produce steam. The water represents the continuous flow of the creator's forgiving love to the people of the earth and the steam is called the sacred breath of the creator. The vapors from the steam penetrate the mind, body, and spirit to expel illness. There is singing and chanting and the sounds of the drum, representing the heartbeat of mother earth, and the shaking of rattles, to summon the spirits to come and care for the people taking part in the ceremony. The elder directs each person to speak about the problem or request that has brought them to the ceremony. While people talk about their struggles, the focus tends to be on others, giving thanks for others, praying for others, and asking for the forgiveness of others in a selfless manner. The theme is consistently about respect. Respect for mother earth and nature, respect for the elders, respect for the traditional ways, respect for fellow inmates/offenders, respect for families, for women, and children, respect for people they have hurt, and a striving toward respect for themselves. As each person talks, the language they speak may vary. An observer would be struck with the level of openness, sincerity, and emotion with which the men talk about themselves, their lives, their behavior, and the people and world around them.

After the first round is completed, the door to the lodge is opened and the cool air comes in and creates a new sensation. In between rounds, the atmosphere is casual and may shift from the serious introspective focus to lighthearted joking (humor is an important part of the process for some elders) and relaxing in preparation for the next round. The ceremony consists of four rounds. More stones are placed in the lodge at the beginning of each round. The length and purpose of each round depends on the reason for the ceremony, the elder's own practices, and the tribe they are from. The number of stones used has symbolic significance and the total number of stones used will depend again on the purpose of the sweat lodge and the elder.

During the ceremony the combination of the heat, changes in temperature, the darkness, the aroma of the burning plants, and the sounds of the music, song, and chanting create an intense atmosphere in which the body, mind, and spirit are barraged with a variety of sensory stimulation. The result is a feeling of release, calm, focus, and clarity. There is a strong sense of group cohesion and togetherness, yet there is an undeniable sensation of each person's own individuality. Upon the conclusion of the sweat lodge ceremony, there is a feeling of serenity. Tensions, anxiety, anger, and fear have been expelled and are said to be left with the grandfathers and grandmothers. They are replaced by a positive energy and a contrast in feelings both of being drained and relaxed yet still invigorated and alert (physically, intellectually, emotionally, and spiritually).

As can be seen, symbols are an important part of aboriginal teaching and ceremony. It is important to note that these symbols are not worshipped but are used for teaching and guidance. Symbols are so heavily relied on as they remain the most effective way for people to express the abstract forces of nature and connect to with the nontangible aspects of our spirit (Hammerschlag, 1988; Kalweit, 1992).

In implementing traditional healing into our program, we have also attempted to structure the healing in such a way as to facilitate interconnectedness. For example, although all the clinic's treatment modalities are sexual offender specific, a decision was made to have the community-based sacred circle open to anyone who wished to attend. Males and females, natives and nonnatives, from our program and other community programs, all attend and are welcome. Having an open sacred circle was seen as important, as we wanted the men in our program to have some treatment/healing experiences in which the common bond among them was not having committed a sexual crime but being a part of a broader group of people, all of whom sharing the commonality of wanting to learn more about their culture and to bring balance to their lives.

In attempting to establish a connectedness with the sweat lodge ceremonies, we chose to conduct the ceremonies on the sacred grounds located at the minimum-security institution. This way, the men in the community program return to the institution and can see where they have come from. They also can support those still incarcerated. The inmates who attend the ceremony are all involved in the institutional sexual offender treatment programs. Their involvement in the sweat lodge with men from the community allows inmates to hear about the struggles associated with living and managing risk in the community (which challenges some of their distorted expectations) and enables them to hear about the success others have had in overcoming adversity and difficulties in the community. Combining men from the institution and the community also allows for a smoother transition from the institutional program to the community program as the men become familiar with each other before the new members are introduced to the community group after their release.

There is an effort to establish continuity between the issues addressed in both the traditional and contemporary treatment approaches. It is not uncommon for the elder to focus on a theme during traditional healing that is also being addressed in individual and group therapy. With this approach men can be working on issues such as victim empathy and anger management in both the traditional and contemporary components of the treatment/healing.

HOME COMMUNITIES

For traditional aboriginals and for many transitional aboriginals, their lives and identities are grounded in their home communities. This is likely where they will return upon their release from prison or at some point either during or after their probation or parole. As indicated earlier, the issues of preparing and supporting an offender to return to his home community is complex because of the diversity of the various communities.

While it is important to play a role in facilitating this transition and making the community aware of pertinent issues related to the offender's treatment, risk, risk factors, and relapse prevention plans, this is not typically easy to achieve. While the public voice of many aboriginal communities asserts their desire and willingness to accept members of their community who have committed sexual offenses back into the community, we have had numerous experiences where the private voice has been a strong opposition to these individuals returning home, or only considering them to return if they have demonstrated significant gains from their involvement in treatment programs like ours, outside of the community. Similar experiences and findings have been reported by LaPrairie (1996) and Native Counseling Services of Alberta (1993). LaPrairie (1996) makes an important distinction between the level of support offenders receive from their families versus the level of support from their home communities. In surveying aboriginal inmates and offenders on parole, she reports that while offenders' families tended to be supportive regardless of their offense, their home communities were less likely to be supportive of them and were more likely to ostracize them if they had committed serious offenses such as sexual or violent crimes. The reasons why many communities report not wanting the offender back in the community involve fear of the offender and his potential to reoffend; concern that offenders are returning to live with dysfunctional families; limited available activities in the communities; the absence of support/treatment programs; and the perception that offenders require intensive counseling with staff who have the training and skill to address the offenders' issues. Even if communities are willing to accept offenders back, for a number of native men who have attended our program feelings of shame and fear of rejection by the community make it difficult for them to return.

Having an offender return to some communities is made exceedingly difficult because of the dysfunctional state of that community. Communities rife with substance abuse, violence, and abuse of all forms simply cannot support the offender. Men who come from these communities must either choose not to return home because they do not want to jeopardize their own gains and place themselves in a high-risk situation or choose to return to environments that have the potential to increase their risk of reoffending in a violent or sexual manner.

While some native communities have not yet faced their problems, others have moved forward with courage, determination, and strength and have begun the healing process for their people as a community. Some of these communities have taken the position of wanting to take responsibility for issues such as sexual abuse and sexual violence and have developed community holistic healing programs in which perpetrators are treated in the community and become the community's responsibility. In this approach, the entire community as well as the offender and his victim(s) work toward healing.

Even in healthy and supportive communities it has still been a challenge to engage the community in the offender's treatment and have them assume some responsibility for learning about and for monitoring and assisting in managing the offender's risk. It is hoped that through ongoing communication, education, and developing a mutual trust and respect that this will occur more readily.

CHALLENGES OF A BLENDED APPROACH

There are a number of challenges in moving toward the blending of contemporary and traditional treatment approaches for aboriginal men who sexually offend. These are important issues that we and other programs must be aware of and work toward resolving if traditional healing is going to be a successful part of the intervention and risk management process for sexual offenders.

There are a number of challenges in working with elders and in evaluating healing gains that will need to be carefully reviewed. As elders become more active in correctional programming, there will need to be consideration given to determining the qualifications of elders and healers who provide traditional healing. Elders do not tend to carry a resumé; therefore, to determine their legitimacy, the community and other elders must be approached and consulted.

The issue of evaluating an offender's progress and gains as a result of their participation in traditional healing will also require much discussion. While many elders practice in an oral tradition, written reports are typically required by institutional case management officers and National Parole Board members, to assist them in commenting on and making decisions about programming required, responsivity to programming, level of accountability and insight, risk for reoffending, and appropriateness for release and release conditions. The issue of report writing by elders is complicated by a number of factors, such as the confidentiality that is an integral part of the traditional ceremony; the elders' tendencies to provide general rather than specific information about how a man is responding to healing; and the elders' focus on growth and positive gains rather than on areas of concern. While it is refreshing and desirable to identify positive qualities, if case management officers, psychologists, and parole board members are going to be able to view traditional programming as a relevant means of addressing risk, there will need to be some way of operationalizing the gains expected to occur from involvement in traditional healing and a means of identifying specific issues that are indicative of progress and risk reduction.

There must also be a means of expressing concern related to those individuals who are not seen as having made gains and who are deemed to be high risk. While culturally it may be common to accept the elder/healer's word out of deference to what is believed to be their highly developed sense of intuitiveness and capacity to assess people, in working with offenders it is unlikely that systems responsible for making decisions related to the release of sexual offenders to the community will accept nonspecific indicators of progress. Research is also need to investigate the efficacy of traditional healing and to determine how this approach influences criminogenic factors, risk, and recidivism.

There is also a need to further investigate both the similarities as well as the differences among aboriginal offenders and between aboriginal and nonaboriginal offenders. In addition, there is a need to further understand how these similarities and differences relate to risk, treatment needs, and responsivity to various treatment approaches.

THE OUTCOME OF A BLENDED APPROACH AND BEYOND

Our experience with an integrated approach to the treatment of aboriginal men who have committed sexual offenses has been a positive one to date. The feedback from men in the treatment program has been supportive and those who have chosen to take part in the traditional component have been highly invested in their participation. Preliminary results of an ongoing outcome study comparing aboriginal men who have participated in the blended approach to those who have only participated in the contemporary approach are encouraging. Within the blended treatment group we have seen a reduction in the number of aboriginal men who have been terminated from and who have dropped out of treatment. There also has been a reduction in the number of aboriginal men suspended while in treatment and a reduction of sexual recidivism.

The men who participate in the blended approach appear to be gaining the best from both worlds. They are learning and developing skills within the traditional approach while simultaneously addressing sexual offender specific issues and other related treatment needs in the contemporary approach. Because these two aspects of treatment work cooperatively, they both support and supplement each other, which further adds to the potential efficacy of this treatment/healing approach.

What we are finding is that there is great potential in the use of both contemporary treatment and traditional healing approaches. The potential of this kind of combined approach has been noted by others (Lee & Armstrong, 1995; Ross, 1992). LaPrairie (1996) states that "the key to effective aboriginal programming is the identification of risk and needs of the offenders, and the blending of the cultural with the mainstream" (p. 127). She further identifies a number of cautions and concerns associated with involving aboriginal offenders in only culturally specific programs without attending other programs specifically designed to address issues related to criminogenic factors and risk.

The blended treatment approach is focused in an attempt to provide the most meaningful interventions to Native Canadian offenders in an effort to prevent/reduce sexual recidivism. In developing and providing programming for native offenders, the aboriginal and nonaboriginal communities have much to learn from one another. If the movement toward culturally relevant programs can stay focused on the necessity to address the range of issues related to an offender's level of risk and their treatment needs, rather than becoming politicized, we will find that we will be better serving the needs of the aboriginal offenders we treat and of all our communities.

REFERENCES

Atkinson, D.R., & Lowe, S.M. (1995). The role of ethnicity, cultural knowledge and conventional techniques in counseling and psychotherapy. In J.G. Ponterotto, J.M. Cases, L.A. Suzuki, & C.M. Alexander (Eds.), *Handbook of multicultural counseling* (pp. 387–414). Thousand Oaks: Sage.

Canadian Centre for Justice Statistics. (1994). *Adult correctional services in Canada.* Cat. 85-211. Statistics Canada.

Cases, L.M., & Casas, A. (1994). The acculturation process and implications for educations and services. In A.C. Matiella (Ed.), *The multicultural challenge in health education* (pp. 23–49). Santa Cruz, CA: ETR Associates.

Choney, S.K., Berryhill-Paapke, E., & Robbins, R.R. (1995). The acculturation of American Indians. In J.G. Ponterotto, J.M. Cases, L.A. Suzuki, & C.M. Alexander (Eds.), *Handbook of multicultural counseling* (pp. 73–92). Thousand Oaks: Sage.

Corey, G. (1990). *Theory and practice of group counseling* (3rd ed.). Pacific Grove, CA: Brooks/Cole.

Correctional Service of Canada. (1993). *The Sweetgrass trail: Aboriginal medicine in the correctional setting.* Ottawa: Health Care Services, Correctional Service Canada.

Couture, J.E. (1995). Multicultural competence: Theory and practice for correctional psychologists. In T.A. Leis, L.L. Motiuk, & R.P. Ogloff (Eds.), *Forensic psychology: Policy and practice in corrections* (pp. 57–68). Ottawa: Correctional Service Canada.

Cowie, G. (1996). *Executive information system data.* Ottawa: Correctional Service Canada.

Ellerby, L. (1994). Community based treatment of aboriginal sexual offenders: Facing realities and exploring possibilities. *Forum on Corrections Research, 6,* 23–25.

Ellerby, J.H. (1995). *Wapi, Yekiya: Sacred healers of the Lakota Souix.* Unpublished paper.

Gelso, C.J., & Fretz, B.R. (1992). *Counseling psychology.* Fort Worth, TX: Harcourt, Brace, Jovanovich.

Gutkin, B., Ellerby, L., Smith, T., & Atkinson, R. (1993, November). *Treating sexual offenders: The impact on clinicians.* A paper presented at the Association for the Treatment of Sexual Offenders, Boston.

Hammerschlag, C.A. (1988). *The dancing healers: A doctor's journey of healing with Native Americans.* San Francisco: Harper Collins.

Harner, M. (1990). *The way of the shaman.* San Francisco: Harper & Row.

Johnson, D.W., & Johnson, F.P. (1994). *Joining together: Group theory and group skills.* Boston: Allyn & Bacon.

Kalweit, H. (1992). *Shamans, healers and medicine men.* Boston: Shambhala.

Kottler, J.A. (1993). *On being a therapist.* San Francisco: Jossey-Bass.

LaPrairie, C. (1996). *A state of aboriginal corrections.* Ottawa: Ministry of the Solicitor General Canada.

LeClair, M. (1996). Profile of aboriginal sex offenders. Ottawa: Correctional Service of Canada.

Lee, C.C., & Armstrong, K.L. (1995). Indigenous models of mental health intervention: Lessons from traditional healers. In J.G. Ponterotto, J.M. Casas, L.A. Suzuki, & C.M. Alexander (Eds.), *Handbook of multicultural counseling* (pp. 414–456). Thousand Oaks, CA: Sage.

Merta, R.J. (1995). Group work: Multicultural perspectives. In J.G. Ponterotto, J.M. Cases, L.A. Suzuki, & C.M. Alexander (Eds.), *Handbook of multicultural counseling* (pp. 567–585). Thousand Oaks, CA: Sage.

Motiuk, L. (1996). *The Aboriginal sexual offender in federal corrections: A profile.* A paper presented at the Aboriginal Sexual Offender: Management and Treatment Conference, Winnipeg, MB.

Motiuk, L., & Belcourt, R. (1996). *Homicide, sexual, robbery and drug offenders in federal corrections: End of 1995 review.* Research Brief B-13. Ottawa: Correctional Service of Canada.

Native Counselling Service. (1993). *Evaluation of Stan Daniales Correctional Centre,* Edmonton, AB.

Pithers, W.D., & Cumming, G.F., Beal, L.S., Young, W., & Turner, R. (1989). Relapse prevention: A method for enhancing behavioral self-management and external supervision of the sexual aggressor. In B. Schwartz (Ed.), *Sexual offenders: Issues in treatment* (pp. 292–310). Washington, DC: National Institute of Corrections.

Ross, R. (1992). *Dancing with a ghost: Exploring Indian reality.* Markham, ON: Octopus Publishing Group.

Ryan, R.A, & Ryan, L. (1989). *Multicultural aspects of chemical dependency treatment: An American Indian perspective.* Unpublished manuscript. Turnaround Adolescent Treatment Program, Vancouver, BC.

Thin Elk, G. (1995). Red road approach. In D. Arbogast (Ed.), *Wounded warrior: A time for healing* (pp. 319–320). Omaha, NB: Little Turtle Publications.

Torrey, E.F. (1986). *Witchdoctors and psychiatrists: The common roots of psychotherapy and its future.* New York: Harper & Row.

Waldram, J. (1992). *Aboriginal offenders at the Regional Psychiatric Centre (Prairies).* Saskatoon, SK: Correctional Service Canada.

28

Treatment of United States American Indians

Dewey J. Ertz

THE AMERICAN INDIAN

The definition of an "American Indian" has undergone several changes over time. In the United States, there are over 500 Indian tribes recognized by either federal or state governments, and many of these tribes have under 1000 members. The Bureau of Indian Affairs under the United States Department of the Interior had developed a definition that identified someone being Indian if their blood quantum was one fourth or greater. The concept of blood quantum continues to be used by many tribal groups, although an individual is generally recognized as being an American Indian if they are enrolled in a tribe regardless of their degree of blood. Tribal enrollment requirements vary greatly, with some tribes enrolling individuals with very small blood quantum, while other tribes require a blood quantum of one fourth or more, and still other tribes base enrollment on factors unrelated to blood percentages.

Using blood quantum to define a person as being "American Indian" views Indian people from primarily a racial standpoint. However, ethnic issues are more important in considering an individual's behavior than is their racial background. A concept that is often used in considering ethnic variables is identification. This term is a combination of how the individual and their family views their heritage. Indian identification follows a continuum from traditional to contemporary, depending on the style and practices the individual adopts. A traditional person would be expected to be fluent or highly knowledgeable of their native language, to practice the ceremonies and belief patterns of their tribal group, and to hold values consistent with the morals of their tribal group. A contemporary individual would be expected to have a lifestyle consistent with the dominant society and to adopt value and behavioral patterns held by that society.

Some Indian people do not identify with either a traditional or contemporary model. They are often referred to as being marginally identified, and May (1989) has demonstrated that these individuals are at greater risk for developing substance abuse and other emotional problems. As can be seen from this short discussion, the definition of an American Indian involves several variables. These variables may be racial or ethnic in origin and it is

Dewey J. Ertz • The Manlove Psychiatric Group, Rapid City, South Dakota 57701.

Sourcebook of Treatment Programs for Sexual Offenders, edited by Marshall et al. Plenum Press, New York, 1998.

necessary to take into account the individual's self-view. This self-view is often derived from the person's family and societal context, and great variations regarding how individuals define themselves as an American Indian can be expected as a result.

Gaining an understanding of this self-view is necessary if providers are to successfully treat American Indian sexual offenders. Bennett (1979) has presented an excellent discussion of the differences between sympathy and empathy when attempting to understand the experiences of an individual from another ethnic group. He defines sympathy as a projection of how you would feel in a similar circumstance onto the other person, while empathy includes managing your feelings to understand how the other person is reacting. Patients in treatment may reject or manipulate a provider's sympathy, thus reducing potential gains. Providers must understand their need to develop empathy as defined above if they are expected to be effective. This skill must be developed by providers regardless of their ethnic identification, and providers who are themselves American Indian often have greater resources to accomplish this responsibility.

The Old Ways

The origin of Indian people has been subject to debate for several years. Contemporary society has generally adopted a view that American Indian people migrated from Asia into North America during periods of past climatic changes. Many American Indian people hold the view that "we were always here," meaning that they do not necessarily agree with the migration theory. Whatever the origin of American Indian people, we do know that they developed specific life patterns and methods of interaction. Information regarding the traditional beliefs and lifestyles of many tribal groups has been lost over years of persecution and forced aculturalization. It is known that American Indian people developed various societal patterns based on the different lifestyles they led.

Rituals were often practiced to reinforce identity development and the boundaries necessary for societal functioning. These rituals frequently involved protection and bonding before the time of conception and specific activities at birth to protect the child throughout his or her life. Ceremonies and practices for naming were common among tribal groups, although certain variations were present. Children were generally viewed as being sacred and special, and child-rearing practices were developed to reinforce these concepts. Danger, violence, and other traumas have changed these processes.

Indian people often have been viewed and identified as being psychologically minded in their worldviews. Beane (1995) has noted that Indian people developed many concepts that are characterized by three marked differences from non-Indian Americans. These differences were that they employed different metaphors, that they did not copyright their ideas, and that their ideas had a longer tradition than those coming from traditional psychology. Another major difference between the American Indian views and that of the dominate American society concerns their behavior management efforts. The dominant society views behavior management as primarily a system of providing consequences. An inappropriate behavior is punished, while appropriate behavior is rewarded or reinforced by various methods. Many Indian cultures saw the use of antecedents as being the primary method of behavior management. Child-rearing practices were aimed at enabling appropriate behaviors, and a high value was placed on the person's ability to make and accept their own decisions.

Five values are noted by Bryde (1971) regarding the cultural interactions he studied among a northern plains tribe. He identifies these as bravery, individual freedom, generosity and sharing, adjusting to nature, and good advice from Indian wisdom. Each of these values had specific impacts on an individual's behavior. Bravery was a process of doing the most difficult thing for yourself, and this would likely vary between individuals. Individual freedom was a concept that implied that each individual had to make their own choices, and it was understood that these choices would be beneficial for both the person and his family or tribal group. Sharing included areas of food and shelter and the areas of praise and shame. If an individual behaved in a shameful manner, it reflected not only on him or her but on the entire family and tribe. Being adjusted to nature meant living in a balance and having a sense of belonging between yourself and your entire environment. Good advice was always present, and specific responsibilities for giving this advice were detailed by the Elders. It was the individual's responsibility to seek out the Elders to gain this advice. Brendtro, Brokenleg, and Van Brockern (1990) present additional information regarding how Indian cultural groups combine child care and daily living activities. They discuss concepts of belonging, mastery, independence, and generosity as being of major importance. They further define a "broken circle" that results when individuals develop distorted means of expressing these values toward others. The concept of mending the circle highlights a view that many current Indian leaders have that identifies cultural destruction and trauma as major concerns for the American Indian population.

The final important issue concerns the differences in spiritual functioning between Western and American Indian societies. Western society tends to identify spiritual functioning as a process of "giving to God." This process involves an individual denying himself or herself certain activities or pleasures, and specific behavioral requirements are usually required. American Indian ways address a concept of "living with God" as being spiritual functioning. Bonding was looked at in all areas, especially with people, the environment, and the Creator. This process emphasizes the idea of being in balance, which is addressed in physical, emotional, intellectual, and spiritual areas.

The Boarding Schools

A major instrument of cultural destruction for American Indian people has been the institution generally referred to as the boarding school. Boarding schools were both church and government managed and they had certain similarities. Individual students were not allowed to speak their own language, with instruction being given to them in English. Most of the early boarding schools were managed so that classroom activities covered half of the day and the rest of the day was dedicated toward work that supported the overall school operation.

Boarding schools were generally rigid in their discipline and many stories are available in Indian families about family members who ran away from the boarding schools. The boarding school setting also placed children at risk to be abused and molested by adults, and this process appears to bear some responsibility for current levels of offender behaviors within the American Indian population. Generations of the same family often attended boarding schools. This process eliminated traditional child-rearing practices and replaced them with Western society's emphasis in using consequences in behavior management. Many American Indian people believe that the legacy of the boarding schools can be found in today's Indian families through abusive discipline systems and through sexual offending.

The boarding schools also followed the tradition of early colonial schools in America. These early schools served the purpose of socializing children into a single culture that was mostly Anglo-Saxon, agrarian, based on religion, concerned with morality, and designed to fill a requirement of literacy for future landowners. This purpose was, and is, in sharp contrast to the educational needs for American Indian students who were losing their land and lifestyle and who were seen as needing to adopt the values and behaviors of American society. As a result, schools often became a battleground where change in identity was enforced and steps needed to be taken to ensure that students did not "run away" from the instruction being offered. The grounds of early boarding schools often became restricted encampments with limited access as a result. These schools developed curriculum that presented traditional Indian beliefs as wrong or inappropriate. A percentage of the students accepted such views, leading to rejection of their traditional value system.

Many of these same beliefs were shared and implemented by public, private, and other day schools attended by Indian people. Parents who spoke their native language often experienced learning difficulties in the school setting. In turn, they elected not to teach their children to speak in their native language so the children could be spared the same stress and embarrassment experienced by the parents. This process is directly related to the loss of native languages being experienced by American Indian people today.

Current Lifestyles and Sexuality

A central theme of this chapter is that unresolved trauma from the families and communities of American Indian people is affecting the current functioning of Indian society. Bunk (1994) considers that in severe cases of traumatization, negative coping styles adopted and passed on to family members can be more devastating than the actual content of the trauma. This process of transmitting negative coping styles appears to have been active in the American Indian population over the past several generations. Inherent in this process is a lack of appropriate sexual boundaries. These traditional boundaries were likely present in past lifestyles, as tribal groups were able to grow and expand. However, these boundaries seem to have been eliminated by the involvement of Western culture, and in many cases they do not appear to have been adequately replaced.

Numbing responses have been cited as one method for coping with trauma (Middleton-Moz, 1989). Such numbing responses can be identified in the Indian population, and they include numbing through anger, substance use, and sexual activities. The process of coping with trauma has become a major need for many Indian people, and this process has the effect of expanding and increasing the severity of the trauma experienced. This is especially true regarding sexual identity, as appropriate prosocial sexual behaviors are not adequately defined.

DEVELOPING THE PROGRAM

The programming efforts that are described here represent an anecdotal record of services provided through the Indian Health Service on a specific reservation. These efforts were not preplanned, but were guided by the needs identified through the client population in a social service/mental health setting.

From Treating Victims to Treating Offenders

In the course of providing mental health services to this population, a strong correspondence was found between patients describing anxiety and depressive symptoms and a history of sexual molestation. This association had also been recognized by the staff members of a local women's shelter. Staff members from both the mental health program and the women's shelter became involved in training at the Giarretto Institute in San Jose, California. As a follow-up to this training, a group was formed in January 1993 to provide treatment and support for adults molested as children (AMAC). A 16-week treatment cycle was completed with eight individuals.

There was an increased demand for these services as community members became knowledgeable of the group. As a result, a second adult group was formed and these groups continued to meet for 16-week cycles 2 hours per group on different weekday evenings. The groups were closed once a cycle began, and invitations to join these groups were extended through the author in his role as a mental health professional. Groups numbered from seven to nine individuals.

In the year following the development of outpatient treatment for adult victims of sexual abuse, the Indian Health Service awarded a contract to Judith V. Becker, PhD, from the University of Arizona, to provide training for the initiation of outpatient therapy programs for adolescent Indian sexual offenders. These program efforts were strongly supported by the community, as several issues regarding youth had been identified and the need for intervention programs among youth was felt to be a priority. Training was provided both in Tucson, Arzona, and through visits to the reservation by Dr. Becker. Assessments were completed, and a group using cognitive–behavioral methods was formed among adolescent offenders that met weekly.

Contact was then initiated through the local alcohol/substance abuse prevention program to inquire about treatment for adolescent victims of sexual abuse. This contact was based on case documentation of adolescents who disclosed a prior history of sexual victimization when they were placed for inpatient substance abuse treatment. Another group was formed that met weekly after school, and several adolescent females were treated in this setting. Males were referred but they did not attend the group sessions. These adolescents displayed a relationship between their substance use problems and their history of having been sexually abused.

Part of the process of developing services for adolescent sexual offenders included court contact and a review of the tribal code regarding sexual offenses. It was found that the tribe did not have a code to prosecute sexual offenses, and that typically these offenses were either referred to the federal agencies with jurisdiction or they were simply dropped. A code to prosecute these offenses was developed and passed by the tribal council, and once this code was in place, prosecution began for both adolescent and adult sexual offenders. As prosecution was completed for adult offenders, a need was identified to provide treatment for these individuals. Such a treatment system was implemented, and referrals were received from both the tribal court and from federal parole officers who were managing adult offenders in the community. This progression of treating adults who were molested as children, then adolescent offenders, followed by adolescent victims, and finally adult offenders, was highly supported and well received throughout all segments of the community. The next step in this process was to begin identifying and providing services to domestic violence offenders, as these offenders often showed similar characteristics to the sexual offenders.

Understanding the American Indian in the Context of Trauma

Two major understandings are necessary regarding the American Indian context of trauma. One of these understandings is that there have been historical issues of grief and loss that have not been adequately addressed or coped with within the American Indian population. These issues have been present on a generational basis and additional difficulties have occurred each generation that added to the trauma.

The second area to be noted is the concept of horizontal violence. Horizontal violence is a process of acting out anger at displaced targets. Within the American Indian population there was and is a strong prohibition of harming other family or tribal members. This prohibition was generally maintained by people leaving the tribal group at various times to live with other family members or with other bands when tension reached the point that nonaggressive behavior could not be maintained. Placement on reservations and substance abuse led to this prohibition being broken, and Indian families are repeatedly assaulted by their own members, with anger and substance usage in today's environment. These assaults involve both elder and child abuse, and they have dramatically altered the tranquility of home and community life.

Special Needs and the Social Environment of Therapy

A major concern in developing programmatic efforts was the ability to have a safe environment for therapy. This environmental safety was primarily an emotional issue, but it can become a physical issue as well. Middleton-Moz (1989) discusses four needs in treating trauma: validation of the events, support persons/systems, validation of emotions, and time. To complete validation requires that the individuals involved feel safety in the support person and persons and within the environment of therapy. Five areas were identified as necessary before the safety issues could be maintained: the knowledge and acceptance of routines, the ability to assist in task completion or other activities, expressing and accepting emotional support, expressing and allowing others to express emotions, and ownership of the overall environment and processes involved.

These areas were operationally employed on a session evaluation form for each of the groups treating victims. This allowed for a continuous focusing on these variables and a review of how well each individual felt these areas were being maintained during the group therapy process. Two rules were structurally identified for the groups. One was that what was said in the group stayed in the group, and the second one was that confidentiality would be an ongoing issue and concern. This attention to detail regarding environmental safety is felt to have had a major contributing factor in the success of the therapy efforts. The offenders were also provided with a session evaluation form that concentrated on their participation, their cooperation, the ability to accept responsibility for their actions, how they treated themselves, and how they treated other individuals. These efforts were felt to have added success because they allowed both victims and offenders in treatment to bond with a system of support rather than with specific individuals.

Gaining and Maintaining Support

A major focus of program support was gained through the mental health program by developing a Council of Elders. This council met on a rotational basis and was primarily developed to address issues in preventing alcohol exposure to fetuses during pregnancy. The council was kept to a small number, and meetings were held in a relaxed atmosphere that involved serving and sharing a meal. This approach began to address issues of why mothers were using alcohol and led to discussions regarding sexual abuse. Elders are a very powerful source of information in many American Indian communities and their utilization is felt to be critical for program success.

Networking represented a second area of gaining and maintaining support. Networking was completed with the tribal prosecutor, with court personnel, and with social service staff. Fragmentation could also be experienced when working within the court system, as reservations often have two systems of judicial jurisdiction. One is the tribal system and the other is the federal system. Frustration was often related to the view that the federal system was either not responsive to needs at the tribal level or that the main goal of this system was incarceration. Changing the tribal code allowed for joint prosecution to be pursued and also allowed for the tribal court to become an advocate for treatment and other intervention efforts. This became a very important process, as the history of Indian people with the United States government includes separation and loss of family members for long periods of time.

The third area of support came from other health care providers. Data from several different sources and populations identify trends that are being found among female victims who were sexually abused in childhood. Overall, female victims appear to be involved with the health care system with several different complaints. These complaints involve depression, anxiety, a potential for eating disorders, posttraumatic stress disorder, other somatic concerns, and dissociation. Specific information regarding the impact of childhood sexual abuse on female American Indians does not currently exist. Treatment and management of medical issues requires the understanding of abuse as a traumatic antecedent of physical and psychological symptoms (Courtois, 1993) and a higher incidence of alcohol use appears to be related to sexual abuse histories among adolescents (Hernandez, 1992).

These relationships were discussed with primary health care providers at the Indian Health Service Hospital where the program was developed, and this allowed the health providers to make referrals for mental health therapy among patients showing depression, anxiety, eating disorders, posttraumatic stress disorder, and somatization. A related concern is the potential to encounter sexual abuse victims or offenders in program staff where networking is taking place. Such individuals generally add stress to the systems and prevent these systems from addressing treatment needs if they have not addressed their own history. The plans or discussions of treatment appear to trigger defense processes and motivate such people to resist implementation of services. The solution for this needs to be planned in each situation and it may include confrontation and offers of personal intervention.

CONTINUING THE PROGRAM

Once the program was established, several efforts needed to be undertaken to continue its development. These efforts included personnel recruitment and retention, developing service priorities and funding, addressing the stressors for therapists and support staff, coping with failures, and developing further solutions and ideas for change. The services reached a termination point when the authors of this chapter relocated into a private practice setting.

Personnel Recruitment and Retention

The process of adding services to treat victims and offenders of sexual abuse increased the demands placed on therapeutic personnel. These demands were both in time and in emotional stamina. Levels of support for these programming efforts seemed to remain consistently high among patients and community members, but the increased demands did decrease the ability of therapeutic personnel to provide services. Family costs were also experienced, as less time was available for family activities and it became difficult to set aside the impact of providing service during leisure activities. Few complaints were received from individuals or families involved in the treatment programming. This was consistent for both victims and offenders. A major issue became apparent as therapeutic staff were accepted by community members. Once this acceptance was gained, the therapeutic staff became a more likely target for horizontal violence and anger. Adequate solutions to the personnel recruitment and retention issues were not developed.

Developing Service Priorities in Funding

The process previously described of discussing a relationship between health care, substance use, and sexual victimization was very helpful in identifying service and funding needs. This process also began to address self-harm and suicidal behaviors among residents of the reservation. Case studies were used to reinforce treatment priorities and to gain funds for auxiliary treatment needs that specific victims had displayed. This information was employed to develop broader intervention strategies aimed at prevention and community presentations were made to various groups. A repeated message was developed and included in these presentations regarding primary prevention. This message was that sexual victimization could be reduced by treating sexual offenders when they are identified in adolescence. The message was well received by the community at large, and this helped generate referrals into the program from family members. These referrals were made for both sexual offenders and victims.

Stressors for Therapists and Support Staff

A major concern in continuing program efforts was to develop appropriate leadership. In order to make changes in community attitudes and structures, someone has to start the process, and this process has to be accepted and maintained. The underlying force in the leadership effort was communicating a sense that sexual abuse was not acceptable on a general society level. The value of assisting individuals in need from traditional Indian culture was employed in this communication. Support was gained from Elders and medicine people who echoed the concept that Indian people who were involved in offending behavior were not in balance. Discussions of traditional Indian spirituality and levels of responsibility were included in the treatment process, and efforts were made to identify traditional forms of social and behavioral control.

Such efforts placed stress on therapeutic staff because expertise was not generally available among staff members regarding many of these traditions. A reliance was made on Elders to gain this information and their support as well as on other specific individuals who had continued to practice traditional Indian ways. These methods were focused on behavioral issues, especially with the offenders being treated. A major concept in these efforts was allowing offenders to identify triggers for their offending behavior from the historical grief and other traumas they had experienced. Alternative behaviors for responding to these triggers were then mandated as part of the relapse prevention program each offender was required to develop.

Coping with Failures

A high priority was placed on understanding that some patients would reoffend. It was also emphasized that this recidivism would not be something that could be predicted, and that the potential for relapse highlighted a need for a more secure level of treatment. The most difficult areas of concern were when court personnel were unable to proceed with prosecution necessary to mandate treatment. This does not appear to be unique in the program being described, and these issues seem to be present regardless of the amount of networking that is accomplished. A coping strategy in dealing with this issue was to understand that there were important differences between the primary purposes of the mental health structure and the primary purposes of the court structure, and to accept that these differences would not always lead to outcomes that both areas could identify as being successful.

Solutions and Ideas

American Indian offenders in this program were repeatedly found to have been victimized themselves. This led to a requirement for these victim issues to be treated as part of the overall offender treatment effort. A method of approaching this task was to have each offender generate an autobiography, which was referred to as a life graph. This process was completed in a booklet form and each patient was instructed to arrange a notebook by year, beginning with their year of birth. Two pages opposite each other were used for each year. Trauma experiences within each year were listed on the left hand page, while the right hand page was employed to list healing or positive experiences. Offenders were encouraged to consult friends and family members to help place life events and certain records were helpful in this process. Records commonly employed were school records and medical records from health clinics. Patients were encouraged to consider anniversary dates including marriages, divorces, births, and deaths. Time was made available within group therapy to discuss and share information from the life graph, and specific examples from the life graph were often shared as major therapy topics. Another part of the life graph was for each patient to detail their own sexual history.

These histories were compared with the behavioral time lines completed when the patient was assessed before coming into the program. This comparison was generally interesting, as additional information was often provided that was important for the overall treatment efforts. Patients were instructed to list information as topics and to use a pencil so that information could be easily moved from year to year. This format was employed because some patients had rather limited writing skills. Other patients would choose to represent topics in alternative forms such as pictures or short poems. Patients were encouraged to use methods that were helpful to them in listing and processing information.

After completion, the life graph was used as a reference point when the relapse prevention program was being designed. On the healing side of the page for each year, several alternative actions were listed to deal with sexual offending problems. The trauma side of the page often helped offenders identify triggers or risk situations. Follow-up contact with offenders suggested that they often referred to the life graph and continued to work on those issues as part of their overall aftercare program. Group session evaluations were also used consistently to help provide feedback to patients regarding their performance and progress.

Another solution developed as part of the programming efforts was an understanding that treatment and prevention efforts were being employed simultaneously. School and social services' staff were often providing primary and secondary prevention information to young children to encourage reporting of inappropriate contacts by others. The early identification and treatment of children and early adolescent offenders was also included as part of primary prevention efforts, since these techniques have the capacity to minimize the number of future victims. The treatment of adult offenders was viewed as a tertiary prevention effort, and this effort was well supported by the overall community. Secondary prevention involved children who had been traumatized, or who had begun to display some early sexual behavior problems. These children were usually referred to by their families, and many times family therapy efforts became part of the treatment.

PROGRAM CONTENT

Three areas will be discussed under program content. They are assessment issues, the content of the cognitive–behavioral methods employed, and solutions for substance use difficulties. Additional program content involving, for example, storytelling techniques were employed, but discussion of them is too lengthy for inclusion in this chapter.

Assessment Issues

Five areas of assessment issues were commonly experienced in implementing the program. These areas were: (1) Indian identification; (2) differences in defining assertive, passive, and aggressive behaviors; (3) nonverbal communication concerns and learning styles; (4) value clarification in a dual system of social control; and (5) how these social systems address the role of shame. The concept of Indian identification will not be discussed further as this discussion was presented earlier in the chapter. However, it was found that Indian offenders often justified their behavior by labeling the behavior as being "traditional." This process was countered with information from Elders and members of the offender's family who defined the offending behaviors as being inappropriate. In addition, each offender was required to choose an identification area for themselves, which was then employed in the treatment process as a model for prosocial behavior.

Several cultural differences were found to exist between American Indian ways and the dominate society regarding behaviors labeled as assertive, passive, or aggressive. These differences may result from behavioral predispositions, differences in socialization patterns, or differences between thought patterns or content. To complete an adequate assessment in these areas, it is first necessary to obtain a behavioral standard through consulting family and other community members and to develop definitions. These definitions are then compared with those given by the offender, and efforts are required to reconcile differences. Providers should be careful to qualify opinions they express in these efforts regarding both source and content, since this involves providing instruction on Indian culture.

The third area of assessment concerns involved stereotyped nonverbal communication patterns attributed to American Indians. One such example is that traditional Indian ways discourage direct eye contact. While this is a true statement in general for several tribal groups, much has changed for Indian people. It is recommended that judgments not be made to explain certain nonverbal patterns displayed during the assessment simply because a person is identified as being American Indian. Communication patterns are also directly related to learning styles, and it is generally stated that Indian people learn in different ways from members of the dominant society. Variables such as color, sound, movement, and vision have been found to be more important than verbal components; however, no single learning style was identified. A need is present to assess the learning variables for each person being evaluated and to choose materials and methods for the cognitive–behavioral programming based on this assessment.

Sexual offender treatment techniques often involve value clarification methods, and this is the fourth assessment issue to be discussed. Differences have been acknowledged between the American Indian societies and that of the dominate society in this chapter, and these differences translate into a dual system of social control for the Indian offender. Clinicians should not assume that there is a particular identification pattern or code that is superior, and as recommended in the discussion of identification it is necessary to allow individuals to choose between which code of conduct they feel is most appropriate for their needs. This choice includes a commitment to follow the code and display appropriate behaviors, and once the choice is made it should be reinforced throughout the treatment process. Providers need to be careful of the issues and beliefs that they bring to the assessment process regarding social rules and appropriate behaviors. This is necessary because providers need to confront thinking errors and value issues that have led to offending.

The final assessment area to be considered is a role of shame in the traditional Indian societies and the dominate society's methods of social control. As noted before in this chapter, traditional Indian values placed an emphasis on sharing shame. This process appears to have increased the responsibilities that individuals had to a wider social group, and it conflicts with the dominate society's tendency to assign blame as a way of removing responsibility. It often seems to traditional Indian people that members of the dominate American society seek to blame other individuals as a way to avoid having responsibility for undesired outcomes. This view is generally absent in the American Indian systems, as the social control network is responsible to assist each individual in making good choices and displaying appropriate behaviors. This value often involves therapy needs for the Indian family that may not be present in dominate society American families.

Cognitive–Behavioral Methods and Relapse Prevention

Very few individuals are skilled in dealing with both the cultural issues of American Indians and with the assessment of sexual offenders. As a result, it is often necessary to employee a team of individuals to complete assessment information. As previously noted, the offender treatment program described in this chapter was modeled from training provided by Judith V. Becker, PhD. Seven components were included in these efforts: satiation, covert sensitization, cognitive restructuring, anger control, social skills, sex education, and relapse prevention. Satiation is an exercise of verbally recording thoughts about inappropriate sexual behavior to reduce arousal levels, and covert sensitization is aimed at developing alternative responses to sexually acting out by addressing potential consequences. Few modifications were found necessary in these two techniques when dealing with American Indian offenders.

Cognitive restructuring involves the evaluation of sexual behavior to correct beliefs that could lead to further inappropriately acting out. This area was found to have several differences when treating American Indian offenders because of different belief patterns. It became necessary to identify these areas as part of the assessment, so appropriate decisions could be made regarding the advisability of outpatient therapy while the person was in the community. Different methods of anger control were also found to exist between the American Indian thought patterns and those of the dominate American society. Both patterns were often discussed in the group format, as individuals attending group had different identification areas. The same was true for socialization patterns and the mastery of appropriate social skills. This area was addressed in much the same way as anger control, with dual discussions from both ethnic points of view. Major differences were not found in addressing sex education, as both the American Indian and the dominate society views of sexuality tend to emphasize personal responsibility and how sex and feelings should work together. A related issue encountered was the lack of information regarding traditional patterns of sexuality and sex education. These patterns appear to have been lost to time by forced aculturalization and no solutions were found to replace this information. A text by Michael, Gagnon, Laumann, and Kolata (1994) was employed as a source of usual sexual behavior for adults in the general American society. Relapse prevention programs were generated on a similar basis regardless of the patients' identification areas, and considerable reference was made to the life graph throughout this process. Both individual and group settings were employed in treatment, and some individuals were treated in a combination of these methods.

Solutions for Substance Use Areas

It is frequently acknowledged that Indian people have severe difficulties with substance use (Herring, 1994). Indian people have recognized these difficulties and efforts have been made to develop treatment approaches that are culturally relevant. Arbogast (1995) provides information on one of the methods referred to as the "red road approach." This is an experiential process that assists people in identifying past traumas and then helps them search for solutions to the emotional pain they continue to project into their daily lives. Besides alcohol use, many offenders in this program were also the children of alcoholics and they presented several intervention needs because of these factors. Brown (1988) was employed as a source of information in defining these efforts, and many of these issues appeared in the life graphs presented by individual patients.

The Swinomish Tribal Community (1991) has identified a general pattern of depression, alcohol abuse, and destructive acting out in American Indian patients seen for mental health intervention. This same triad was routinely encountered through the present program, and the cognitive–behavioral methods noted above were used to treat substance abuse as part of the overall program. This was found to be preferable to fragmentation and referral to other program sources, and it appeared to be more appropriate to employ such a holistic philosophy. This philosophy is repeatedly represented in traditional beliefs of many American Indian tribal groups.

SUMMARY

The definition of who is an American Indian presents certain inconsistencies across tribal groups. This definition sometimes uses racial components such as blood quantum, and is also recognized to contain many ethnic issues. The ethnic issues are more important to understand and document in the assessment and treatment of the American Indian sexual offender. American Indian people have a long history that has been dedicated to beliefs and cultural patterns that differ from the dominate American society. They have suffered many traumas, which include boarding schools, exploitation, and loss of traditional language and behavioral patterns.

This chapter describes a treatment program that emerged from an adult outpatient mental health case load. The program began by treating adult victims, and then addressing the assessment and treatment of adolescent sexual offenders. The program continued by treating adolescent victims who were showing acting out and substance use problems, and it helped bring about changes in the tribal law enforcement code to include sexual offenses. With the change in the tribal code, adult offenders were also referred for assessment and treatment.

Providing services to the American Indian sexual offender requires an understanding of the historical grief and other violent behavioral patterns that have affected American Indian people. These events were defined under the general heading of trauma, and the need for a safe therapeutic environment was emphasized. Elders and other community people became a major source of support for these programming efforts. Assistance was received from other programming areas and administrative staff as the linkage between sexual victimization, health care, substance use, and other acting out behaviors was made. This process required considerable leadership efforts, and the demands placed on therapeutic personnel increased as this process continued.

Treating American Indian sexual offenders required the development of techniques that allowed services to address both their offending issues and other issues of victimization they had experienced directly or indirectly. The life graph procedure was developed to help address this issue, and cognitive–behavioral programming was also applied to areas of substance use and dependence. A specific program was implemented for treating sexual offenders as designed and instructed by Judith V. Becker, PhD. Areas of cultural differences were found to exist in the assessment process and in certain areas of the treatment programming. Major changes were not found to be necessary in implementing satiation, covert sensitization, and sex education components. The areas of cognitive restructuring, anger control, and social skills presented several cultural differences. Relapse prevention programs were developed within the framework of using the life graph system and by having offenders specify a system of social control they felt was most appropriate for them as an individual.

The use of therapy teams for assessment and treatment is advocated. There are two basic purposes for employing a team setting. One purpose is to provide support for the therapeutic staff, while the other purpose is to provide the expertise necessary in understanding Indian culture and sexual offending. Clinicians are also encouraged to develop their techniques for treating American Indian sexual offenders on the basis of needs presented by the offenders and to avoid taking specific stances regarding a superiority of either the American Indian or the dominate society's methods of social control. Appropriate definitions of prosocial behaviors can be developed for each offender through employing this approach, and the potential for positive treatment outcomes is increased.

ACKNOWLEDGMENTS. Dr. Ertz is a member of the Cheyenne River Sioux Tribe in South Dakota. The opinions expressed in this chapter are those of the author and do not necessarily reflect the views of the Indian Health Service.

REFERENCES

Arbogast, D. (1995). *Wounded warriors—A time for healing*. Omaha, NE: Little Turtle Publications.

Beane, S. (1995, April). *Broadening our perspectives in service to families*. Paper presented at the National Indian Family Preservation Conference, Phoenix, AZ.

Bennett, M.J. (1979). Overcoming the golden rule: Sympathy and empathy. In D. Nimmo (Ed.), *Communication yearbook three* (pp. 407–422). Austin, TX: International Communication Association.

Brendtro, L.K., Brokenleg, M., & Van Bockern, S. (1990). *Reclaiming youth at risk: Our hope for the future*. Bloomington, IN: National Educational Services.

Brown, S. (1988). *Treating adult children of alcoholics: A developmental perspective*. New York: Wiley.

Bryde, J.F. (1971). *Modern Indian psychology*. Vermillion: Institute of Indian Studies, The University of South Dakota.

Bunk, P.D. (1994, July). *Influence of parental coping on the psychological development of children following severe traumatization*. Abstract presented at the 13th International Congress of the International Association for Child and Adolescent Psychiatry and Allied Professionals, San Francisco, CA.

Courtois, C.A. (1993). Adult survivors of sexual abuse. *Primary Care, 20*, 433–446.

Hernandez, J.T. (1992). Substance abuse among sexually abused adolescents and their families. *Journal of Adolescent Health, 13*, 658–662.

Herring, R.D. (1994). Substance use among Native American Indian youth: A selected review of causality. *Journal of Counseling and Development, 72*, 578–584.

May, P.A. (1989). Alcohol abuse and alcoholism among American Indians: An overview. In T.D. Watts, & R. Wright (Eds.), *Alcoholism in minority populations* (pp. 96–119). Springfield, IL: Charles C. Thomas.

Michael, R.T., Gagnon, J.H., Laumann, E.O., & Kolata, G. (1994). *Sex in America*. Boston: Little, Brown and Company.

Middleton-Moz, J. (1989). *Children of trauma: Rediscovering our discarded self*. Deerfield Beach, FL: Health Communications.

Swinomish Tribal Community. (1991). *A gathering of wisdoms*. LaConner, WA: Swinomish Tribal Mental Health Project.

29

Australian Aborigines

Cultural Factors Pertaining to the Assessment and Treatment of Australian Aboriginal Sexual Offenders

Denise M. Cull and David M. Wehner

This chapter discusses the evolution of a sexual offender treatment program for the Aboriginal population in the state of Western Australia, Australia. The plight of the Australian Aboriginal has much in common with the Maori population of New Zealand, the Indians and Inuit of North America, and other indigenous populations. The initial section will briefly review the cultural and historical path of the Aborigines since colonization. This will provide the context for the establishment of a culturally appropriate sexual offender treatment program for Aboriginal men. The second section will detail the process of coming to terms with our inability to meaningfully assist the majority of this client group and our work with the Aboriginal community to develop a relevant approach to intervention with genuine opportunities to effect behavior change. The third section will describe the types of program offered and how they are implemented. The fourth section will discuss the critical importance of release to supportive environments and posttreatment follow-up. We offer our thoughts on this topic not as the "right path," but as a path we have traveled. We encourage others seeking to provide treatment services to indigenous populations to follow those paths that are most likely to assist their clientele.

COLONIZATION

Some stayed bush. Some went urban. Some went both ways. Many got lost.

Prior to the arrival of European settlers, the Aboriginals of Australia were a highly functional people who enjoyed a self-reliant subsistence, maintained clearly identifiable social groups and boundaries, lived life with meaning and purpose, and had a strong

Denise M. Cull • Victim and Offender Assessment and Treatment Services Ltd., Claremont, Western Australia 6010. **David M. Wehner** • Sex Offender Treatment Unit, Ministry of Justice, Northbridge, Western Australia 6003.

Sourcebook of Treatment Programs for Sexual Offenders, edited by Marshall et al. Plenum Press, New York, 1998.

identity based around spirituality, collectivism, kinship, and personal competence and ability (Pickett, 1994). It was the world's oldest continuously maintained culture (Flannery, 1994).

Under the 1788 English proclamation that Australia was *terra nullius* (an empty land), a process of colonization ensued that systematically assaulted and attempted to dismantle Aboriginal culture. The Europeans took the view that Aboriginals were an inferior people who lacked intelligence and whose culture was primitive and not worthy of being sustained.

Using the concept of English law and the array of force behind it, Aboriginal laws and customs were subordinated. Statutory measures aimed at the protection and control of Aboriginal people legalized the removal of their children from the family unit with a view to assimilating the children into Western culture. Reserves and missions were established and, eventually, Aboriginals were prohibited from entering into white communities, prohibited from cohabiting with non-Aboriginal people, and prohibited from consuming alcohol (Dudgeon & Mitchell, 1991; Pickett, 1994).

The paternal treatment of the Aboriginal culture continued throughout the 19th century and well into the 20th century. It was not until 1944 that Aboriginals were allowed limited citizenship rights. Under the Native Citizens Rights Act, individual Aboriginals were accorded the normal rights of citizenship including the right to drink provided that they could establish that they had adopted a civilized life, were not infected with leprosy or syphilis, could speak English, and were capable of managing their daily lives (Pickett, 1994). An additional proviso stipulated that Aboriginals who acquired citizenship could have no contact or association with family members who were ineligible for citizenship. These restrictions were not fully removed until full citizenship rights were granted in 1963. Only as recently as 1972 were Aboriginal people allowed a role in the governmental decision-making processes that affected them. Under the enactment of the Aboriginal Affairs Planning Authority Act, it became a statutory requirement that the Aboriginal people be consulted in all matters pertaining to their welfare.

The colonization process and its legal adjuncts had removed the Aboriginal from their traditional and spiritual base: the land. They lost their right to self-determination and their freedom to move about was curtailed. Their social and legal customs were undermined. In many instances, their children were taken from them. The woven fabric of Aboriginal kinship and social life became fragmented. Their normal methods of sharing and exchange were disrupted. Gradually, the use of alcohol became the commodity that facilitated the social exchange process (Kelly, 1993, 1994).

The period of "settlement" included the mistreatment, brutalization and, occasionally, the slaughter of Aborigines. The various laws enacted to control them frequently led to physical confrontations that almost inevitably led to the settlers acquiring that which they wanted—whether it was Aboriginal land, Aboriginal labor, Aboriginal women, or Aboriginal children (Atkinson, 1990a,b; Wilson, 1982). After decades of being subjected to this process, the cumulative effect resulted in collective disempowerment, with feelings of inadequacy, self-doubt, worthlessness, and self-hatred. Many Aboriginal people came to identify with the negative self-image that Western culture imposed on them (Pickett, 1994). The sense of pain, grief, and loss accompanying the loss of one's homeland, social status, and independence would be overwhelming for any individual, let alone an entire race. In this context the emergence of substance abuse, self-harm, neglect, and depression is not surprising. Nor are its concomitants: homicide, manslaughter, domestic violence, and sexual abuse (Wilson, 1982).

Various researchers and criminal justice agencies attest to the fallout. Aboriginal people are 20 times more likely to be arrested than non-Aboriginal people (Royal Commission into Aboriginal Deaths in Custody, 1991). They are also ten times more likely to be imprisoned. In August 1988, 29% of the 28,566 people held in some form of custody were Aboriginal, although they comprised only 1.5% of the national population. The number of Aboriginal people in prison between June 1987 to June 1991 increased by 25%. This increase was far greater than the increase in non-Aboriginal imprisonment (Paxman, 1993).

During the process of colonization, Aboriginal women frequently suffered physical and sexual abuse at the hands of white men (Daylight & Johnstone, 1986). However, as the process of cultural deterioration escalated, it became increasingly common for Aboriginal men (frequently affected by alcohol or other substances) to sexually assault and rape Aboriginal women and children. This development, and the horrific impact on the victims and on the Aboriginal community in general, has been well documented (Atkinson, 1990c; Bell, 1991; Bolger, 1991; Daylight & Johnstone, 1986). The lives of Aboriginal women and children have not only been brutally affected by white colonization, they have been further crushed and curtailed by the actions of Aboriginal men. The process has been aided and abetted by the perpetrators of these offenses who have claimed that traditional law sanctions much of their physical and sexual assaults (Lloyd & Rogers, 1993) and by a criminal justice system (defense lawyers and sentencing judges) prepared to support the proposition. An example of this collusion can be found in the sentencing remarks of His Honor, Justice Millhouse in the South Australian Supreme Court (*R. v. Wangkadi Munghilli*, 1991). Evidence was led that three men who were accused of the incestuous rape of an Aboriginal woman had acted in accordance with tribal law. Following conviction, the Honorable Judge stated in the sentencing remarks "There is no crime of rape known in your community. Forcing a woman to have sexual intercourse is not socially acceptable but it is not regarded with the seriousness as it is by white people" (p. 2). Lloyd and Rogers (1993) and Bolger (1991) provide substantial detailed evidence that such biased and unfounded commentaries are not unique events in Australian Jurisprudence.

Both Atkinson (1990a,b) and Bolger (1991) have criticized the justifications put forth by Aboriginal and non-Aboriginal men in support of the view that physical and sexual violence against Aboriginal women and children is sanctioned in customary law. In their review of sexual crimes against women, Lloyd and Rogers (1993) add support to this view on behalf of an array of Aboriginal groups and agencies representing the interests of the Aboriginal community. All of these researchers highlight the fact that most Aboriginal men and women are very clear on what constitutes correct social and sexual relationships and the types of relationships that fall outside the strictures of the kinship system and customary law. The vast majority of sexual assaults, rape, incestuous acts, and all child sexual assault are not supported within normal Aboriginal cultural and legal practices. Under Aboriginal law perpetrators of sexual offenses may be subjected to a range of punishments including banishment, spearing, or death.

The Aboriginal people have experienced a 200-year assault on their culture. The effect of this sustained attack has left their spiritual, social, and moral sense of connectedness impoverished, which, in turn, has resulted in extensive boundary breaching of both the white man's law and their own law. The problem is exacerbated by their marginalization in Australian society and their inability to establish economic security. This observation does not constitute an excuse for offending behavior but serves as a statement of fact. Without oppression, physical and sexual violence would still occur within this culture, as is the case with nearly all cultural groups. Regardless of the degree of provocation or sense of hopelessness, perpetrators of such aggression must be held accountable and bear responsibility for addressing their offensive behavior.

It is accepted that any attempt to alter the current rate of physical and sexual assault must include an awareness of the larger issues that facilitated the present crisis and an acknowledgment that they too must also be addressed. This, in fact, has begun to occur with the passage of land rights and racial hate legislation; the ongoing push to reduce substance abuse; and concerted efforts to improve education, job opportunities, community health, and housing. Only a holistic approach will suffice.

IDENTIFYING THE PROBLEM

Finding Our Way

In 1990, the Sex Offender Treatment Unit in Western Australia established a procedure for assessing and treating all sexual offenders who were under the supervision of the Ministry of Justice. Problems typically associated with the implementation of a new intervention inevitably emerged, most of which were gradually addressed and resolved without significant difficulty.

An area of ongoing concern, however, soon became evident within the process of assessing Aboriginal sexual offenders. An apparent cultural collision between this particular offender group and the non-Aboriginal (frequently female) staff from the Sex Offender Treatment Unit was preventing the assessment and treatment process from being appropriately and adequately implemented.

From our experience we realized that Aboriginal sexual offenders were encountering extreme embarrassment, shame, or anger when asked to speak of their offenses within the formal assessment environment. Often they would not attend when called for the assessment interview, or, once aware of the nature of the interview, would either (1) be cooperative but refuse to speak of their offending behavior; or (2) refuse, or be unable, to engage in any form of contact with the staff member concerned. Only occasionally did we encounter an Aboriginal sexual offender who was eager to participate in the assessment procedure and willing to carry it through to the treatment phase.

From time to time the Aboriginal offender would speak of his shame or other reasons for his refusal to discuss the specifics of his offending behavior, or of sexual matters generally. More often we encountered denial or an intense expression of anger. Sometimes the offender became mute—stuck within the difficulty of having no response.

The denial of responsibility for the offending behavior was frequently presented as a blunt statement of fact with an unwillingness, sometimes refusal, by the offender to discuss any aspect of the behavior associated with the conviction. The mute offender would become lost in his difficulty and offer nothing beyond a very clear desire to be elsewhere. The angry offender would typically direct his quite intense feelings toward the perceived presumption of the interviewer—or of "the system"—that we might even attempt to understand the cultural specificities of the Aboriginal offender group.

As a consequence of these difficulties, the outcome for the Aboriginal sexual offenders became very apparent when reviewed for parole suitability. Given that release to parole was heavily influenced by the offender having satisfactorily addressed the issues pertaining to his offending behavior, the need to seriously consider the case for the Aboriginal sexual offender was clearly significant and in the interests of both the community and the offender.

Having been unwilling or unable to participate in treatment, these men, with very few exceptions, collectively were becoming identified as a group highly likely to remain incarcerated beyond their earliest expected date of release. A quite noticeable experience of helplessness and hopelessness, not inconsistent with their personal and cultural history, was emerging. As a consequence, some definable issues for prisoner management became evident, not the least of which was the effect on the prison muster. The increasing number of angry prisoners who were becoming quite voluble in their claims of discrimination and injustice was similarly of concern for administrators. The validity of their complaints was accepted by senior management on advice from the Sex Offender Treatment Unit.

As a consequence, a working party was formed whose brief it was to review the cross-cultural issues and difficulties and to determine what, if anything, we could offer this particular offender group. The working party comprised four staff members from the Sex Offender Treatment Unit and two professional Aboriginal people who worked in related areas.

Pursuing the Process

The first task of the working party was to address a range of questions of concern and to clarify the more specific issues with which we were commonly confronted when attempting to assess and occasionally treat Aboriginal sexual offenders. These questions and issues included:

1. How much validity could or should be placed on the claim that cultural implications negated the need for sexual offender treatment programs for Aboriginal sexual offenders?
2. How much credence should be given to the assertions that non-Aboriginal female staff members either could not or should not attempt to understand the multiplicity of issues that allegedly underpinned sexual behavior per se and/or sexual offending within the Aboriginal culture?
3. Should our standard assessment protocol and treatment design be modified to cater to the cultural differences, most particularly with regard to the use of psychometric instrumentation?
4. How valid was the claim that Aboriginal shame was so great it would inhibit both the assessment and the treatment process?
5. Does the geographic territory with which the Aboriginal sexual offender identifies (predetermined according to tribal ancestry or familial settlement) determine a range of different attributions toward the sexual offense and would these differences undermine treatment issues?
6. Were some sexual offenses committed by Aboriginals considered normative within their culture, thereby negating the need for treatment, or were such claims, in fact, a new range of cognitive distortions and avoidance strategies hidden under the umbrella of cultural difference?
7. Would the high levels of illiteracy with this particular client group prevent meaningful intervention?
8. Similarly, should an Aboriginal sexual offender be excluded from treatment due to cognitive impairment, frequently the result of the abuse of alcohol or other substances?

The aims and objectives of the working party were to ascertain the validity of these issues and to determine how, if at all, we might attempt to meet what appeared to be a quite daunting challenge.

Making Connections

The next task for the working party was to enter into a program of self-education in order to quell our ignorance and to ascertain the validity of the issues that had been identified. The information and advice provided by the members of the working party who were of the Aboriginal culture were extremely valuable and highly respected. Their interest, preceded by initial caution, resulted in significant contact being made with other members of local Aboriginal communities, some of whom occasionally attended our meetings. From them we began to clarify and explore the issues with which we were regularly confronted. They facilitated our contact with members of the less-readily accessible Aboriginal communities, emphasizing the significance of talking with and listening to these people, most of whom had something important to offer. Under their direction, a questionnaire was devised that was taken into the communities by Aboriginal workers who raised the issues with the tribal elders. The nature of the information being sought related to both deviant and nondeviant sexual behavior within Aboriginal tribal communities.

As a consequence, the message that we began to consistently hear was that members of the communities despaired for the future of the men who committed these and other serious offenses; they despaired for the integrity of the Aboriginal culture in its pure form, and for the well-being of the Aboriginal families who needed the men to be home taking their role in the community. However, they also desperately wanted women and children to be safe.

The Aboriginal people with whom we made contact were typically eager to establish a collaborative approach to resolving the many problems we had jointly identified. However, in wanting to work with us, they also wanted some assurance as to our integrity. They wanted their voice to be heard along with ours. Within the context of our contacts, we became aware that our motives, our openness, and our capacity to respect their ways was continually being assessed.

Through these early connections, it is our understanding that information pertaining to our attempts to provide a solution to the problem spread from one community to another. We were advised that we had been accepted and could be trusted; that our concern was accepted as genuine; and that we had something to offer that would help, not only to bring their menfolk home, but also help them learn how to live differently and bring safety to the community. History, however, has taught the Aboriginal people to be wary of "white man's interventions," and we could never presume that, once accepted, our line of communication might not be revoked at any time, should we give cause through our intervention and attempts at mediation.

The process of making contact moved from the metropolitan area into the various regional centers. Links were made with some of the tribal communities who sent their leaders to listen, to (sometimes) talk, but certainly to always be assessing our motives. A delicate process ensued, each step forward requiring a consultation and consolidation phase with members of the Aboriginal communities. Mistakes were inadvertently made. We believe we learned from those errors of judgment and we appreciate the tolerance and understanding that these people gave to our sometimes inadequate attempts to understand their cultural norms.

During our discussions, the originally identified issues were continually raised, the general consensus on each being described below. These are necessarily generalizations; as with any group study, individual differences will inevitably be presented. The information gleaned was extremely valuable and always viewed within the wider cultural context and the destructive events since 1788.

Should We Attempt to Treat Aboriginal Sexual Offenders?

The outcome of the communication process embarked on by the working party clearly reinforced and supported our perception of the need to proceed with assessment and treatment procedures. In doing so, we clearly had the acceptance and the encouragement of the wider Aboriginal community. Their support was integral to the acceptance of our efforts by the offenders themselves. Sexual deviance was not accepted within their culture.

Gender Issues

Contrary to general belief, the alleged difficulty for Aboriginal men in speaking of sexual matters with female staff members is not supported by the Aboriginal community as a valid objection on cultural grounds. In fact, in Aboriginal communities, many sexual matters are considered to be "women's business," with the women having responsibility for issues pertaining to this area.

Furthermore, as a consequence of having persisted with our efforts to assist this offender group, we have found that, given a supportive and safe environment, the Aboriginal sexual offender generally will not be too greatly troubled by the presence of a female staff member—either during the assessment process or treatment itself. Exceptions, of course, will always present themselves. All treatment groups are co-facilitated by a male and a female for very sound reasons. The same reasoning applied to Aboriginal sexual offenders. While some Aboriginal sexual offenders experience difficulty speaking of sexual issues with females, so too do some non-Aboriginal sexual offenders. We acknowledge, however, that the extent of the difficulty is more frequently greater with the Aboriginal offender. It is the task of the interviewer, or the group facilitator, to facilitate the flow of information with sensitivity and persistence. The safety of the community necessarily overrides individual discomfort.

Psychometric Instrumentation

Information provided by Aboriginal psychologists and other similarly trained professionals confirm the difficulties in using psychometric testing procedures with this particular client group. While the Multiphasic Sex Inventory and the Minnesota Multiphasic Personality Inventory–2 are our instruments of choice for assessment purposes, neither of these are intended for use with a culture of this nature. We have been advised that when required to respond to questions through selection of true–false or multiple choice answers, a majority of Aboriginals would do so in a manner that invalidates the outcome. Furthermore, the language and terminology is frequently inappropriate with this particular client group and, with the possible exception of those well-educated Aboriginals who have assimilated fully into the non-Aboriginal community, most would experience difficulty in attempting to respond according to the expectations of the test. The need for flexibility within any assessment situation certainly applies with Aboriginal sexual offenders. Consequently, the administration of psychometric instrumentation has occurred sparingly and cautiously with this particular population.

Issues of Shame

Shame is widely acknowledged as being deeply experienced by many Aboriginal men who have been convicted of sexual offending; however, while the experience is valid, it should not necessarily be problematic to treatment. Given a safe and sensitive treatment environment, the offender can usually be supported through the experience of shame.

The fact that shame is so readily experienced may impede the more clinically defined assessment process. Consequently, extreme sensitivity needs to be used when speaking of the offending issues at that time. A willingness to modify the standard assessment procedure is necessary. Once the issue of treatment suitability has been determined, it is important in some instances not to proceed beyond the point of essential relevance by attempting to obtain full factual details of the extent and breadth of the sexually deviant activity (a significant departure from the normal assessment process). This can be dealt with far more appropriately and sensitively within the context of treatment or in a pretreatment interview with the people who in fact will be the treatment facilitators.

While shame certainly is an issue, it need not and in fact should not preclude any offender of any culture from the opportunity of treatment. We have been encouraged by Aboriginal consultants to not waiver in the task when this issue is presented and to proceed (with cultural awareness), trusting that shame will take care of itself within the treatment environment. All interested parties agree that community safety is a priority over individual discomfort.

Territoriality

With the progression of time and our persistent attempts to assess and treat the Aboriginal sexual offender, we have observed a number of them who can cope satisfactorily with standard assessment procedures and who adjust well to the mainstream treatment options. These men typically have lived within a metropolitan or rural–urban environment and have basic literacy skills.

Aboriginals who most typically experience difficulty with the assessment or standard treatment procedures tend to be those who choose to live on the fringe of both cultures. While their bonding within their own subculture is cohesive and particularly strong, they often present as troubled people, on the edge of two quite different cultures. Assessment for treatment suitability can be difficult for these men, as they are frequently unsettled and angry and ready to challenge the "white man's law" and its applicability to them. Participation in any of the mainstream sexual offender treatment programs can be effective, given a willingness to apply themselves to addressing the offending behavior; very few, however, have chosen to take advantage of the opportunity in the past. Frequently, the tendency has been for them to regard themselves as "different" and to promote the belief that treatment is unnecessary or that it would not be suitable for their particular needs. This issue was integral to the decision to provide culturally appropriate programs.

Tribal and/or desert Aboriginal people typically live their lives ensconced within the cultural traditions of their people. They have their own system of law that is respected and rigidly enforced. Many of these men cannot participate in any of the standard treatment programs, and consequently face the duality of both Aboriginal and white man's punishment without accessing any form of assistance that would reduce the risk of reoffense.

Culturally Specific Issues in Sexual Deviance

Sexual offending against children is never condoned within any Aboriginal community. Cultural customs do exist in some tribal communities, however, that would cross legal principles of European law. For instance, some young females are promised in marriage to older men, when they enter puberty. Many of the initiation rituals associated with "going through the law" for adolescent males would be considered sexually inappropriate or deviant within non-Aboriginal cultures. A process of "payback" is accepted within the Aboriginal culture with, for example, the rape of a sister entitling the brother or other male family member to reciprocate against the perpetrator's relevant family member. These acts must be sanctioned by tribal elders. Some culturally specific beliefs (for example, that women who drink with the men are "available" for sex) may have become normalized over time; however, these are not necessarily sanctioned by the community or the tribal elders.

While acknowledging the reality of these culturally accepted practices in some Aboriginal communities, participation in treatment can still assist the offender to address issues pertaining to his lifestyle generally, to challenge distortions that may exist surrounding the behavior, and to consider the impact of his actions on the victim or young participant. Although the practice may possibly be considered acceptable in Aboriginal law, the offender is encouraged to look closely at the motives for his involvement in the activity.

From our discussions with members of the Aboriginal communities, we have been encouraged to persist with challenging many of these alleged culturally specific practices. The need for a sensitive and sometimes cautious approach to the challenge is accepted as necessary and realistic if the treatment intervention is to have any impact. Challenge from within the group by his Aboriginal peers is frequently the most effective means of determining whether a participant is attempting to distort his particular offense situation.

Illiteracy

Literacy levels are frequently problematic with this offender group. With the exception of the intensive treatment option, the treatment groups are able to accommodate to the special needs of the illiterate participant. By facilitating the assessment of treatment needs early in the sentence, the offender may choose to access educational opportunities during his incarceration as he is awaiting treatment, which by design is scheduled for the latter stage of the sentence plan. The intensity and depth of therapeutic exploration within the full-time treatment option necessitates extensive written work and an ability to read without too much difficulty. People falling short of this standard are encouraged to improve their literacy skills and on entering treatment are paired with another program participant who will aid and support this individual in the completion of his reading and homework assignments.

Cognitive Impairment

Cognitive impairment is a significant challenge for both Aboriginal and non-Aboriginal sexual offenders and this remains to be addressed fully within the resource constraints of the Sex Offender Treatment Unit. There is available a specific intervention program directed at intellectually impaired sexual offenders within the metropolitan area; however, the culturally specific difficulties continue to be relevant for the Aboriginal sexual offender population who experience the additional impediment of being cognitively impaired.

As a direct result of the consultation process, two culturally specific treatment programs have been established: a permanent Aboriginal position within the Sex Offender Treatment Unit has been created, and two Aboriginal contractors have been recruited to co-facilitate the treatment programs. With the availability of these new options, a far greater number of sexual offenders from this particular cultural group now have appropriate opportunities to address their offending behavior.

CURRENT PROGRAMS

Aboriginal Men Find Their Way

Aboriginal sexual offenders now have access to a variety of treatment options within Western Australia. During the assessment process, the various treatment options are discussed with each offender. They include participation in the intensive treatment program (5 days per week for 6 months), participation in a prerelease treatment program (3 hours per week for 6 months), or participation in a community-based treatment program (3 hours per week for 8 months). These programs operate within a continuum of care model (Marshall, Eccles, & Barbaree, 1993), with those offenders posing the greatest degree of risk receiving additional treatment. Therefore, some offenders may complete treatment at all three venues, while others may complete treatment at only one venue. For those Aboriginals who choose the mainstream option, we endeavor to place more than one Aboriginal offender within the group to facilitate comfort, support, and culturally relevant challenging within the group environment.

In addition to the risk assessment, all offenders are also assessed for their ability to participate meaningfully at a nominated treatment venue. The intensive treatment program requires a comparatively higher rate of literacy, familiarization with Western culture, fluent English-speaking ability, and normal intellectual ability. The prerelease and community-based programs are suitable for nearly all individuals, except those who have extremely limited English-speaking ability, little or no knowledge of Western culture, and extremely limited intellectual ability.

Many Aboriginal men have met the requisite criteria to participate in these programs, but we acknowledge that both the content and process were at times not sensitive to cultural issues. As a consequence, the working party was formed, leading to the introduction of culturally specific treatment groups. Aboriginal men who meet mainstream program requirements are offered the opportunity to participate in those programs or in the culturally specific program. There are a small number of Aboriginal men who meet the entrance criteria for the intensive treatment program and are considered to be at extremely high risk of reoffending. These men are not offered access to the culturally specific program in the first instance. They may access that option, however, following participation in the intensive treatment program.

There are two treatment venues (Broome Regional Prison and Greenough Regional Prison), both of which are well outside the main metropolitan area, offering the culturally specific programs. Both operate as prerelease programs and meet for 3 hours per week over a 6-month period. All group members, and at least one of the group facilitators, are Aboriginal.

As with mainstream sexual offender treatment programs offered by the Ministry of Justice in Western Australia, the intervention process is driven by the relapse prevention model of treatment (Pithers, Marques, Gibat, & Marlatt, 1983). This model is well described within the literature (Freeman-Longo & Knopp, 1992; Marlatt & Gordon, 1985; Pithers & Cumming, 1995) and will not be detailed here. The basic tenet of the model is that people develop maladaptive behaviors in response to internal and external stressors. In order to gain control over the target behavior(s), the individual needs to acquire an understanding of the life experiences that have influenced the maladaptive behavior and the thoughts, feelings, and actions that promote and maintain that behavior. He must then identify those situations in which the unwanted behavior is most likely to occur and devise alternative prosocial responses that will assist him to maintain control over his urge to engage in activity that may lead to relapse.

In adapting the relapse prevention model to the Aboriginal population, special care is given to ensuring that the underlying concepts are explained in culturally relevant terminology, including the use of audiovisual aids depicting Aboriginal people. Particular emphasis is given to discussion of family histories. Many Aboriginal men were taken away from their family of origin in childhood and raised in church-based missions administered by non-Aboriginals. Alternatively, they were raised by foster families (typically non-Aboriginal). Many also were raised in impoverished conditions where violence and substance abuse were rife. For these men substance abuse and aggression may have been normative, and it is essential to understand whether they wish to continue to subscribe to that "norm." The treatment implications are obvious.

The participants' reactions to their childhood situations are equally important. Although the majority of men have difficulty in expressing their feelings, this difficulty is more pronounced with Aboriginal men. It is essential that these men be given repeated opportunities at self-expression. This can be facilitated by having them describe people or activities that are of interest to them and gradually to ask them to identify the feelings associated with those activities. This process can proceed in stages to where they eventually discuss unpleasant issues. As previously discussed, care must always be given to issues involving feelings of shame for the individual.

Group participants are encouraged to describe life processes or thoughts associated with their inappropriate behavior in a variety of ways (e.g., use of a translator, use of artwork, or use of audiotapes). In our experience we have found "buddy" systems are much more frequently utilized with this client group. Sometimes a fellow participant is utilized to help a colleague talk through his experiences and feelings prior to sharing them with the group or committing them to paper. On some occasions a colleague or a group facilitator may be requested to write down the content of an offender's story.

Within the relapse prevention framework at Broome and at Greenough, particular emphasis is given to the role of substance abuse in acts of violence and sexual aggression. It is our experience that the vast majority of inappropriate aggression occurs during a state of intoxication. Group participants will offer a wide variety of explanations for their use of drugs and alcohol. A common theme is that substance abuse is an integral aspect of family and social life. Each individual is encouraged to explore the costs and benefits of this lifestyle. For those intending to alter their lifestyle, a very significant amount of time is spent supporting the offender in constructing appropriate postrelease activities and behaviors. Constructing alternative behavioral responses that can be consistently applied in the external environment in the face of high-risk situations is the most difficult task for these clients.

POSTRELEASE

Negotiating the Future

The importance of posttreatment follow-up is repeatedly stressed by experts in the management of sexual offending behavior (Pithers & Cumming, 1995). New behaviors learned within the relative isolation of the prison environment or within an ongoing community group are inevitably strongly tested when the client returns to his usual environment and routine. Offenders of all cultures have consistently stated that the threats to maintenance of treatment gains are nearly always stronger than they had envisaged. Their ability to call on third-party support has been crucial to resisting invitations to reoffend. For this reason, treatment maintenance groups have been established. Attendance at these groups affords offenders the opportunity to meet with a supportive group and to discuss the various issues that may lead to potential offending situations. These groups work well for both Aboriginals and non-Aboriginals in the metropolitan area. However, resource limitations and the tyranny of distance (Western Australia encompasses 2,525,500 km^2) precludes our ability to offer this service to outlying areas. For rural locations, emphasis is placed on coordinating postrelease follow-up with local supervising corrections officers and, where relevant, the community leaders or tribal elders.

As previously indicated, many Aboriginal sexual offenders have grown up and lived in environments where substance abuse and various forms of aggression are the norm. Returning to such an environment, in and of itself, constitutes a high-risk situation. Others may have a relatively stable and supportive home environment but come under pressure to engage in risk-taking behavior with extended family members or friends. To resist engaging in the various activities of these groups carries the risk of ostracism. Without appropriate social support the offender could easily become socially isolated. The various options are not encouraging. The offender could: (1) return to his former high risk-lifestyle; (2) associate with his friends and relatives but not share in destructive activities, which, of course, will result in social isolation; or (3) find an entirely different social environment, which may well involve leaving the family of origin. Given the strength of kinship and the extended family system, as well as the significant spiritual association with their land, all of these choices are fraught with difficulty. Additional to his specific social situation, the offender frequently faces a number of the usual challenges: finding employment, housing, health services, and so forth. The need for ongoing support (and the offender's willingness to use it) is critical and will frequently strongly influence whether or not he commits further offenses.

In discussing postrelease plans, it is essential to alert the client to the realities that confront him. This process can be significantly aided by inviting previous program participants, who have successfully completed treatment and returned to the community, to meet with the current client prior to his release and share their experiences of the difficulties encountered upon their release from prison.

CONCLUSIONS

The initial consultation process has long been finished. The support and encouragement received from Aboriginal elders, leaders, and community members at all levels have been extremely valuable. Throughout the course of providing information and enhancing our knowledge, an even more important process has been facilitated at a different, more subtle, level. While we sought guidance from them, they sought credibility and integrity from us. We believe that, at each step of the way, our efforts, our approaches, our mistakes, and our naivety were continually being assessed by those with whom we connected. Could they trust us? Were we prepared to listen to them? Was this merely lip service covering a political imperative? How seriously did we really want to understand the issues?

We believe this process occurred at each point of contact and has been mirrored within the prison environment over the past 5 or 6 years as we have gone about our task of assessing and treating sexual offenders. We have been watched, changes have been observed and noted, and our reliability and trustworthiness have been continually under scrutiny. It would appear the word has spread that as individuals we are "OK," and that what we are doing is acceptable. However, the greatest reflection of the credibility of the program has been demonstrated by the greatly increased number of Aboriginal men who have taken the step and chosen to participate in the assessment and treatment process. Prior to these changes, less than 30% of convicted Aboriginal sexual offenders were engaged. Currently, 68% choose to participate in treatment. Their word and the demonstrated change in behavior apparently have been accepted by their Aboriginal peers that what we offer is worthwhile.

REFERENCES

Atkinson, J. (1990a). Violence in Aboriginal Australia: Colonalization and gender. Part 1. *The Aboriginal and Islander Health Worker, 14*(2), 5–21.

Atkinson, J. (1990b). Violence in Aboriginal Australia: Colonalization and gender. Part 2. *The Aboriginal and Islander Health Worker, 14*(3), 4–27.

Atkinson, J. (1990c). Violence against Aboriginal women: Reconstitution of customary law—The way forward. *Aboriginal Law Bulletin, 2,* 6–9.

Bell, D. (1991). Inter-racial rape revisited. *Womens Studies International Forum, 14,* 385–412.

Bolger, A. (1991). *Aboriginal women and violence: A report for the Criminology Research Council and the Northern Territory Commissioner of Police.* Darwin, NT: Australian National University, North Australian Research Unit.

Daylight, P., & Johnstone, M. (1986). *Women's business: Report of the Aboriginal Women's Task Force.* Canberra: Australian Government Publishing Service.

Dudgeon, P., & Mitchell, R. (1991, September). *Internalized racism and drug abuse: Some consequences of racial oppression in Australia.* Paper presented at the Australian Psychological Society Conference. Adelaide, South Australia.

Flannery, R. (1994). *The future eaters.* Chatswood, NSW: Reed Books.

Freeman-Longo, R.E., & Knopp, F.H. (1992). State of the-art sex offender treatment: Outcome and issues. *Annals of Sex Research, 5,* 141–160.

Kelly, K. (1993). *Contextualizing the problem of Aboriginal alcohol abuse.* Unpublished honors thesis, Department of Psychology and Sociology, James Cook University of North Queensland, Townsville.

Kelly, K. (1994, September). *De-myth-tifying Aboriginal use of alcohol.* Paper presented at the Conference of the Council of Remote Area Nurses of Australia, Cairns, Queensland.

Lloyd, J., & Rogers, N. (1993, October). *Crossing the last frontier: Problems facing Aboriginal women—victims of rape in Central Australia*. Paper presented at the Conference on Without Consent: Confronting Adult Sexual Violence, Melbourne, Victoria.

Marlatt, G.A., & Gordon, J.R. (1985). *Relapse prevention*. New York: Guilford Press.

Marshall, W.L., Eccles, A., & Barbaree, H.E. (1993). A three-tiered approach to the rehabilitation of incarcerated sex offenders. *Behavioral Sciences and the Law, 11*, 441–455.

Paxman, M. (1993). Women and children first. *Alternatives Law Journal, 18*, 153–157.

Pickett, H. (1994). *An historical overview of models of addiction*. W.A. Alcohol and Drug Authority and Centre for Aboriginal Studies, Curtin University, Western Australia.

Pithers, W.D., & Cumming, G.F. (1995). Relapse prevention: A method for enhancing behavioral self management and external supervision of the sexual aggressor. In B.K. Schwartz & H.R. Cellini (Eds.), *The sex offender: Corrections, treatment and legal practise* (pp. 20-2–20-32). Kingston, NJ: Civic Research Institute.

Pithers, W.D., Marques, J.K., Gibat, C.C., & Marlatt, G.A. (1983). Relapse prevention with sexual aggressors: A self-control model of treatment and maintenance of change. In J.G. Greer & I.R. Stuart (Eds.), *The sexual aggressors: Current perspectives on treatment* (pp. 214–239). New York: Van Nostrand Reinhold.

R. v. Wangkadi Munghilli. (1991). Unreported. South Australian Supreme Court: Port Augusta.

Royal Commission into Aboriginal Deaths in Custody. (1991). *Final Report*. Canberra: Australian Government Publishing Service.

Wilson, P.R. (1982). *Black death, white hands*. Sydney, NSW: Allen and Unwin.

30

Treatment for Hispanic Sexual Offenders

Pablo E. Moro

Arlington County, Virginia, is a diverse community of over 184,000 residents, approximately 14% of whom are Hispanic immigrants. Most of the newcomers are from Central America, the majority being from El Salvador. The Arlington County Juvenile Sexual Offenders Program is a community-based program that is part of the county's Child and Family Services Division. It treats adolescent sexual offenders and abuse-reactive children (children who molest), as well as provides evaluations for adult sexual offenders. The program includes offender-specific treatment services for low- to medium-risk offenders and incorporates an interagency approach to the provision/delivery of services. It focuses on enhancing community safety by identifying the more serious sexual offenders who require out-of-community placement in a secure environment; by providing intervention/prevention for lower-risk offenders who are able to remain in the community while receiving offender-specific treatment to prevent the development of more serious offending behavior; and by ensuring continuity of care/enhancing community safety by continuing treatment for those offenders released from state correctional centers and who return to the community. The program includes risk assessment (sexual aggression assessment) and psychoeducational groups, as well as ongoing group, family, multifamily, and individual therapy to English- and Spanish-speaking clients. It uses a cognitive–behavioral approach and works in collaboration with other child-serving agencies in the community. The majority of referrals originate from the juvenile court and most clients have already been adjudicated for sex crimes. Close contact is maintained with other agencies working with the offenders such as probation, school, social services, the police department, and so forth. The program also provides consultation and training to other community agencies.

ASSESSMENT AND TREATMENT

The first step for all clients who are referred to the program is to receive a risk assessment (sexual aggression assessment). This evaluation serves to identify whether the

Pablo E. Moro • Arlington County Juvenile Sexual Offenders Program, Child and Family Services Division, Arlington, Virginia 22205.
Sourcebook of Treatment Programs for Sexual Offenders, edited by Marshall et al. Plenum Press, New York, 1998.

client presents a pattern of deviant sexual behavior and how serious the problem is and it makes clear recommendations about treatment and any other interventions that may be necessary. Those clients who are determined to be lower risk and appropriate for a community-based setting are accepted into the program. This only occurs if and when the juvenile court supports the clinical assessment and the client is court ordered to "successfully" complete treatment.

Treatment consists of four different phases, each including a number of components. Offenders graduate from the program when they complete the four phases and show significant positive changes at home, school, and in social situations. They are expected to be honest, responsible, understand their sexual offending problem, and demonstrate the ability to manage it.

History of the Program

The program was created to address a gap in community services. Through training and direct clinical experience, it was recognized that specialized services were necessary to work effectively with perpetrators. When sexual offenders were referred for therapy, they posed challenges to the therapists. Therapists found it difficult to treat offenders using "traditional psychotherapy" and questioned its effectiveness. In an attempt to better serve the needs of the community, it was decided that the adolescent population would be prioritized. This was done because it was believed that there would be better success with adolescent offenders and it would prevent them from becoming adult offenders. To do this, the mental health center pursued grant funding through the Department of Criminal Justice Services. Intensive staff training was established as an important component to program development and a national expert was contracted to provide ongoing consultation. Another integral component was the establishment of an interagency advisory board made up of various agencies (i.e., mental health, substance abuse, health services, school, police department, social services, and commonwealth attorney, juvenile probation, and a regional representative of the state from the Department of Youth and Family Services, a liaison to the grantor). Its purpose was to draft and oversee protocol, policy, and procedures and to elicit collaborative ownership.

Funding

The grant funding received by the center was one full-time employee position for 4 years, with the county assuming 50% of the funding for the fourth year of operation and incorporating 100% of the funding into its budget upon the fifth year. Being a "one full-time employee" program brought risky implications. The risk of having a program so small is that it was initially viewed as too specialized, serving too few clients. It became necessary to demonstrate that sexual offender treatment was rather an integrated component of a larger child and family unit, which in fact served many clients. The program relied a great deal on the other agencies to support the continued offender treatment. It also had to bring to light its preventative value, which included: (1) financial savings in preventing costly residential placements by providing appropriate community interventions for youth; and (2) a result of treatment being the prevention of the development of adult perpetrators. Overall, the program had to prove there was mutual recognition of the need of such a service, that it was qualitative, and that it would have a cost savings effect. This need was supported by the fact that the program focused on community safety by identifying those high-risk sexual offenders. Such a service had not been available and proved to be one of the significant assets of the program.

Importance of the Assessments

One of the most unexpected factors at the start of the program was the importance of the risk assessment (sexual aggression assessment). By using such a thorough evaluation, client risk level is identified. This tool is of significant use in identifying high-risk offenders and in enhancing community safety. The problem was that a large percentage of the perpetrators were higher risk, and thus could not be treated in the program. Of all the cases referred, about 25% of the offenders were higher risk and needed to be treated in a residential facility. This made the leverage used by the court a crucial aspect in appropriately evaluating sexual offenders as well as being able to provide the necessary treatment.

SYSTEMS ISSUES

Referrals

In the first year of operation, there were numerous obstacles to overcome. One of the first obstacles was receiving sufficient referrals. Even though several agencies had been involved in the creation of the program, the number of referrals was very low. Part of the problem revolved around the fact that offenders had to be adjudicated and court ordered in order to receive sexual offender treatment in this program during the first 2 years of its operation. In many cases, adolescents did not make it that far through the court system. Referring agencies often did not realize that charges had to be pressed against the offender and that the case needed to go through the court. There was also ambivalence by the referring agencies because of the length of time the court process often takes, whether such a process was really necessary, and whether the offender should go through such an experience. In some cases, referrals without the crucial leverage of legal litigation were attempted with the hope that the case would automatically be taken. The consequence was that the program was not viewed as practical or time efficient and few referrals were made.

There was a misperception that this was a "catch-all program" that took all cases related to sexual acting out. Often, these cases would not fit an appropriate referral. In many situations, whether adolescent or adult, there was hope that the case would somehow be taken automatically, even without court litigation or a strong suspicion that abuse had taken place. Additionally, there was an inclination to refer Spanish-speaking clients because of the limited resources available and because of the knowledge that the treating therapist was Hispanic.

As important as it was to build a good reputation, boundaries had to be established in selecting clients. The parameters of the program were expanded to create a balance that could serve other agencies without jeopardizing the program. For example, while designed as a juvenile program, adults were accepted for assessments. More importantly, efforts were made to serve as consultants to any case of sexual abuse. To do this required the flexibility of being accessible to discuss cases (at times extensively) and/or visit other community agencies.

Location and Space

Finding space at the mental health center was a task in and of itself. Inadequate office space had been a problem for years. Finding space required sharing offices, which meant that hours had to be fit in to somehow not conflict with other therapists who were using the same space. For the offender program, it was even more complicated because it was preferable that a separate area be used. Optional sites within the Department of Human Services were considered, but factors such as easy access to children and insufficient security were deterrents. As open as other therapists were to treating sexual offenders, there remained a sense of uneasiness and concern about this population. Some of the concern had to do with the possibility that incest cases (perpetrator–victim) might have unplanned contact with one another in the lobby or the hallway. It was unclear how the perpetrators or the victims would react to such a situation. To avoid potential contact with perpetrators, therapists who were treating victims were notified of the date and time when sessions were held and scheduled their clients accordingly.

Another concern materialized in the sharing of offices: This concerned the possibility that non-sexual-offender clients might react to viewing the treatment materials displayed in the office such as treatment books, flip charts that identify treatment components, cognitive distortions, cycle of abuse, relapse prevention, and so forth. Because of this, whenever the office was not in use, the materials had to be covered.

Community Outreach

Another problem presented during the start up of the program was the lack of knowledge in the community about the services. This meant that the staff had to make numerous presentations to a variety of professionals. When doing this, it was difficult to present juvenile sexual offenders as clients needing treatment and explain the court process necessary to assure they received this help. While there were many reactions and opinions about sexual offenders, there were two that stood out. It was questioned whether "treatment" was too easy and a way out for offenders instead of punishing them for their behavior. There were also doubts about the difference between sexual offender treatment and psychotherapy. In some situations, it was difficult for people to accept that there was a difference. In other cases, the court process combined with sexual offender treatment was seen as punitive. Overall, it seemed that despite any information or knowledge given, many professionals had their own judgments and prejudices about sexual offenders, and it was clear that it would be very difficult to influence the stereotypes that existed.

In this early stage, the program placed much emphasis on providing training to community agencies. The advisory board developed a work plan for informing these agencies. As a result, presentations were carried out in a systematic and repeated manner to the police department, probation counselors, schools, social services, and commonwealth attorneys.

Stereotypes

It is important to be aware that just because the terms *Hispanic*, *Latin American*, or *Latino* are used in the United States, they do not fairly describe all Spanish-speaking people. Even though the word *Latino* is known, when asked about their heritage, immigrants are not likely to say "Hispanic" or "Latino." They will say Bolivian, El Salvadorian, Peruvian, and so forth. We had to be sensitive to the reality that there are over 20 Spanish-speaking countries with different histories, dialects, ideas, and beliefs. While the Spanish language in these countries is similar, these are independent nations that have their own customs. Often, Spanish-speaking people are grouped together as Hispanics or Latin Americans. Having knowledge about the different cultures can be quite valuable in understanding the clients we treat.

A major challenge seen in working with Hispanic sexual offenders was the perception by the community that this ethnic group was more frequently involved in sexual offenses. The stereotype of Latinos as sexist womanizers and "machistas" who have no respect for women was prevalent. When sexual harassment took place, it was often too quickly assumed that the perpetrator was Hispanic. Unfortunately, such views were common and unfairly portrayed Latino culture in a negative light without considering the cultural issues involved.

In the struggle to become culturally informed, it was common to see the system react in two opposing and extreme views about Hispanic offenders. One attitude was to ignore and minimize the behavior. This was more than the "boys will be boys" idea. It was an attitude based on the idea that because the culture was *machista*, sexist, and male dominant, inappropriate sexual acts by males were to be expected. The other view was one that suggested offending behavior in general was to be expected in Latinos. The common perception of Hispanics as *machistas* made them easily targeted as sexual predators.

This attitude seems to interfere with the ability of other agencies to fairly assess a situation. The program continues to struggle with this belief and the fact that about half of the referrals are Latino clients, when Hispanics make up only about 14% of the population in Arlington County. A possible explanation for this is that Latino families have difficulty with the accessibility to services, which could prevent contact with the court. They may not receive adequate representation when a family member commits a sexual offense. Hispanic families in the program tend to show a lack of understanding and knowledge of American culture and society. This is not to deny that many clients referred are guilty, but to point out that along the way the adolescent could have received some intervention that may have prevented the offense from taking place or perhaps received better legal representation. It is important to note that for many Latino offenders, our program is the first mental health intervention they have received in their lives. This is in contrast to middle-class American children who may be more likely to get some kind of early intervention, which could prevent the offending from progressing.

Community Issues

The reality in Northern Virginia is that there are a limited number of programs or a continuum of care services for sex offenders. If an offender is lower risk, the Arlington program can provide the necessary intervention in most cases. Problems occur, however, if the offender is incestuous or is one who is acting out at home and needs a more structured environment. There is a lack of alternative housing for offenders that would allow placement in a community-based program rather than a residential setting. Group homes are not available for offenders, many having shut their doors because of the liability issues and risks involved. As a result, therapeutic foster homes have been used in some cases, although these are very difficult to find and tend to be very costly. They also require much effort in educating foster parents who are not likely to have knowledge of sexual offenders.

Relatives have been used as alternative placements, bringing about many concerns. Usually, the parents select the home and there is very little information available about the relatives. The relatives also tend to be reluctant to get involved in the program and may not provide the necessary monitoring of the offenders. In the end, such homes have shown to be more risky and problematic. This is an area of continued concern and there appears to be little interest in either opening doors to offenders in group homes or in creating such a group home.

The child-serving systems are not prepared to provide support for families that come from very traumatized backgrounds. Agencies easily become overwhelmed by the juvenile Hispanic sexual offender, who brings with him a host of traumas in multiple areas of his life. One incest family by itself may require numerous interventions. The identified needs can include but are not limited to: the adolescent who sexually abused someone in the family; his sibling/victim who was abused; the father who may have an alcohol problem and/or may be physically abusive with his wife; the mother who is likely to have her own history of sexual abuse and is battered by her husband; and a lack of sociocultural adjustment adds to their stressors and the whole family is often in a state of disequilibrium.

There is a lack of comprehensive services for the offender and the offender's family. Because of this, it is rare that the entire dysfunctional incestuous family can be treated, at least by the same mental health provider. In these kinds of cases, either only part of the family is treated or the treatment is divided among several providers. While in most cases working with other therapists who are working with the same family is not an issue, it can create complications in situations in which the other therapist(s) has little training in working with sexual offenders. When only part of the family can be treated, it raises concerns of how the other untreated family members could affect the recovery of the offender. To complicate matters more, treatment will likely be long term, costly, and most of the families are unable to pay for it. Several of these families alone are enough to overwhelm any mental health provider.

TREATMENT ISSUES

Traumatic Experiences

In our work with sexual offenders, we have found that it is very common for the offenders to have experienced some kind of trauma. The most frequent traumas seen in the program are neglect and sexual and physical abuse. In working with Hispanic sexual offenders, there are two additional traumatic areas frequently evident: (1) living through a civil war and a chaotic social environment; and (2) undergoing harmful separations during childhood, particularly when coming to live in the United States.

Many of the Central American countries have endured extensive periods of instability, violence, and suffering. In many cases, significant atrocities took place that the young offenders and their families encountered. These included witnessing the torture of others, including family members, watching people being taken away, seeing dead bodies in the street, or knowing about the death of a loved one. In some cases, the offenders may have witnessed rapes or other abuses. At the very least, there was usually a fear of the unknown, a fear that perhaps they or one of their family members would be harmed. This was a life of constant tension and unpredictability of the future.

Separation issues seem to be very common with the Hispanic offenders. Within our program, parents were frequently separated from their children at an early age and most of the adolescents did not have fathers who took responsibility for them. Mothers were often left to care for their child, usually with the help of their parents or relatives. The fathers often had little contact with their sons and offered minimal emotional or financial support. Additionally, when trouble broke out in their native land, many families desperately tried to flee the country, having little preparation to do so. In most cases, it was not possible for all of them to leave together. This meant that the mother would come to the United States first to establish herself and slowly bring the rest of the family. As she worked and saved money, she would send these savings home to bring one or two of her children at a time to the United States. This process often took years and brought many hardships for the families. Once the children came to join the family in the United States, they often had a great deal of resentment against their mothers for leaving them behind and the mothers often experienced strong guilt feelings. Commonly, adolescents have expressed feelings of being conflicted about leaving home behind, being happy and angry to be with their mothers, having difficulty adapting to a totally different culture, and finding even more changes in their families. Generally, the mother had remarried and the adolescent had a new father and new siblings. He no longer received the attention he recalled getting and became envious of his siblings, who seemed to take all of his mother's time. In the incestuous cases in the program, it has been found that much of this anger is redirected against the offender's new little sister or brother, who the offender ends up sexually abusing.

Cultural Issues

The majority of Hispanic clients in the program have come from homes of origin where they lived very simple lives in rural areas of their country. Their lifestyle was slow, and the common means of supporting a family was working the land. A large number were illiterate or had received minimal schooling by the time they came to the United States. One of the first problems the therapists in the program encounter is the ability to communicate with the adolescent or his parents, even in Spanish. As with each country, there are many words used that are unrecognizable and certainly cannot be found in a Spanish language book. It is a challenge to explain to a family that their son is a sexual offender, is a risk to the community, and to the other siblings, and that he needs to be separated from the family or that he has to be incarcerated. The court process itself, which can be confusing to Americans, is often overwhelming to immigrant families. These families crave some explanation or clarification that they may never receive, even with a Spanish-speaking translator. This is not to blame the court but to point out that there are few people with cross-cultural experience working with these challenging families.

There are characteristics that are generally evident in Latino sexual offenders. A common ritual or passage to manhood experienced by our program participants is having sex with a prostitute during early adolescence. Sex with prostitutes has been found to vary in frequency, although it tends to continue, even if randomly, into adulthood and marriage. This sexual experience appears to often be accepted and considered to be part of normal life. This behavior was evident in the case of a perpetrator in the program who had sexually assaulted a younger same-sex peer, and his parents decided that his father would take him to a prostitute to teach him to be a "man."

There are many situations seen in which families live in overcrowded quarters. In such cases, it is more likely that the adolescents have seen or heard their parents or relatives in sexual situations. Adolescents often would admit that at a very early age, they watched some relative having sex. In some incestuous families, the adolescent reported that he and a cousin or brother would try sexual acts with their younger sister or brother or cousin.

In numerous cases, the families of the offenders are poor and have jobs that require them to work for much of the day, leaving the children alone at home. This means that they are left in the care of an older relative or are unsupervised for long periods of time. There seems to be a pattern in which they have been more vulnerable to victimization by others.

Assessment

When a therapist attempts to get certain psychological tests such as the Minnesota Multiphasic Personality Inventory (MMPI) or some tool such as the Multiphasic Sex Inventory (MSI) for use with Hispanic offenders, they will typically find them useless. The education level in these testing tools is too high, ends up confusing the adolescents, and does not provide the data needed. It should also be noted the MSI is available in audiotapes, which can be helpful in some cases. However, the Spanish used is Castilian, or specifically from Spain, and may not be appropriate for many clients.

Treatment

In creating the first group of adolescent offenders, there were complications that occurred. These had to do with putting all of the Hispanic clients together in the same group. In meetings with the family and juveniles, the communication was mostly in Spanish. Therapists assumed that all Latino clients could be placed in the same group. The problem came about with adolescents who were bilingual and had spent several years living in the United States. This group expressed themselves better in English and preferred to speak English. Once in the group, communication was difficult with other group members who were more recent immigrants and who did not speak English well and could only express themselves in Spanish. It should also be noted that there were differences found that went past the language barrier itself. The attitude, behavior, and expression of the recent immigrants (1 to 5 years) and those who had maintained close ties with their own culture was quite different from the Hispanic adolescents who had lived in the United States longer or had assimilated into American culture. In many ways, those who spent more years living in the United States were similar to American youth. When these clients were placed in a Spanish-speaking group, they did not blend in together as well as they did with the English-speaking clients.

In a group setting, the Latino clients are typically more cohesive and supportive of each other than are non-Hispanic adolescents in a similar group situation. There seems to be a genuine concern for each other and an effort to make sure the group works together. It is unclear if this is because of their common background (country of origin, language, new immigrants) and/or because Hispanics are more community-oriented people. It also may be that having a Hispanic therapist contributed to the cohesiveness of the group. This raises the question of how the group would have reacted to a Spanish-speaking American therapist and what other differences, if any, would be evident.

Another important characteristic that is different and is seen with the Hispanic offenders is their ability to confront each other. They usually are more willing than non-Hispanics to point out and discuss the lack of responsibility or distorted thinking presented by someone in the group. It is also uncommon for a Latino offender to act in a defiant manner. They show much *respeto* (respect) even during very tense and emotional situations.

During the assessment process and throughout treatment, the Latino clients are usually found to be more honest and forthcoming with information about themselves, which was

not expected. In contrast, American offenders typically struggle when talking about masturbation and deviant sexual fantasies, whereas Hispanic clients usually openly discuss such
topics individually or in a group situation. This is also true of situations in which clients
disclose their deviant sexual behavior to their parents. It seems that once in the program,
they develop a sense of trust that facilitates volunteering a great deal about themselves.

Working with the Family

In our experience, when it comes to situations in which the Latino family is threatened,
they are extremely protective of the family unit and of allowing anyone in. In cases of
sexual abuse, it is unlikely for a parent to report the abuse. In most of the cases seen in the
program, the abuse allegations came from outside the family (school, neighbor, etc.). In the
few cases in which a parent reported that their son had abused a younger sibling, there was
significant criticism from relatives. This pressure from the relatives often continued
throughout the time that the adolescent was in treatment. The Latino families seem to
believe that turning in your own to the police is wrong and goes against their cultural value
of unconditional support.

The common ways families deal with sexual abuse varies, depending on the victim. If
it is within the family, the older brother is likely to "get a beating." The parents may in
some cases seek the advice of an elder in their community (e.g., a priest) who is respected. It
is important to note that there may be little communication between the parents and son
(perpetrator), and that the family may end up not doing much more than trying to tell their
daughter or son (victim) to make sure to tell next time and/or to take care of themselves and
not to be alone with the perpetrator.

This protection of family secrets can be troublesome when trying to find out about a
history of incest in the extended family. Parents are reluctant to give such important
information and it is often not until many months into the treatment that they indirectly
disclose that there had been incidents of a relative who had "played too much with the
children" and that everyone had known that they probably should not leave their children
with this person.

The tendency of the family to protect the perpetrator may be the biggest problem for
those providing the treatment. Parents are unable to give such awful details about their
children. Therapists need to keep in mind that for the parent, the child is a reflection of
themselves. If anyone were to find out that their son committed such an act, it would look
terrible for them as parents and as a family. Offenders themselves are generally more
reliable in providing valuable facts about pornography use, family secrets, or other abuse
allegations.

Respeto (respect), a central value of Hispanic culture, which means respect for elders
and those in authority, is a common issue in dealing with the family. During therapy,
parents are very polite and cooperative and will likely agree to what a therapist may say.
This does not mean they are going to follow through. This is actually a superficial
cooperation, because the parents do not want to be "disrespectful." In an evaluation, the
parents often present their son and family as normal. They may leave out important
information about the family or acting out behavior by their son. They may also reassure the
therapist that their son does not have a sexual offending problem. In order to get past this
barrier, it is imperative that the therapist is able to join with the family and to educate them
about the benefits of their cooperation in their son's treatment.

Treatment may be more effective if the first few sessions with such a family is informal, to give the parents an opportunity to relax. The fact that they are having to come to therapy at all is threatening by itself. It is even worse that the therapist is someone who specializes in sexual offending. This can be a good opportunity to ask the family about their native land and learn from them. It is not unusual to have all children show up for the meeting, as well as an uncle or aunt or grandparent. These first few meetings can set the stage for how invested parents will become. Making the therapy formal will often distance the parents and will hurt the needed alliance that is most beneficial in the recovery of the offenders.

For most of the people from rural backgrounds, therapists can be seen as psychic counselors. The family does not understand the profession and would probably believe that to see a therapist, one must be crazy. Mental health professions are not well understood. To make matters worse, at least one parent may work two jobs, making it difficult to have both participate. Usually, only the mother will show up and will be reluctant to consistently attend treatment. A court order is very helpful, although it can bring suspicion and resentment against the system.

To be able to join with the parents and have them support their son's treatment can bring the most success. This, however, means that the therapist should present him- or herself in a very open and nonthreatening manner. The object at first will be to make them feel as comfortable and as safe as possible. Explaining the court process and answering questions can serve significantly at this time. It may also require helping the family with other problems they may have as immigrants, which usually involves taking the time to explain things such as school, jobs, assistance, or anything that may not be related to their son having a sexual offending problem. It may require referrals to other agencies or perhaps doing some of the simple legwork that they are unable to do on their own. The therapist should also stress from the beginning that they do not work for the court, that they are on the family's side, but that together, they have to work on creating safety. Still, it is difficult for the parents who have a son who is a sexual offender, which will bring into question what they did wrong as parents. In this situation, the therapist can find many ways to alleviate the strain on the parents and again have them accept treatment. The therapist can initially take the blame off the parents by using the television or the media as potential sources that influenced offending behavior. They can also talk about the changing society and increasing presence of sex and violence. The adaptation to the new culture and shock it created to their child can also be explained. Last, it should be made clear to parents that they are not coming to treatment, but that they are coming to education classes or courses to learn about this problem and not because they are poor parents or are in need of therapy. It may appear that this only promotes distorted thinking. However, the program has found that by having the parents invested, it is easier for them to later disclose about their son and the family, as well as have an open mind to accepting their responsibility in their son's deviant sexual behavior.

Lack of Materials

A source of much frustration at the start of the program was that insufficient materials were available for working with Latino sexual offenders. Except for one small workbook, most of the resources were in English. Even using the available workbook in Spanish was a problem because it was geared for adults and required a certain degree of schooling. Available material required a language and culture translation, which was time consuming. The additional complication of the lack of education of the clients made it difficult to use the different treatment components with the Spanish-speaking offenders. For example, the cycle of abuse can be translated, but there is the problem of understanding each of its parts and the time it requires to teach it, particularly for an outpatient program that only meets on a weekly basis. As a result, the program had to take the time to reshape these different components, such as the cycle, to best meet the needs of the clients. Materials from workbooks and conferences have typically not been useful or have had to be changed to be used in the program.

EFFECTS ON THERAPISTS

The work with the offenders from Central America offered a rude awakening to the horrors of civil war. Little is known about these countries and few are aware of their past or present history. It was and still is difficult to believe how the families and their children have survived emotionally. One of the problems when encountering such clients is that when the program first started, there were times that the therapist fell in to the trap of feeling sorry for the perpetrators. Doing this undermined and rationalized the seriousness of the sexually abusive behavior as well as had the potential to affect clinical decisions and interventions.

The staff also felt a sense of helplessness because of how needy the families were and the reality that the program was limited in how much it could do for them. Each family required a significant amount of energy. Taking too much time and effort with one case took away from what could be given to others. Finding a balance in the services to all families in the program was and is an ongoing frustrating struggle.

For the Hispanic therapist, caution had to be used in order to not overidentify with this clientele. With a majority of Hispanic cases coming to the program, the clinician sometimes found himself on the defensive, attempting to explain why so many "Hispanics" were perpetrators. There also was a sense of disappointment and anger when finding out there was yet another Latino sexual offender and that the statistics would continue to overrepresent the Hispanic culture. It was important to make sure such feelings did not influence the clinical judgment used in treating these clients.

CONCLUSIONS

The Arlington County Juvenile Sexual Offender Program has had a great deal of success. This, however, has come as a result of careful planning, support, diplomacy, and effort. Over the years, there were numerous situations in which it seemed that the program would fold or that treating sexual offenders appropriately in the system was not possible. The presence of experts in this field (Jonathan Ross and Dr. John Hunter) helped to guide the program in the right direction. Along the way, their clinical experience was of critical value. The Advisory Board also played an important role in the program in the collaborative work with other agencies. A key aspect that may have made the largest difference was the support from the court. There is no doubt that much of the reputation of the program came about by gaining the confidence of the court. One element of this success was the referrals made by the probation officers and the second, and more significant, element was the court's willingness to comply with the recommendations made by the program. The willingness of the court to accept what may appear to be unusual requests (violations for attendance problems, lack of participation, following treatment guidelines, etc.) provided the necessary leverage to encourage offenders along the way in their treatment.

Successful sexual offender treatment is clearly not just carried out in the office, but with the collaboration of other agencies. Treatment has been a team effort involving various systems. However, to work with these various systems, which may not always be open to others, required an open attitude, communication, flexibility, and a great deal of patience.

31

Community-Based Sexual Offender Treatment for Inner-City African-American and Latino Youth

Robin L. Jones, Mark X. Winkler, Elymar Kacin, William N. Salloway, and Marsha Weissman

INTRODUCTION

There is considerable evidence that traditional psychological interventions are less success-ful with minority and socioeconomically disadvantaged populations than with Caucasian and middle-class clients (e.g., Berry & Annis, 1988; Boyd-Franklin, 1989; Comaz-Diaz & Griffith, 1988; Sartorius, Pedersen, & Marsella, 1984; Suc & Sue, 1990). For example, minority clients are less likely to voluntarily seek psychological treatment in traditional settings, less likely to attend appointments, and less likely to complete treatment with a positive outcome in such settings. Thus, there is a distinct need for mental health and social service programs to develop and nurture treatment contexts that are responsive to clients' cultural backgrounds and economic circumstances. This is especially relevant to programs that serve criminal justice populations, owing to the disproportionate number of minorities in the criminal justice system and the compulsory nature of participation required by mandated treatment.

The Project for Rape and Abuse Prevention (Project RAP), located in New York City, is a community-based program for adolescent sexual offenders. Since the vast majority of youth and families referred to the program are African American or Latino, efforts have been made to develop services that directly meet the needs of a youthful inner-city minority population. Indeed, the planning and development of Project RAP has created an ideal opportunity to pilot creative initiatives in this area. The model and context of Project RAP are now described, as well as the characteristics of the clients served.

Robin L. Jones, Mark X. Winkler, Elymar Kacin, William N. Salloway, and Marsha Weissman • Project RAP, Center for Community Alternatives, New York, New York 10011.
Sourcebook of Treatment Programs for Sexual Offenders, edited by Marshall et al. Plenum Press, New York, 1998.

PROGRAM DESCRIPTION AND CONTEXT

Project RAP offers a combination of intensive offense-specific therapy and case management supervision for 13- to 17-year-old male sexual offenders. It is one of several programs at the Center for Community Alternatives (CCA), a private, nonprofit organization that develops and promotes alternatives to incarceration. Project RAP is staffed by a clinical director, two case managers, and a part-time therapist. It offers a 12-month intensive phase and a 12-month follow-up for 16 to 20 families each year. Most referrals come from the courts and probation. Exclusion criteria are limited to factors that clearly contraindicate community-based treatment, such as severe learning difficulties or an excessively high-risk assessment profile. After a comprehensive assessment of the youth's suitability for services, a "client-specific" treatment plan is prepared for the court. Project RAP staff are available in court to advocate for a youth's release to the program. Most youth enter Project RAP as an alternative to detention or as an alternative to incarceration (i.e., placement in a juvenile institution). Finally, the program provides regular progress reports to the court or probation.

The therapy component of Project RAP consists of offense-specific and life skills group sessions for the youth, support and education groups for parents and guardians, adjunctive individual or family therapy, and follow-up relapse prevention groups. The case management component consists of court advocacy, crisis intervention, assistance with school and residential resources, home visits, monitoring a curfew, and accessing other services. Several additional opportunities are available to the youth through other programs at the CCA, including a human immunodeficiency virus (HIV) peer education program for youth, biweekly "Choices Unlimited" workshops where regular guest speakers offer inspirational/motivational material, and drug testing (urinalysis) of RAP participants where needed.

CLIENT CHARACTERISTICS

Since its inception in early 1994, Project RAP has worked intensively with 31 male youth and their families. All but 10% have been either black (65%, mostly African American and a few Afro-Caribbean) or Latino (25%, predominantly from Puerto Rico or the Dominican Republic). The overrepresentation of minorities exists in spite of a growing awareness in the field that sexual offending cuts across all ethnic groups and socioeconomic levels, and reflects the disproportionate numbers of minority youth in the juvenile justice system.

All youth in Project RAP have been male, with a mean age of 15.1 years, ranging from 12.8 to 17.0 years old when referred. Three quarters of the sample were convicted of sodomy (35%) or rape in the first degree (20%), or attempted rape/sodomy (20%). The remainder were convicted of lesser charges such as sexual abuse in the first or second degree, some which had been bargained down from more serious charges, to facilitate a plea of guilty and avert a trial. The majority of cases were processed within the Family Court system; however, 22% of the youth were convicted as juvenile offenders in the Supreme Court (adult criminal justice system) and potentially faced very long custodial sentences. Fifty-two percent of the families referred to Project RAP had a past or current open case with the city's child welfare agency.

Exactly half the sample had committed their crimes against male victims and half against female victims. Male victims tended to be younger (mean 6.9 years) than female victims (mean 9.1 years). Seventy-one percent of the sample abused siblings, nieces, nephews, or cousins, including partial or nonblood kin in blended family situations. The remainder had abused children or peers who were known to them but unrelated. Two thirds of the youth were convicted for molesting a single victim, 20% had molested two, and 13% had molested three or more victims. One in every five of the youth offended in conjunction with a codefendant, and one in every three utilized direct physical force in the commission of the crime. Ten percent of the sample had been offending for a year or longer when apprehended.

One in every five of the youth had a history of prior arrest for nonsexual allegations in all but one case. Fifty-two percent had been suspended or expelled from one or more schools on account of behavior problems, and 29% were in special education classes. Ten percent were functionally illiterate when referred.

In terms of family characteristics, 57% of the youth still lived with one or both parents (45% with their mother, 6% with their father and 6% with both parents). The others lived either with relatives or in group homes or residential drug treatment centers. Biological fathers shared the household with 12% of the youth in our sample, and a further 29% still had some form of access to their biological fathers within their communities. This illustrates that although the fathers were often not present in the household, they were still somewhere within the youth's social sphere in almost half the cases. Further, one third of the youth's households included some form of "father figure" other than the youth's biological father, for example, an uncle or a stepfather.

Almost all Project RAP youth (91%) had a history of parental loss, primarily through separation or divorce, but in some cases due to parental incarceration, death, or abandonment. In half the cases at least one parent had a known criminal history, and 63% of parents had a past or present substance abuse problem, principally alcohol, heroin, or crack cocaine. For most cases in which the drug problem was ongoing, the parent was either unavailable or unprepared to follow through on drug treatment. Sixty percent of the youth had witnessed chronic violence within the home, and half disclosed having experienced physical abuse.

At the time of writing, 40% of the youth had disclosed a history of sexual abuse in their own lives; however, a significant number are still early in treatment, and this figure is likely to increase. Of special significance is that the same proportion of youth reported female abusers (17%) as male abusers (17%). Seven percent reported a history of abuse by both males and females. A range of female perpetrators were reported, including older female cousins, babysitters, mothers' friends, and women in their 20s or 30s whom the youth at least superficially viewed as "girlfriends." Since our sample consists predominantly of incest and incestlike offenders, it may be that abuse of boys by female perpetrators is an especially strong predisposing factor toward adolescent incest offending.

A number of positive resources were available to the youth and families in our sample, either in the community or extended family. This is in spite of the fact that four of every five of the youth lived in neighborhoods where drug sales and other criminal activity frequently took place. A little over half of the youth's households were supported by a parent in full-time employment, and 26% of the parents or guardians were furthering their education through part- or full-time study. Forty-five percent of the parents or guardians reported having access to at least one supportive person within their family or social network who knew about the youth's offense; interestingly, the closest support person was not always the spouse or partner of those in a permanent relationship. A quarter of parents or guardians had strong connections with spiritual resources in the community such as churches or mosques.

In terms of positive resources available to the youth, upon referral 35% were already involved in organized after-school or weekend activities, none that provided access to high-risk environments for reoffending. These included part-time work, church or mosque activities, sports teams, art programs, or youth social clubs. Several youth also showed considerable unrealized talents in these and additional areas such as "rapping," "rhyming," and writing poetry. Many youth not involved in positive activities when referred showed a strong interest in developing their talents should a suitable resource be identified in their community.

Collectively, these client characteristics demonstrate considerable personal, social, environmental, and economic problems for the population served by Project RAP. They also demonstrate some resiliencies and strengths, of which intervention strategies also need to be cognizant.

A cognitive–behavioral approach combined with group and family therapy underpins the Project RAP treatment approach. A range of adaptations in the areas of staffing, program environment, assessment, and treatment methods have expanded the model to facilitate direct responsiveness to the specific needs of an inner-city minority client group. Collectively, these adaptations are consistent with the multisystems approach for black families advocated by Boyd-Franklin (1989). They are also consistent with guidelines on cultural sensitivity in the Revised Report from the National Task Force on Juvenile Sex Offending (1993). Initiatives and adaptations in the four areas mentioned above will be examined in turn, together with problems, solutions, and further suggestions.

STAFFING CONSIDERATIONS

Project RAP is a small multiethnic team. Since the clinical director was hired in early 1994, past and present staff (including interns) have generally been balanced among African American, Afro-Caribbean, Caucasian, and Latino and also equally balanced for male–female representation. These proportions are consistent with the ethnicity of all CCA staff.

The diversity of staff in all CCA programs has significantly protected Project RAP from problems that commonly arise in workplaces when a predominantly Caucasian staff works with predominantly minority clients. Such problems may include insufficient cross-cultural expertise among Caucasian staff, underrepresentation, marginalization or burnout of minority persons on staff, and the monocultural definition and application of treatment models (Pedersen, 1988). These are important concerns for sexual offender treatment programs, since very personal family and sexual matters are especially likely to be culturally influenced.

The following sections offer suggestions to prevent such problems and are offered on the basis of our experience, as well as on the team's view of the "ideal" responses if sufficient resources could be made available.

Increase Culture-Specific Knowledge of All Staff

Staff can be encouraged to read and discuss clinical and applied cross-cultural and ethnic psychology literature and to examine ways in which new principles and practices can be built into existing treatment approaches. While direct applications to sex offender treatment are only just beginning to emerge in the published literature, generic cross-cultural material still offers many possibilities that can be adapted for use with sexual offenders. This parallels the process by which aspects of generic psychotherapy and family therapy continue to inform many aspects of sexual offender treatment. Very useful cross-cultural resources include Berry and Annis (1988) on ethnic psychologies, Boyd-Franklin (1989) on interventions with black families, Comaz-Diaz and Griffith (1988) on cross-cultural mental health, McGoldrick, Pearce, and Giordano (1982) on ethnicity and family therapy, Pedersen (1988) on multicultural awareness, Sue and Sue (1990) on cross-cultural counseling, and Taylor-Gibbs and Huang (1989) on interventions with minority children and youth.

Staff can also be encouraged to read and discuss contemporary and historical socio-political literature. This may be especially helpful for increasing the understanding of the nonminority staff about the experiences and perspectives of minority individuals, in turn allowing empathy to more effectively bridge the cultural gap between therapist and client. It also facilitates more genuine dialogue between minority and nonminority staff on racial and cultural issues and their impact in the workplace, on clients and colleagues alike. A vast range of titles are available in the areas of African-American studies and Hispanic studies.

Programs and agencies also can encourage staff to join cross-cultural and multi-cultural counseling or therapy organizations, to facilitate learning, dialogue, and training opportunities. Multicultural trainers could be invited into the workplace to provide staff training workshops on diversity issues. Such workshops need to offer a variety of angles and starting points. For example, in many organizations minorities are underrepresented in management and overrepresented among line staff, and thus issues and perceptions of what is needed may diverge along hierarchical lines. In these instances, McGoldrick et al. (1982) point to the particular need for management staff to be targeted for diversity training, since attitude change at that level will most rapidly reduce institutional barriers affecting minority staff and clients alike. Training opportunities need to be repeated and cumulative, to reinforce efforts and ensure maintenance and generalization of the concepts learned (Pedersen, 1988).

Cultural sensitivity and expertise could be included as a performance indicator in annual staff performance reviews, and upward feedback as well as downward feedback could be built into the evaluation system. Upward feedback could be especially valuable in workplaces where most line staff are minorities and most managers are Caucasian.

Seek Culture-Specific Supervision

Another area of suggestions to improve culture-specific expertise in the workplace is in the area of staff supervision. Senior staff could seek culture-specific supervision and consultation to guide decision making and policy development, through peer supervision with minority colleagues within and beyond the organization, and/or regular consultation with a multiethnic committee or council with special expertise in multicultural consulting.

Peer supervision opportunities need to be created in the workplace so that cultural issues and concerns for both clients and staff can be safely and routinely discussed. This will be especially necessary as efforts to increase minority staff representation meet with success, since new expectations, values, and beliefs regarding minority clients' needs and program policies may increase accordingly.

Project RAP staff have utilized some of these methods to address diversity issues.

Staff regularly read and discuss cross-cultural clinical material and have established regular weekly staff meetings in an off-site location conducive to relaxed, expansive discussions of program and case-related issues. The multicultural nature of both the team and the client group has meant that cultural issues and concerns are routinely raised, since they are part of the backdrop to many of the other matters that need to be addressed. Many times different perceptions of the same incident have been productively discussed, with the understanding that different members of the team are likely to be able to see or "sense" different things based on their own experience and expertise, some of which is culturally determined. A mutual learning process has therefore been facilitated.

A similar initiative has been to organize 1-day "retreats" every 4–6 months for the team. A work-related focus has been combined with a social or cultural event. The retreat is focused on refining the program's mission statement, reviewing the large-scale goals, and brainstorming ways to narrow the gap between the "ideals" and the realities within the limits of scarce resources. Notably, several of the more creative adaptations to program structure and content originated from discussions at retreats or staff meetings off-site. The retreats have also facilitated cultural expertise within the team not just by direct means (e.g., discussion) but also by strengthening the relationships between staff members of a culturally diverse team and increasing trust and communication.

Develop Culturally Diverse Teams

Cross-cultural studies of culture-matching in therapy indicate that treatment outcome tends to be better when the ethnicity of the therapist is similar to or matches the ethnicity of the client. It appears not to be race or skin color per se that determines this finding, but rather the depth of knowledge and understanding of the client's cultural norms, values, and concerns that the therapist can bring to the situation (Comaz-Diaz & Griffith, 1988). Therefore, another avenue to address the need for culturally skilled staff is to increase the representation and influence of minority people at all levels in the workplace. In addition to offering a direct, immediately visible cultural connection for minority clients, strong minority representation in the workplace provides another direct source of cross-cultural learning for nonminority staff.

A common institutional barrier to increasing minority influence in the workplace is the underrepresentation of minorities among graduates with masters and doctoral level qualifications. Several suggestions are offered to prevent this barrier from overwhelming efforts to increase minority presence in senior and influential positions in the workplace.

Mechanisms to help identify suitably qualified minority applicants could be enhanced through bilingual recruitment efforts and recruitment through minority professional organizations such as the Association for Black Social Workers and the Association for Black Psychologists, as well as community organizations that have a strong affiliation with the black and Latino communities. *The Black Resource Guide* (1991) provides comprehensive nationwide listings of resources and organizations. Word of mouth through existing minority colleagues may be especially helpful.

Sufficient value needs to be placed on culture-specific knowledge when hiring. Boyd-Franklin (1989) asserts that culture-specific knowledge and experience need to be treated as a prerequisite (rather than a desirable extra) for positions in programs with a high proportion of minority clients. It needs to be ranked alongside education and work history. If staff roles and responsibilities are defined in keeping with this emphasis, particular jobs may then be especially likely to attract minority candidates. For example, Project RAP case management positions are defined in ways that naturally play to the strengths of many minority candidates, such as mentoring and outreach dimensions, and the provision of bilingual services.

Existing minority staff members could be offered incentives to continue their studies if they do not already have graduate degrees. The workplace could offer flexible work hours, as well as clinical opportunities and supervision by appropriately qualified existing staff, so the current job can accommodate internship requirements. It may also be helpful to work closely with colleges and universities, especially those with high minority student ratios or strong cultural studies departments, and offer student placements for existing clinically oriented programs.

ENVIRONMENTAL CONSIDERATIONS

It is very important to adapt program settings to be environmentally accessible, attractive, and responsive to an inner-city minority youthful population. The setting needs to communicate that it is specifically for them, rather than just another part of an impersonal social or criminal justice bureaucracy. Project RAP's environment has been conducive for the youth and appears to have contributed to a high attendance rate. Although community based, many of CCA's initiatives could be adapted for use in residential settings.

Location and Transport

If possible, the program needs to be located within the youths' own community. If not, travel monies may need to be reimbursed. In Project RAP, subway tokens are made available, and at times it has also been necessary to utilize case managers as escorts to and from the agency for youth who are in restrictive residential treatment settings.

Decor and Layout

It is extremely helpful to have design and decoration details that cater to the interests of a multicultural client group. Helpful touches at CCA include having bilingual reception staff, telephone messages and signs in more than one language, posters and displays on the walls reflecting aspects of African-American, Caribbean, and Latino culture, and magazines in the waiting area that are intended for a minority readership. A play area is available for small children, and a range of activities is available for the teens including games, computers, a workout machine, TV/VCR, and music in one of the multipurpose rooms.

Food and Drink

Offering food and drink can be very helpful for increasing client rapport and comfort levels, for example, before or after groups or partway through a long assessment. It is also especially important for the teenagers, not only because their stage of development determines that they are constantly hungry, but also because not all the families can afford to give the youth enough money to buy something substantial to eat at school during the day. CCA has a fully equipped kitchen, and meals or snacks can be made available to clients at short notice. The parents of the youth in Project RAP have been especially grateful for their teenagers being fed when they attend after school, and the youth and parents alike have appreciated choices of food that acknowledge their cultural values, likes, and dislikes.

Security

The programs at CCA have operated very much from a position of trust and individual responsibility concerning security. While obvious precautions are taken, the open plan layout of the agency has mitigated against a high-security atmosphere. Stealing or other breaches of trust by clients have been rare; most incidents or losses have been due to the actions of persons not affiliated with the agency's programs. In view of all programs having a criminal justice population most whom have felony convictions, it is particularly noteworthy that the atmosphere of trust has been largely respected.

Project RAP youth generated their own set of rules for conduct, which included refraining from bringing drugs, alcohol, or weapons into the agency, and ensuring that clients and staff are treated with respect.

ASSESSMENT

Several adaptations to standard assessment procedures are necessary to address the additional needs of inner-city minority clients. Some adaptations relate to how the standard intake and clinical interview process is handled and others concern the definition and breadth of the assessment itself. The combination of therapy and case management dimensions in Project RAP has facilitated the development of a broad assessment approach.

Clinical Interviewing Considerations

Establishing rapport with youthful sexual offenders and their families at the outset is not an easy process. It is a difficult balancing act to offer oneself as a potential advocate but also as accountable to the court with a responsibility to the community at large. It is also difficult to establish rapport when the family has been mandated to the program and is not really seeking treatment by free choice. When we add to this the fact that most Project RAP clients are socioeconomically disadvantaged and are minorities, some further considerations need to be taken into account when undertaking a clinical assessment.

The families are likely to have had some negative experiences with the criminal justice and welfare systems, and this may contribute to an initial sense of wariness or distrust. Language barriers may also exist. Culturally influenced attitudes to authority, beliefs about therapy, and values about family and sexuality will demand a certain level of culture-specific knowledge and skill, especially if the clinician is of a different ethnicity than the client and family. For families who moved to the United States from elsewhere such as the Caribbean or Central America, acculturation pressures and their impact on the family will need to be assessed. Spiritual beliefs and practices may also be important.

Project RAP has attempted to address these issues within the assessment process in a range of ways, presented in the following sections as suggestions.

Provide Flexible Hours

Project staff are flexible about appointment times and scheduling, since the parent or guardian may be trying to juggle a large number of obligations, and those who work may have already been docked a considerable amount of pay on account of court-related absences. Whenever possible the intake interviews and psychometric testing for the Project

RAP intake are done in a single day, or across an afternoon and evening, to minimize the number of appointments required.

Have a Multicultural and Bilingual Intake Team

A clinician and a case manager generally undertake the first part of the assessment interview together. This makes it possible for the family to have at least one person involved in the intake process who is from a similar ethnic or cultural background to themselves. An especially positive response has been noted from African-American parents or guardians when it is evident to them that African-American staff will be involved in the youth's case. The presence of a bilingual member of staff has been met very positively by Latino parents. For may families, even if the parents do speak some English, the information they provide in their native language is infinitely more rich, emotionally expressive, and meaningful.

Having bilingual intake staff is far preferable to communicating through interpreters, especially if the interpreter is a family member or relative of the youth. It is entirely inappropriate for the interpreter to be a child (even though the younger family members are the most likely to be fluently bilingual), since family roles and hierarchies will be distorted and the material that needs to be discussed in the interview is often not appropriate for children to hear from their parents. Finally, using interpreters takes considerably more time, often yields meanings that are only approximate, and makes rapport difficult to establish. Therefore, it is by far the preferred option to have fully bilingual members on the intake team.

Be Sparing in the Use of Psychometric Instruments

Many psychometric instruments are inappropriate to use with minority clients, since psychological constructs are often defined in very culture-specific terms. This problem is especially amplified for clients whose first language is not English or for those with literacy problems. Some minority clients may have negative associations with the concept of pencil-and-paper testing owing to prior failure experiences in the education system. Others may have difficulty with the concept of there being "no right or wrong answers." It is important to be able to distinguish culture-specific from culture-general concepts when deciding how and what to measure, and to confine one's choice of instruments to those which have been normed and validated cross-culturally (Lonner, 1990).

Provide Information Early and Demystify Therapy

Many families referred to Project RAP have lacked adequate information regarding the court process, therapy, and clinicians. Often they have viewed therapy and mental health services as serving only those who are severely psychiatrically disordered, and have therefore avoided such stigmatized avenues of assistance in the past unless all other sources of help—especially extended family networks, friends, and spiritual resources—have been exhausted.

Therefore, starting the intake process with educational information about the purpose and scope of the assessment has helped dispel myths or misconceptions, for example, the fear that the interviewer or others will define the youth or family as "crazy." At Project RAP this information has generally been offered in the context of a meeting between the parents, youth, clinician, and case manager together on the family's arrival at the office.

Issues discussed have included limited confidentiality, the program's dual role as advocate and agent of the court, the exact program requirements of parents and youth, the nature and extent of community-based supervision offered by case managers, and the purpose and content of the therapy components of the program. It has been the experience of Project RAP that the families respond positively to a frank, direct approach such as this.

Extend Respect and Include Fathers

Because of the likelihood that the family will have had negative experiences with the system in the past, it is especially important to extend respect to clients in direct, concrete ways. For example, it is exceedingly important to contact and speak with each involved family member directly, rather than relying on intermediaries or messages. This has been especially so with black and Latino fathers who are not present in the home but who are still involved in the youth's life. The fathers of Project RAP youth have usually wanted to have input into decisions about their son's case, but have often needed the program staff to reach out to them first, to invite them to participate, and to let them know their opinion is desired.

In the efforts of Caucasian staff to extend respect and build credibility with minority clients, it is important to develop self-awareness about one's style and approach. An especially common mistake is referred to by Boyd-Franklin (1989) as "missionary racism"; a situation in which a well-intentioned white clinician unknowingly patronizes his or her black clients by subtly conveying that she or he (the therapist) is there to "rescue" the poor black client.

Expect a Range of Attitudes toward Authority

Minority youth and their parents or guardians are likely to respond in a variety of ways to the clinician's position of power and authority over them in the assessment situation. Those who have had bad experiences with the criminal justice or human service systems may respond with hostility or suspicion. While efforts to make the environment positive and inclusive for minority clients may decrease this tendency, it is very important for program staff to expect their credibility and authority to be tested and challenged, sometimes in ways that include an implied or stated racial dimension. For example, Caucasian staff may be challenged about their ability to understand or relate to the circumstances of minority families, and minority staff may be accused of having "sold out" to the system. In expecting these kinds of challenges as part of the process of earning credibility, staff will be more able to respond nondefensively and explore these issues in a nonconfrontational way.

Minority families who have immigrated to the United States within the most recent generation may, in contrast, unquestioningly confer respect on program staff by virtue of their title and position. An important dynamic to be aware of in these instances is the tendency of some clients to answer "yes" or to agree with the interviewer whether or not they understand the question. This may be part of their effort to be cooperative and reveals a reluctance to confront the interviewer by asking for clarification.

Another related issue may be the expectation that the interviewer, as a perceived expert, will advise and dispense information that will "cure" the youth's sexual offending problem, much as a doctor might prescribe medicine for a physical ailment. Identifying behavioral control (rather than cure) as the goal of treatment will help the family form a more accurate perception of what is to follow. This may be achieved by educating the parent about the social learning approach to understanding and treating the problem of sexual offending.

Assess Acculturation Pressures Directly

An important dynamic to assess with families who have recently immigrated to the United States is the presence and impact of intergenerational differences in the rate of acculturation. Children will always adjust more rapidly, not only in terms of language, but also the norms, values, and behaviors of their new environment. Often, dynamics in these areas are directly or indirectly related to the youth's sexual offense. For example, intergenerational conflicts about family values and sexual matters appear to be especially common among first-generation families referred to Project RAP. Problems arising from family disintegration and abject poverty are especially common in first- and second-generation families who have not managed to succeed in education and employment since migrating to the United States.

For example, an assessment of a sibling incest situation might reveal that a single mother is isolated in the new country, does not have the usual range of extended family available to contribute to child care, works two jobs to send money back to family in her country of origin, and is therefore overly dependent on her son to care for his younger sisters. She may also be reluctant to give her son freedom owing to fears about negative street influences. The youth may resent his lack of freedom and his child-care responsibilities, and respond to this by sexually abusing his sister. An assessment of the conflicting acculturation pressures on each family member is therefore crucial and will provide the groundwork for family-based interventions that are responsive to these matters.

Assess Spiritual Affiliations and Resources

Minority families may have very strong links with religious institutions, and spirituality may be one of their most important sources of strength, comfort, and social support. Religious institutions may also be a source of positive peer and adult role models for the youth. Therefore, it is important to assess the family's social and personal resources in this area, and to see whether spiritual support can be integrated into the treatment plan. For example, in several Project RAP cases, the homes of church elders were considered as possible residential resources for youth who had committed incest offenses, and therefore could not remain in the home.

Be Aware of Flexible Family Definition and Roles

Many minority families have a much broader definition of family membership than typical Caucasian families. There may be little distinction between nuclear and extended family. Child-raising responsibilities may be spread laterally and vertically across the family tree. Genetically unrelated persons may be viewed as close family members (e.g., godparents, mentor figures), and children may be born and raised within families where their parents are not married but where both still contribute. Household membership may span three or even four generations. Genograms can be an especially useful assessment tool after rapport has been established.

These features reflect a collectivist rather than individualistic values orientation, which in some cases may be a continuation of cultural traditions from the country of origin, while in others may have developed out of necessity. For example, economic survival in the inner city may depend on pooling scarce resources. Crucial family members may be missing owing to death, incarceration, substance abuse problems, or work obligations. An assessment of the family's functioning may require interviews or telephone contact with a broad range of persons. An assessment of the youth's level of resilience and difficulties adjusting to traumatic loss may also be needed, as these issues may have a bearing on his offending.

The more expansive definition of family described above also has implications for role definitions within the family. In some cases clearly defined, rigid roles (e.g., the overall authority of the strongest parental figure) may coexist with flexible, creatively defined roles (e.g., the adolescent as cooperative "child," responsible helper in raising younger siblings, confidante for a lonely parent, and/or financial contributor to the household with an after-school job). The flexibility of roles has often been cited as one of the main adaptations to adversity that has allowed poor inner-city families to survive. An awareness of this is important during the assessment. In some instances the way the youth's role has been defined may have inadvertently contributed to the motivation or opportunity to offend; for example, by affording him considerable unsupervised access to children. By the same token, the flexibility of family roles may also offer alternative solutions. A youth who works after school to contribute financially to a female-headed household may gain self-esteem and a healthy sense of responsibility, so long as his mother maintains a parental relationship with him that is both nurturing and authoritative, in which care is taken not to treat him like an adult male "equal" in the home.

Be Aware of Cultural Influences on Sexual Attitudes and Beliefs

Cultural background may have considerable influence on a client's attitudes and values about sexuality. The extent to which the client feels able or prepared to discuss explicit sexual matters is most likely to have an immediate impact on the assessment process. The age, gender, and language of the interviewer may also have an influence on the client's comfort level. If clients are clearly uncomfortable discussing sexual matters, it is useful to explore the meaning and significance of their discomfort. Weighing the long-term benefits of being open (such as getting help for the offender and stopping the abuse) against the short-term costs of breaking a "taboo" may also help clients to disclose necessary sexual information.

Breadth of Assessment

It is generally acknowledged that sexual offender assessment information needs to be gathered and compared across multiple sources (e.g., Ryan & Lane, 1991; Steen & Monnette, 1989). Our experience with a youthful minority inner-city population has drawn attention to the need for assessment to also extend into the larger community, to include an assessment of the home and neighborhood environment, the school, and the presence and impact on the family of other systems. While not all of these variables directly contribute to the risk assessment of the youth with respect to sexual offending, they are equally important because they help identify potential environmental and systemic barriers that, if unaddressed, may result in failure to attend or engage in treatment.

Assessment methods used at Project RAP to address these factors are summarized in the following sections. These are undertaken in addition to standard assessment strategies, such as reviewing legal documents, clinical interviewing, and psychometric testing, where appropriate.

Home Visits

One or more home visits are routinely undertaken as part of the Project RAP assessment procedure. Often more than one household needs to be visited because, consistent with the flexible definitions of family described above, several households may share responsibility for the youth. Home visits are necessary in order to assess victim safety issues, space, privacy and basic resource concerns, consistency and quality of supervision of the youth, presence of other children, and the like. Often the gravity of a family's situation regarding poverty or the urgency of need for other services can only be accurately gauged from a visit since, on account of shame, or fears about the agency's response, parents or guardians may conceal this information when interviewed at the office. Such information is in turn vital to decisions about the suitability of the youth's proposed living environment, especially in view of the nature of his offense. In cases where the living situation is assessed as unsatisfactory, Project RAP case managers work to identify suitable alternatives, seeking first within the extended family network and then residential options through child welfare services if necessary.

It is noteworthy that staff have rarely had to remove a youth to another living situation on the basis of information gathered from home visits; usually if the home environment is unsuitable, this has been established already by the time the youth is referred to Project RAP. However, the visits have frequently allowed additional service needs for the family to be identified and have also helped pinpoint extended family situations that need to become "off limits" for the youth because of the presence of children, inadequate supervision, or adult substance abuse.

Assess the Neighborhood Environment

Home visits also allow the case manager to gain a firsthand impression of the neighborhood in which the youth lives. Potential barriers and resources can then be identified and addressed. For example, a strong base of cultural resources in the neighborhood may provide a "cushion" and many avenues of support for an acculturating family, whereas if the neighborhood has been negatively influenced by a street drug trade and other hallmarks of poverty, an awareness of this can add special significance to the evening curfew imposed by the program. It can also increase staff credibility in addressing both the risk of negative peer influence with the youth and the fears parents may hold for their children's safety when they are outside of the apartment. Parents' reality-based fears in this regard often lead to severe or seemingly excessive restrictions on their teenage children. This dynamic needs to be discussed in the program because in some instances it has inadvertently contributed to the youth's offense behavior.

Seeing the youth's neighborhood also allows several more practical concerns to be assessed, such as accessibility to public transport and proximity to positive resources such as supportive extended family, after-school programs, or sport and recreation facilities.

The question has often been raised about the safety of staff venturing into these neighborhoods, especially given that in households where parents or guardians work, visits are often undertaken in the evening. We have enforced a policy that staff undertake home visits in pairs and use an agency car whenever possible. It has helped that case managers have generally already been familiar with some of the city's poorer neighborhoods. To date, no incidents have occurred when staff have undertaken home visits.

Visit the School

Regular school visits are another part of the Project RAP brief, and if the youth is attending school at the time he is referred, an initial visit is included as part of the assessment process. While much school-related information can be gained by telephone, again there is an important qualitative aspect that can only be gleaned from a personal visit. Since many inner-city schools are severely underresourced, a visit may identify more clearly issues such as overcrowding, lack of safety, or other factors that are likely to exacerbate problems and interfere with the youth's learning. Truancy and cutting class, learning difficulties, being "left back," and disruptive or aggressive behaviors in school are the norm for many of the youth in Project RAP and are of considerable concern not only because they undermine the youth's future educational and life opportunities, but also because these behavioral problems could be sufficient for a violation of probation or for the court to remand the youth to jail.

A thorough assessment of the school situation by Project RAP case managers has identified needs such as a review of the appropriateness of special education placements, transfers to alternative schools, enrollment in after-school tutoring programs, or training for school personnel on how to set appropriate limits and boundaries on sexual acting out behavior in the classroom. Addressing these needs early has, in turn, helped these youth to be effectively maintained in the community rather than having to be incarcerated or placed in a more restrictive setting.

Assess the Involvement and Impact of Other Systems

Several other systems will be involved with the youth's family as a matter of course. The family or supreme court, probation or parole, child welfare services, and victim services may all be involved. These systems are all in addition to the systems the family routinely has to negotiate, such as the school, the parent's workplace, or the public assistance system for parents who are disabled or do not work. Also, in many cases health, housing, or insurance concerns may be affecting the family. As a consequence, many families who are referred to Project RAP are already overwhelmed or frustrated by the demands of other systems.

Awareness of this can assist with assessment in several ways. First, it underscores the importance of maintaining a positive, welcoming environment at the agency so the family's experience of dealing with the program can stand in contrast to some of their other system-related experiences. Second, it can prepare staff for the possibility of hostility or negativity from the parents on first meeting, especially given that their cooperation with a referral to the program is often either mandated or in other ways required of them under duress. Third, an awareness of the other systems involved with the family should become the basis for interdisciplinary sharing of information, with the family's consent. This should be the cornerstone of any sexual offender assessment, as well as the effective monitoring of treatment response thereafter.

TREATMENT

Many adaptations to youth and parent interventions follow naturally from the staffing, environmental, and assessment issues discussed earlier in this chapter, including cofacilitation of all groups by a clinician and a case manager, to effect gender and cultural diversity. This has also allowed case managers to be closely informed about therapeutic issues for the families on their caseloads and to learn group therapy skills. A bilingual staff member is available in parent groups to translate for those who speak only Spanish, and a completely Spanish-speaking parent group will be developed if enough Latino families are referred. Food and drink are made available at parent and youth groups, and subway tokens are dispensed to cover the cost of travel. Several more specific adaptations to youth and parent interventions are summarized in the following sections.

Therapy for the Youth: Adaptations

The clients meet weekly for a 2-hour cognitive–behavioral offense-specific therapy group, which covers issues such as accountability for offenses, victim empathy, sex education, social skills, anger management, and relapse prevention. This fairly generic model of sexual offender treatment has been tailored specifically to the needs of minority inner city youth in a range of ways described as follows.

The Use of Active Methods

While active, participatory strategies are particularly appropriate for adolescent treatment approaches in general, they are especially useful with inner-city minority youth, some whose school difficulties have produced low reading levels or whose behavioral difficulties include impulsivity. The African-American and Latino youth have shown a particular liking for role plays, *in vivo* exercises, stories, and pictures or diagrams, as well as methods that are affectively expressive. For example, they have responded well to Johnson's (1996) "tree life cycle" analogy for the offense cycle and related treatment concepts, and they have enjoyed developing their own conflict resolution–anger management scenarios on the basis of street or home experiences. These active methods have drawn attention to the need for group facilitators to be familiar with street terms and slang and to be able to contextualize "street smart" behaviors when they emerge in the group setting.

Peer Education Component

The youth groups are "open" groups, and thus clients enter and graduate from the program at different times. While this has sometimes made it difficult to cover all the necessary material, it has also created many opportunities to teach the more experienced group members peer education skills for the benefit of new group members. The youth in Project RAP have responded positively to peer education opportunities. Not only has it reinforced familiar ground in a verbal, experiential way, it has also taught them some prosocial ways to interact with peers and has helped build self-esteem and group cohesion.

Special Focus Areas

The unique circumstances and problems facing urban minority youth point to several areas of special need in offense-specific therapy efforts. Four that have been especially important for Project RAP youth are the need for issues of grief and traumatic loss to be directly addressed, the need for creative anger management–violence prevention strategies that carry street credibility, the need to address the youths' considerable vulnerability and exposure to negative peer pressure, and in some cases the need to take into account the presence of vast intergenerational value differences within the family on account of differential rates of acculturation. In these and other areas of intervention, a practical emphasis on generating alternatives and choices has been especially important, to help combat the sense of helplessness and the external locus of control commonly seen in these youth and families in response to poverty.

Life Skills Component

A successful addition to the treatment component of Project RAP has been a weekly life skills group, run and coordinated by case managers. This is separate from the offense-specific group, and focuses on assisting the youth negotiate systemic barriers that, if left unaddressed, increase their risk of further criminal behavior. These barriers include under-education, underemployment, lack of positive community resources, and an accompanying pervasive sense of disempowerment and alienation. Therefore, the life skills group focuses on teaching job-readiness skills, increasing literacy and communication skills, and developing positive activities and interests so that leisure time can be productively used.

The life skills group has been well-attended by the youth, and they have had an active role in determining its content. The job-readiness aspect has been especially popular and, staff resources allowing, the next step will be to secure a small source of funding so that this aspect of the life skills group can be extended into a community-based summer job placement program. With their case manager's guidance, the youth would then be able to offer themselves as a free labor resource for local merchants and business persons in their own communities in exchange for on-the- job training and a stipend paid by CCA.

Efforts toward improving the client's literacy and communication skills have also been creatively addressed in this group. For example, the clients have worked on play readings, speeches, debates, and letter-writing tasks on topics that are of direct interest or concern within their own communities.

While the life skills group does not address offense issues specifically, it has had some very direct positive implications for the overall program. Since this group teaches clients skills that are overwhelmingly needed in the African-American and Latino communities, this component has instantly increased the credibility of the program in the eyes of both the youth and their parents, therefore increasing their commitment to Project RAP as a whole. It has also given the clients opportunities to spend quality time with staff and each other on issues that are not offense related, thus helping the youth develop positive, nonthreatening associations about attending the agency. Finally, it has directly mitigated several factors strongly associated with delinquency risk.

"Rites of Passage" and Celebrations

Project RAP youth have been very enthusiastic about creating and celebrating birthdays, graduations, and other significant "landmarks" during their involvement in the program. An acknowledgment of "rites of passage" is consistent with Afrocentric ideals (Mincey, 1994) and provides a positive response to the general lack of recognition many of these youth feel in their lives. Project RAP staff are attempting to make the clients increasingly responsible for planning these celebrations for each other and including parents and significant others in events such as the youth's graduation at the end of the 12-month program.

Follow-up Options

Efforts are made prior to the clients' graduation to refer them to other positive community-based resources. However, in view of the scarcity of equality resources available to many of the youth, the continuing availability of open-ended services at CCA has been especially important. As part of their probationary sentence, the youth are mandated to attend monthly relapse prevention groups for 1 year following their graduation from the 12-month intensive phase. They are also encouraged to continue attending the life skills group and Choices Unlimited workshops on a voluntary basis. They also have the opportunity to join two further activities: a Youth Advisory Council, which offers the agency feedback and suggestions from the clients' perspective, and an HIV peer education training program, which offers a small stipend in exchange for delivering HIV education to youth in residential and community settings.

Therapy for Parents, Guardians, and Other Family Members

A range of fairly generic parent and family therapy needs have been identified in the adolescent sexual offender treatment literature, including processing reactions to the offense, learning about offense dynamics, addressing victim safety and empathy issues, restructuring sexual boundaries and patterns of communication within the family, enhancing parenting skills, and applying the principles of relapse prevention (e.g., Ryan & Lane, 1991; Steen & Monnette, 1989). For the African-American and Latino families in Project RAP, some more specific patterns of need are evident within these areas. For example, intergenerational patterns of abuse have been evident in some of the families, pointing to the need for treatment of a range of extended family members. Specific deficits in parenting skills have often been evident in the areas of positive expressions of emotion and nurturance and conflict resolution and negotiation skills with adolescent children, especially on sexuality issues. Acculturation has caused family roles and hierarchies to be disrupted for first-generation families migrating to the United States. Parental substance abuse, relationship problems, and/or social isolation have often been present. The need for parents to tolerate and process considerable amounts of anger and anxiety is a feature for most of the families, owing to their economic, social and environmental circumstances, and the impact of racism.

In an effort to address issues such as these, Project RAP originally offered an open-ended biweekly parent education and group, with additional family therapy as needed. The intended benefits of the parent group included the dispensing of information, the opportunity to regularly update the parents about the youth's progress and behavior in the program, the opportunity to maintain face-to-face contact with parents, and the provision of a source of social support and validation for the parents. However, the open-ended nature of the group meant that parents entered and completed the group at different times. This, in conjunction with the fact that meetings were held only once every 2 weeks, appeared to be causing a lack of cohesion and continuity in the group.

The greatest single problem with the parent group has been inconsistent attendance. The parent group was especially poorly attended by the fathers and/or other male figures in the clients' lives. Many parents and guardians expressed the view that the program's demands upon their time were an imposition and an inconvenience, and many were reluctant to recognize that family intervention is a necessary aspect of an effective response to youthful sexual offending. Some parents felt that their attendance somehow implied they were responsible for the youth's offending behavior. Their sensitivity to the possibility of being blamed has been particularly difficult to dispel and may reflect a combination of the parents' own sense of guilt and their difficulty in trusting a program that is connected with the criminal justice system.

Common reasons for poor attendance offered by the parents themselves have included work obligations, lack of alternative child care for single parents with young ones at home, and feelings of anger toward the youth who committed the offense. The latter point reveals the degree to which the staff and parents have differed in their conceptualization of the purpose of the group: It is almost as though the parent believes that she or he attends the group as a favor to the youth and that missing sessions is a form of punishment for the youth, rather than seeing the group as being a source of information and support for themselves, which is especially important if they are having problems with the youth's behavior. Finally, in some cases a continuing substance abuse problem contributed to the parent or guardian's absence.

Practical considerations such as holding groups in the evenings, providing food, drink, and subway tokens, reminder letters and phone contacts, and calling absentees, although appreciated, have not been sufficient to consistently engage the parents. More coercive efforts such as having the probation officer contact the parent and reinforce the importance of attendance have had, if anything, a negative impact.

Project RAP's response to the problem of poor parent attendance has been to offer a broader range of intervention options. Adaptations to parent therapy are summarized in the following sections.

Option 1: Closed Biweekly Parent Group (12 Months)

The biweekly parent group has been made a "closed" group in an attempt to increase parent's sense of commitment and ownership of it. This modification has improved the attendance rate.

Option 2: Closed Weekly Parent Group (3 Months)

The project also created a closed parent group that meets weekly. After 3 months, the parents will decide whether they wish to continue the group, switch to individualized family therapy, or continue their contact with the program in some other way. Another feature is that it has been left for the parents to decide what kind of group it will be and what topics will be discussed. The parents decided that the group should be part educational and part supportive. Attendance in this group has been remarkably better than the biweekly group. Further, the quality and depth of discussions have been greater. Therefore, the biweekly group will soon be phased out and replaced with a second weekly parent group, at a different time and day of the week.

Option 3: Family Therapy On-Site

Family therapy in addition to (or instead of) the parent group has been offered to some parents. Staff resources are insufficient to extend this offer to all parents in the program. The choice of who gets these services is based largely on the degree to which the family needs the additional attention and the likelihood that they will take advantage of the opportunity. Family therapy has been offered by existing clinical staff in the program and also by family therapy interns from a local postmasters program at a local university with which Project RAP has developed a mutually beneficial relationship. Interns working with the project are already clinically trained and receive external supervision from licensed family therapists. Particular efforts have been made to attract bilingual and African-American interns.

Option 4: Therapy Options in the Family's Neighborhood

Some parents are unable or unwilling to attend any of the parent intervention options offered on-site at Project RAP. In most of these instances, family members are severely affected by other problems such as substance abuse or poor health. Efforts have been made in these cases to refer the parent to an appropriate resource within their own community or neighborhood, in the hope that they will cooperate with something closer to home. Generally, the most obvious areas of need for these families are parental substance abuse treatment and/or therapy for the victim of the youth's offending in intrafamilial abuse cases. Project RAP staff have had little success with parents following up on substance abuse referrals, even if they are accompanied to the clinic. Success has been somewhat better with parents following up on referrals for their children who have been victimized and at least marginally involving themselves in therapy with their child.

Option 5: Involving the Fathers

There is a clear need to develop a specific outreach component for fathers and other significant men in the youth's lives. Men rarely attend the groups for parents and guardians, and the mothers and female relatives in attendance have frequently identified the emotional and/or physical absence of fathers as a contributing to the youth's emotional or behavioral problems, which in many cases feeds directly into vulnerability to further offending. Current possibilities being explored include increasing positive contact between fathers and sons through activities organized in conjunction Project RAP, perhaps on the basis of all-male planning workshops with the fathers or with the fathers and youth together. The youth and their female caregivers have expressed strong support for these ideas.

PRELIMINARY OUTCOME DATA AND CONCLUDING COMMENTS

The youth attendance rate at Project RAP group sessions has been exceptional, averaging 86%. Outcome data for Project RAP, while promising, need to be treated as preliminary, since the program is still very new. The period of time "at risk" for all youth who have received services, past or present, currently averages 9 months, and ranges from 1 to 20 months. So far the program has had an attrition and incarceration rate of 9.5%. None of the youth have been rearrested for sexual allegations, and while 30% of the youth have been rearrested for other reasons (mainly misdemeanors), only 13% of these cases have resulted in a conviction.

In view of the generally poor response of minorities to psychological interventions and the considerable crime-related risks and vulnerabilities these youth face in their homes and communities, these preliminary indicators certainly look positive. When asked how they account for their high attendance and responsiveness, the youth have most often cited the open atmosphere and "feel" of the agency and the quality of their relationships with their case managers. Therefore, it does appear that some of the staffing and environmental adaptations described above have had the desired impact. From a program design perspective, the interweaving of the case management/intensive supervision component through all aspects of the program has been a very important foundation for expanding a traditional cognitive–behavioral approach to become more directly responsive to cultural and socioeconomic concerns.

REFERENCES

Berry, J.W., & Annis, R.C. (Eds.). (1988). *Ethnic psychology: Research and practice with indigenous peoples, immigrants, refugees and sojurners.* Amsterdam, Holland: Swetz and Zeitlinger.

The Black Resource Guide. (1991). Washington, DC: R. Benjamin Johnson and Jacqueline L. Johnson.

Boyd-Franklin, N. (1989). *Black families in therapy: A multisystems approach.* New York: Guilford Press.

Comaz-Diaz, L., & Griffith, E.H. (Eds.). (1988). *Clinical guidelines in cross cultural mental health.* New York: Wiley.

Johnson, S. (1996). *An effective approach to a more thorough treatment repertoire for African-American clients.* Workshop presented at the 12th Annual Conference of the National Adolescent Perpetrator Network, Minneapolis, Minnesota.

Lonner, W.J. (1990). An overview of cross cultural testing and assessment. In R.W. Brislin (Ed.), *Applied cross-cultural psychology* (pp. 56–76). Newbury Park, CA: Sage.

McGoldrick, M., Pearce, J., & Giordano, J. (Eds.). (1982). *Ethnicity and family therapy.* New York: Guilford Press.

Mincey, R. (1994). *Nurturing young black males: Challenges to institutions, agencies and social policy.* Washington, DC: The Urban Institute.

Pedersen, P.B. (1988). *A handbook for developing multicultural awareness.* Alexandria, VA: American Association for Counseling and Development Press.

Revised Report from the National Task Force on Juvenile Sex Offending. (1993). The National Adolescent Perpetrator Network. *Juvenile and Family Court Journal, 44,* 40–42.

Ryan, G., & Lane, S. (1991). *Juvenile sex offending: Causes, consequences and correction.* New York: Lexington Books.

Sartorius, N., Pedersen, P.B., & Marsella, A.J. (1984). *Mental health services: The cross-cultural context.* Newbury Park, CA: Sage.

Steen, J.C., & Monnette, B. (1989). *Treating adolescent sex offenders in the community.* Springfield, IL: Charles C. Thomas.

Sue, D.W., & Sue, D. (Eds.). (1990). *Counseling the culturally different: Theory and practice* (2nd ed.). New York: Wiley.

Taylor-Gibbs, J., & Huang, L.N. (Eds.). (1989). *Children of color: Psychological interventions with minority youth.* San Francisco, CA: Jossey-Bass.

32

Conclusions and Future Directions

William L. Marshall, Yolanda M. Fernandez,
Stephen M. Hudson, and Tony Ward

This volume has brought together treatment programs for sexual offenders from around the world. While it remains true that most of the well-developed and established programs are in North America (United States and Canada), the present volume reveals that similar programs have appeared with increasing frequency over the past 10 years in the United Kingdom, the Netherlands, Australia, and New Zealand. Furthermore, it is evident that both Western (Marshall & Frenken, in press) and Eastern Europe (Dunovsky, Weiss, & Trojan, 1997), as well as South Africa (Marshall, 1996) and Bermuda (Marshall, 1993) are developing treatment for sexual offenders.

Two of the interesting features of this remarkable recent growth concerns the facts that: (1) these programs predominantly derive from the same conceptualization of treatment; and (2) they are being applied to increasingly diverse populations. Most of the programs described in this volume are based on a cognitive–behavioral approach that is guided by a relapse prevention framework. The beliefs, attitudes, and perceptions of sexual offenders are being challenged using a supportive but firm approach that respects the dignity of the client while offering alternative, more prosocial views of the offense and the victims. Care providers are trained in skills that are meant to equip offenders with the capacity to meet their needs in more appropriate ways, and clients are taught to apply these skills to avoid or abort an identified relapse process.

Interestingly, while the majority of the programs outlined in this book utilize relapse prevention concepts in treatment [i.e., the internal management component as described by Pithers (1990)], a significant number do not describe elaborate postdischarge supervision (i.e., the external management component). Most seem to make some effort to provide postdischarge support of some kind, but quite often this does not involve (even in the institutionally based programs) the extensive supervision provided in the "model" relapse prevention programs outlined by both Marques and colleagues (Marques, 1984; Marques, Day, Nelson, & Miner, 1989) and Pithers and colleagues (Pithers, 1990; Pithers, Martin, &

William L. Marshall and Yolanda M. Fernandez • Department of Psychology, Queen's University, Kingston, Ontario, Canada K7L 3N6. **Stephen M. Hudson and Tony Ward** • Department of Psychology, University of Canterbury, Christchurch, New Zealand.

Sourcebook of Treatment Programs for Sexual Offenders, edited by Marshall et al. Plenum Press, New York, 1998.

Cumming, 1989). Whether these elaborate maintenance programs advocated by relapse prevention advocates produce significantly better results than either treatment alone or some minimal support and supervision remains to be seen, although the evidence to date is not encouraging (Marshall & Anderson, 1996). Indeed, it remains to be unequivocally demonstrated that treating sexual offenders produces reductions in recidivism, although our view (Marshall, Jones, Ward, Johnston, & Barbaree, 1991) is that there are good grounds for optimism.

One thing is certainly clear from the present volume: there are many well-established treatment programs around the world, so it should only be a matter of time until outcome studies become available in sufficient number to answer these important questions about efficacy. With the development of specific programs for offenders at different levels of risk (see Chapter 5, this volume), for offenders with specific characteristics or disabilities (see Part II, this volume), and for offenders from particular cultural backgrounds (see Part III, this volume), we may be able to more accurately discern with whom our treatment programs are most effective.

In any case, the programs presented in this volume represent exciting developments in the treatment of sexual offenders and it is especially encouraging to see such an expansion of programs in this time of fiscal restraint. We hope all readers will be as encouraged as we are and will find information in the programs that will assist them in their own work.

REFERENCES

Dunovsky, J., Weiss, P., & Trojan, O. (Eds.). (1997). *Child sexual abuse and sexual violence*. Prague: Czech Ministry of Labor and Social Affairs.

Marques, J. K. (1984). *An innovative treatment program for sex offenders: Report to the legislature*. Sacramento, CA: California State Department of Mental Health.

Marques, J.K., Day, D.M., Nelson, C., & Miner, M.H. (1989). The Sex Offender Treatment and Evaluation Project: California's Relapse Prevention Program. In D.R. Laws (Ed.), *Relapse prevention with sex offenders* (pp. 247–267). New York: Guilford Press.

Marshall, W.L. (1993, April). *The prosecution, treatment, and case management of sex offenders*. Paper presented at the Professional Seminar on Sex Offenders, Hamilton, Bermuda.

Marshall, W.L. (1996, April). *Treatment and its effectiveness with incarcerated sexual offenders*. Paper presented to South African Correctional Services, Johannesburg.

Marshall, W.L., & Anderson, D. (1996). An evaluation of the benefits of relapse prevention programs with sexual offenders. *Sexual Abuse: A Journal of Research and Treatment, 8*, 290–221.

Marshall, W.L., & Frenken, J. (Eds.). (in press). *North American and European approaches to sexual offending: Converging trends*. Thousand Oaks, CA: Sage.

Marshall, W.L., Jones, R., Ward, T., Johnston, P., & Barbaree, H.E. (1991). Treatment outcome with sex offenders. *Clinical Psychology Review, 11*, 465–485.

Pithers, W.D. (1990). Relapse prevention with sexual aggressors: A method for maintaining therapeutic gain and enhancing external supervision. In W.L. Marshall, D.R. Laws, & H.E. Barbaree (Eds.), *Handbook of sexual assault: Issues, theories, and treatment of the offender* (pp. 343–361). New York: Plenum Press.

Pithers, W.D., Martin, G.R., & Cumming, G.F. (1989). Vermont Treatment Program for Sexual Aggressors. In D.R. Laws (Ed.), *Relapse prevention with sex offenders* (pp. 292–310). New York: Guilford Press.

Index

ISBN 0-306-45730-X

90000